Posttraumatic Stress Disorder

From Neurobiology to Treatment

Posttraumatic Stress Disorder

From Neurobiology to Treatment

EDITED BY

J. Douglas Bremner

Departments of Psychiatry & Behavioral Sciences and Radiology,
Emory University School of Medicine, and the Atlanta VA Medical Center,
Atlanta, GA, USA

WILEY Blackwell

Published by John Wiley & Sons, Inc., Hoboken, New Jersey

Published simultaneously in Canada

For general information on our other products and services or for technical support, please contact our Customer Care Department within the United States at (800) 762-2974, outside the United States at (317) 572-3993 or fax (317) 572-4002.

Wiley also publishes its books in a variety of electronic formats. Some content that appears in print may not be available in electronic formats. For more information about Wiley products, visit our web site at www.wiley.com.

Library of Congress Cataloging-in-Publication Data:

Posttraumatic stress disorder (Bremner)
 Posttraumatic stress disorder : from neurobiology to treatment / [edited by] J. Douglas Bremner.
   p. ; cm.
 Includes bibliographical references and index.
 ISBN 978-1-118-35611-1 (hardback)
 I. Bremner, J. Douglas, 1961- , editor. II. Title.
 [DNLM: 1. Stress Disorders, Post-Traumatic. 2. Stress, Psychological. WM 172.5] RC552.P67
 616.85′21–dc23

                                                                                          2015036889

Cover image: © Katie Nesling/Getty
Printed and bound in Malaysia by Vivar Printing Sdn Bhd

1   2016

Contents

v

List of contributors

Karl-Juergen Bär, M.D
Department of Psychiatry and Psychotherapy, University Hospital, Jena, Germany

Elisabeth Binder, Ph.D
Department of Translational Research in Psychiatry, Max Planck Institute of Psychiatry, Munich, Germany

J. Douglas Bremner, M.D
Departments of Psychiatry & Behavioral Sciences and Radiology, Emory University School of Medicine, and the Atlanta VA Medical Center, Atlanta, GA, USA

Christopher Cain, Ph.D
Department of Child and Adolescent Psychiatry, New York University School of Medicine, New York, NY, and The Emotional Brain Institute, Nathan S. Kline Institute for Psychiatric Research, Orangeburg, NY, USA

Carolina Campanella, Ph.D
Department of Psychiatry & Behavioral Sciences, Emory University, Atlanta, GA, USA

Nicolaos Daskalakis, Ph.D
Department of Psychiatry, Icahn School of Medicine at Mount Sinai, New York, NY, USA

Lori Davis, M.D
Department of Psychiatry, University of Alabama-Birmingham and the Tuscaloosa VA Medical Center, Tuscaloosa, AL, USA

David Diamond, Ph.D
Departments of Psychology and Molecular Pharmacology & Physiology, University of South Florida, Tampa, FL, USA

Molly J. Dickens, Ph.D
Department of Integrative Biology, University of California, Berkeley, Berkeley, CA, USA

Robert Drugan, Ph.D
Department of Psychology, University of New Hampshire, Durham, NH, USA

Bernet M. Elzinga, Ph.D
Institute for Psychological Research, Section Clinical Psychology, Leiden University, The Netherlands

Dora B. Guzman, M.S
Department of Psychiatry & Behavioral Science, School of Medicine, and Yerkes National Primate Research Center, Emory University, Atlanta, GA, USA

Mark Hamner, M.D
Department of Psychiatry, Medical University of South Carolina, and The Charleston VA Medical Center, Charleston, SC, USA

Brittany Howell, Ph.D
Institute of Child Development, University of Minnesota, Minneapolis, MN, USA

Amy Lehrner, Ph.D
Department of Psychiatry, Icahn School of Medicine at Mount Sinai, New York, NY, USA

Emeran Mayer, M.D
UCLA School of Medicine, Los Angeles, CA, USA

Leah A. McGuire, Ph.D
Center for Attention and Learning, Department of Psychiatry, Lenox Hill Hospital, North Shore LIJ Health System, New York, NY, USA

Divya Mehta, Ph.D
Department of Translational Research in Psychiatry, Max Planck Institute of Psychiatry, Munich, Germany

Christian J. Merz, Ph.D
Institute of Cognitive Neuroscience, Cognitive Psychology, Ruhr-University, Bochum, Germany

Brad Pearce, Ph.D
Department of Epidemiology, Rollins School of Public Health, Atlanta, GA, USA

Sarah C. Reitz, M.D
Department of Psychosomatic Medicine and Psychotherapy, Central Institute of Mental Health Mannheim, Medical Faculty Mannheim, Heidelberg University, Mannheim, Germany

Michael Romero, Ph.D
Department of Biology, Tufts University, Medford, MA, USA

Mar Sanchez, Ph.D
Department of Psychiatry & Behavioral Science, School of Medicine, and Yerkes National Primate Research Center, Emory University, Atlanta, GA, USA

Christian Schmahl, M.D
Department of Psychosomatic Medicine and Psychotherapy, Central Institute of Mental Health Mannheim, Medical Faculty Mannheim, Heidelberg University, Mannheim, Germany

Lars Schwabe, Ph.D
Institute for Psychology, Department of Cognitive Psychology, University of Hamburg,
Hamburg, Germany

Arieh Y. Shalev, Ph.D
Department of Psychiatry, New York University School of Medicine, Langone Medical
Center, New York, NY, USA

Nathaniel P. Stafford, B.S
Department of Psychology, University of New Hampshire, Durham, NH, USA

Regina Sullivan, Ph.D
Department of Child and Adolescent Psychiatry, New York University School of
Medicine, New York, NY, and The Emotional Brain Institute, Nathan S. Kline Institute
for Psychiatric Research, Orangeburg, NY, USA

Viola Vaccarino, M.D, Ph.D
Department of Epidemiology, Emory University Rollins School of Public Health, and
Department of Internal Medicine (Cardiology), Emory University School of Medicine,
Atlanta, GA, USA

Timothy A. Warner, B.A
Department of Psychology, University of New Hampshire, Durham, NH, USA

Rachel Yehuda, Ph.D
Department of Psychiatry, Icahn School of Medicine at Mount Sinai, New York, NY, USA

Anthony S. Zannas, Ph.D
Department of Translational Research in Psychiatry, Max Planck Institute of Psychiatry,
Munich, Germany

Phillip R. Zoladz, Ph.D
Department of Psychology, Sociology, & Criminal Justice, Ohio Northern University, Ada,
OH, USA

Introduction

J. Douglas Bremner

Since the establishment of posttraumatic stress disorder (PTSD) as a psychiatric diagnosis for the first time in 1980 by the American Psychiatric Association's (APA) manual for psychiatric disorders, the *Diagnostic and Statistical Manual* III (Saigh & Bremner, 1999), there has been an expansion of research on the effects of traumatic stress on the individual. Basic science research on the effects of stress on brain circuits and systems has complemented clinical research. Together, this increased understanding of stress has been beneficial for the treatment of PTSD. This volume brings together some of the most authoritative researchers and authors on the topic of traumatic stress in both the basic science and clinical dimensions, and relates this to a better understanding of treatment approaches for PTSD.

The diagnosis of PTSD requires exposure to an event which involves a threat to one's life or self-integrity. In addition, the diagnosis requires the presence of symptoms in three clusters, including intrusions, avoidance and hyperarousal, and the presence of clinically significant distress or impairment. The diagnosis requires at least one symptom in the intrusion category, three in the avoidance category, and two in the hyperarousal category. Intrusive symptoms include recurrent intrusive memories, nightmares, feeling as if the event were recurring, and feeling a lot worse with reminders of the event, and having increased physiological reactivity with the event. Avoidant symptoms include avoidance of reminders of the event, avoidance of thoughts and feelings related to the event, trouble remembering an important aspect of the trauma, decreased interest in things, feeling detached or cut off from others, emotional numbing, and a sense of a foreshortened future. Hyperarousal symptoms include a difficulty falling or staying asleep, irritability or outbursts of anger, difficulty concentrating, hypervigilance, and exaggerated startle response.

Symptoms of PTSD are a behavioral manifestation of stress-induced changes in brain structure and function. Stress causes acute and chronic changes in neurochemical systems and specific brain regions, which result in long-term changes in brain "circuits" involved in the stress response.

The premise of our understanding of the effects of stress on neurobiology is based on animal models. The chapters in this volume outline how stress affects important stress-sensitive circuits, including norepinephrine, the cortisol/hypothalamic–pituitary–adrenal (HPA) axis, dopamine, serotonin, neuropeptides, the glutamatergic/excitatory amino acids systems, and the gamma-aminobutyric acid (GABA)/benzodiazepine systems, as well as numerous other neuropeptidal and neurohormonal systems.

A critical field of study that has important public health implications is the interaction between early life stress and brain development. Two key chapters address this, and outline brain areas involved in the stress response, including the hippocampus, amygdala, and medial prefrontal cortex. Other chapters review the effects of stress on memory, including both animal models of showing the effects of stress on the hippocampus, which plays an important role in short-term memory, and mechanisms of new learning, including long-term potentiation, as well as studies in PTSD of neuropsychological testing of memory and brain imaging of the hippocampus. Finally, later chapters review brain imaging studies in PTSD, and the effects of both pharmacotherapy and psychotherapy on brain function in PTSD. Later chapters also review the important topics of the effects of stress and PTSD on cardiovascular health and other physical parameters, and the role of genetic factors in the development of PTSD.

Posttraumatic stress disorder is a common condition that can be associated with considerable morbidity and mortality and is often only partially treated with current therapies. The chapters in this volume outline how PTSD is associated with long-term changes in the brain and stress-responsive systems. Changes in brain areas including the amygdala, hippocampus, and frontal cortex, can lead to memory problems, maintenance of abnormal fear responses and other symptoms of PTSD. A better understanding of neurobiological changes in PTSD will inform the development of new treatments for this disabling disorder. Integrating basic science and clinical approaches to stress and PTSD, as is done in this volume, has the greatest potential impact for patients with PTSD.

Reference

Saigh PA, Bremner JD (1999). The history of posttraumatic stress disorder. In: Saigh PA, Bremner JD, eds. *Posttraumatic Stress Disorder: A Comprehensive Text*. Needham Heights, MA: Allyn & Bacon, pp. 1–17.

SECTION I
Preclinical sciences of stress

CHAPTER 1

Posttraumatic stress disorder: from neurobiology to clinical presentation

Arieh Y. Shalev[1] & J. Douglas Bremner[2]

[1] *Department of Psychiatry, New York University School of Medicine, Langone Medical Center, New York, NY, USA*
[2] *Departments of Psychiatry & Behavioral Sciences and Radiology, Emory University School of Medicine, and the Atlanta VA Medical Center, Atlanta, GA, USA*

1.1 PTSD: prevalence, risk factors, and etiology

Posttraumatic stress disorder (PTSD) is a chronic, disabling, and prevalent anxiety disorder. It is triggered by exposure to a psychologically traumatic event, yet only a minority of those exposed actually develop the disorder. Trauma characteristics, as well as genetic, biological, and psychosocial risk factors, contribute to the occurrence of PTSD among survivors of traumatic events. PTSD, therefore is a prime example of gene-environment and psycho-biological interaction. There is a large amount of research in animals on the effects of stress on neurobiology. This has been translated into clinical neuroscience research in PTSD patients. The overarching goal is for our understanding of the neurobiology of the stress response and the long-term effects of stress on stress-responsive systems to inform treatment approaches to PTSD patients. The chapters in this volume, from researchers in all areas of the stress field, including basic scientists as well as research and clinical psychologists and psychiatrists, illustrate the advances in the field that have continued to move from neurobiology to treatment of PTSD. This chapter serves as an introduction to the volume and gives a broad overview of the field.

Posttraumatic stress disorder was first recognized as a distinct psychiatric disorder in the third edition of the American Psychiatric Association's (APA) *Diagnostic and Statistical Manual of Mental Disorders* (DSM-III; APA, 1981). Subsequent studies have established – and slightly modified – the disorder's symptom structure, evaluated its natural course, and assessed the disorder's biological features. The DSM-IV-TR has been in use for many years, and PTSD symptoms based on that are shown in Box 1.1; however, recently the DSM-5 was released (APA, 2014), and the changes from DSM-IV-TR are described later in this chapter.

Box 1.1 *Diagnostic and statistical manual of mental disorders-IV-TR* criteria for posttraumatic stress disorder.

A. The person has been exposed to a traumatic event in which both of the following were present:

1 The person experienced, witnessed, or was confronted with an event that involved actual or threatened death or serious injury, or a threat to the physical integrity of self or others.
2 The person's response involved intense fear, helplessness, or horror. Note: In children this may be expressed, instead, by disorganized or agitated behavior.

B. The traumatic event is persistently re-experienced in one (or more) of the following ways:

1 Recurrent and intrusive distressing recollections of the event, including images, thoughts, or perceptions. Note: In young children, repetitive play may occur in which themes or aspects of the trauma are expressed.
2 Recurrent distressing dreams of the event. Note: In children, there may be frightening dreams without recognizable content.
3 Acting or feeling as if the traumatic event were recurring (includes a sense of reliving the experience, illusions, hallucinations, and dissociative flashback episodes, including those that occur on awakening or when intoxicated). Note: In young children, trauma-specific re-enactment may occur.
4 Intense psychological distress at exposure to internal or external cues that symbolize or resemble an aspect of the traumatic event.
5 Physiological reactivity on exposure to internal or external cues that symbolize or resemble an aspect of the traumatic event.

C. Persistent avoidance of stimuli associated with the trauma and numbing of general responsiveness (not present before the trauma), as indicated by three (or more) of the following:

1 Efforts to avoid thoughts, feelings, or conversations associated with the trauma.
2 Efforts to avoid activities, places, or people that arouse recollections of the trauma.
3 Inability to recall an important aspect of the trauma.
4 Markedly diminished interest or participation in significant activities.
5 Feeling of detachment or estrangement from others.
6 Restricted range of affect (e.g., unable to have loving feelings).
7 Sense of a foreshortened future (e.g., does not expect to have a career, marriage, children, or a normal life span).

D. Persistent symptoms of increased arousal (not present before the trauma), as indicated by two (or more) of the following:

1 Difficulty falling or staying asleep.
2 Irritability or outbursts of anger.
3 Difficulty concentrating.

4 Hypervigilance.
5 Exaggerated startle response.

E. Duration of the disturbance (symptoms in criteria B, C, and D) is more than 1 month.

F. The disturbance causes clinically significant distress or impairment in social, occupational, or other important areas of functioning.

Specify if:
Acute – if duration of symptoms is less than 3 months.
Chronic – if duration of symptoms is 3 months or more.
With delayed onset – if onset of symptoms is at least 6 months after the stressor.

Posttraumatic stress disorder frequently follows a chronic course and can be associated with recurrences related to exposure to multiple traumas. In addition, PTSD is frequently comorbid with other psychiatric conditions, such as anxiety disorders, depression and substance abuse (Kessler et al., 1995).

Posttraumatic stress disorder is hypothesized to involve the brain's emotional-learning circuitry, and the various brain structures (e.g., prefrontal lobes) and neuroendocrine systems (e.g., the hypothalamic–pituitary–adrenal [HPA] axis) that modulate the acquisition, retention, and eventual extinction of fear conditioning (Bremner & Charney, 2010).

The purpose of this chapter is to bridge the gap between neurobiology and treatment of PTSD that is covered in more detail in the many chapters in this volume related to these topics. This chapter will address issues concerning the acquisition and course of PTSD, including physiological and neuroendocrine factors; recognition and impairment; recent studies of psychotherapy and pharmacotherapy and their effects on neurobiology as well as symptom response; and suggest some directions for research.

1.1.1 The syndrome

Formally, PTSD is defined by the co-occurrence of three clusters of symptoms (*re-experiencing, avoidance*, and *hyperarousal*) in an individual who had undergone a traumatic event (Box 1.1).

Symptoms of *re-experiencing* consist of intrusive, uncontrollable and involuntary instances of re-living the traumatic event, with feelings of fear and panic, and with corresponding physiological responses such as palpitation, sweating or muscular tension. Such "intrusive" experiences often occur upon exposure to cues that remind the person of the traumatic event, but they also occur spontaneously, such as during nightmares or periods of relaxed attention.

Avoidance in PTSD includes phobic avoidance (i.e., of cues and situations that resemble the traumatic event) along with extended avoidance and numbing, expressed as restricted range of affects, diminished interest in previously significant activities, feelings of detachment and estrangement from others and a sense of foreshortened future. The latter clearly resemble symptoms of depression, and may explain the frequent overlap between PTSD and depression.

Symptoms of *PTSD hyperarousal* include insomnia, anger, difficulties concentrating, hypervigilance and exaggerated startle. Importantly, these symptoms are unrelated to specific reminders of the traumatic event, and constitute an unrelenting and pervasive background of tension and irritability, affecting the patient's entire life.

In the recently released DSM-5, symptoms of PTSD have remained mostly the same, but the trauma definition no longer requires feelings of fear, helplessness, or horror in conjunction with the trauma (APA, 2014). In addition, new qualifying symptoms were added. As can be seen from Box 1.1, symptoms must be present for at least 1 month for a formal diagnosis of PTSD to be made. If symptoms are present for less than 3 months, the disorder is termed "acute," while symptoms enduring beyond 3 months are considered "chronic" PTSD.

The *symptom criteria* of PTSD have been rather consistent across successive revisions of the DSM. The few changes that were made concerned manifestations of guilt, which figured in DSM-III, and were omitted from subsequent editions, and the presence of bodily responses upon exposure to reminders of the traumatic event, a diagnostic criterion which has been moved from the "hyperarousal" cluster into the "re-experiencing" cluster. More recently, DSM-5 added a new criterion of negative alterations in cognition and mood, which comprises symptoms such as a persistent and distorted blame of self or others, and a persistent negative emotional state. A new symptom of reckless or destructive behavior was also added as part of the hyperarousal symptom cluster.

In contrast, the appraisal of the *traumatic event* has changed considerably. The original description of PTSD, in DSM-III, was clearly influenced by the consequences of the Vietnam war, and therefore defined the traumatic event as being out of the range of normal human experiences and capable of provoking distress among most subjects exposed. This perception has been eroded by studies that showed that PTSD could develop in the aftermath of frequently occurring traumata, such as road traffic accidents or physical assault (Shalev et al., 1988). Consequently, the current definition of a traumatic event is very permissive indeed and applies to a large array of situations and events. DSM-IV-TR required both *exposure* to a threatening event and *intense response* in the form of fear, horror, or helplessness in order for an event to formally qualify as "traumatic." The requirement of the latter was dropped in the most recent version, DSM-5. Overall the DSM-5 has loosened the criteria for PTSD, so that a much larger proportion of the population is expected to meet criteria for PTSD under the new definition (APA, 2014).

The risk of developing PTSD varies according to the type of trauma. The disorder's lifetime prevalence rates among civilians has been estimated at 1.3–7.8% (Davidson et al., 1991; Kessler et al., 1995). A higher lifetime PTSD prevalence of around 30% has been reported for Vietnam veterans and female victims of rape in retrospective epidemiological studies (Kulka et al., 1990; Resnick et al., 1993). In common with many other psychiatric disorders, a higher prevalence of PTSD occurs in women than in men (Kessler et al., 1995).

1.1.2 Natural course, vulnerability and risk factors

Many trauma survivors develop transient and self-remitting forms of PTSD. Prospective studies have shown 66% recovery from fully expressed PTSD among survivors of motor vehicle accidents (Kessler et al., 1995), and 66% recovery within 1 year of a traumatic event of 236 survivors of miscellaneous civilian events who had PTSD 1 month after the traumatic event (Shalev et al., 1993b). However, the recovery curve of PTSD reaches a plateau after 72 months (Solomon et al., 1989), with most cases of recovery occurring during the first year that follows the traumatic event. Recovery from chronic PTSD is often incomplete (Pelcovitz et al., 1994; Shalev et al., 1993b), and those who recover remain vulnerable to subsequent stress.

Prospective studies have also shown that the symptoms of early and "recoverable" PTSD resemble those seen months and years later in people who remain ill (van der Kolk et al., 1996). Moreover, subjects who continue to suffer from PTSD seem to express the *same intensity* of symptoms that they have expressed shortly after the traumatic event. The phenotype, therefore, appears to remain over time, whereas the nature of the underlying mechanisms might change. This is in line with a general model of learning (Andreski et al., 1998), according to which neuronal mechanisms that mediate the *acquisition of new behavior* are not the same as those involved in its subsequent practice. Reversibility during the latter phase is obviously more difficult than during acquisition, and this may explain the prolonged and treatment-resistant nature of chronic PTSD.

In its chronic form, PTSD is often complicated by co-occurring depression. The nature of the association between PTSD and depression is unclear, with some studies suggesting that depression develops as a secondary consequence of PTSD (Solomon et al., 1989; Turnbull, 1998) and others suggesting that the two may be independent consequences of traumatic events, and develop simultaneously (Pelcovitz et al., 1997). In addition to depression, substance abuse is commonly reported in survivors of traumatic events with PTSD, physical health often declines, and social relationships can be adversely affected (Bremner et al., 1996c). Thus, chronic PTSD is very disabling, with symptoms affecting patients' well-being, interpersonal relationships and vocational capacity. PTSD is associated with a significant loss of role functioning, as expressed by absence from work or unemployment (Shalev et al., 1996).

1.1.3 Understanding the occurrence of PTSD

There are two competing models for understanding the occurrence and the persistence of PTSD among some survivors. The first model assumes that PTSD is triggered by an abnormal *initial* response to traumatic stress, affecting memory consolidation and aversive learning (Chilcoat & Breslau, 1998; Fesler, 1991). This view is supported by findings of intense autonomic response during the traumatic event (Shalev et al., 1988, 1998). These initial "unconditioned" responses were thought to reinforce aversive learning via excessive adrenergic drive and through a failure to mount sufficient amounts of the protective stress hormone cortisol (Yehuda & Antelman, 1993). The model points to the need to address the very early bodily and emotional responses to a traumatic event in order to prevent PTSD.

The alternative model postulates that PTSD is significantly affected by factors that follow the traumatic event and is, therefore, a "disorder of recovery." In a recent meta-analysis of risk factors for PTSD, for example, deficient recovery environment and adversity following trauma were found to be the major risk factors for subsequent PTSD (Brewin et al., 2000). A prospective study has also shown that abnormal startle response – a typical symptom of PTSD – develops within the first few months after the traumatic event in individuals who continue to express PTSD symptoms (Shalev et al., 2000). These findings are in line with the *progressive sensitization* model of PTSD, according to which the occurrence and persistence of PTSD symptoms progressively alter the central nervous system (CNS). It suggests that preventive interventions be conducted during the acquisition phase of the disorder (i.e., the first few months following exposure).

Finally, the likelihood of developing PTSD is significantly affected by factors that precede the traumatic event. For example, a twin study of Vietnam veterans (Goldberg et al., 1990; True et al., 1993) showed a significant contribution of inherited vulnerability PTSD symptoms following combat. Inherited factors also affect the likelihood of being exposed to combat (Goldberg et al., 1990; True et al., 1993). Other vulnerability factors include lifetime occurrence of psychiatric disorders, cumulated exposure to traumatic events and adversities during childhood, lower education levels and adverse family environments.

Thus, PTSD should be seen as the compounded result of several risk factors, in the presence of which a traumatic event triggers a cascade of biological, mental and interpersonal processes leading to chronic PTSD.

Recent studies of the extinction of fear responses raise the previously discussed possibility that PTSD might be the result of a failure to extinguish an initial fear response (Bremner & Charney, 2010). Functional brain imaging studies, reviewed later in this chapter, have explored the role of medial prefrontal structures in PTSD.

1.1.4 Delayed and chronic forms of PTSD

The onset of PTSD can be delayed for years. In a large study by Solomon et al. (1989) looking at individuals who presented for treatment within 6 years of the Lebanon war, 10% were considered delayed onset, 40% were delayed help-seeking, 33% were exacerbation of subclinical PTSD, 13% were reactivation of recovered PTSD, and the remaining 4% had other psychiatric disorders. This is confirmed in the study by Shalev et al. (1996), in which 5.1% of patients were truly delayed-onset PTSD and the rest were mainly PTSD patients who recovered and were then reactivated by another event.

Most cases of PTSD recover within 1 year, and after 6 years recovery without treatment is unlikely (Kessler et al., 1995). However, up to 40% of patients with acute PTSD end by having a chronic condition. Chronic PTSD is prolonged and may be unremitting, and subject to reactivation upon exposure to stressors. In addition, it can be disabling and associated with substantial comorbidity. The risk of developing secondary comorbid disorders is related to a number of factors, including the severity of the trauma, gender, family history, past history and the complexity of the PTSD reaction. Chronic PTSD is linked with abuse of alcohol, drugs and prescription medications (Kulka et al., 1990). It is also associated with an increase in suicidal behavior, although studies have not documented an increase in completed suicide (Krysinska & Lester, 2010). The percentages of individuals with PTSD who have at least one other lifetime disorder is 88.0% for men and 79.0% for women. The major comorbid disorder seen with PTSD is depression, occurring in 47.9% of men and 48.5% of women. Other comorbid disorders include dysthymia, simple phobia and generalized anxiety disorder.

1.1.5 Disability associated with PTSD

The chronic form of PTSD is often debilitating. The disability associated with PTSD includes work impairment, change in life trajectories, impaired social relations, marital instability and perpetuation of violence. This represents a burden not only to the individual but also to society.

In a study based on analysis of the National Comorbidity Survey (NCS) data, which examined the effects of mental disorders on work impairment, work loss (defined as missing a full day of work) and work cut-back (either missing part of a day or working less efficiently than usual) during the previous month were 0.8 and 2.8 days/month, respectively (Kessler & Frank, 1997). The amount of work impairment associated with PTSD was the same as that associated with major depression but less than that associated with panic disorder (Kessler & Frank, 1997).

In term of disability to life events caused by PTSD in the NCS data, there is an increased risk of making suicide plans (odds ratio [OR] = 2.4; 95% confidence interval [CI] : 1.7–3.3) and an increased risk of attempting suicide (OR = 6; 95% CI : 3.4–10.7) for patients suffering from PTSD. In addition, marital instability, unemployment and increased use of outpatient care contribute greatly to the burden to society (Kessler, 2000). It remains unclear whether similar effects exist in other countries, although the NCS analyses showed that the most extreme adverse effects of traumatic events were associated with complex ongoing traumas that occur in childhood, such as parental violence, alcoholism or depression. Such experiences interfere with lifelong patterns of interpersonal relationships and the process of mastering basic educational skills.

In the study by Stein et al. (2000b), patients with PTSD reported significantly more functional impairment than patients without mental disorders. In addition, patients with PTSD made greater use of healthcare resources than non-mentally ill patients and encountered considerable functional impairment.

A study of the quality of life with PTSD reported greater impairment at baseline for subjects with PTSD relative to those with major depression and obsessive-compulsive disorder on several domains of the 36-item Short-Form Health Survey (Malik et al., 1999). Similarly, in a study of PTSD among civilians, significant impairment was associated with PTSD as seen on the Sheehan Disability Scale, which measures the total work, family and social/leisure disability, and the Vulnerability to the Effects of Stress Scale (Connor et al., 1999). Considerable improvement to this disability with PTSD was achieved through treatment in both these studies.

1.1.6 Comorbidity

Chronic PTSD is linked with abuse of alcohol, drugs and medication (Chilcoat & Breslau, 1998; Kessler, 2000). In common with many other anxiety disorders, PTSD is often complicated by secondary depression (60–80% of patients), particularly if the condition has not been treated. Patients will therefore present in either primary or secondary care with comorbid depression, which complicates the recognition of PTSD *per se*, and prevents the primary diagnosis from being made. Despite some of the symptoms of PTSD being shared with major depression, the clinician should be alerted by the presence of intrusive recollections and pervasive avoidance of a trauma. In addition, when PTSD is complicated by secondary depression, the symptom profile tends to differ from that of major depression, with less psychomotor retardation or agitation (Ballenger et al., 2000). In the study of PTSD in the primary care medical setting by Stein et al. (2000b), 11.8% of primary care attendees met diagnostic criteria for either full or partial PTSD.

Comorbidity with major depression (61% of cases of PTSD) and generalized anxiety disorder (39%) was common, but less so with social phobia (17%) and panic disorder (6%). Substance-use disorder comorbidity (22%) was also fairly common.

Patients who suffer from the effects of chronic interpersonal violence are more likely to have chronic PTSD, and the symptom profile is likely to be more complex and often involves severe forms of dissociation not found in more typical cases of PTSD. The profile is so distinct it has been argued for the creation of a separate diagnosis to characterize this response known as "complex PTSD" (Herman, 1992; Zlotnick et al., 1996) or "disorders of extreme stress not otherwise specified" (van der Kolk et al., 1996; Pelcovitz et al., 1997). Although this diagnosis is not included in the DSM-IV due to the fact that the vast majority of patients with this symptom cluster also meet criteria for PTSD, it is nonetheless clear that a complex PTSD subtype exists. This subtype is more chronic and disabling than other cases of PTSD, and it is particularly common among patients who were exposed at an early age to chronic traumatic interpersonal violence.

1.2 Neurobiology of PTSD

The neurobiology of the stress response involves mechanisms related to bodily survival and adaptation to change. Stress is associated with various types of learning, including the learning of conditioned fear responses and autobiographical memory formation. While these adaptations can have survival value, a failure of another type of learning – the turning off of the fear response (or extinction) when no longer needed – can lead to pathology, including symptoms of PTSD. The breadth of the topic can be appraised by examining the time frames of some of the typical responses. The latter extend from fragments of seconds (e.g., for defense reflexes such as auditory startle), to several seconds (for sympathetic activation), tens of minutes (for activation of the HPA axis), hours (for early gene expression), days (for memory consolidation) and months (for permanent changes in the CNS to occur) (Post, 1992).

Furthermore, at each stage, the biological responses to mental stressors are heavily modulated by appraisal (e.g., of the threat and of one's own resources; Lazarus & Folkman, 1984), controllability, and attribution of meaning, and by the relative success in coping with tasks related to survival and learning. Prior experiences and beliefs are also powerful modulators of the mental and therefore the biological response to adversities. Most adverse mental health consequences of traumatic events result from our immense ability to learn, remember, and reshape our behavior (and the underlying CNS functioning) on the basis of new – including catastrophic – experiences. The meaning conveyed to one's action (e.g., cowardice, heroism), as well as the meaningfulness of a group effort (e.g., unnecessary war) can either soothe and down-regulate fear responses or maintain and reinforce them (Holloway & Ursano, 1984).

Stress results in acute and chronic changes in neurochemical systems and specific brain regions, which result in long-term changes in brain "circuits" involved in the stress response (Bremner, 2011; Vermetten & Bremner, 2002a,b). Brain regions that are felt to play an important role in PTSD include the hippocampus, the amygdala, and the medial prefrontal cortex. Cortisol and norepinephrine are two neurochemical systems that are critical in the stress response.

1.2.1 Cortisol and norepinephrine

The corticotropin-releasing factor (CRF)/HPA axis system plays an important role in the stress response (Chrousos & Gold, 1992) (see Chapter 11). CRF is released from the hypothalamus, with stimulation of adrenocorticotropin hormone (ACTH) release from the pituitary, resulting in glucocorticoid (cortisol in man) release from the adrenal, which in turn has a negative feedback effect on the axis at the level of the pituitary, as well as central brain sites including the hypothalamus and hippocampus. Cortisol has a number of effects that facilitate survival and triggers other neurochemical responses to stress, such as the noradrenergic system via the brainstem locus coeruleus (Melia & Duman, 1991). Other responses include an activation of brain areas related to perceiving and responding to the environment. Other players in the immediate response include nuclei controlling facial expression, breathing rhythm, startle response, and parasympathetic modulation of heart rate. This cluster of responses is controlled by the central nucleus of the amygdala – a powerful modulator of fear responses (Davis, 1992; LeDoux, 1993, 1996).

Stress also results in activation of the noradrenergic system, centered in the locus coeruleus. Noradrenergic neurons release transmitter throughout the brain which is associated with an increase in alerting and vigilance behaviors, critical for coping with acute threat (Abercrombie & Jacobs, 1987; Bremner et al., 1996a,b).

Studies in animals have shown that early stress has lasting effects on the HPA axis and norepinephrine (Plotsky & Meaney, 1993). These effects could be mediated by an increase in synthesis of CRH messenger RNA (mRNA) following stress (Makino et al., 1995). Exposure to chronic stress results in potentiation of noradrenergic responsiveness to subsequent stressors and increased release of norepinephrine in the hippocampus and other brain regions (Abercrombie & Jacobs, 1987). It has been theorized that a failure to mount appropriate levels of cortisol during traumatic events may lead to prolonged adrenergic activation and thereby increase the risk of developing PTSDs (Yehuda, 1998). Abnormally low cortisol levels following trauma were, in fact, reported in vulnerable rape victims and in road accident survivors who were at higher risk for developing PTSD (McFarlane et al., 1997; Resnick et al., 1995), but the causal link with PTSD has not been established. A combination of adrenergic activation and low levels of cortisol has been shown to significantly increase emotional learning in animals (Bohus, 1984; Munck et al., 1984). Importantly, the hormonal stress response seems to "go wrong" in individuals whose prior life experience was particularly stressful (Resnick et al., 1995) – yet this also requires further confirmation. The intensity of biopsychological responses to traumatic events increases in circumstances that are uncontrollable and inescapable (Anisman et al., 1981; Breier, 1989; Seligman & Meier, 1967).

1.2.2 Biology of learning and adaptation in PTSD

Immediate alarm responses are followed, in the brain, by a cascade of metabolic and genomic (i.e., expression of new genes) events (Post, 1992). Importantly, the cascade of neuronal changes includes areas of the brain that are not directly involved in stress response. Particularly interesting is the activation of protein synthesis in brain areas related to learning and memory, such as the hippocampus and the amygdala (e.g., Davis, 1994) (see Chapter 6). Newly synthesized proteins in these areas constitute the biological basis of long-term memories of stressful events.

The distribution of these biological changes in the brain suggests that there are two types of memory traces of stressful events: explicit memories (i.e., verbal and retrievable) and implicit memories (e.g., changes in habits, conditioned responses). This is very important, because non-verbal, implicit memories of traumatic events may shape future behavior in the absence of conscious elaboration and verbal recall (e.g., by causing bodily alarm and emotional fear responses upon exposure to reminders of the traumatic event). Experimental work in animals has shown that a subtype of emotional memories, based on "quick and dirty" processing of sensory information, is acquired and stored in the lateral and basal nuclei of the amygdala (LeDoux, 1993, 1995). LeDoux has also shown that such "emotional" learning (indeed, fear conditioning) is relatively immune to change. Memory traces stored in the basal and lateral nuclei of the amygdala are subsequently used to interpret new sensory signals as to their aversive nature, such that when a stimulus is interpreted as immediately threatening, the central nucleus of the amygdala is activated (see earlier) and the fear response is put in motion.

Despite the persistence of emotional learning, the behavioral expression of fear conditioning can be inhibited by the activity of cortical areas of the brain (Morgan et al., 1993; Morgan & LeDoux, 1995). This is, in fact, what happens when aversive or conditioned responses subside; the information is not forgotten or erased, but rather put under inhibitory control (Quirk et al., 2006). Brain areas involved in such inhibitory control include sensory association areas, areas in the frontal lobe and the hippocampus. Memories of traumatic events, therefore, are not suppressed, but rather controlled and neglected, such that they have no behavioral expression. Subsequent traumatization may activate such memories, yet the strategy of controlling the effect of aversive learning may also be stronger in individuals who recover from traumatic events. Exposure to stressful events, therefore, may either "sensitize" or "immunize" survivors (Solomon et al., 1987).

Further experimental work has shown that aversive memories, at the level of the amygdala, can be reinforced by elevated plasma levels of the stress hormone epinephrine (Cahill & McGaugh, 1998; McGaugh, 1985, 2000). An initial hypersecretion of the epinephrine could be involved in an exaggeration and a consolidation of fear-related memories of the traumatic event (Cahill et al., 1994; McGaugh et al., 1990). Moreover, the intensity of the adrenergic "stress" response can also foster emotional (and amygdala-mediated) learning at the expense of rational or declarative, hippocampus-mediated learning (Metcalfe & Jacobs, 1996). Supportive evidence for the link between an initial autonomic activation and subsequent PTSD has been found in a study of patients presenting to the emergency room after a trauma (Shalev et al., 1998). Heart rate levels upon admission were higher in subjects who subsequently developed PTSD. In another study of trauma survivors, the physiological response of heart rate, skin conductance and electromyography (*frontalis*) to mental imagery recorded a short time following the trauma was shown to differentiate between those who went on to develop PTSD and those who did not (Shalev et al., 1993a). Trauma survivors admitted to the emergency room, who subsequently went on to develop PTSD had higher heart rates at the emergency department and 1 week later, but not after 1 and 4 months (Shalev et al., 1988). PTSD patients can re-access their trauma memories as often as 100 times a day, and elicit these physiological reactions each time. PTSD patients possibly continue to reinforce the initial impact of the trauma by reactivating it in this way. PTSD patients have also been reported to differentiate from normal survivors by poor habituation of skin conductance to a repetition of loud startling noises (Shalev et al., 1992). This may represent a primary defect of the CNS that continues to identify and classify the loud tones as threatening in people with PTSD. PTSD patients, therefore, continue to react, rather than rejecting the noises as redundant information and stopping the reaction to them. In a prospective study of 239 trauma survivors (Shalev et al., 2000), the auditory startle response of all the trauma survivors is normal at 1 week. The response of those patients who go on to develop PTSD becomes abnormal between 1 and 4 months after the trauma, suggesting that this is the critical period during which the CNS adapts its response to ambiguous stimuli (such as loud noises) and determines whether PTSD develops.

There are two important questions for the clinician to address when trying to recognize the vulnerable patients who will develop PTSD: why does trauma lead to PTSD for them rather than some other psychiatric disorder or no disorder at all; and what are the risk factors for determining these patients? The acute stress response is universal and non-predictive of PTSD. Moreover, as mentioned, patients who develop PTSD fail to show a remission of these acute symptoms and show abnormally increased heart rates several days after the trauma, as well as other abnormal physiological responses such as the increased startle response. It would therefore appear that PTSD might develop as a failure of the body to reverse the acute stress response.

Preclinical and clinical studies have shown alterations in memory function following traumatic stress as well as changes in a circuit of brain areas, including hippocampus, amygdala, and medial prefrontal cortex, that mediate alterations in memory (Bremner, 2003, 2010, 2011; Bremner & Charney, 2010; Garakani et al., 2011). The hippocampus, a brain area involved in verbal declarative memory, is very sensitive to the effects of stress (see Chapter 6). Stress in animals was associated with alterations in neuronal structure in the CA3 region of the hippocampus (which may be mediated by hypercortisolemia, decreased brain-derived neurotrophic factor, and/or elevated glutamate levels) and inhibition of neurogenesis (Magarinos & McEwen, 1995; Nibuya et al., 1995; Sapolsky et al., 1990). As reviewed in Chapter 6, high levels of glucocorticoids seen with stress were also associated with deficits in new learning (Diamond et al., 1996; Luine et al., 1994). Antidepressant treatments block the effects of stress and/or promote neurogenesis in the hippocampus (Nibuya et al., 1995; Santarelli et al., 2003), including phenytoin (Watanabe et al., 1992), tianeptine, dihydroepiandosterone, and fluoxetine (Czeh et al., 2001; D'Sa & Duman, 2002; Duman, 2004; Duman et al., 2001; Garcia, 2002; Lucassen et al., 2004; Malberg et al., 2000; McEwen & Chattarji, 2004), which may represent, at least in part, the mechanism of action of the behavioral effects of antidepressants (Santarelli et al., 2003; Watanabe et al., 1992; although see Henn & Vollmayr, 2004). Changes in the environment have also been shown to modulate neurogenesis in the dentate gyrus of the hippocampus, and slow the normal age-related decline in neurogenesis (Gould et al., 1999; Kempermann et al., 1998).

Chapter 11 of this volume reviews the long-term dysregulation of the HPA axis associated with PTSD. Findings include low or normal baseline levels of cortisol (Yehuda et al., 1991, 1995a) with two studies using multiple serial measurements in plasma showing a loss of normal diurnal rhythm and decreases at specific times of the day (Bremner et al., 1997; Yehuda et al., 1994), elevations in CRF (Baker et al., 1999; Bremner et al., 1997), increased negative feedback of the HPA axis after dexamethasone challenge (Stein et al., 1997; Yehuda et al., 1993) and increased cortisol response to stress, especially trauma-specific stressors (Elzinga et al., 2003).

1.2.3 Cognitive function and brain structure in PTSD

Studies in PTSD are consistent with changes in cognition and brain structure (see Chapter 12 in this volume for a review of brain imaging studies in PTSD). Multiple studies have demonstrated verbal declarative memory deficits in PTSD

(Brewin, 2001; Buckley et al., 2000; Elzinga & Bremner, 2002; Golier & Yehuda, 1998). Patients with PTSD secondary to combat (Bremner et al., 1993a; Golier et al., 1997; Uddo et al., 1993; Vasterling et al., 1998; Yehuda et al., 1995b), rape (Jenkins et al., 1998), the Holocaust (Golier et al., 2002; Yehuda et al., 1995b), and childhood abuse (Bremner et al., 1995a; Bremner et al., 2004; Moradi et al., 1999) were found to have deficits in verbal declarative memory function based on neuropsychological testing with a relative sparing of visual memory and IQ (Barrett et al., 1996; Bremner et al., 1993a, 1995a; Gil et al., 1990; Gilbertson et al., 2001; Golier et al., 1997, 2002; Jenkins et al., 1998; Moradi et al., 1999; Roca & Freeman, 2001; Sachinvala et al., 2000; Uddo et al., 1993; Vasterling et al., 1998, 2002; Yehuda et al., 1995b). Other types of memory disturbance studies in PTSD include gaps in memory for everyday events (dissociative amnesia; Bremner et al., 1993b), deficits in autobiographical memory (McNally et al., 1994), an attentional bias for trauma-related material (Beck et al., 2001; Bryant & Harvey, 1995; Cassiday et al., 1992; Foa et al., 1991; Golier et al., 2003; McNally et al., 1990, 1993; McNeil et al., 1999; Moradi et al., 2000; Thrasher et al., 1994) and frontal lobe-related impairments (Beckham et al., 1998). These studies show that PTSD is associated with deficits in verbal declarative memory (Elzinga & Bremner, 2002).

Studies have also shown a smaller volume of the hippocampus in PTSD (Bremner & Vermetten, 2012). Vietnam veterans with PTSD were originally shown to have 8% smaller right hippocampal volume based on magnetic resonance imaging (MRI) relative to controls matched for a variety of factors such as alcohol abuse and education (Bremner et al., 1995b). These studies, which are described in detail in Chapter 12 of this volume, were later extended to adults with PTSD from childhood abuse, but not children with PTSD. Other studies in PTSD have found smaller hippocampal volume and/or reductions in N-acetyl aspartate, a marker of neuronal integrity. Meta-analyses, in which data are pooled from all of the published studies, found smaller hippocampal volume for both the left and the right sides, equally in adult men and women with chronic PTSD, and no change in children (Kitayama et al., 2005; Smith, 2005; Woon et al., 2010). Several studies have shown that PTSD patients have deficits in hippocampal activation while performing a verbal declarative memory task (Astur et al., 2006; Bremner et al., 2003; Shin et al., 2004b).

In addition to the hippocampus, other brain structures have been implicated in a neural circuitry of stress, including the amygdala and prefrontal cortex. Animal studies also show that early stress is associated with a decrease in branching of neurons in the medial prefrontal cortex (Radley et al., 2004). Studies in PTSD found smaller volumes of the anterior cingulate based on MRI measurements (Kitayama et al., 2006; Rauch et al., 2003). Structural imaging studies in PTSD are reviewed in more detail in Chapter 12.

1.2.4 Neural circuits in PTSD

Brain imaging studies have shown alterations in a circuit, including medial prefrontal cortex (including anterior cingulate), hippocampus and amygdala, in PTSD (Bremner, 2011). Exposure to traumatic reminders in the form of traumatic slides and/or sounds or traumatic scripts was associated with an increase in PTSD symptoms and most consistently decreased blood flow and/or failure of activation in the medial prefrontal cortex/anterior cingulate, as well as decreased hippocampal function in some studies, as reviewed in more detail in Chapter 12. Exposure to specific fearful stimuli or fear conditioning resulted in increased amygdala function (Bremner et al., 1999, 2005; Rauch et al., 1996, 2000, 2006; Shin et al., 1997, 2004a) Studies have shown that treatment with medication, including the antidepressant paroxetine and phenytoin, and various psychotherapies and behavioral therapies, increase hippocampal volume in PTSD patients and reverse medial prefrontal cortical dysfunction.

In summary, dysfunction of a circuit involving the medial prefrontal cortex hippocampus and amygdala underlies symptoms of PTSD. Imaging studies are reviewed in more detail in Chapter 12.

1.3 Synthesis of findings: from neurobiology to treatment of PTSD

Traumatic stress has a broad range of effects on brain function and structure, as well as on neuropsychological components of memory. Brain areas implicated in the stress response include the amygdala, hippocampus, and prefrontal cortex. Neurochemical systems including cortisol and norepinephrine play a critical role in the stress response. These brain areas play an important role in the stress response. They also play a critical role in memory, highlighting the important interplay between memory and the traumatic stress response. Studies outlined in the chapters in this volume show that translation of basic science studies of the effects of stress on brain and behavior to clinically relevant aspects of approaches to PTSD treatment can potentially add to the treatment of PTSD.

Studies in patients with PTSD show alterations in brain areas implicated in animal studies, including the amygdala, hippocampus, and prefrontal cortex, as well as in neurochemical stress response systems, including cortisol and norepinephrine. Treatments that are efficacious for PTSD show a promotion of neurogenesis in animal studies, as well as a promotion of memory and increased hippocampal volume in PTSD. Studies also show an improvement with treatment in brain circuits underlying PTSD symptoms.

Intervening soon after the trauma is critical for long-term outcomes, because, with time, traumatic memories become indelible and resistant to treatment (Meadows & Foa, 1999). Early treatments are not necessarily effective. For instance, studies have shown that critical incident stress debriefing (CISD) can be associated with a worsening of outcome relative to no treatment at all (Mayou et al., 2000). Pharmacological treatment of chronic PTSD has shown efficacy originally for imipramine, amitriptyline and phenalzine and later for brofaramine, paroxetine and sertraline (see Chapter 16). Selective serotonin reuptake inhibitors (SSRIs) are now recommended as first-line treatment for PTSD (Ballenger et al., 2004; Davidson, 2000, 2004; Davis et al., 2001; Foa et al., 1999; Stein et al., 2000a). The utility of early treatment is also demonstrated by animal studies showing that pretreatment before stress with antidepressants reduces chronic behavioral deficits related to stress (Petty et al., 1992; Sherman & Petty, 1982). Antidepressants, including both norepinephrine and SSRIs, as well as gabapentine and phenytoin, promote nerve growth (neurogenesis) in a part of the brain called the hippocampus, while stress inhibits neurogenesis (see Chapter 6). The chapters in this volume outline all aspects of research in PTSD, from epidemiology to the science of stress to evidence-based approaches to treatment. It is hoped that in future an integrated line of research will ultimately bear fruit in terms of successful new treatments for patients suffering from this crippling disorder and their families.

References

Abercrombie ED, Jacobs BL (1987) Single-unit response of noradrenergic neurons in the locus coeruleus of freely moving cats. I. Acutely presented stressful and non-stressful stimuli. *J Neurosci* 7, 2837–2847.

American Psychiatric Association (APA) (1981) *Diagnostic and Statistical Manual of Mental Disorders*, 3rd edn. American Psychiatric Association Press.

American Psychiatric Association (APA) (2014) *Diagnostic and Statistical Manual-5 (DSM-5)*. American Psychiatric Association Press.

Andreski P, Chilcoat H, Breslau N (1998) Post-traumatic stress disorder and somatization symptoms: a prospective study. *Psychiatry Res* 79, 131–138.

Anisman H, Ritch M, Sklar LS (1981) Noradrenergic and dopaminergic interactions in escape behavior: analysis of uncontrollable stress effects. *Psychopharmacology* 74, 263–268.

Astur RS, St Germain SA, Tolin D et al. (2006) Hippocampus function predicts severity of post-traumatic stress disorder. *Cyberpsychol Behav* 9, 234–240.

Baker DG, West SA, Nicholson WE et al. (1999) Serial CSF corticotropin-releasing hormone levels and adrenocortical activity in combat veterans with posttraumatic stress disorder. *Am J Psychiatry* 156, 585–588.

Ballenger JC, Davidson JR, Lecrubier Y et al. (2000) Consensus statement on posttraumatic stress disorder from the International Consensus Group on Depression and Anxiety. *Clin Psychiatry* 61, 60–66.

Ballenger JC, Davidson JR, Lecrubier Y et al. (2004) Consensus statement update on post-traumatic stress disorder from the international consensus group on depression and anxiety. *J Clin Psychiatry* 65 Suppl 1, 55–62.

Barrett DH, Green ML, Morris R et al. (1996) Cognitive functioning and posttraumatic stress disorder. *Am J Psychiatry* 153, 1492–1494.

Beck JG, Freeman JB, Shipherd JC et al. (2001) Specificity of Stroop interference in patients with pain and PTSD. *J Abnorm Psychology* 110, 536–543.

Beckham JC, Crawford AL, Feldman ME (1998) Trail making test performance in Vietnam combat veterans with and without posttraumatic stress disorder. *J Trauma Stress* 11, 811–819.

Bohus B (1984) Humoral modulation of learning and memory processes: physiological significance of brain and peripheral mechanisms. In: A Delacour (Ed.), The Memory System of the Brain. World Scientific, Singapore, pp. 337–364. In: Delacour A (ed.) *The Memory System of the Brain World Scientific, Singapore, pp* 337–364. World Scientific, Singapore, pp. 337–364.

Breier A (1989) Breier A (1989). Experimental approaches to human stress research: assessment of neurobiological mechanisms of stress in volunteers and psychiatric patients. *Biol Psychiatry* 26: 438–462.

Bremner JD (2003) Long-term effects of childhood abuse on brain and neurobiology. *Child Adolesc Psychiat Clin NA* 12, 271–292.

Bremner JD (2010) Imaging in CNS disease states: PTSD. In: Borsook D, Beccera L, Bullmore E et al. (eds) *Imaging in CNS Drug Discovery and Development: Implications for Disease and Therapy.* Springer, Basel, Switzerland, pp. 339–360.

Bremner JD (2011) Stress and human neuroimaging studies. In: Conrad CD (ed.) *The Handbook of Stress: Neuropsychological Effects on the Brain.* Wiley-Blackwell.

Bremner JD, Charney DS (2010) Neural circuits in fear and anxiety. In: Stein DJ, Hollander E, Rothbaum BO (eds) *Textbook of Anxiety Disorders*, 2nd edn. American Psychiatric Publishing, Arlington, VA, pp. 55–71.

Bremner JD, Krystal JH, Southwick SM et al. (1996a) Noradrenergic mechanisms in stress and anxiety: I. *Preclinical studies. Synapse* 23, 28–38.

Bremner JD, Krystal JH, Southwick SM et al. (1996b) Noradrenergic mechanisms in stress and anxiety: II. *Clinical studies. Synapse* 23, 39–51.

Bremner JD, Licinio J, Darnell A et al. (1997) Elevated CSF corticotropin-releasing factor concentrations in posttraumatic stress disorder. *Am J Psychiatry* 154, 624–629.

Bremner JD, Narayan M, Staib LH et al. (1999) Neural correlates of memories of childhood sexual abuse in women with and without posttraumatic stress disorder. *Am J Psychiatry* 156, 1787–1795.

Bremner JD, Randall PR, Capelli S et al. (1995a) Deficits in short-term memory in adult survivors of childhood abuse. *Psychiatry Res* 59, 97–107.

Bremner JD, Randall PR, Scott TM et al. (1995b) MRI-based measurement of hippocampal volume in patients with combat-related posttraumatic stress disorder. *Am J Psychiatry* 152, 973–981.

Bremner JD, Scott TM, Delaney RC et al. (1993a) Deficits in short-term memory in post-traumatic stress disorder. *Am J Psychiatry* 150, 1015–1019.

Bremner JD, Southwick SM, Darnell A et al. (1996c) Chronic PTSD in Vietnam combat veterans: Course of illness and substance abuse. *Am J Psychiatry* 153, 369–375.

Bremner JD, Steinberg M, Southwick SM et al. (1993b) Use of the Structured Clinical Interview for DSMIV-Dissociative Disorders for systematic assessment of dissociative symptoms in posttraumatic stress disorder. *Am J Psychiatry* 150, 1011–1014.

Bremner JD, Vermetten E (2012) The hippocampus and post-traumatic stress disorders. In: Bartsch T (ed.) *The Clinical Neurobiology of the Hippocampus: An integrative view.* Oxford University Press, USA, New York, NY, pp. 262–272.

Bremner JD, Vermetten E, Nafzal N et al. (2004) Deficits in verbal declarative memory function in women with childhood sexual abuse-related posttraumatic stress disorder (PTSD). *J Nerv Ment Dis* 192, 643–649.

Bremner JD, Vermetten E, Schmahl C et al. (2005) Positron emission tomographic imaging of neural correlates of a fear acquisition and extinction paradigm in women with childhood sexual abuse-related posttraumatic stress disorder. *Psychol Med* 35, 791–806.

Bremner JD, Vythilingam M, Vermetten E et al. (2003) MRI and PET study of deficits in hippocampal structure and function in women with childhood sexual abuse and posttraumatic stress disorder. *Am J Psychiatry* 160, 924–932.

Brewin CR (2001) A cognitive neuroscience account of post-traumatic stress disorder and its treatment. *Behav Res Ther* 39, 373–393.

Brewin CR, Andrews B, Valentine JD (2000) Meta-analysis of risk factors for posttraumatic stress disorder in trauma-exposed adults. *J Consulting Clin Psychol* 68, 748–766.

Bryant RA, Harvey AG (1995) Processing threatening information in posttraumatic stress disorder. *J Abnorm Psychology* 104, 537–541.

Buckley TC, Blanchard EB, Neill WT (2000) Information processing and PTSD: A review of the empirical literature. *Clin Psychol Rev* 28, 1041–1065.

Cahill L, McGaugh JL (1998) Mechanisms of emotional arousal and lasting declarative memory. *Trends Neurosci* 21, 294–299.

Cahill L, Prins B, Weber M et al. (1994) Beta-adrenergic activation and memory for emotional events. *Nature* 371, 702–704.

Cassiday KL, McNally RJ, Zeitlin SB (1992) Cognitive processing of trauma cues in rape victims with posttraumatic stress disorder. *Cog Therap Res* 16, 283–295.

Chilcoat HD, Breslau N (1998) Posttraumatic stress disorder and drug disorders: testing causal pathways. *Arch Gen Psychiatry* 55, 913–917.

Chrousos GP, Gold PW (1992) The concepts of stress and stress system disorders: Overview of physical and behavioral homeostasis. *JAMA* 267, 1244–1252.

Connor KM, Sutherland SM, Tupler LA et al. (1999) Fluoxetine in post-traumatic stress disorder. Randomised, double-blind study. *Br J Psychiatry* 175, 17–22.

Czeh B, Michaelis T, Watanabe T et al. (2001) Stress-induced changes in cerebral metabolites, hippocampal volume, and cell proliferation are prevented by antidepressant treatment with tianeptine. *Proc Natl Acad Sci USA* 98, 12796–12801.

D'Sa C, Duman RS (2002) Antidepressants and neuroplasticity. *Bipolar Disorder* 4, 183–194.

Davidson JR (2000) Pharmacotherapy of posttraumatic stress disorder: treatment options, long-term follow-up, and predictors of outcome. *J Clin Psychiatry* 61, 52–56.

Davidson JR (2004) Long-term treatment and prevention of posttraumatic stress disorder. *J Clin Psychiatry* 65, 44–48.

Davidson JRT, Hughes D, Blazer DG (1991) Post-traumatic stress disorder in the community: an epidemiological study. *Psychol Med* 21, 713–721.

Davis LL, English BA, Ambrose SM et al. (2001) Pharmacotherapy for post-traumatic stress disorder: a comprehensive review. *Expert Opin Pharmacother* 2, 1583–1595.

Davis M (1992) The role of the amygdala in fear and anxiety. *Annu Rev Neurosci* 15, 353–375.

Diamond DM, Fleshner M, Ingersoll N et al. (1996) Psychological stress impairs spatial working memory: Relevance to electrophysiological studies of hippocampal function. *Behav Neurosci* 110, 661–672.

Duman RS (2004) Depression: a case of neuronal life and death? *Biol Psychiatry* 56, 140–145.

Duman RS, Malberg JE, Nakagawa S (2001) Regulation of adult neurogenesis by psychotropic drugs and stress. *J Pharmacol Exp Ther* 299, 401–407.

Elzinga BM, Bremner JD (2002) Are the neural substrates of memory the final common pathway in PTSD? *J Affect Disord* 70, 1–17.

Elzinga BM, Schmahl CS, Vermetten E et al. (2003) Higher cortisol levels following exposure to traumatic reminders in abuse-related PTSD. *Neuropsychopharmacology* 28, 1656–1665.

Fesler FA (1991) Valproate in combat-related posttraumatic stress disorder. *J Clin Psychiatry* 52, 361–364.

Foa EB, Davidson JRT, Frances A et al. (1999) The expert consensus guideline series: treatment of posttraumatic stress disorder. *J Clin Psychiatry* 60, 4–76.

Foa EB, Feske U, Murdock TB et al. (1991) Processing of threat related information in rape victims. *J Abnorm Psychology* 100, 156–162.

Garakani A, Murrough J, Mathew SJ et al. (2011) The neurobiology of anxiety disorders. In: Charney DS, Nestler EJ (eds) *Neurobiology of Mental Illness*.

Garcia R (2002) Stress, metaplasticity, and antidepressants. *Current Molecular Medicine* 2, 629–638.

Gil T, Calev A, Greenberg D et al. (1990) Cognitive functioning in posttraumatic stress disorder. *J Trauma Stress* 3, 29–45.

Gilbertson MW, Gurvits TV, Lasko NB et al. (2001) Multivariate assessment of explicit memory function in combat veterans with posttraumatic stress disorder. *J Trauma Stress* 14, 413–420.

Goldberg J, True WR, Eisen SA et al. (1990) A twin study of the effects of the Vietnam war on posttraumatic stress disorder. *JAMA* 263, 1227–1232.

Golier J, Yehuda R (1998) Neuroendocrine activity and memory-related impairments in posttraumatic stress disorder. *Dev Psychopathol* 10, 857–869.

Golier J, Yehuda R, Cornblatt B et al. (1997) Sustained attention in combat-related posttraumatic stress disorder. *Integr Physiol Behav Sci* 32, 52–61.

Golier JA, Yehuda R, Lupien SJ et al. (2003) Memory for trauma-related information in Holocaust survivors with PTSD. *Psychiatry Res* 121, 133–143.

Golier JA, Yehuda R, Lupien SJ et al. (2002) Memory performance in Holocaust survivors with posttraumatic stress disorder. *Am J Psychiatry* 159, 1682–1688.

Henn FA, Vollmayr B (2004) Neurogenesis and depression: etiology or epiphenomenon? *Biol Psychiatry* 56, 146–150.

Herman JL (1992) Complex PTSD: A syndrome in survivors of prolonged and repeated trauma. *J Trauma Stress* 5, 377–391.

Holloway HC, Ursano RJ (1984) The Vietnam veteran: memory, social context and metaphor. *Psychiatry* 47, 103–108.

Jenkins MA, Langlais PJ, Delis D et al. (1998) Learning and memory in rape victims with posttraumatic stress disorder. *Am J Psychiatry* 155, 278–279.

Kempermann, G., Kuhn, H. G., & Gage, F. H. (1998). Experience-induced neurogenesis in the senescent dentate gyrus. *Journal of Neuroscience* 18, 3206–3212.

Kessler RC (2000) Posttraumatic stress disorder: the burden to the individual and to society. *J Clin Psychiatry* 61, 4–12.

Kessler RC, Frank RG (1997) The impact of psychiatric disorders on work loss days. *Psychol Med* 27, 861–873.

Kessler RC, Sonnega A, Bromet E et al. (1995) Posttraumatic stress disorder in the national comorbidity survey. *Arch Gen Psychiatry* 52, 1048–1060.

Kitayama N, Quinn S, Bremner JD (2006) Smaller volume of anterior cingulate cortex in abuse-related posttraumatic stress disorder. *J Affect Disord* 90, 171–174.

Kitayama N, Vaccarino V, Kutner M et al. (2005) Magnetic resonance imaging (MRI) measurement of hippocampal volume in posttraumatic stress disorder: A meta-analysis. *J Affect Disord* 88, 79–86.

Krysinska K, Lester D (2010) Post-traumatic stress disorder and suicide risk: a systematic review. *Archives of Suicide Research* 14, 1–23.

Kulka RA, Schlenger WE, Fairbank JA et al. (1990) *Trauma and the Vietnam War Generation: Report of Findings from the National Vietnam Veterans Readjustment Study*. Brunner/Mazel, New York.

Lazarus RS, Folkman S (1984) *Stress, Appraisal and Coping*. Springer, New York.

LeDoux JE (1995) Setting stress into motion: brain mechanisms of stimulus evaluation. I In: Friedman JM, Charney DS, Deutch AY (eds) *Neurobiological and Clinical Consequences of Stress*. Lipincott-Raven, Philadelphia, pp. 125–134.

LeDoux JE (1996) *The Emotional Brain: The Mysterious Underpinnings of Emotional Life*. Simon & Schuster, New York, NY.

LeDoux JL (1993) In search of systems and synapses. *Ann NY Acad Sci* 702, 149–157.

Lucassen PJ, Fuchs E, Czeh B (2004) Antidepressant treatment with tianeptine reduces apoptosis in the hippocampal dentate gyrus and temporal cortex. *Eur J Neurosci* 14, 161–166.

Luine V, Villages M, Martinex C et al. (1994) Repeated stress causes reversible impairments of spatial memory performance. *Brain Res* 639, 167–170.

Magarinos AM, McEwen BS (1995) Stress-induced atrophy of apical dendrites of hippocampal CA3c neurons: involvement of glucocorticoid secretion and excitatory amino acid receptors. *Neuroscience* 1, 89–98.

Makino S, Smith MA, Gold PW (1995) Increased expression of corticotropin-releasing hormone and vasopressin messenger-ribonucleic acid (messenger RNA) in the hypothalamic paraventricular nucleus during repeated stress-association with reduction in glucocorticoid messenger-RNA levels. *Endocrinology* 136, 3299–3309.

Malberg JE, Eisch AJ, Nestler EJ et al. (2000) Chronic antidepressant treatment increases neurogenesis in adult rat hippocampus. *J Neurosci* 20, 9104–9110.

Malik ML, Connor KM, Sutherland SM et al. (1999) Quality of life and posttraumatic stress disorder: a pilot study assessing changes in SF-36 scores before and after treatment in a placebo-controlled trial of fluoxetine. *J Trauma Stress* 12, 387–393.

Mayou RA, Ehlers A, Hobbs M (2000) Psychological debriefing for road traffic accident victims. Three-year follow-up of a randomised controlled trial. *Br J Psychiatry* 176, 589–593.

McEwen BS, Chattarji S (2004) Molecular mechanisms of neuroplasticity and pharmacological implications: the example of tianeptine. *Eur Neuropsychopharmacol* 14 Suppl 5, S497–502.

McFarlane AC, Atchison M, Yehuda R (1997) The acute stress response following motor vehicle accidents and its relations to PTSD. *Ann NY Acad Sci* 821, 437–441.

McGaugh JL (1985) Peripheral and central adrenergic influences on brain systems involved in the modulation of memory storage. *Ann NY Acad Sci* 444, 150–161.

McGaugh JL (2000) Memory – A century of consolidation. *Science* 287, 248–251.

McGaugh JL, Introini-Collison IB, Nagahara AH et al. (1990) Involvement of the amygdaloid complex in neuromodulatory influences on memory storage. *Neurosci Biobehav Rev* 14, 425–431.

McNally RJ, English GE, Lipke HJ (1993) Assessment of intrusive cognition in PTSD: Use of the modified Stroop paradigm. *J Trauma Stress* 6, 33–41.

McNally RJ, Kaspi RJ, Riemann BC et al. (1990) Selective processing of threat cues in posttraumatic stress disorder. *J Abnorm Psychology* 99, 398–402.

McNally RJ, Litz BT, Prassas A et al. (1994) Emotional priming of autobiographical memory in posttraumatic stress disorder. *Cogn Emot* 8, 351–367.

McNeil DW, Tucker P, Miranda R et al. (1999) Response to depression and anxiety Stroop stimuli in posttraumatic stress disorder, obsessive-compulsive disorder and major depressive disorder. *J Nerv Ment Dis* 187, 512–516.

Meadows EA, Foa EB (1999) Cognitive-behavioral treatment of traumatized adults. In: Saigh PA, Bremner JD (eds) *Posttraumatic Stress Disorder: A Comprehensive Text*. Allyn & Bacon, Needham Heights, MA, pp. 376–390.

Melia KR, Duman RS (1991) Involvement of corticotropin-releasing factor in chronic stress regulation of the brain noradrenergic system. *Proc Natl Acad Sci USA* 88, 8382–8386.

Metcalfe J, Jacobs WJ (1996) A "hot-system/cool-system" view of memory under stress. *PTSD Research Quarterly* 7, 1–3.

Moradi AR, Doost HT, Taghavi MR et al. (1999) Everyday memory deficits in children and adolescents with PTSD: performance on the Rivermead Behavioural Memory Test. *J Child Psychol Psychiatr* 40, 357–361.

Moradi AR, Taghavi R, Neshat-Doost HT et al. (2000) Memory bias for emotional information in children and adolescents with posttraumatic stress disorder: A preliminary study. *J Anxiety Disord* 14, 521–534.

Morgan CA, LeDoux JE (1995) Differential contribution of dorsal and ventral medial prefrontal cortex to the acquisition and extinction of conditioned fear in rats. *Behav Neurosci* 109, 681–688.

Morgan CA, Romanski LM, LeDoux JE (1993) Extinction of emotional learning: Contribution of medial prefrontal cortex. *Neurosci Lett* 163, 109–113.

Munck AP, Guyre PM, Holbrook NJ (1984) Physiological functions of glucocorticoids in stress and their relation to pharmacological actions. *Endocr Rev* 5, 25–44.

Nibuya M, Morinobu S, Duman RS (1995) Regulation of BDNF and trkB mRNA in rat brain by chronic electroconvulsive seizure and antidepressant drug treatments. *J Neurosci* 15, 7539–7547.

Pelcovitz D, Kaplan S, Goldenberg B et al. (1994) Post-traumatic stress disorder in physically abused adolescents. *J Am Acad Child Adolesc Psychiatry* 33, 305–312.

Pelcovitz D, van der Kolk B, Roth S et al. (1997) Development of a criteria set and a Structured Interview for Disorders of Extreme Stress. *J Trauma Stress* 10, 3–16.

Petty F, Kramer G, Wilson L (1992) Prevention of learned helplessness: in vivo correlation with cortical serotonin. *Pharmacol Biochem Beh* 43, 361–367.

Plotsky PM, Meaney MJ (1993) Early, postnatal experience alters hypothalamic corticotropin-releasing factor (CRF) mRNA, median eminence CRF content and stress-induced release in adult rats. *Mol Brain Res* 18, 195–200.

Post RM (1992) Transduction of psychosocial stress into the neurobiology of recurrent affective disorder. *Am J Psychiatry* 149, 999–1010.

Quirk GJ, Garcia R, Gonzalez-Lima F (2006) Prefrontal mechanisms in extinction of conditioned fear. *Biol Psychiatry* 60, 337–343.

Radley JJ, Sisti HM, Hao J et al. (2004) Chronic behavioral stress induces apical dendritic reorganization in pyramidal neurons of the medial prefrontal cortex. *Neuroscience* 125, 1–6.

Rauch SL, Shin LM, Phelps EA (2006) Neurocircuitry models of posttraumatic stress disorder and extinction: human neuroimaging research--past, present, and future. *Biol Psychiatry* 60, 376–382.

Rauch SL, Shin LM, Segal E et al. (2003) Selectively reduced regional cortical volumes in post-traumatic stress disorder. *Neuroreport* 14, 913–916.

Rauch SL, van der Kolk BA, Fisler RE et al. (1996) A symptom provocation study of posttraumatic stress disorder using positron emission tomography and script-driven imagery. *Arch Gen Psychiatry* 53, 380–387.

Rauch SL, Whalen PJ, Shin LM et al. (2000) Exaggerated amygdala response to masked facial stimuli in posttraumatic stress disorder: a functional MRI study. *Biol Psychiatry* 47, 769–776.

Resnick HS, Kilpatrick DG, Dansky BS (1993) Prevalence of civilian trauma and posttraumatic stress disorder in a representative national sample of women. *J Consult Clin Psychol* 61, 984–991.

Resnick HS, Yehuda R, Pitman RK et al. (1995) Effect of previous trauma on acute plasma cortisol level following rape. *Am J Psychiatry* 152, 1675–1677.

Roca V, Freeman TW (2001) Complaints of impaired memory in veterans with PTSD. *Am J Psychiatry* 158, 1738.

Sachinvala N, vonScotti H, McGuire M et al. (2000) Memory, attention, function, and mood among patients with chronic posttraumatic stress disorder. *J Nerv Ment Dis* 188, 818–823.

Santarelli L, Saxe M, Gross C et al. (2003) Requirement of hippocampal neurogenesis for the behavioral effects of antidepressants. *Science* 301, 805–809.

Sapolsky RM, Uno H, Rebert CS et al. (1990) Hippocampal damage associated with prolonged glucocorticoid exposure in primates. *J Neurosci* 10, 2897–2902.

Seligman MEP, Meier SF (1967) Failure to escape traumatic shock. *J Exp Psychol* 74, 1–9.

Shalev AY, Freedman S, Peri T et al. (1988) Prospective study of post-traumatic stress disorder and depression following trauma. *Am J Psychiatry* 155, 630–637.

Shalev AY, Orr SP, Peri T et al. (1992) Physiologic responses to loud tones in Israeli patients with posttraumatic stress disorder. *Arch Gen Psychiatry* 49, 870–875.

Shalev AY, Orr SP, Pitman RK (1993a) Psychophysiologic assessment of traumatic imagery in Israeli civilian patients with posttraumatic stress disorder. *Am J Psychiatry* 150, 620–624.

Shalev AY, Peri T, Brandes D et al. (2000) Auditory startle response in trauma survivors with posttraumatic stress disorder: A prospective study. *Am J Psychiatry* 157, 255–261.

Shalev AY, Peri T, Canetti L et al. (1996) Predictors of PTSD in injured trauma survivors: A prospective study. *Am J Psychiatry* 153, 219–225.

Shalev AY, Sahar T, Freedman S et al. (1998) A prospective study of heart rate responses following trauma and the subsequent development of posttraumatic stress disorder. *Arch Gen Psychiatry* 55, 553–559.

Shalev AY, Schreiber S, Galai T (1993b) Early psychiatric responses to traumatic injury. *J Trauma Stress* 6, 441–450.

Sherman AD, Petty F (1982) Additivity of neurochemical changes in learned helplessness and imipramine. *Behav Neurol Biol* 35, 344–353.

Shin LM, Kosslyn SM, McNally RJ et al. (1997) Visual imagery and perception in posttraumatic stress disorder: A positron emission tomographic investigation. *Arch Gen Psychiatry* 54, 233–237.

Shin LM, Orr SP, Carson MA et al. (2004a) Regional cerebral blood flow in the amygdala and medial prefrontal cortex during traumatic imagery in male and female Vietnam veterans with PTSD. *Arch Gen Psychiatry* 61, 168–176.

Shin LM, Shin PS, Heckers S et al. (2004b) Hippocampal function in posttraumatic stress disorder. *Hippocampus* 14, 292–300.

Smith ME (2005) Bilateral hippocampal volume reduction in adults with post-traumatic stress disorder: a meta-analysis of structural MRI studies. *Hippocampus* 15, 798–807.

Solomon Z, Garb R, Bleich A et al. (1987) Reactivation of combat-related posttraumatic stress disorder. *Am J Psychiatry* 144, 51–55.

Solomon Z, Kotler M, Shalev A et al. (1989) Delayed post-traumatic stress disorders. *Psychiatry* 52, 428–436.

Stein DJ, Zungu-Dirwayi N, van der Linden GJ et al. (2000a) Pharmacotherapy for posttraumatic stress disorder. *Cochrane Database Systematic Review* 4, CD002795.

Stein MB, McQuaid JR, Pedrelli P et al. (2000b) Posttraumatic stress disorder in the primary care medical setting. *Gen Hosp Psychiatry* 22, 261–269.

Stein MB, Yehuda R, Koverola C et al. (1997) Enhanced dexamethasone suppression of plasma cortisol in adult women traumatized by childhood sexual abuse. *Biol Psychiatry* 42, 680–686.

Thrasher SM, Dalgleish T, Yule W (1994) Information processing in post-traumatic stress disorder. *Behav Res Ther* 32, 247–254.

True WR, Rice J, Eisen SA et al. (1993) A twin study of genetic and environmental contributions to liability for posttraumatic stress disorder symptoms. *Arch Gen Psychiatry* 50, 257–264.

Turnbull GJ (1998) A review of post-traumatic stress disorder. Part I: Historical development and classification. *Injury* 29, 87–91.

Uddo M, Vasterling JJ, Braily K et al. (1993) Memory and attention in posttraumatic stress disorder. *J Psychopathol Beh Assess* 15, 43–52.

van der Kolk BA, Pelcovitz D, Roth S et al. (1996) Dissociation, somatization, and affect dysregulation: the complexity of adaptation to trauma. *Am J Psychiatry* 153, 83–93.

Vasterling JJ, Brailey K, Constans JI et al. (1998) Attention and memory dysfunction in posttraumatic stress disorder. *Neuropsychology* 12, 125–133.

Vasterling JJ, Duke LM, Brailey K et al. (2002) Attention, learning, and memory performance and intellectual resources in Vietnam veterans: PTSD and no disorder comparisons. *Neuropsychology* 16, 5–14.

Vermetten E, Bremner JD (2002a) Circuits and systems in stress. I. Preclinical studies. *Depress Anxiety* 15, 126–147.

Vermetten E, Bremner JD (2002b) Circuits and systems in stress. II. Applications to neurobiology and treatment of PTSD. *Depress Anxiety* 16, 14–38.

Watanabe YE, Gould H, Cameron D et al. (1992) Phenytoin prevents stress and corticosterone induced atrophy of CA3 pyramidal neurons. *Hippocampus* 2, 431–436.

Woon FL, Sood S, Hedges DW (2010) Hippocampal volume deficits associated with exposure to psychological trauma and posttraumatic stress disorder in adults: a meta-analysis. *Prog Neuropsychopharmacol Biol Psychiatry* 34, 1181–1188.

Yehuda R (1998) Psychoneuroendocrinology of post-traumatic stress disorder. *Psychiatr Clin North Am* 21, 359–379.

Yehuda R, Antelman SM (1993) Criteria for rationally evaluating animal models of posttraumatic stress disorder. *Biol Psychiatry* 33, 479–486.

Yehuda R, Kahana B, Binder-Brynes K et al. (1995a) Low urinary cortisol excretion in holocaust survivors with posttraumatic stress disorder. *Am J Psychiatry* 152, 982–986.

Yehuda R, Keefe RS, Harvey PD et al. (1995b) Learning and memory in combat veterans with posttraumatic stress disorder. *Am J Psychiatry* 152, 137–139.

Yehuda R, Southwick SM, Krystal JH et al. (1993) Enhanced suppression of cortisol with low dose dexamethasone in posttraumatic stress disorder. *Am J Psychiatry* 150, 83–86.

Yehuda R, Southwick SM, Nussbaum EL et al. (1991) Low urinary cortisol in PTSD. *J Nerv Ment Dis* 178, 366–369.

Yehuda R, Teicher MH, Levengood RA et al. (1994) Circadian regulation of basal cortisol levels in posttraumatic stress disorder. *Ann NY Acad Sci*, 378–380.

Zlotnick C, Zakriski AL, Shea MT et al. (1996) The long-term sequelae of sexual abuse: support for a complex posttraumatic stress disorder. *J Trauma Stress* 9, 195–205.

CHAPTER 2

The epidemiology of posttraumatic stress disorder in children and adolescents: a critical review

Leah A. McGuire

Center for Attention and Learning, Department of Psychiatry, Lenox Hill Hospital, North Shore LIJ Health System, New York, NY, USA

2.1 Introduction

The term *epidemiology* refers to the "study of health and morbidity in human populations" (Saigh et al., 1999, p. 18). Epidemiological analyses typically examine the prevalence, causes, risk factors, distribution, and control of disorders/diseases in populations, as well as possible associations between two or more disorders/diseases. With regard to child and adolescent posttraumatic stress disorder (PTSD), epidemiological research provides essential information about traumatic stress responses (Kessler et al., 1995) and about the risk associated with traumatic exposure in youth (Kilpatrick et al., 2003). Such information may enhance understanding of the etiology and treatment of child-adolescent PTSD (Angold et al., 1999). In addition, PTSD prevalence approximations may influence policymakers with regard to the allocation of resources for prevention and treatment. Given the importance of epidemiological research, this chapter examines the epidemiology of PTSD with respect to child and adolescent populations. Consistent with guidelines established by the American Psychological Association (APA, 2013a), the term *children* is used to refer to persons aged 12 and younger, and the term *adolescents* is used to refer to individuals between 13 and 21 years of age.

2.2 Studies involving general population surveys

Government data and surveys indicate that exposure to traumatic events is common (Breslau et al., 1991, 1998; Kessler et al., 1995; Norris, 1992; Resnick et al.,

Posttraumatic Stress Disorder: From Neurobiology to Treatment, First Edition.
Edited by J. Douglas Bremner.
© 2016 John Wiley & Sons, Inc. Published 2016 by John Wiley & Sons, Inc.

1993). Approximately 66% of the US population is exposed to a traumatic stressor during their lives. Moreover, approximately 20% of Americans are exposed to traumas on an annual basis (Breslau et al., 1991; Kessler et al., 1995). A 2005 report from the American Red Cross indicated that its staff responded to 72,883 disasters. The Red Cross report also indicated that 92.0% of the disaster populations that were examined were fire victims.

Experiencing traumatic events can elicit varying rates of PTSD in adults. The *Diagnostic and Statistical Manual of Mental Disorders*, Fourth Edition (DSM-IV; APA, 1994) specified that the prevalence of PTSD varied from 1.0% to 14.0% amongst American adults. The DSM-IV-TR (APA, 2000) reported an 8.0% prevalence of PTSD amongst US adults. The DSM-5 (APA, 2013a) projected lifetime risk for PTSD, using DSM-IV criteria, at age 75 years to be 8.7%. Further, 12-month prevalence among American adults was found to be approximately 3.5%. All three versions of the DSM provide different prevalence rates for individuals who may be at risk for developing the disorder (APA, 2013a). The DSM-IV, DSM-IV-TR and DSM-5 did not specify PTSD prevalence rates with regard to children and adolescents.

2.3 Prevalence of exposure to traumatic events in youth populations

Within the context of research assessing PTSD in adolescents, Breslau et al. (1991) reported that 6.0% of male adolescents and 11.3% of female adolescents had a lifetime history of PTSD. However, there is a paucity of information available regarding the risk for PTSD with reference to different types of trauma exposure in children and adolescents (Copeland et al., 2007). Due to the scarcity of community-based studies investigating the prevalence of PTSD in youth (Giaconia et al., 1995), studies have focused on determining prevalence rates for PTSD in epidemiological surveys following child and adolescent exposure to traumatic events.

Government statistics indicate that children experience a disproportionate number of traumatic events each year. For example, between 1992 and 1994, Americans aged 12–24 years suffered approximately half of all violent crimes committed, despite comprising less than a quarter of the United States population at that time (United States Department of Justice, 1997). Similarly, the United States Department of Justice's (2006a) national crime statistics indicated that, between 1973 and 2005, teens and young adults consistently experienced the highest rates of violent crime in the nation. Additionally, the 2004 National Crime Victimization Survey (United States Bureau of Justice, 2007) reported that 24 million American residents over the age of 12 were victims of violent and/or property crimes. Specifically, adolescents aged 12–19 years reported higher rates of victimization than did adults. While male adolescents were more frequently the victims of violent crimes, female adolescents were more likely to have reported that they were rape victims.

The United States Department of Transportation (2006b) reported that in 2005 approximately 640 American children were injured each day in motor vehicle accidents. Similarly, a 2006 report from the New York State Department of Motor Vehicles indicated that approximately 10.3% of motor vehicle accident victims were under the age of 17 years. Specifically, 7,867 youths aged 17 years or less were seriously hurt or died in motor vehicle accidents that year. Additionally, the United States Department of Transportation (2007) reported that more 16- to 20-year-old individuals were killed in motor vehicle accidents each year between 1996 and 2005 than Americans in any other age group.

Kessler et al.'s (1995) National Comorbidity Survey observed that 60.7% of males and 51.2% of females aged 15–24 years in the United States reported that they had experienced at least one traumatic incident during their lives. Analogously, Kilpatrick and Saunders (1997) performed a representative survey involving 4,023 American youths aged 12–17 years, and determined that 39.4% of the sample witnessed at least one incident involving interpersonal violence. It was also reported that 17.4% of the sample were victims of serious physical assaults, and 8.1% were sexually assaulted. Likewise, Schwab-Stone et al. (1995, 1999) administered written surveys to 5,348 adolescents in an urban public school system. More than one-third (36.0%) of the adolescents reported having directly experienced at least one type of violent act. In addition, 18.0% of the adolescents reported having been chased by a gang or individual, and 18.0% reported having been threatened with physical harm. Between 5.0% and 10.0% reported events such as being attacked or stabbed with a knife, being beaten or mugged, being seriously wounded, or being shot. In 1994 and 1996, 46.0% and 39.0% of adolescents, respectively, reported that they had seen someone shot or shot at. At both data collection points, more than 25.0% of the adolescents reported having seen someone being attacked or stabbed with a knife.

Finkelhor et al. (2005) assessed a nationally representative sample of 2,030 youths aged 2–17 years using the Developmental Victimization Survey (DVS) in order to examine exposure to 34 forms of victimization experiences. Results indicated that 71.0% of the participants experienced at least one incident involving victimization during a 1-year period. Further, nearly 70.0% of victimized children reported that they had experienced multiple traumatic experiences, with an average of three different kinds of victimization reported on the Juvenile Victimization Questionnaire (JVQ; Hamby et al., 2004).

Studies have demonstrated that trauma exposure is commonly related to subsequent psychiatric impairment in childhood. For example, Copeland et al. (2007) examined the prevalence of exposure to traumatic events and the range and frequency of PTSD symptoms within a community sample of 1,420 children using annual child and parent reports on the Child and Adolescent Psychiatric Assessment (CAPA; Angold & Costello, 2000). They utilized a representative sample of children aged 9, 11, and 13 years at intake and followed up with them annually through 16 years of age. Copeland et al. found that approximately two-thirds of the participants reported having been exposed to one or more traumatic events by 16 years of age. It was also reported that approximately 14% of these cases had some symptoms of PTSD. Less than 0.5% of the children met the full criteria to diagnose PTSD by DSM-IV standards (APA, 1994). PTSD symptoms were predicted by previous exposure to multiple traumas, anxiety disorders, and family adversity, with the highest rates of symptoms being correlated with violent or sexual trauma. This study served to demonstrate that exposure to traumatic events is common in the general population of children and adolescents. However, exposure to traumatic events does not often result in PTSD symptoms, except after multiple traumas or a history of anxiety.

In a related study, Breslau et al. (2004) estimated the cumulative occurrence of traumatic events and PTSD, using the DSM-IV (APA, 1994) criteria, in a high-risk sample of urban youth. The sample ($n = 2,311$) was recruited in 1985 through 1986 at entry into the first grade of a public school system in a large mid-Atlantic city. Participants were interviewed about history of trauma and PTSD in 2000 through 2002 when their mean age was 21 years ($n = 1,698$). The lifetime prevalence of exposure to assaultive violence was greater for males (62.6%) than for females (33.7%). However, females had a higher risk of PTSD than males following assaultive violence, but not following other traumas.

2.4 Community surveys assessing child-adolescent PTSD prevalence

Given the reported rates of exposure to traumatic events, it is important to recognize that children and adolescents who are traumatized may be at risk for PTSD and for related disorders. In addition to the studies and government statistics that reported prevalence rates for exposure to traumatic incidents, community surveys have reported PTSD prevalence rates following a wide range of traumatic incidents. For example, Giaconia et al. (1995) documented the prevalence of PTSD in a sample of 384 adolescents who were participating in an ongoing longitudinal study. The sample was drawn from a predominantly Caucasian working-class community in the northeastern United States. The study was initiated when the youths were 5 years old, and data were collected at ages 9, 15, and 18 year. When participants reached the age of 18 years, structured clinical interviews using the National Institute of Mental Health Diagnostic Interview Schedule III-R (DIS-III-R; Robins et al., 1989) indicated that 165 participants (43.0% of the sample) reported having experienced a trauma by the age of 18 that met the

DSM-III-R (APA, 1987a) traumatic event criteria. The most commonly reported trauma involved learning about another's sudden death or accident (13.0%). Frequently reported traumas also included having seen someone hurt or killed (12.8%) or having experienced personal injury (10.4%). Less prevalent traumas included physical assault (6.5%), rape (2.1%), being threatened (2.1%), and natural disasters (1.3%). Giaconia et al. (1995) indicated that 14.5% of individuals who reported that they had experienced a trauma met criteria for a lifetime diagnosis of PTSD, which comprised 6.3% of the total sample. The authors additionally indicated that PTSD prevalence estimates for rape (50.0%) were markedly higher than physical assault (12.0%) and natural disasters (0.0%) prevalence rates.

In another study, Cuffe et al. (1998) examined the prevalence of PTSD in a community-based sample of 490 12th-grade students in a school district in suburban South Carolina. Using an author-devised, semi-structured clinical interview, Cuffe et al. concluded that 15.0% ($n = 80$) of the participants had experienced a traumatic event. Of these, 12.4% met DSM-IV (APA, 1994) criteria for PTSD. In the overall sample, 3.0% of females and 1.0% of males had PTSD. Cuffe et al. (1998) further reported that there was a significantly increased risk of PTSD among females, rape or child sexual abuse victims, and youths who witnessed an accident or medical emergency.

Perkonigg et al. (2000) examined the lifetime and 12-month prevalence rates of trauma exposure and PTSD in a sample of 3,021 individuals between the ages of 14 and 24 years. The Munich Composite International Diagnostic Interview (M-CIDI; Wittchen & Pfister, 1997) was used to assess traumatic events and PTSD. Overall, 21.4% of the sample endorsed having at least one traumatic event (i.e., the person experienced, witnessed, or was confronted with an event or events that involved actual or threatened death or serious injury, or a threat to the physical integrity of self or others). Only 17.0% of the sample additionally satisfied the A2 criterion for DSM-IV (APA, 1994) PTSD by reporting that at the time of trauma exposure, participants had feelings of horror and/or helplessness. With reference to participants who met both A1 and A2 criteria, 7.8% met full criteria for PTSD diagnosis. This corresponded to a lifetime prevalence of 1.3%.

Utilizing data from the National Survey of Adolescents, Kilpatrick et al. (2003) reported the prevalence of PTSD in a nationally representative sample of 4,023 adolescents between 12 and 17 years of age. Youth endorsements on the National Women's Study modified PTSD module (Kilpatrick et al., 1989) indicated that 4.8% of the participants met DSM-IV (APA, 1994) criteria for PTSD. Specifically, 3.7% of male adolescents and 6.3% of female adolescents met DSM-IV PTSD criteria. Furthermore, it was found that three-quarters of participants who were diagnosed with PTSD had one or more comorbid diagnoses. Kilpatrick et al.

(2003) further indicated that sexual assault, physical assault, and having witnessed violence were associated with an increased risk of PTSD that was comorbid with a major depressive episode or substance abuse/dependence. After controlling for the presence of comorbid disorders, 1.4% ($n = 55$) of the sample had PTSD without comorbidity.

Breslau et al. (2006) performed a longitudinal investigation involving 713 children and adolescents from a variety of socioeconomic backgrounds. The DIS-III-R (Robins et al., 1989) was administered to the participants when they were aged 6, 11, and 17 years, and a lifetime prevalence of 75.9% for trauma exposure was observed. They also reported significantly higher rates of exposure to trauma among urban youth (86.0%) as compared with suburban youth (65.3%). Moreover, a lifetime PTSD prevalence rate of 8.3% was indicated for the sample. Males reported more frequent exposure to traumatic events relative to females (79.2% vs. 72.9%).

Storr et al. (2007) also completed a long-term study examining trauma exposure and PTSD prevalence among urban children and adolescents. Initially, the PTSD module of the Composite International Diagnostic Interview (CIDI; World Health Organization [WHO], 1997) was administered to 2,311 first-grade students from 19 public schools within the same district. Evaluations were made 15 years later, sampling 1,698 participants (794 males, 904 females; mean age = 21 years) from the original cohort. There were two classifications of traumatic events: assaultive violence (i.e., rape, sexual assault excluding rape, and being badly beaten) and non-assaultive violence (i.e., major road traffic accidents, disasters, and life-threatening illness). Storr et al. (2007) reported that 82.5% of the sample had a lifetime prevalence of exposure to a DSM-IV-qualifying traumatic event, 47.2% experienced one or more traumatic events that involved assaultive violence, and 91.0% of individuals who experienced assaultive violence additionally experienced at least one non-assaultive, violent traumatic experience. Moreover, the authors reported that male children and older adolescents had higher prevalence rates for exposure to assaultive violence as compared with females and younger adolescents. Storr et al. (2007) also observed a lifetime PTSD prevalence rate of 8.8%.

In examining community-based surveys collectively, prevalence estimates for youth exposure to traumatic incidents ranged from 21.4% to 82.5%. With regard to the entire sample, lifetime prevalence rates for PTSD ranged from 1.3% to 8.8%. The outcomes of the community-based research and government data suggest that American youths are at risk for trauma exposure and that the majority of the cases that were exposed to traumatic events did not evidence PTSD. Traumatic experiences in the majority of cases that were studied did not lead to PTSD. See Table 2.1 for a summary of community-based surveys.

Table 2.1 Community surveys assessing child-adolescent posttraumatic stress disorder (PTSD) prevalence.

Study	Measure(s)	Sample size	Age	Elapsed time	Trauma exposure prevalence	PTSD prevalence
Giaconia et al. (1995)	DIS-R-III	$n = 384$	5 years	13 years	43.0%	14.5%
Cuffe et al. (1998)	Author devised, semi-structured clinical interview	$n = 490$	12th grade		15.0%	12.4%
Perkonigg et al. (2000)	M-CIDI	$n = 3,021$	14–24 years		21.4%	1.3%
Kilpatrick et al. (2003)	National Women's Study PTSD module	$n = 4,023$	12–17 years		No percentage reported; nationally representative sample of US adolescents	4.8%
Breslau et al. (2006)	DIS-III-R	$n = 713$	6 years	0, 5, and 11 years	75.9%	8.3%
Storr et al. (2007)		$n = 2,311$ at start, $n = 1,698$ at follow-up	1st grade	15 years	82.5%	8.8%

DIS-III-R, National Institute of Mental Health Diagnostic Interview Schedule III-R; M-CIDI, The Munich Composite International Diagnostic Interview.

2.5 Childhood/adolescent PTSD rates according to type of trauma

Studies have examined clinical samples to estimate the prevalence of PTSD following a broad range of traumatic events. A majority of this research has considered youth PTSD estimates in the general areas of war-related events, criminal victimization, natural disasters, and life-threatening accidents. The subsequent sections consider PTSD rates as a function of trauma type.

2.5.1 War settings

Research involving child and adolescent emotional distress due to war-related events has been extensively studied. Research has assessed prevalence estimates of child-adolescent PTSD following exposure to violence in the Middle East (e.g., Ahmad et al., 2000; Almqvist & Broberg, 1999; Saigh et al., 1997), Asia (e.g., Kinzie et al., 1986, 1989; Sack et al., 1993, 1994) and Africa (e.g., Bayer et al., 2007; Schaal & Elbert, 2006). War-related research determined PTSD prevalence rates ranging from 7.6% to 87.0%. Table 2.2 summarizes data regarding prevalence of child-adolescent PTSD following war-related trauma exposure.

2.5.2 Criminal victimization

Investigators have also examined child and adolescent PTSD prevalence rates following a variety of criminal acts. Examined collectively, the reported PTSD prevalence rates following criminal victimization without sexual contact ranged from 0.0% to 60.4%. Sexual assault incidents were associated with PTSD prevalence rates ranging from 9.0% to 63.5%. (Table 2.3) summarizes epidemiological research regarding PTSD prevalence among youth following various types of criminal victimization.

2.5.3 Disasters/accidents

Disasters and accidents are frequently unanticipated traumatic events that may lead to injury or mortality. Burkle (1996) indicated that 13.0% of American citizens reported having experienced a natural or human-induced disaster during their lifetimes. The National Comorbidity Survey (Breslau et al., 1998) indicated that approximately 19.0% of men and 15.0% of women sampled were exposed to a natural disaster at least once in their lifetimes. Many researchers have examined posttraumatic stress reactions of children and adolescents following natural disasters and accidents (Jones-Alexander et al., 2005; Kolaitis et al., 2003; Laor et al., 2002; McDermott et al., 2005; Pynoos et al., 1993; Yule et al., 2000).

The results of these studies clearly indicated that a large number of youths may be severely psychologically affected following exposure to disasters and accidents. PTSD prevalence rates among the reviewed natural disasters and accidents studies ranged from 0.0% to 95.0%. Table 2.4 summarizes studies regarding the prevalence of PTSD subsequent to natural disasters and accident-related traumas.

2.6 Child-adolescent PTSD and comorbid disorders

Comorbidity refers to the "co-occurrence of two or more psychiatric conditions in the same individual" (Saigh & Bremner, 1999, p. 31). Comorbidity affects the conceptualization, assessment and course of treatment of psychiatric populations (Fairbank et al., 1995). PTSD is associated with comorbid disorders (Faustman & White, 1989; Kulka et al., 1990). Research with adults demonstrates that many

Table 2.2 Studies of child-adolescent posttraumatic stress disorder (PTSD) in war settings.

Study	Measure(s)	Gender	Age	Elapsed time	PTSD prevalence
Middle East conflicts					
Saigh (1988)	DSM-III Author-devised interview	12 females	Mean age 18.2 years	63 days prior to stressor exposure and 316 days after stressor exposure	63 days before: 0.0% 316 days after: 8.3%
Saigh (1989a)	DSM-III Children's PTSD Inventory	42 males, 50 females	Mean age 13 years	Not reported	29.3%
Saigh (1989b)	DSM-III Children's PTSD Inventory	403 males, 437 females	Age range 9–12 years	1–2 years	32.5%
Saigh et al. (1997)	DSM-III Children's PTSD Inventory	48 males, 47 females	Mean age 17.5 years	Mean = 4.2 years, range 4.2–21 years	Stress-exposed = 46.70% Overall sample = 14.70%
Schwarzwald et al. (1993)	CPTSDI-RI	227 males, 265 females	Grades 5, 7 and 10	Not reported	Grade: males/females Grade 5, 24.5/22.4%; grade 7, 3.4/7.9%; grade 10, 1.6/7.0%
Almqvist & Broberg (1999)	DSM-IV-based clinical interview	29 males, 10 females	Mean age 8 years 4 months	3.5 years	18.0%
Ahmad et al. (2000)	HTQ, PTSS-C	24 males 21 females	Mean age 12.3 years Mean age 12.4 years	5 years	87.0%
Khamis (2005)	DSM-IV-based clinical interview	523 males 477 females	Mean age 14.2 years	Not reported	34.1%
Thabet et al. (2009)	SCID – PTSD module	200 males, 212 females	Mean age 13.7 years	Not reported	30.8%
Khamis (2012)	DSM-IV structured clinical interview	Gaza: 150 males, 150 females South Lebanon: 123 males, 177 females	Gaza, mean age 12.8 years South Lebanon, mean age: 14.2 years	Not reported	25.7% collectively
Lavi & Solomon (2005)	CPTSD-RI	358 males, 371 females	Age range 11.5–15 years	Not reported	Disputed territories, 27.6%; Jerusalem, 12.4%; Gilo, 11.2%

(continued)

Table 2.2 *(Continued)*

Study	Measure(s)	Gender	Age	Elapsed time	PTSD prevalence
Kaufman-Shriqui et al. (2013)	CPSS	n = 167; 49.0% male	Mean age: 5.3 years	Not reported	21.0%
Elbedour et al. (2007)	CPTSD-I	121 males, 108 females	Mean age 17.1 years	Not reported	68.9%
Pat-Horenczyk et al. (2007)	UCLA PTSD Reaction Index	192 males, 217 females	Mean age 16.44 years	22 months of recurrent attacks	Direct exposure, 13.6%; near-miss, 7.7%; overall sample, 7.6%
Southeast Asian Conflicts					
Kinzie et al. (1986)	DSM-III Diagnostic Interview	25 males, five females	Mean age 14 years	2.5 years	50.0%
Sack et al. (1993)	DSM-III-R DICA	Not reported (n = 19)	Mean age 23.0 years	12–18 years	12 years, 52.0%; 15 years, 47.0%; 18 years, 32.0%
Kinzie et al. (1989)	DSM-III-R DIS	16 males, 11 females	Mean age 20 years	5.5 years	48.0%
Sack et al. (1994)	K-SADS-E DICA	104 males, 105 females	Mean age 19.8 years	13 years	Current, 18.2%; lifetime, 21.5%
Hubbard et al. (1995)	DSM-III-R Clinical Interview	29 males, 30 females	Mean age 19.5 years	15 years	Current, 24.0%; lifetime, 59.0%
Savin et al. (1996)	DSM-III-R DICA	89 males, 10 females	Age range 18–25 years	10 years	Point, 26.3; lifetime, 31.3%
African conflicts					
Schaal & Elbert (2006)	CIDI Event Scale	33 males, 35 females	Mean age 17.72 years	~10 years	44.0%
Bayer et al. (2007)	CPTSD-RI	141 males, 28 females	Mean age 15.3 years	Demobilized, 2.3 months Time spent as child soldiers, 38.3 months	34.9%

DSM, *Diagnostic and Statistical Manual of Mental Disorders*; CPTSDI-RI, Children's PTSD Inventory-Reaction Index; HTQ, Harvard Trauma Questionnaire; PTSS-C, Posttraumatic Stress Symptoms in Children; SCID, Structured Clinical Interview for DSM-IV; CPSS, Child PTSD Symptom Scale; DICA, Diagnostic Interview for Children and Adolescents ; DIS, Diagnostic Interview Schedule; K-SADS-E, Kiddie-SADS-E; CIDI, Composite International Diagnostic Interview.

Table 2.3 Studies of child-adolescent posttraumatic stress disorder (PTSD) following criminal victimization.

Study	Measure(s)	Gender	Age	Elapsed time	PTSD prevalence
School shootings					
Pynoos et al. (1987)	PTSD Reaction Index	80 males 79 females	Age range 5–13 years; mean age 9.2 years	1 month 14 months	60.4% 29.0%
Schwarz & Kowalski (1991)	DSM-III, DSM-III-R, DSM-IV criteria	32 males, 32 females	Mean age 8.6 years	6–14 months	27.0%
Vila et al. (1999)	Kiddie-SADS-L	14 males, 12 females	Age range 6.0–9.5 years	1 month 2 months 4 months 7 months 18 months	11.5% 15.4% 3.8% 7.7% 3.8%
Various traumas					
Fitzpatrick & Boldizar (1993)	Perdue Posttraumatic Stress Scale	102 males, 119 females	Mean age 11.9 years	Not reported	27.0%
Berman et al. (1996)	PTSD-RI	52 males, 44 females	Age range 14–18 years; mean age 16.4 years	Not reported	34.5%
Berton & Stabb (1996)	CM-PTSD, Keane PTSD Scale	21 males, 78 females	Mean age 17 years	Not reported	29.0%
Steiner et al. (1997)	DSM-III-R PDI-R	85 males	Mean age 16.6 years	Not reported	31.7%
Lipschitz et al. (2000)	DSM-IV Child PTSD Checklist	90 females	Mean age 17.3 years	Not reported	Stress-exposed, 14.4%; overall sample: 13.0%
Jaycox et al. (2002)	Child PTSD Symptom Scale	(*n* = 1,004) 48.8% female	Mean age 11.4 years	Not reported	29.4%

(*continued*)

Table 2.3 (*Continued*)

Study	Measure(s)	Gender	Age	Elapsed time	PTSD prevalence
Abram et al. (2004)	DISC-IV	532 males, 366 females	Age range 10-18 years	Not reported	11.2%
Foster et al. (2004)	TSCC	84 males, 62 females	Mean age 13.16 years	Not reported	Males, 11.5%; females, 11.8%
Horowitz et al. (2005)	UPID	11 males, 17 females	Mean age 11.7 years	Not reported	50.0%
Seedat et al. (2004)	Child PTSD Checklist	South Africa: n = 1140; 43.3% male Kenya: n = 901; 41.9% male	Mean age 15.8 years	Not reported	Lifetime, 14.8%
Alderfer et al. (2009)	FAD, SCID-NP	n = 144; 52.0% female	Mean age 14.6 years	1–12 years post-cancer treatment Mean 5.3 years	8.3%
Luthra et al. (2009)	K-SADS	91 males, 66 females	Mean age 12.2 years	Not reported	19.0%
Frounfelker et al. (2013)	DSM-IV-TR Axis 1 diagnosis	37 males, 47 females	Age range 16–21 years	Not reported	36.0%
Landolt et al. (2013)	UCLA-RI	3,551 males, 3,236 females	Mean age 15.5 years	Not reported	4.2%
Physical and sexual assault					
McLeer et al. (1988)	DSM-III-R structured interview	Six males, 25 females	Mean age 8.4 years	Not reported	48.4%
Merry & Andrews (1994)	DISC-2	11 males, 55 females	Mean age 8 years	12 months	63.5%
Wolfe et al. (1994)	DSM-III-R checklist	21 males, 69 females	Mean age 12.4 years	Not reported	48.9%

Study	Measure	Sample	Age	Duration	Prevalence
Cauffman et al. (1998)	DSM-III-R PDI-R	96 females	Mean age 17.2 years	Not reported	Point, 48.9; lifetime, 65.3%
Ackerman et al. (1998)	DICA-R	73 males, 131 females	Age range 7–13 years	At least 4 weeks	Overall sample, 34.0%; sexual abuse alone, 31.8%; physical abuse alone, 25.4%; both sexual and physical abuse, 51.9%
Silva et al. (2000)	KID-SCID	39 males, 20 females	Mean age 9.95 years	Not reported	Sexual abuse, 15.0%; physical abuse, 21.0%; witnessed domestic violence, 17.0%
Linning & Kearney (2004)	C-PTSDI	22 males, 33 females	Mean age 12.65 years	2 years	67.3%
Stewart et al. (2004)	Author designed victimization measure and DSM-IV PTSD	n = 374; 54% male, 46% female	Mean age 17.1 years	Not reported	17.7%
D'Augelli et al. (2006)	DISC	275 males, 253 females	Mean age 17.03 years	Not reported	Stress-exposed, 9.0%
Broman-Fulks et al. (2006)	National Women's Study PTSD Module	2,002 males, 1,904 females	Mean age 14.5 years	Not reported	Non-disclosers, 24.0%; short-delay disclosers, 22.0%; long-delay disclosers, 13.0%

DSM, *Diagnostic and Statistical Manual of Mental Disorders*; PTSDI-RI, PTSD Inventory-Reaction Index; CM-PTSD, Civilian Mississippi Scale for PTSD; PDI-R, Psychiatric Diagnostic Interview, Revised; DISC, Diagnostic Interview Schedule for Children; TSCC, Trauma Symptom Checklist for Children; FAD, Family Assessment Device; SCID, Structured Clinical Interview for DSM-IV; DICA, Diagnostic Interview for Children and Adolescents.

Table 2.4 Child-adolescent posttraumatic stress disorder (PTSD) research following natural disasters/accidents.

Study	Measure(s)	Gender	Age	Elapsed time	PTSD prevalence
Earthquakes					
Pynoos et al. (1993)	DSM-III-R Clinical Interview	Not reported (n = 111)	Mean age 12.8 years	1.5 years	70.3%
Najarian et al. (1996)	DICA-R	37 males, 37 females	Age range 11–13 years	2.5 years	High exposure, 33.0%; relocated, 28.0%; low exposure, 4.0%
Hsu et al. (2002)	SCL-90-R, ChIPS	141 males, 182 females	Mean age 13.3 years	6 weeks	21.7%
Laor et al. (2002)	DSM-III-R Reaction Index	135 males, 168 females	Mean age 8.5 years	4–5 months	20.8%
Kolaitis et al. (2003)	CPTSD-RI	55 males, 60 females	Grades 4, 5 and 6	6 months	78.0%
Yorbik et al. (2004)	DSM-IV Checklist	17 males, 18 females	Mean age 9.2 years	>30 days	Overall sample, 40.0%; aged 2–6 years, 0.0%; aged 7–11 years, 56.3%; aged 12–16 years, 50.0%
Bulut et al. (2005)	SBC-PTSDI	Not reported	Grades 4 and 5	11 months	High impact, 73.2% Low impact, 73.7%
Roussos et al. (2005)	UCLA PTSD-RI	847 males, 1,090 females	Age range 9–18 years	3–4 months	4.5%
Bal & Jensen (2007)	CPTSD-RI	141 males, 152 females	Mean age 11.2 years	Not reported	Moderate, 31.4%; severe: 24.2%; very severe, 3.8%
Bokszczanin (2007)	Revised Civilian PTSD Scale	213 males, 320 females	Age range 11–21 years Younger mean age, 13.6 years Older mean age 17.8 years	28 months	17.7%
Ziaaddini et al. (2009)	Structured PTSD Questionnaire, Davidson Trauma Scale	183 males, 283 females	Mean age 15.9 years	10 months	66.7%

Study	Measure	Sample	Age	Time points	Rate
Wang et al. (2011)	PCL-S	1,327 males, 1,473 females	Mean age 15.2 years	Not reported	21.8%
Zhang et al. (2012)	PCL-C, BDI	237 males, 311 females	Mean age 16.9 years	6 months 12 months 18 months	9.7% 1.3% 1.6%
Ying (2013)	CPSS	n = 3,052, 53.5% female	Mean age 13.3 years	Not reported	8.6%
Hurricanes and floods					
Goenjian et al. (2001)	CPTSD-RI	81 males, 77 females	Mean age 13 years	6 months	High impact, 90.0%; medium impact, 55.0%; low impact, 14.0%
Brown (2013)	UCLA PTSD Reaction Index Revision-1 – OTHERS	n = 426, 51.0% female	Mean age 11 years	3 months, 13 months, 19 months, 25 months	~25.0% recovering, youths initially reporting significant PTSD symptoms, 4.0% chronic symptom trajectory
Motor vehicle accidents					
DiGallo et al. (1997)	CPTSD-RI	38 males, 19 females	Mean age 10.2 years	12–15 weeks	49.0%
Zink & McCain (2003)	DICA-R	85 males, 58 females	Mean age 10.8 years	2 and 6 months	2 months, 18.0%; 6 months, 10.0%
Meiser-Stedman et al. (2005)	ADIS	60 males, 33 females	Mean age 13.9 years	6 months	12.5%
Landolt et al. (2005)	CPTSD-RI	37 males, 31 females	Mean age 9.8 years	4–6 weeks, 12 months	4–6 weeks, 16.2%; 12 months, 17.6%
Jones-Alexander et al. (2005)	CPTSD-I, PCL-C	11 males, 10 females	Mean age 12.7 years	1 month	23.0%
Schäfer et al. (2006)	DIPS	42 males, 30 females	Mean age 13.6 years	1 week, 3 months	1 week, 0.0%; 3 months, 0.0%
Wildfires					
McDermott et al. (2005)	PTSD-RI, SDQ	n =222, 54.9% female	Mean age: 12.5 years	6 months	Moderate: 12.1% Severe: 7.5% Very severe: 1.5%

(continued)

Table 2.4 (*Continued*)

Study	Measure(s)	Gender	Age	Elapsed time	PTSD prevalence
Transportation accidents					
Yule et al. (2000)	CAPS	Not reported	Not reported	6 months, 5–8 years	6 months, 90.0%; 5–8 years, 51.7%
Zink & McCain (2003)	CBCL, DICA-R	58 males, 85 females	Mean age 10.8 years	2 months post-injury 6 months post-injury	18.0% 10.0%
Mirzamani et al. (2006)	PSS	Not reported	Not reported	18 months	84.2%
Meiser-Stedman et al. (2008)	PTSD structured interviews Clinician administered PTSD Scale – Child and Adolescent version	n = 114, 47.4% female	Mean age 6.7 years	2–4 weeks 6 months	11.5% 13.9%

DSM, *Diagnostic and Statistical Manual of Mental Disorders*; DICA, Diagnostic Interview for Children and Adolescents; SCL-90-R, Symptom Checklist-90-Revised; ChIPS, Children's Interview for Psychiatric Syndromes; SBC-PTSDI, Sefa Bulut Child - Posttraumatic Stress Disorder Inventory; CPTSD-RI, Children's PTSD-Reaction Index; PCL, PTSD Checklist; BDI, Beck Depression Inventory; CPSS, Child PTSD Symptom Scale; DICA, Diagnostic Interview for Children and Adolescents; ACIS, Anxiety Disorders Interview Schedule; DIPS, Diagnostisches Interview bei psychischen Störungen; SDQ, Strengths and Difficulties Questionnaire; CAPS, Clinician Administered PTSD Scale; CBCL, Child Behavior Checklist; PSS, Post-Traumatic Stress Disorder Symptom Scale.

individuals with PTSD qualify for at least one co-occurring psychiatric diagnosis (Brady et al., 2000).

Consistent with adult PTSD research findings, youths with PTSD may also qualify for one or more comorbid disorders. Depressive disorders, substance-use disorders, and other anxiety disorders are the most common comorbid diagnoses found among children and adolescents. The studies that were reviewed indicated the following comorbid prevalence estimates: 7.7–18.4% (panic disorder), 35.1–41.6% (separation anxiety disorder), and 15.0–39.0% (unspecified anxiety disorders). Table 2.5 summarizes the epidemiological findings involving comorbidity specific to the stressor types mentioned earlier in this chapter.

2.7 Risk factors associated with child-adolescent PTSD

Studies have also assessed risk factors for the development of child-adolescent PTSD. These risk factors include gender; age; race/ethnicity/national origin; psychopathology among first-degree relatives; child characteristics; earlier histories involving traumatic stressors; intensity of and proximity to exposure to traumatic event; type of traumatic stressor; duration and number of traumatic experiences; time span between trauma exposure and diagnostic evaluation; and relationship between victims and perpetrators. Many risk factors reviewed found inconsistent relationships between the risk factor and the prevalence of child-adolescent PTSD. This section will review the literature and associations for each factor.

2.7.1 Gender
There have been inconsistent findings with reference to gender as a risk factor for PTSD. Some studies have indicated a greater rate of PTSD in trauma-exposed females than in males. Specifically, Fitzpatrick and Boldizar (1993) determined that female crime victims experienced more numerous and severe PTSD symptoms in comparison to criminally victimized males. Analogously, Perkonigg et al. (2000) found that women were more likely to experience trauma and meet criteria for PTSD. For example, Schaal and Elbert (2006) indicated that Rwandan females who were exposed to war-related events developed PTSD at more than double the rate of males (60.0% vs. 27.0%, respectively). Similarly, Pat-Horenczyk et al. (2007) reported that more women evidenced probable PTSD than males (9.5% vs. 5.4%, respectively) following missile attacks. D'Augelli et al. (2006) reported that more females (15.0%) than males (4.0%) developed PTSD after being attacked due to their sexual orientation. Research by Ziaaddini et al. (2009) indicated that Iranian girls were about three times more likely than boys to meet diagnostic criteria for PTSD after an earthquake.

Table 2.5 Child-adolescent posttraumatic stress disorder (PTSD) and comorbid disorders.

Study	Diagnostic measure	Prevalence of comorbid disorder with PTSD
War-related traumas		
Kinzie et al. (1986)	SADS	Panic disorder, 15.0%
		Unspecified depressive disorders, 85.0%
		Unspecified anxiety disorders, 35.0%
Kinzie et al. (1989)	SADS	Panic Disorder, 7.7%
		Unspecified affective disorders, 37.0%
Sack et al. (1993)	K-SADS-E	Conduct disorder, 0.0%
		Unspecified anxiety disorders, 15.0%
		Major depressive disorder, 60.0%
Sack et al. (1994)	K-SADS-E	Conduct disorder, 10.5%
		Panic disorder, 10.5%
Hubbard et al. (1995)	KID-SCID	Major depressive disorder, 21.0%
		Generalized anxiety disorder, 21.0%
		Social anxiety disorder, 21.0%
Servan-Schreiber et al. (1998)	Structured interview	11.5% major depressive disorder
Husain et al. (2008)	PTSD Reaction Index, IES, CBCL-TRF	68.6% with significant attention problems (interviewer report)
		79.0% with significant attention problems (SR)
Various traumas		
Perkonigg et al. (2000)	M-CIDI	Depressive disorders, 68.5%
		Agoraphobia with or without panic disorder as well as substance use or dependence, 70.6%
Saigh et al. (2002)	CPTSDI	Internalizing behavior problems, 62.5%; externalizing behavior problems, 45.8%
Physical/sexual assault		
McLeer et al. (1994)	KSADS-E	ADHD, 23.1%
		Panic disorder, 18.4%
		ADHD and conduct disorder, 11.5%
Famularo et al. (1996)	DICA-C-R	Unspecified anxiety disorders, 39.0%
		ADHD, 37.0%
		Unspecified mood disorders, 32.0%
		ODD and conduct disorder, 24.0%
Reebye et al. (2000)	DICA-R	CD, 17.0%
Kilpatrick et al. (2003)	NWS PTSD module	Major depressive episode: boys, 47.3% girls, 70.6%
		Substance abuse/dependence: boys, 29.7%; girls, 24.2%
Abram et al. (2007)	DISC-IV	Affective disorder, 17.0%
		Anxiety disorder, 38.0%
		ADHD/behavioral disorder, 43.0%
		Substance abuse disorder, 79.0%

K-SADS, Kiddie-SADS; SCID, Structured Clinical Interview for DSM-IV; IES, Impact of Event Scale; CBCL-TRF, Child Behavior Checklist-Teacher Report Form; M-CIDI, Munich Composite International Diagnostic Interview; CPTSDI, Children's PTSD Inventory; DICA, Diagnostic Interview for Children and Adolescents ; NWS, National Women's Study; DISC, Diagnostic Interview Schedule for Children; ADHD, attention deficit hyperactivity disorder; ODD, Oppositional Defiant Disorder; CD, conduct disorder.

Conversely, Khamis (2005) found that Palestinian males who experienced ongoing violence had a higher prevalence of PTSD (20.0%) in comparison to violence-exposed females (14.1%). Overall, it may be said that many of these studies reported no significant gender differences with regard to the prevalence of child-adolescent PTSD (e.g., Ackerman et al., 1998; Ahmad et al., 2000; Broman-Fulks et al., 2007; Elbedour et al., 2007; Fairbank et al., 1995; Foster et al., 2004; Goenjian et al., 1995; Hubbard et al., 1995; Realmuto et al., 1992; Saigh, 1988, 1997; Schwarzwald et al., 1994; Seedat et al., 2004; Silva et al., 2000; Yasik et al., 2012; Yorbik et al., 2004). Although the relationship between gender and PTSD is not always obvious, it is probable that gender is somehow related to the development and/or expression of PTSD (Rojas & Pappagallo, 2004).

2.7.2 Age

Studies have also looked at age as a possible risk factor for PTSD. Although a number of investigations suggested that older youths had higher prevalence rates of PTSD (Garrison et al., 1993; Schwarz & Kowalski, 1991), other studies found that younger youths are more susceptible to PTSD (Bokszczanin, 2007; Schwarzwald et al., 1993). Research by Wolfe et al. (1994) indicated that sexually abused adolescents had a significantly higher prevalence of PTSD (56.5%) as compared with sexually abused children (32.1%). Analogously, Ahmad et al. (2000) found that, subsequent to a violent military occupation, Kurdish youths with an older mean age were more likely to evidence PTSD than younger youths. Yorbik et al. (2004) reported that no children aged 6 years and younger developed PTSD after a massive earthquake in Turkey. In contrast, 56.3% of children aged 7–11 years and 50% of children aged 12–16 years met criteria for the disorder.

Schwarzwald et al. (1993) found higher prevalence estimates of PTSD among Israeli fifth graders who were exposed to a Scud missile attack relative to seventh and tenth graders (25.4%, 3.4% and 1.6%, respectively). These findings were relatively consistent at a 1-year follow-up (Schwarzwald et al., 1993). Similarly, Bokszczanin (2007) reported that older male youths were less likely to develop PTSD following a flood than younger males. Finally, many studies reported no age differences relative to PTSD prevalence estimates (Landolt et al., 2005; Lavi & Solomon, 2005; Schaal & Elbert, 2006). In summary, there is a lack of conclusive evidence that age is a risk factor for PTSD in children.

2.7.3 Race/ethnicity/national origin

There are also conflicting results regarding the relationship between race/ethnicity/national origin and PTSD in children and adolescents. Research in this area is complicated by the fact that there are varying definitions of race, ethnicity, and culture (Rojas & Pappagallo, 2004).

Some investigations have found significant relationships between race, ethnicity and/or place of national origin and PTSD diagnosis. For example, March et al. (1998) reported that African-American youths had higher rates of PTSD than Caucasian youths following an industrial explosion. Additionally, Jones et al. (2002) reported that Mexican-American children developed PTSD at significantly higher rates than youths from any other ethnic background after a California wildfire. Galea et al. (2003) observed that Dominican and Puerto Rican children were more likely than Hispanic youths to present with symptoms of probable PTSD following the September 11, 2001 attacks. LaGreca et al. (1996) determined that African-American and Hispanic children developed significantly higher rates of PTSD than Caucasian children following exposure to Hurricane Hugo. However, Garrison et al. (1995) and Shannon et al. (1994) found nonsignificant differences between these groups.

Other investigations have found nonsignificant relationships between ethnicity/race/national origin and PTSD in children and adolescents. PTSD studies involving criminal victimization have indicated that race and ethnicity were not significantly related to the development of PTSD (Abram et al., 2004; Famularo et al., 1996; Lawyer et al., 2006; Linning & Kearney, 2004; Lipschitz et al., 1999). Further, reports examining PTSD after natural disasters indicated nonsignificant variations when race was used as a predictor (Garrison et al., 1993; Langley & Jones, 2005; Shannon et al., 1994; Shaw et al., 1995). Finally, DeVries et al. (1999) and Zink and McCain (2003) reported that ethnicity and race were not related to PTSD among child-adolescent motor vehicle accident victims.

2.7.4 Psychopathology among first-degree relatives

There are reports in the literature suggesting that the prevalence of PTSD among stress-exposed youths is related to parental psychopathology. For example, Sack et al. (1993) found that Cambodian youths whose parents met criteria for PTSD had significantly higher PTSD prevalence rates (22.3%) in comparison to youths whose parents did not have PTSD (12.9%). Ahmad et al. (2000) also found a significant relationship between child and parent PTSD symptoms. Similarly, a study of individuals exposed to California wildfires by Jones et al. (2002) reported that parent PTSD symptoms were significantly correlated with child symptoms. A study by Linning and Kearney (2004) indicated that parental psychopathology significantly correlated with PTSD estimates among maltreated children.

2.7.5 Child characteristics

Studies have also looked at the relationships between intelligence quotient (IQ) in children and PTSD (Breslau et al., 2006; Saigh et al., 2006). Breslau et al.

(2006) found that a child's IQs at the age of 6 years was significantly related to PTSD development following a traumatic stressor later in life. Specifically, children with an IQ that fell at least one standard deviation above the mean (i.e., IQ ≥ 115 points) had a decreased risk for developing PTSD relative to children with an IQ placed below the mean (i.e., IQ ≤ 100 points). Breslau et al. (2006) also reported that children who received teacher ratings that indicated heightened externalizing behavior problems in the first grade had an increased risk for developing PTSD if they were exposed to a traumatic event. In a similar vein, Saigh et al. (2006) compared the Wechsler Intelligence Scale for Children–III (WISC–III; Wechsler, 1991) scores of traumatized youths with PTSD with the scores of trauma-exposed and non-exposed comparison groups without PTSD. All groups were free of additional major childhood psychiatric disorders. The PTSD group scored significantly lower than the comparison groups on verbal subtests, but not on performance subtests. The scores of the trauma-exposed PTSD negatives and non-exposed controls were not significantly different. While this study clearly denotes that lower verbal IQ was associated with child PTSD, the authors cautioned that they employed a cross-sectional design and that estimates of pre-trauma intelligence were not available. These studies suggest that high IQ may have a protective effect on the development of PTSD, although the cognitive consequences of trauma and PTSD may also contribute to lower IQ in PTSD patients.

2.7.6 Earlier histories involving traumatic stressors

Some of the findings that were reviewed herein suggested that early traumatic experiences that were followed by subsequent trauma exposures increased vulnerability to the disorder. For example, Garrison et al. (1993) determined that exposure to abuse or assault prior to Hurricane Andrew was associated with PTSD after the hurricane. A study of female children and adolescents who had experienced various forms of community violence by Lipschitz et al. (2000) determined that a prior history of child abuse and physical neglect was predictive of significantly greater rates of PTSD. Likewise, Saigh (1988) indicated that multiple exposures to war-related traumatic events were predictive of PTSD. Conversely, Jones et al. (2002) found that stress exposure before a fire was not associated with PTSD.

2.7.7 Intensity of and proximity to exposure to traumatic event

Research has indicated that the proximity to and intensity of stress exposure are associated with PTSD prevalence rates. For example, Schwarzwald et al. (1994) determined that Israeli children who were rocketed by Scud missiles developed higher rates of PTSD (24.9%) than children that did not experience such attacks

(12.9%). Likewise, Goenjian et al. (1995, 2001) indicated that physical proximity to the epicenter of an Armenian earthquake or eye of an American hurricane was correlated with the development of PTSD in youth. These authors also reported higher PTSD estimates among children living in close geographic proximity to the events. Additionally, Pat-Horenczyk et al. (2007) determined that 13.6% of Israeli youths who were exposed to a war-related terrorist attack met criteria for PTSD. These authors also reported that children who had near-miss experiences had a 7.7% rate of PTSD. Hsu et al. (2002) indicated that the prevalence of PTSD was significantly elevated among students who were physically injured (43.2%) following an earthquake as compared with children who were not hurt (12.9%). Similarly, Kolaitis et al. (2003) and Roussos et al. (2005) reported that child-adolescent development of PTSD was significantly associated with personal injury and home damage after a Greek earthquake. Finally, Schaal and Elbert (2006) interviewed Rwandan children who witnessed brutal parental executions and reported that 61.0% met the criteria for PTSD. This estimate is in marked contrast to a rate of 33.0% among youths who did not see their parents' deaths.

Conversely, Koplewicz et al. (1994) found that PTSD prevalence rates among youths who experienced high and low life threat during the 1993 World Trade Center bombing were comparable (66.0% and 69.0%, respectively), and therefore determined that the level of stress exposure was not predictive of PTSD. Shaw et al. (1995) also indicated that there was no significant association between PTSD rates and proximity of exposure to Hurricane Andrew. Also contrary to expectations, Saigh et al. (2002) indicated that stressor severity did not predict PTSD prevalence, and Landolt et al. (2005) and DeVries et al. (1999) reported that physical injury status did not predict PTSD. Likewise, Saigh et al. (2004) reported that preschool youths aged 3–5 years who were within 1 mile of the World Trade Center and exposed to one or more traumatic events prior to the bombing did not have PTSD. Additionally, this cohort did not differ significantly with regard to probable PTSD diagnoses in comparison to preschool youths who were 2–14 miles away and not exposed to traumatic events. Moreover, endorsements from the trauma-exposed group on the Posttraumatic Stress Disorder Checklist (PCL; Weathers et al., 1993), Beck Depression Inventory-II (BDI-II; Beck et al., 1996), and Beck Anxiety Inventory (BAI; Beck, 1990) did not differ significantly from those made by children who were not exposed to traumatic events.

2.7.8 Type of traumatic stressor

Research has also demonstrated that different avenues of trauma exposure were associated with different rates of PTSD. Saigh's (1991) study of 230 stress-exposed Lebanese youths with PTSD determined that 25.2%, 55.6%, 5.6%, and 13.5% had been traumatized through direct traumatic experiences (e.g., gunshot victims), observation (e.g., observing parental execution), information transmission (e.g., being told about the traumatic experiences of a parent or sibling), or combinations of such experiences. Lawyer et al. (2006) reported that 20.3% of sexually assaulted children had PTSD, in comparison to 15.1% of physically assaulted children. Similarly, a study by McLeer et al. (1994) indicated that the prevalence of PTSD among sexually abused children (42.3%) was significantly greater than that among non-sexually abused children (8.7%).

2.7.9 Duration and number of traumatic experiences

Studies have examined the association between duration and frequency of exposure to traumatic events and PTSD rates. A study by Wolfe et al. (1994) found significantly higher rates of PTSD among sexually abused children who experienced maltreatment for more than 1 year relative to youths who were abused for less time. Berton and Stabb (1996) determined that domestic or community violence exposure, as denoted by child self-reports, was correlated with PTSD rates. Analogously, Ackerman et al. (1998) reported a higher prevalence of PTSD among youths who were sexually and physically abused (54.9%) than among children who reported either sexual (31.8%) or physical abuse (22.4%). With regard to a sample of sexually abused youths, Ruggiero et al. (2000) indicated that increased frequency and duration of sexual abuse significantly predicted PTSD. With reference to children and war traumas, Ahmad et al. (2000) found that duration of captivity was positively correlated with PTSD. Further, Seedat et al. (2004) and Schaal and Elbert (2006) reported that child exposure to three or more war-related traumatic events was associated with increased risk for PTSD in comparison to youths who experienced one trauma. On the other hand, Bayer et al. (2007) reported a nonsignificant association between PTSD and the amount of time spent as a child soldier during the African wars. In summary, most studies showed a positive correlation between trauma duration and frequency, although some studies showed no such association.

2.7.10 Time span between trauma exposure and diagnostic evaluation

The studies reviewed reported inconsistent findings with reference to the duration of time between trauma exposure and clinical diagnosis of children and adolescents. Pynoos et al. (1987) indicated that 60.4% of youths met diagnostic criteria for PTSD when assessed 1 month after a school-based shooting. The rate dropped to 29.0% at a 14-month follow-up. Likewise, Saigh (1988) determined that 75.0% ($n = 9$) of war-exposed Lebanese youths developed PTSD 37 days after experiencing a major war-related traumatic experience in Beirut. In contrast, a single case (8.3%) met PTSD criteria 316 days after trauma exposure. Sack et al. (1993) reported that PTSD estimates among Cambodian refugee youths declined from 50.0% to 48.0% to 38.0% at evaluations that were respectively conducted 5, 8, and 11 years after the Pol Pot-led genocide. Analogously, Vila et al. (1999) reported PTSD prevalence rates of 15.4% among youth hostages 2 months after a school-based shooting, and prevalence rates of 3.8% 18 months after the event. Finally, Bayer et al. (2007) reported that those who had been liberated from duty as child soldiers for less than 2 months experienced higher PTSD prevalence rates than those who had been liberated for more than 2 months. In contrast, a study by Landolt et al. (2005) found that while 16.2% of children who experienced motor vehicle accidents met criteria for PTSD 4–6 weeks after the accidents, 17.6% evidenced PTSD 1 year later. In sum, most studies show that PTSD rates decline with time following the trauma exposure.

2.7.11 Relationship between trauma victims and perpetrators

Findings by McLeer et al. (1988) indicated that 75.0% children who were the victims of paternal abuse showed evidence of PTSD. In a later study, McLeer et al. (1994) reported that 25.0% of the participants who were abused by trusted adults had PTSD relative to 10.0% of the children who had been abused by strangers. Both studies found that youths who were abused by an older child did not develop PTSD. In contrast, Ackerman et al. (1998) examined a sample of abused children and reported that the relationship between physically abused children and perpetrators was not predictive of PTSD.

2.8 Summary

The literature reviewed in this chapter demonstrates that although young people are frequently exposed to a variety of traumatic events, the majority of them do not develop PTSD. The research also indicates that a host of traumatic stressors can induce PTSD in children and adolescents. Tables 2.2–2.4 present an overview of PTSD rates as a function of different trauma types. Within this context, PTSD rates ranged from 0.0% to 95.0%. Marked differences were also evident within trauma categories. Specifically, war-related traumas reflected prevalence rates ranging from 7.6% to 87.0%, criminal victimization rates ranged from 9.0% to 63.5%, and disaster and accident studies ranged from 0.0% to 90.0%.

The reported differences with respect to PTSD prevalence among young people may be accounted for by numerous factors, including differences in diagnostic measures; samples; severity and type of traumatic experiences, and the interval of time between psychological assessment and trauma exposure. First, a variety of measures and methods reflecting three different sets of diagnostic criteria (i.e., DSM-III, DSM-III-R, and DSM-IV) were used. The variations in criteria indicated by the different versions of the DSM may have been associated, in part, with the range in PTSD prevalence rates. Secondly, the measures used to diagnose

PTSD varied. More specifically, these measures differed in relation to format, as individually administered semi-structured interviews and/or structured clinical interviews, parental ratings, teacher ratings, group self-report measures, and PTSD symptom checklists were used. Overall, 40 tests were used to denote PTSD. It is very important to note that psychometric properties of these measures vary. In fact, many of the tests that were used lack proof to support reliability and validity. Of particular concern is the failure to document content validity (i.e., concordance between DSM PTSD criteria and test items). For example, the content validity of the Reaction Index (Frederick et al., 1992) that was used in 14 studies that were reviewed has been questioned (Saigh, 1992), as this test does not reflect all of the criteria for PTSD as denoted by the DSM-IV, such as functional impairment. The failure to assess functional impairment may have increased the base rates for PTSD in the studies that relied on this test to measure PTSD. Additionally, there was great variability between studies with respect to the participants' demographic characteristics. Finally, as the majority of published reports indicate that PTSD tends to remit over time (e.g., Sack et al., 1993; Saigh, 1988; Vila et al., 1999), the changing PTSD estimates across studies may be associated with differing time spans between actual trauma exposure and clinical evaluation.

It should also be noted that PTSD frequently presents with major comorbid disorders (Faustman & White, 1989; Goenjian et al., 1995, 2001; Kessler et al., 1995; Kilpatrick et al., 2003; Kinzie et al., 1986; Kulka et al., 1990; McLeer et al., 1994). As having PTSD and a major comorbid disorder (e.g., substance dependence, major depressive disorder) may influence the selection and course of treatment for PTSD (Hubbard et al., 1995; Saigh et al., 2002), researchers need to consider carefully how these disorders may affect the efficacy of interventions.

Studies investigating the influence of factors that were related to the onset of the disorder indicated various degrees of concordance. First, inconsistencies were noted relative to gender and age. Six studies reported that females had higher PTSD prevalence than males (D'Augelli et al., 2006; Fitzpatrick & Boldizar, 1993; Pat-Horenczyk et al., 2007; Perkonigg et al., 2000; Schaal & Elbert, 2006; Ziaaddini et al., 2009), and one study indicated that males had higher rates (Khamis, 2005). However, an even larger number of studies (15) failed to observe a relationship between gender and PTSD (Ackerman et al., 1998; Ahmad et al., 2000; Broman-Fulks et al., 2007; Elbedour et al., 2007; Foster et al., 2004; Goenjian et al., 1995; Hubbard et al., 1995; Realmuto et al., 1992; Saigh, 1988; Saigh et al., 1997; Schwarzwald et al., 1994; Seedat et al., 2004; Silva et al., 2000; Yorbik et al., 2004). With regard to age, while six studies determined that older children had higher prevalence rates for PTSD (Ahmad et al., 2000; Garrison et al., 1993, 1995; Schwarz & Kowalski, 1991; Wolfe et al., 1994; Yorbik et al., 2004), two studies indicated that younger children had a higher PTSD prevalence (Bokszczanin, 2007; Schwarzwald et al., 1993), and three did not identify an association between age and PTSD (Landolt et al., 2005; Lavi & Solomon, 2005; Schaal & Elbert, 2006).

There were conflicting results regarding the relationship between race/ethnicity/national origin and PTSD in children and adolescents. While some studies found significant relationships between race, ethnicity and/or national origin and PTSD diagnosis or symptoms (March et al., 1998; Jones et al., 2002; Galea et al., 2003; LaGreca et al., 1996), other studies found nonsignificant differences between these groups (Abram et al., 2004; DeVries et al., 1999; Famularo et al., 1996; Garrison et al., 1993; Langley & Jones, 2005; Lawyer et al., 2006; Linning & Kearney, 2004; Lipschitz et al., 1999; Shannon et al., 1994; Shaw et al., 1995; Zink & McCain, 2003). Five of the studies investigating the association between child PTSD and parental psychological distress (Ahmad et al., 2000; Jones et al., 2002; Khamis, 2005; Linning & Kearney, 2004; Sack et al., 1993) determined that parental psychopathology was associated with PTSD in children.

With regard to child characteristics, the studies reviewed demonstrated that children with an IQ that was at least one standard deviation above the mean (i.e., IQ ≥ 115 points) had a decreased risk for developing PTSD (Breslau et al., 2006; Saigh et al., 2006) and children who received teacher ratings that indicated heightened externalizing behavior problems in the first grade had an increased risk for developing PTSD if they were exposed to a traumatic event (Breslau et al., 2006). Four studies suggested that prior trauma exposure, especially where PTSD developed, and exposure to post-trauma stressors increase an individual's vulnerability to the disorder (Garrison et al., 1993; Lipschitz et al., 2000; Saigh, 1988; Sack et al., 1993), while one study found that neither pre- nor post-stress exposure was associated with PTSD (Jones et al., 2002).

Nine studies examining the relationship between stressor severity and PTSD indicated that greater intensity is predictive of the disorder (Goenjian et al., 1995, 2001; Hsu et al., 2002; Kolaitis et al., 2003; Pat-Horenczyk et al., 2007; Pynoos et al., 1987; Roussos et al., 2005; Schaal & Elbert, 2006; Schwarzwald et al., 1994). Six studies indicated that there was no relationship between the stressor severity and prevalence of PTSD (DeVries et al., 1999; Koplewicz et al., 1994; Landolt et al., 2005; Saigh et al., 2002; Shaw et al., 1995).

Research has also demonstrated that the type of trauma exposure may present as a risk factor (Lawyer et al., 2006; Famularo et al., 1996; McLeer et al., 1994; Saigh, 1991). For instance, traumas that were intentionally induced by others were marked by higher PTSD prevalence rates. With reference to the number and duration of traumatic experiences, seven studies indicated that longer and/or more frequent exposure to traumatic events was associated with higher rates of PTSD (Ackerman et al., 1998; Ahmad et al., 2000; Berton & Stabb, 1996; Ruggiero et al., 2000; Schaal & Elbert, 2006; Seedat et al., 2004; Wolfe et al.,

1994). In contrast, one study (Bayer et al., 2007) found that there was no relationship between frequency and duration of exposures and PTSD.

Many studies indicated that PTSD estimates varied as a function of the time between trauma exposure and assessment (Bayer et al., 2007; Pynoos et al., 1987; Sack et al., 1993; Saigh, 1988; Vila et al., 1999). In effect, the literature indicates that PTSD prevalence decreased over time. Two studies investigating the relationship between trauma victims and perpetrators indicated that young people who were the victims of abuse by trusted adults had higher rates of PTSD in comparison to those who were abused by strangers (McLeer et al., 1988, 1994). In contrast, one study (Ackerman et al., 1998) reported that the relationship between physically abused children and perpetrators was not predictive of PTSD.

Overall, epidemiological research demonstrates that numerous young people are exposed to one or more traumatic events during the course of their lives. Precisely estimating trends over time is an ongoing challenge, as evidenced by the inconsistencies in the literature (Finkelhor & Jones, 2004). Further, prevalence rates have not yet been determined relative to the amended DSM-5 PTSD criteria. Certainly, the generalizability of the PTSD prevalence estimates that were reported herein relative to the new DSM-5 PTSD classification is difficult to estimate, as the new criteria differ significantly from the DSM-IV PTSD criteria (APA, 2013b). As such, there is a need for prospective research that enhances understanding of correlates, prevalence, and expression of child-adolescent PTSD and a pressing need to study the prevalence of the disorder as measured by the DSM-5.

Acknowledgement

This chapter is based on the life's work and intellectual inspiration of Professor Philip A. Saigh, Ph.D. It is the result of work completed under his mentorship and guidance, and I am truly grateful for his invaluable expertise and insight.

References

Abram KM, Teplin LA, Charles DR, et al. (2004) Posttraumatic stress disorder and trauma in youth in juvenile detention. *Archiv Gen Psychiatry* 61, 403–410.

Abram KM, Washburn JJ, Teplin LA et al. (2007 et al. Posttraumatic stress disorder and psychiatric comorbidity among detained youths. *Psychiatr Serv* 58, 1311–1316.

Ackerman PT, Newton JE, McPherson WB et al. (1998) Prevalence of posttraumatic stress disorder and other psychiatric diagnoses in three groups of abused children (sexual, physical, and both). *Child Abuse Neglect* 22, 759–774.

Ahmad A, Sofi MA, Sundelin-Wahlsten V et al. (2000) Posttraumatic stress disorder in children after the military operation "Anfal" in Iraqi Kurdistan. *Eur J Child Adol Psychiatry* 9, 235–243.

Alderfer MA, Navsaria N, Kazak AE (2009) Family functioning and posttraumatic stress disorder in adolescent survivors of childhood cancer. *J Family Psychol* 23, 717–725.

Almqvist K, Broberg AG (1999) Mental health and social adjustment in young refugee children 3 ¹/₂ years after their arrival in Sweden. *JAMA* 38, 723–730.

American Psychiatric Association (1994) *Diagnostic and Statistical Manual of Mental Disorders*, 4th edn. APA, Washington, DC.

American Psychiatric Association (2000) *Diagnostic and Statistical Manual of Mental Disorders*, 4th edn. (text revision). APA, Washington, DC.

American Psychiatric Association (2013a) *Diagnostic and Statistical Manual of Mental Disorders*, 5th edn. APA, Washington, DC.

American Psychiatric Association (2013b) *Highlights of Changes from the DSM-IV TR to DSM 5*. APA, Washington, DC.

Angold A, Costello, EJ (2000) The Child and Adolescent Psychiatric Assessment (CAPA) *JAMA* 39, 39–48.

Angold A, Costello EJ, Erkanli A (1999) Comorbidity. *J Child Psychol Psychiatry* 40, 57–87.

Bal A, Jensen, B (2007) Post-traumatic stress disorder symptom clusters in Turkish child and adolescent trauma survivors. *Eur Child Adol Psychiatry* 16, 449–457.

Bayer CP, Klasen F, Adam H (2007) Association of trauma and PTSD symptoms with openness to reconciliation and feelings of revenge among former Ugandan and Congolese child soldiers. *JAMA* 298, 555–559.

Beck, AT (1990) *Beck Anxiety Inventory (BAI)*. Psychcorp, San Antonio, TX.

Beck AT, Steer RA, Brown, GK (1996) *Beck Depression Inventory-II (BDI-II)*. Psychcorp, San Antonio, TX.

Berman SL, Kurtines WM, Silverman WK et al.(1996) The impact of exposure to crime and violence on urban youth. *Am J Orthopsychiatry,* 66, 329–336.

Berton MW, Stabb, SD (1996) Exposure to violence and post-traumatic stress disorder in urban adolescents. *Adolescence* 31, 489–498.

Bokszczanin, A (2007) PTSD symptoms in children and adolescents 28 months after a flood: Age and gender differences. *J Traum Stress* 20, 347–351.

Brady KT, Killeen TK, Brewerton T et al. (2000) Comorbidity of psychiatric disorders and posttraumatic stress disorder. *J Clin Psychiatry* 61, 22–32.

Breslau N, Davis GC, Andreski P et al. (1991) Traumatic events and posttraumatic stress disorder in an urban population of young adults. *Archiv Gen Psychiatry* 48, 216–222.

Breslau N, Kessler R C, Chilcoat HD et al. (1998) Trauma and posttraumatic stress disorder in the community. The 1996 Detroit Area Survey of Trauma. *Archiv Gen Psychiatry* 55, 626–632.

Breslau N, Lucia VC, Alvarado GF (2006) Intelligence and other predisposing factors in exposure to trauma and posttraumatic stress disorder: A follow-up study at age 17 years. *Archiv Gen Psychiatry* 63, 1238–1245.

Breslau N, Wilcox HC, Storr CL et al. (2004) Trauma exposure and posttraumatic stress disorder: a study of youths in urban America. *J Urban Health* 81, 530–544.

Broman-Fulks JJ, Ruggiero KJ, Green BA et al.(2006) Taxometric investigation of PTSD: Data from two nationally representative samples. *Behav Therap* 37, 364–380.

Broman-Fulks JJ, Ruggiero KJ, Hanson RF et al. (2007) Sexual assault disclosure in relation to adolescent mental health: Results from the National Survey of Adolescents. *J Clin Child Adol Psychol* 36, 2, 260–266.

*Brown C, Lai BS, Thompson JE et al.(2013) Posttraumatic stress disorder symptom trajectories in Hurricane Katrina affected youth. *J Affective Disord* 147, 198–204.

Bulut S, Bulut S, Tayli A (2005) The dose of exposure and prevalence rates of post-traumatic stress disorder in a sample of Turkish children eleven months after the 1999 Marmara earthquakes. *School Psychol Int,* 26, 55–70.

Burkle FM (1996) Acute-Phase Mental Health Consequences of Disasters: Implications for Triage and Emergency Medical Services. *Annal Emerg Med* 28, 119–128.

Cauffman E, Feldman S, Waterman J, Steiner, H (1998) Posttraumatic stress disorder among female juvenile offenders. *Am J Acad Child Adol Psychiatry* 37, 1209–1216.

Copeland WE, Keler G, Anglold A et al. (2007) Traumatic events and posttraumatic stress in childhood. *Archiv Gen Psychiatry* 64, 577–584.

Cuffe SP, Addy CL, Garrison CZ et al. (1998) Prevalence of PTSD in a community sample of older adolescents. *J Am Acad Child Adol Psychiatry* 37, 147–154.

D'Augelli AR, Grossman AH, Starks, M. T (2006) Childhood gender atypicality, victimization, and PTSD among lesbian, gay, and bisexual youth. *J Interpers Viol* 21, 1–21.

DeVries, A. P. J, Kassam-Adams N et al. (1999) Looking beyond the physical injury: Posttraumatic stress disorder in children and parents after pediatric traffic injury. *Pediatrics*, 104, 1293–1299.

DiGallo A, Barton J, Parry-Jones, W. L (1997) Road traffic accidents: Early psychological consequences in children and adolescents. *Br J Psychiatry* 170, 358–362.

Elbedour S, Onwuegbuzie AJ, Ghannam J et al. (2007) Posttraumatic stress disorder, depression, and anxiety among Gaza Strip adolescents in the wake of the second uprising (Intifada). *Child Abuse Neglect* 31, 719–729.

Fairbank JA, Schlenger WE, Saigh PA et al. (1995) An epidemiologic profile of post-traumatic stress disorder: Prevalence, comorbidity, and risk factors. In: Friedman MJ, Charney DS, Deutch AY (eds) *Neurobiological and clinical consequences of stress: From normal adaptation to post-traumatic stress disorder*. Lippincott, Williams & Wilkins, Philadelphia, PA, pp. 415–427.

Famularo R, Fenton T, Kinscherff R, Augustyn, M (1996) Psychiatric comorbidity in childhood posttraumatic stress disorder. *Child Abuse Neglect* 20, 953–961.

Faustman WO, White PA (1989) Diagnostic and psychopharmacological treatment characteristics of 536 inpatients with posttraumatic stress disorder. *J Nervous Mental Disord* 17, 154–159.

Finkehor D, Hamby SL, Ormrod RK et al. (2005) The Juvenile Victimization Questionnaire: Reliability, validity, and national norms. *Child Abuse Neglect* 29, 383–412.

Finkelhor D, Jones LM (2004) *Explanations for the decline in child sexual abuse cases*. Office of Juvenile Justice and Delinquency Prevention, Washington, DC.

Fitzpatrick KM, Boldizar JP (1993) The prevalence and consequences of exposure to violence among African-American youth. *JAMA* 32, 424–430.

Foster JD, Kuperminc GP, Price AW (2004) Gender differences in posttraumatic stress and related symptoms among inner-city minority youth exposed to community violence. *J Youth Adol* 33, 59–69.

Frederick CJ, Pynoos RS, Nader KO (1992) Child Post-Traumatic Stress Reaction Index (CPTS-RI). Calvin J. Frederick, PhD Psychological Services, Los Angeles, CA.

Frounfelker R, Vorhies Klodnick V, Mueser KT, Todd, S (2013) Trauma and posttraumatic stress disorder among transition-age youth with serious mental health conditions. *Int Soc Traum Stress Studies* 26, 409–412.

Galea S, Vlahov D, Resnick H et al. (2003) Trends of probable post-traumatic stress disorder in New York City after the September 11 terrorist attacks. *Am J Epidemiol* 158, 514–524.

Garrison CZ, Bryant ES, Addy CL et al. (1995) Posttraumatic stress disorder in adolescents after Hurricane Andrew. *JAMA* 34, 1193–1201.

Garrison CZ, Weinrich MW, Hadin SB et al. (1993) Posttraumatic stress disorder in adolescents after a hurricane. *J Epidemiol* 138, 522–530.

Giaconia RM, Reinherz HZ, Silverman AB et al. (1995) Traumas and posttraumatic stress disorder in a community population of older adolescents. *JAMA* 34, 1369–1380.

Goenjian AK, Molina L, Steinberg AM et al. (2001) Posttraumatic stress and depressive reactions among Nicaraguan adolescents after Hurricane Mitch. *Am J Psychiatry* 158, 788–794.

Goenjian AK, Pynoos RS, Steinberg AM et al. (1995) Psychiatric comorbidity in children after the 1988 earthquake in Armenia. *JAMA* 34, 1174–1184.

Hamby SL, Finkelhor D, Ormrod RK, Turner, H. A (2004) *The Juvenile Victimization Questionnaire (JVQ): Child Self-Report Version*. Crimes against Children Research Center, Durham, NH.

Horowitz K, McKay M, Marshall, R (2005) Community violence and urban families: Experiences, effects, and directions for intervention. *Am Orthopsychiatr Assoc* 75, 356–368.

Hsu C, Chong M, Yang P, Yeh, C (2002) Posttraumatic stress disorder among adolescent earthquake victims in Taiwan. *JAMA* 41, 875–81.

Hubbard J, Realmuto GM, Northwood AK et al. (1995) Comorbidity of psychiatric diagnoses with posttraumatic stress disorder in survivors of childhood trauma. *JAMA* 34, 1167–1173.

Husain SA, Allwood MA, Bell DJ (2008) The relationship between PTSD symptoms and attention problems in children exposed to the Bosnian war. *Journal of Emotional Behav Disord* 16, 52–62.

Jaycox LH, Stein BD, Kataoka SH et al. (2002) Violence exposure, posttraumatic stress disorder, and depressive symptoms among recent immigrant school children. *JAMA* 41, 1104.

Jones RT, Ribbe DP, Cunningham PB et al. (2002) Psychological impact of fire disaster on children and their parents. *Behav Modif* 26, 163–186.

Jones-Alexander J, Blanchard EB, Hickling, E. J (2005) Psychophysiological assessment of youthful motor vehicle accident survivors. *Appl Psychophysiol Biofeedback* 30, 115–123.

Kaufman-Shriqui V, Werbeloff N, Faroy M et al. (2013) Posttraumatic stress disorder among preschoolers exposed to ongoing missile attacks in the Gaza war. *Depression Anxiety* 30, 425–431.

Kessler RC, Sonnega A, Bromet E et al. (1995) Post-traumatic stress disorder in the national comorbidity survey. *Archiv Gen Psychiatry* 30, 776–783.

Khamis, V (2005) Post-traumatic stress disorder among school age Palestinian children. *Child Abuse Neglect* 29, 81–95.

Khamis, V (2012) Impact of war, religiosity and ideology on PTSD and psychiatric disorders in adolescents from Gaza Strip and South Lebanon. *Social Sci Med* 74, 2005–2011.

Kilpatrick DG, Resnick HS, Saunders BE et al. (1989) *The National Women's Study PTSD module*. National Crime Victims Research and Treatment Center, Medical University of South Carolina, Charleston, SC.

Kilpatrick DG, Ruggiero KJ, Acierno R et al. (2003) Violence and risk of PTSD, major depression, substance abuse/dependence, and comorbidity: Results from the national survey of adolescents. *J Consult Clin Psychol* 71, 692–700.

Kilpatrick DG, Saunders BE (1997) *Prevalence and Consequences of Child Victimization: Results from the National survey' of adolescents*. Final report. US Department of Justice, Office of Justice Programs, National Institute of Justice, Washington, DC.

Kinzie JD, Sack W, Angell R et al. (1989) A three-year follow-up of Cambodian young people traumatized as children. *J Am Acad Child Adol Psychiatry* 28, 501–504.

Kinzie JD, Sack WH, Angell R, Manson, S (1986) The psychiatric effects of massive trauma on Cambodian children: Part I. The children. *J Am Acad Child Adol Psychiatry* 25, 370–376.

Kolaitis G, Kotsopoulus J, Tsiantis J et al. (2003) Posttraumatic stress reactions among children following the Athens earthquake of September 1999. *Eur Child Adol Psychiatry* 12, 273–280.

Koplewicz HS, Vogel JM, Solanto MV et al. *Child and Parent Response to the World Trade Center bombing*. Poster session presented at the American Academy of Child and Adolescent Psychiatry, New York, NY.

Kulka RA, Schlenger WE, Fairbank JA et al. (1990) *Trauma and the Vietnam War generation*. Brunner/Mazel, New York, NY.

LaGreca A, Silverman W, Vernberg E et al. (1996) Posttraumatic stress symptoms in children after Hurricane Andrew: A prospective study. *J Consult Clin Psychol* 64, 712–723.

Landolt MA, Vollrath M, Timm K et al. (2005) Predicting posttraumatic stress symptoms in children with road traffic accidents. *JAMA* 44, 1276–1283.

Landolt MA, Schnyder U, Maier T et al. (2013) Trauma exposure and posttraumatic stress disorder in adolescents: A national survey in Switzerland. *J Traum Stress* 26, 209–216.

Langley A, Jones, R. T (2005) Post-traumatic symptomatology in adolescents following wildfire: The role of coping strategy and efficacy. *Fire Technol* 12, 587–599.

Laor N, Wolmer L, Kora M et al. (2002) Posttraumatic, dissociative and grief symptoms in Turkish children exposed to the 1999 earthquakes. *J Nerv Mental Dis* 190, 824–832.

Lavi T, Solomon, Z (2005) Palestinian youth of the Intifada: PTSD and future orientation. *JAMA* 44, 1176–1183.

Lawyer SR, Resnick HS, Galea S et al. (2006) Predictors of peritraumatic reactions and PTSD following the September 11th terrorist attacks. *Psychiatry* 69, 130–141.

Linning LM, Kearney, C. A (2004) Posttraumatic stress disorder in maltreated youth. *J Interpers Viol* 19, 1087–1101.

Lipschitz DS, Rasmusson AM, Anyan W et al. (2000) Clinical and functional correlates of posttraumatic stress disorder in urban adolescent girls at a primary care clinic. *JAMA* 39, 1104–1111.

Lipschitz DS, Winegar R, Hartnick E et al. (1999) Posttraumatic stress disorder in hospitalized adolescents: Psychiatric comorbidity and clinical correlates. *JAMA* 38, 385–392.

Luthra R, Abramovitz R, Greenberg R et al. (2009) Relationship between type of trauma exposure and posttraumatic stress disorder among urban children and adolescents. *J Interpers Viol* 24, 1919–1927.

March JS, Amaya-Jackson L, Murray MA et al. (1998) Cognitive behavioral psychotherapy for children and adolescents with posttraumatic stress disorder after a single incident stressor. *JAMA* 37, 585–593.

McDermott BM, Lee EM, Judd M et al. (2005) Posttraumatic stress disorder and general psychopathology in children and adolescents following a wildfire disaster. *Can J Psychiatry* 50, 137–143.

McLeer SV, Callaghan M, Henry D et al. (1994) Psychiatric disorders in sexually abused children. *JAMA* 33, 313–319.

McLeer SV, Deblinger E, Atkins MS et al. (1988) Posttraumatic stress disorder in sexually abused children. *JAMA* 27, 650–654.

Meiser-Stedman R, Yule W, Smith W et al. (2005) Acute stress disorder and posttraumatic stress disorder in children and adolescents involved in assaults and motor vehicle accidents. *Am J Psychiatry* 162, 1381–1383.

Meiser-Stedman R, Smith P, Yule W et al. (2008) The posttraumatic stress disorder diagnosis in preschool- and elementary school-age children exposed to motor vehicle accidents. *Am J Psychiatry* 165, 1326–1337.

Merry S, Andrews, L. K (1994) Psychiatric status of sexually abused children 12 months after disclosure of abuse. *JAMA* 33, 939–944.

Mirzamani M, Mohammadi, M & Besharat, M (2006) Post-traumatic stress disorder symptoms of children following the occurrence of Tehran city park disaster. *J Psychol* 140, 181–186.

Najarian LM, Goenjian AK, Pelcovitz D et al. (1996) Relocation after a disaster: Posttraumatic stress disorder in Armenia after the earthquake. *JAMA* 35, 374–383.

Norris, F. H (1992) Epidemiology of trauma: Frequency and impact of different potentially traumatic events on different demographic groups. *J Consult Clin Psychol* 60, 409–418.

Pat-Horenczyk R, Peled O, Miron T et al. (2007) Risk-taking behaviors among Israeli adolescents exposed to recurrent terrorism: Provoking danger under continuous threat? *Am J Psychiatry* 164, 66–72.

Perkonigg A, Kessler RC, Storz S et al. (2000) Traumatic events and posttraumatic stress disorder in the community: Prevalence, risk factors and comorbidity. *Acta Psychiatr Scand* 101, 46–59.

Pynoos R, Frederick C, Nader K (1987) Life threat and posttraumatic stress in school-age children. *Archiv Gen Psychiatry* 44, 1057–1063.

Pynoos R, Goenjian A, Tashjian M et al. (1993) Posttraumatic stress reactions in children after the 1988 Armenian earthquake. *Br J Psychiatry* 163, 239–247.

Realmuto GM, Masten A, Carole LF et al. (1992) Adolescent survivors of massive childhood trauma in Cambodia: Life events and current symptoms. *J Traum Stress* 5, 589–599.

Reebye P, Moretti MM, Wiebe VJ et al. (2000) Symptoms of posttraumatic stress disorder in adolescents with conduct disorder: Sex differences and onset patterns. *Can J Psychiatry* 45, 746–751.

Resnick HS, Kilpatrick DG, Dansky BS et al. (1993) Prevalence of civilian trauma and posttraumatic stress disorder in a representative national sample of women. *J Consult Clin Psychol* 61, 984–991.

Robins LN, Helzer JE, Cottler et al. (1989) *NIMH Diagnostic Interview Schedule, Version III Revised.* Washington University Department of Psychiatry, St. Louis, MO.

Rojas V, Pappagallo, M (2004) Risk factors for PTSD in children and adolescents. In: Silva RR (ed.) *Posttraumatic Stress Disorders in Children and Adolescents: Handbook.* Norton, New York, NY, pp. 38–59.

Roussos A, Goenjian AK, Steinburg AM et al. (2005) Posttraumatic stress and depressive reactions among children and adolescents after the 1999 earthquake in Ano Liosia, Greece. *Am J Psychiatry* 162, 530–537.

Ruggiero K, McLeer SV, Dixon JF (2000) Sexual abuse characteristics associated with survivor psychopathology. *Child Abuse Neglect* 24, 951–964.

Sack WH, Clarke G, Him C et al. (1993) A 6-year follow-up study of Cambodian refugee adolescents traumatized as children. *JAMA* 32, 431–437.

Sack WH, McSharry S, Clarke GN et al. (1994) The Khmer Adolescent Project. I. Epidemiologic findings in two generations of Cambodian refugees. *J Nerv Mental Dis* 182, 387–395.

Saigh, P. A (1988) Anxiety, depression, and assertion across alternating intervals of stress. *J Abnormal Psychol* 97, 338–342.

Saigh, P. A (1989a) The validity of the DSM-III posttraumatic stress disorder classification as applied to children. *J Abnormal Psychol* 98, 189–192.

Saigh, P. A (1989b) The development and validation of the Children's Posttraumatic Stress Disorder Inventory. *Int J Special Ed* 4, 75–84.

Saigh, P. A (1991) The development of posttraumatic stress disorder following four different types of traumatization. *Behav Res and Ther* 29, 213–216.

Saigh, P. A (1992) History, current nosology, and epidemiology. In Saigh PA (ed) *Posttraumatic Stress Disorder: A Behavioral Approach to Assessment and Treatment.* Allyn & Bacon, Needham Heights, MA, pp. 1–27.

Saigh, P. A (1997) *The Children's Posttraumautic Stress Disorder Inventory.* City University of New York Graduate School, New York, NY.

Saigh PA, Bremner, J. D (1999) History of posttraumatic stress disorder. In: Saigh PA, Bremner JD (eds) *Posttraumatic Stress Disorder: A Comprehensive Textbook.* Allyn and Bacon, Needham Heights, MA, pp. 51–84.

Saigh PA, Mroueh A, Bremner JD (1997) Scholastic impairments among traumatized adolescents. *Behav Res Ther* 35, 429–436.

Saigh PA, Mroueh A, Bremner JD (1999) History of posttraumatic stress disorder. In: Saigh PA, Bremner JD (eds) *Posttraumatic Stress Disorder: A Comprehensive Textbook.* Allyn and Bacon, Needham Heights, MA, pp. 51–84.

Saigh PA, Yasik AE, Mitchell P, Abright R. A (2004) The psychological adjustment of a sample of New York City preschool children 8–10 months after September 11, 2001. *Psychol Trauma* 3, 109–116.

Saigh PA, Yasik AE, Oberfield RO et al. (2006) The intellectual performance of traumatized children and adolescents with or without posttraumatic stress disorder. *J Abnormal Psychol* 115, 332–340.

Saigh PA, Yasik AE, Oberfield RO et al. (2002) An analysis of the internalizing and externalizing behaviors of traumatized urban youth with and without PTSD. *J Abnormal Psychol* 111, 462–470.

Saigh PA, Sack W, Yasik et al. (1999) Child-adolescent posttraumatic stress disorder: Prevalence, risk factors, and comorbidity.In: Saigh PA, Bremner JD (eds) *Posttraumatic Stress Disorder: A Comprehensive Textbook*. Allyn and Bacon, Needham Heights, MA, pp. 18–43.

Savin D, Sack WH, Clarke GN et al. (1996) The Khmer adolescent project: III. a study of trauma from Thailand's Site II refugee camp. *JAMA* 35, 384–391.

Schaal S, Elbert, T (2006) Ten years after the genocide: Trauma confrontation and posttraumatic stress in Rwandan adolescents. *J Traum Stress*, 19, 95–105.

Schäfer I, Barkmann C, Riedesser P, Schulte-Markwort, M (2006) Posttraumatic syndromes in children and adolescents after road traffic accidents – a prospective cohort study. *Psychopathology*, 39,159–164.

Schwab-Stone M, Ayers TS, Kasprow W et al. (1995) No safe haven: A study of violence exposure in an urban community. *JAMA* 34, 1343–1352.

Schwab-Stone M, Chen C, Greenberger E et al. (1999) No safe haven II: The effects of violence exposure on urban youth. *JAMA* 38, 359–367.

Schwarz ED, Kowalski JM (1991) Posttraumatic stress disorder after a school shooting: Effects of symptom threshold selection and diagnosis by DSM-III, DSM-III-R, and projected DSM-IV. *Am J Psychiatry* 148, 592–597.

Schwarzwald J, Weisenberg M, Solomon Z et al. (1994) Stress reaction of school-age children to the bombardment by scud missiles: A one-year follow-up. *J Traum Stress* 7, 657–667.

Schwarzwald J, Weisenberg M, Waysman M et al. (1993) Stress reactions of school-age children to the bombardment by Scud missiles. *J Abnormal Psychol* 102, 404–410.

Seedat S, Nyamai C, Njenga F et al. (2004) Trauma exposure and post-traumatic stress symptoms in urban African schools: survey in Cape Town and Nairobi. *Br J Psychiatry* 184, 169–175.

Servan-Schreiber D, Lin BL, Birmaher, B (1998) Prevalence of posttraumatic stress disorder and major depressive disorder in Tibetan refugee children. *J Am Acad Child Adol Psychiatry* 37, 874–879.

Shannon ME, Lonigan CJ, Finch AJ et al. (1994) Children exposed to disaster: I. Epidemiology of post-traumatic symptoms and symptom profiles. *JAMA* 33, 80–93.

Shaw JA, Applegate B, Tanner S et al. (1995) Psychological effects of Hurricane Andrew on an elementary school population. *JAMA* 34, 1185–1192.

Silva RR, Alpert M, Munoz DM et al. (2000) Stress and vulnerability to posttraumatic stress disorder in children and adolescents. *Am J Psychiatry* 157, 1229–1235.

Steiner H, Garcia IG, Matthews, Z (1997) Posttraumatic stress disorder in incarcerated juvenile delinquents. *JAMA* 36, 357–365.

Stewart AJ, Steiman M, Cauce AM et al. (2004) Victimization and posttraumatic stress disorder among homeless adolescents. *J Am Acad Child Adol Psychiatry* 43, 325–331.

Storr CL, Ialongo NS, Anthony JC, Breslau, N (2007) Childhood antecedents of exposure to traumatic events and posttraumatic stress disorder. *Am J Psychiatry* 164, 119–125.

Thabet AA, Ibraheem AN, Shivram R et al. (2009) Parenting support and PTSD in children of a war zone. *Int J Soc Psychiatry* 55, 226–237.

United States Department of Justice (1997) *Age patterns of victims of serious violent crime* (Bureau of Justice Statistics Report NCJ 162031). USDJ, Washington, DC.

United States Department of Justice (2006a) A National Crime Victimization Survey, 2005 (Bureau of Justice Statistics Report NCJ 215244) USDJ, Washington, DC.

United States Department of Justice (2007) A national crime victimization survey, 2004 (Bureau of Justice Statistics Report NCJ 227669). USDJ, Ann Arbor, MI.

United States Department of Transportation (2006b) 2005 Children Traffic Safety Fact Sheet (National Highway Traffic Safety Administration Report DOT HS 810 618). USDJ, Washington, DC.

United States Department of Transportation (2007) *Estimates Of Motor Vehicle Traffic Crash Fatalities And People Injured* (National Highway Traffic Safety Administration Report DOT HS 810 755) USDJ, Washington, DC.

Vila G, Porche L, Mouren-Simeoni M (1999) An 18-month longitudinal study of posttraumatic disorders in children who were taken hostage in their school. *Psychosom Med* 61, 746–754.

Wang L, Long D, Zhongquan L, Armour, C (2011) Posttraumatic stress disorder symptom structure in Chinese adolescents exposed to a deadly earthquake. *J Abnorm Child Psychol* 39, 749–758.

Weathers F, Litz BX, Herman DS et al. *The PTSD Checklist (PCL): Reliability, validity, and diagnostic utility*. Presented at the International Society of Traumatic Stress Studies, San Antonio, TX.

Wittchen, H-U, Pfister H (1997) *DIA-X-Interviews: Manual fur Screening-Verfahren und Interview*. Swets & Zeitlinger, Frankfurt, Germany.

Wolfe WA, Sas L, Wekerle C (1994) Factors associated with the development of posttraumatic stress disorder among child victims of sexual abuse. *Child Abuse Neglect* 18, 37–50.

World Health Organization (1997) *Composite International Diagnostic Interview — Version 2.1*. World Health Organization, Geneva, Switzerland.

Yasik AE, Saigh PA, Oberfield RO et al. (2012) Self-reported anxiety among traumatized urban youth. *Traumatology* 18, 47–55.

Ying L, Wu X, Lin C, Chen, C (2013) Prevalence and predictors of posttraumatic stress disorder and depressive symptoms among child survivors 1 year following the Wenchuan earthquake in China. *Eur Child Adol Psychiatry* 22, 567–575.

Yorbik O, Akbiyik DI, Kirmizigul P et al. (2004) Posttraumatic stress disorder symptoms in children after the 1999 Marmara earthquake in Turkey. *Int J Ment Health* 33, 46–58.

Yule W, Bolton D, Udwin O et al. (2000) The long-term psychological effects of a disaster experienced in adolescence: The incidence and course of PTSD. *J Child Psychol Psychiatry Allied Disc* 41, 503–511.

Ziaaddini H, Nakhaee N, Behzadi, K (2009) Prevalence and correlates of PTSD among high school students after the earthquake disaster in the City of Bam, Iran (Post traumatic stress disorder report). *Am J Appl Sci* 6, 130.

Zhang Z, Ran MS, Li YH et al. (2012) Prevalence of post-traumatic stress disorder among adolescents after the Wenchuan earthquake in China. *Psychol Med* 42, 1687–1693.

Zink KA, McCain, GC (2003) Post-traumatic stress disorder in children and adolescents with motor vehicle-related injuries. *J Special PediatrNurs* 8, 99–106.

CHAPTER 3

Early life stress and development: preclinical science

Dora B. Guzman[1], Brittany Howell[2] & Mar Sanchez[1]

[1] *Department of Psychiatry & Behavioral Science, School of Medicine, and Yerkes National Primate Research Center, Emory University, Atlanta, GA, USA*
[2] *Institute of Child Development, University of Minnesota, Minneapolis, MN, USA*

3.1 Overview

Significant advances have been made in the last decade using animal models of early life stress, which have impacted our understanding of how early traumatic experiences "get under the skin" and result in psychopathology and psychiatry disorders, such as anxiety, depression, or substance abuse. The field has progressed from the initial demonstrations of long-term negative impact of early trauma on physiological and behavioral development and individual variability in vulnerability due to genetic risks (the "gene × environment" concept), to the more recent identification of a multitude of biological mechanisms through which early adverse experiences can alter brain, behavioral, and physiological development of the infant and the child. These biological mechanisms that translate early stress/trauma into developmental changes go beyond the impact of stress hormones and stress-induced systemic and brain inflammation, and include alterations in the gut and vaginal microbiomes that lead to neurotransmitter changes in the infant's brain, and epigenetic modifications that translate experiences into molecular changes not only in somatic cells of the individual, but also in her/his germ line, leading to the transmission of stress-induced traits and memories from generation to generation.

Critical paradigm shifts have also taken place, with an increased focus on: animal models with ecological and ethological validity that allow us to examine the basic processes of experience-induced developmental adaptations to the environment that result in pathology; resilience factors; and adolescence viewed as another critical period of behavior and brain reorganization, which opens windows of opportunity and vulnerability. At the same time there has been an explosion of research into sex differences and models of female-biased disorders.

Posttraumatic Stress Disorder: From Neurobiology to Treatment, First Edition.
Edited by J. Douglas Bremner.
© 2016 John Wiley & Sons, Inc. Published 2016 by John Wiley & Sons, Inc.

Due to the space limitations, we will only review some highlights from rodent and non-human primate (NHP) animal models that provide examples into biological mechanisms that translate early adversity into psychopathology. The idea is simple: the early environment programs physiological and brain development to support behaviors, cognitive and biological processes that help the offspring (and future generations) adapt to that environment. Therefore, the plasticity of neurobehavioral development has an evolutionary role as it helps species adapt to changing environments. However, some of these adaptations for survival come at a high cost, also resulting in pathology. Among the many aspects of the early environment, one has a particularly critical importance for mammalian species, including rodents, NHPs and humans: maternal care. Thus, this chapter places a special emphasis on animal models that examine the developmental impact of mother–infant relationship disruption, and the mechanisms by which maternal care regulates the development of brain circuits particularly relevant for emotional and stress regulation, which are very sensitive to early life stress.

And finally, there are early critical/sensitive periods that serve as windows of opportunity for adaptation to the environment but that, by the same token, also serve as windows of vulnerability. Thus, if the experience is too aversive, as happens for early traumatic experiences such as childhood maltreatment, it will lead to maladaptive developmental trajectories, including psychopathology and physiological alterations. Preclinical research using animal models of early life adversity are critical to understanding the common principles and mechanisms underlying the relationship between early experience and outcomes in humans. The following sections will present an overview of this relationship.

3.2 Early life stress and the hypothalamic–pituitary–adrenal (HPA) axis

Early life stress alters the development of neurobiological systems, leading to later risk for psychopathology (Gunnar & Vazquez, 2006; Yehuda et al., 2001). Much of the literature examining the biological mechanisms underlying this link has focused on the HPA axis, because it is activated during the stress experience (Heim et al., 2000; Sanchez et al., 2005) and can cause long-term neurobiological changes via genomic mechanisms (Barr et al., 2003; Kinnally et al., 2011). Briefly, stressful stimuli activate neurons in the paraventricular nucleus (PVN) of the hypothalamus that release corticotropin-releasing factor (CRF) into the anterior pituitary which, in turn, releases adrenocorticotropic hormone (ACTH) into the blood circulation (see Chapter 11). In the adrenal cortex, ACTH induces the synthesis and release of glucocorticoids (corticosterone in rodents, cortisol in primates), highly catabolic steroid hormones. Limbic regions such as the amygdala and hippocampus, as well as the ventromedial prefrontal cortex (PFC), regulate

HPA axis activity through indirect projections to the hypothalamic PVN, where corticotropin-releasing hormone neurons are located, and they also express glucocorticoid receptors (GRs), mediating glucocorticoid negative feedback (Bauman et al., 2004; Ichise et al., 2006; Jackowski et al., 2011; Rilling et al., 2001). Stressors, including trauma experienced early in life, activate the HPA axis and associated brain areas, including the cortico-limbic structures mentioned earlier (ventromedial PFC, amygdala, hippocampus). Other neurobiological systems, such as the sympathetic nervous system, are also activated during threatening situations; thus, chronic stress or traumatic experiences early in life can impact the way these stress-response systems mature, leading to extreme emotional and stress reactivity and other psychopathologies.

3.3 Rodent models of early life stress/trauma

Adverse experiences that occur in the early stages of life, such as childhood maltreatment, poverty, exposure to violence and other forms of chronic psychosocial stress, can have lasting impacts on the individual. Early adversity/stress is a major risk factor for later physical health and emotional regulation problems, including a higher risk for the development of psychopathology, such as anxiety and mood disorders or substance abuse.

Most rodent models of early stress/trauma use the experimental disruption of the powerful dam–pup relationship, through either prolonged maternal separations or maternal deprivation, because these adverse experiences produce robust developmental impacts on brain, behavioral, and stress physiology systems that parallel those reported in human populations with trauma-related psychopathology (Marco et al., 2011; Molet et al., 2014; Sanchez et al., 2001). The biological rationale behind the broad use of maternal separation/deprivation during the early postnatal period (birth through postnatal day 14) in these models is based on the remarkable developmental changes in HPA axis and fear regulation during this period, where the dam plays a critical role as an external regulator of the pup's behavior and physiology, keeping both its neuroendocrine stress responses and fear low (Rincon-Cortes & Sullivan, 2014; Sanchez et al., 2001). Therefore, both prolonged pperiods of maternal separation (3–24 hours) and deprivation result in detrimental behavioral outcomes, including higher fear and anxiety, reduced exploration, anhedonia and social and cognitive deficits such as increased aggression and impulsivity (Kaffman & Meaney, 2007; Sanchez et al., 2001).

Although these experimental manipulations in early developmental periods have provided critical information about the biological mechanisms translating maternal behaviors into pup development, they do not fully model the chronicity of early adverse/traumatic experiences in humans, which include childhood maltreatment, poverty and exposure to violence. Recent experimental manipulations have been designed to capture sustained stress that leads to persistent alterations in maternal care by limiting physical resources such as nesting material and cage bedding (Molet et al., 2014). The result of this impoverished cage environment is incompetent maternal care, with delivery of a very fragmented, erratic and unpredictable sensory stimulation and nursing of pups (Baram et al., 2012; Ivy et al., 2008), as well as maternal physical abuse (trampling and rough handling of pups) (Roth & Sullivan, 2005; see also Chapter 3 and 4).

A second model involves experimental manipulations that mimic attachment to an abusive caregiver through maternal odor-shock conditioning (Roth & Sullivan, 2005; Sullivan & Lasley, 2010). This model leads to similar neurobehavioral outcomes as the limited physical resources model, including social deficits (e.g., maternal care), depressive-like behaviors, altered fear responses and disrupted HPA axis and amygdala function (Baram et al., 2012; Rincon-Cortes & Sullivan, 2014). Some of these behavioral, neural, and neuroendocrine alterations seem to be mediated by epigenetic modifications in the brain-derived neurotrophic factor (*BDNF*) gene that result in reduced expression of BDNF in the PFC of abused offspring (Roth et al., 2009).

3.4 Non-human primate models of early life stress/trauma

Non-human primate models offer critical advantages for research translation to humans. Macaque species, in particular, are widely used to study the neurobehavioral and biological impact of early adverse/traumatic experiences because of their phylogenetic, social, neurobiological, and physiological similarities with humans (Barbas, 2000; Croxson et al., 2005; Pryce, 2008; Reep, 1984; Sanchez et al., 2000; Suomi, 2005; Thiebaut de Schotten et al., 2012) and similar temporal and anatomical patterns of brain and behavioral development (Diamond, 1991; Gibson, 1991; Huttenlocher & Dabholkar, 1997). The rhesus macaque (*Macaca mulatta*) is a highly social Old World primate species that is able to adapt to a variety of environments. Rhesus monkeys live in large groups with strict dominance hierarchies that produce a stable, matriarchal social organization. The matrilineal hierarchies are primarily maintained through both contact and non-contact aggression from dominant to subordinate females (Berstein, 1976; Berstein & Gordon, 1974; Berstein et al., 1974) and an animal's social rank determines its access to various resources, such as food and sexual partners (Sade, 1967). In addition to the potential chronic exposure to hierarchy-induced social stress, rhesus monkeys constitute good models of early adversity/trauma due to the fact that they form very strong mother–infant bonds which, as in humans, last beyond weaning (Sanchez, 2006; Sanchez et al., 2001; Suomi, 2005). Thus, this

NHP model has provided critical evidence of the developmental impact of adverse caregiving experiences similar to those experienced in humans and potential mechanisms involved in the development of psychopathologies, e.g., depression and anxiety disorders such as post-traumatic stress disorder (PTSD) (Howell & Sanchez, 2011; Nelson & Winslow, 2008; Parker & Maestripieri, 2011; Sanchez, 2006; Sanchez et al., 2001; Sanchez & Pollak, 2009; Stevens et al., 2009).

3.4.1 Social isolation

An important demonstration of the translational impact of NHP models is Harlow's seminal work in the 1950s using experimental manipulations of the early-rearing environment of rhesus monkey infants, which led to attachment theory (Ainsworth 1969, 1979; Bowlby, 1965; Harlow, 1958; Suomi et al., 1971) and to a switch in our society to the encouragement of warm and sensitive caregiving early in life. Harlow and colleagues first demonstrated that disruptions of the early social environment caused long-term effects on primate development, particularly in social behaviors. Rhesus infants reared in partial social isolation – where infants were separated from their mothers and social groups at birth and only had auditory, visual, and olfactory contact with conspecifics – showed long-term behavioral deficits, including stereotyped movements, self-injury, hyper-aggression, and inability to recognize social cues and develop normal social relationships (Suomi et al., 1971). Complete social isolation resulted in even more severe behavioral deficits as well as an increased fear and anxiety responses (Harlow et al., 1965; Seay & Gottfried 1975). More recent studies have tried to dissect the specific role of the mother by removing her at birth or early in infancy and rearing the infant with other peers (peer-rearing), which resulted in many of the neurobehavioral alterations described above, including elevated anxiety and levels of stress hormones (Dettmer et al., 2012), increased alcohol consumption in juveniles (Higley et al., 1991), cognitive deficits associated with reduced size of the corpus callosum (Sanchez et al., 1998) and broad gene expression changes caused by epigenetic (DNA methylation) modifications (Provençal et al., 2012).

   Although these manipulations have been critical to understanding the powerful role of the mother and social experiences on social, emotional, and endocrine development of infant primates, they are also drastic and artificial manipulations with limited ecological and ethological validity, except possibly for some forms of extreme social deprivation (as seen in some children reared in orphanages).

3.4.2 Maternal separation

To address the issue of ethological validity, maternal separation has been used in NHP species in a similar way to rodents. Maternal separation is a potent stressor in rhesus infants that produces an initial increase of behavioral activity and distress vocalizations, and intense HPA axis activation (Bayart et al., 1990; Harlow et al., 1971; Sanchez et al., 2005). Repeated maternal separation during rhesus infancy leads to long-lasting increased stress reactivity, flattened diurnal cortisol rhythm, and elevated anxiety (Sanchez et al., 2005). But there is evidence of critical sensitive periods to these separations in rhesus, consistent with reports in children. More adverse effects were observed in rhesus infants that experienced earlier maternal separation compared with later time points, including aberrations of social and fear behaviors (O'Connor & Cameron 2006).

Interestingly, studies in marmosets, which are a biparental species, have shown that paternal care is also critical for proper primate neurobehavioral development. Using parent–infant daily separations from postnatal day (PND) 2–28, these studies showed long-term impact during adolescence, including increased stress and behavioral reactivity, and cognitive deficits, e.g., reduced motivation for reward, increased sensitivity to perceived loss of control, and problems with behavioral inhibition and reversal learning (Dettling et al., Dettling, Feldon and Pryce, 2002b; Pryce et al., 2004a,b). Parent–infant separation also impacts the development of neural circuits and physiological systems related to psychopathology, including the HPA axis, the PFC, and the hippocampus (Arabadzisz et al., 2010; Law et al., 2008, 2009).

Removal of the mother from her infant, whether transient or permanently, alters the mother–infant relationship, which is critical for normal development, and hinders the ability of the mother to buffer the infant's reactivity to threat (Erickson et al., 2005; Sanchez et al., 2001, 2005). Interestingly, the vulnerability to early adversity is sex-dependent, with female infants showing higher separation-induced cortisol elevations than males (Bayart et al., 1990; Sanchez et al., 2005) as well as stronger long-term impact, at least in terms of the blunted diurnal cortisol rhythm detected during the juvenile period (Sanchez et al., 2005). These results suggest that female rhesus infants may be more vulnerable to repeated maternal separations than males.

3.4.3 Variable foraging demand

Although the NHP models described above have demonstrated the critical role of parental care for primate neurobehavioral development, they are based on experimental manipulations that lack ecological validity. These NHP species do not experience these alterations in parental care in the wild, making it difficult to translate the meaning of the biological mechanisms involved to human experiences. Thus, we will now discuss more naturalistic NHP models with ecological and ethological validity. The variable foraging demand (VFD), for example, exploits a species-typical behavior in bonnet macaques (*Macaca radiata*), by randomly varying the foraging demands of the mother to disrupt her normal maternal and social behaviors. The VFD involves arbitrary fluctuations of the food supply, from free access to food – where little foraging is required – to times when food is limited and extensive foraging is needed to fulfill dietary needs, strongly affecting the mother–infant relationship, which constitutes a major stressor for the infants (Andrews & Rosenblum 1994; Rosenblum & Paully 1984). The VFD condition led to a reduction of time that it took for mothers to respond to infant solicitations for maternal care – without impacting nutrition or physical health in the mother or the infant – and infants became more fearful and hyper-responsive to both behavioral and physiological stimuli (Andrews & Rosenblum 1994; Coplan et al., 1996). Infants also displayed higher distress during separation from their mother and lower levels of social play and exploration compared with controls (Andrews & Rosenblum 1994; Rosenblum & Paully 1984). This model has a stronger ecological and ethological validity than those described earlier because the manipulation consists on an unpredictable availability of environmental resources that, in turn, affects maternal behavior, as in humans.

The impact extends to the juvenile and adolescent periods, with VFD animals showing reduced affiliation, social incompetence, and increased fear and social subordination while in a new social group (Andrews & Rosenblum 1994). VFD also causes long-term neurobiological alterations, including elevated levels of the stress neuropeptide CRF in cerebrospinal fluid (CSF) of both mother and infant (Coplan et al., 2005) and increased CSF concentrations of 5-hydroxyindoleacetic acid, the main serotonin (5HT) metabolite (Mathew et al., 2002). In addition, the VFD model results in long-term alterations in brain regions involved in emotional and stress regulation, including PFC and limbic regions such as the amygdala and hippocampus (Coplan et al., 1996, 1998, 2001, 2010; Jackowski et al., 2011; Mathew et al., 2003), suggesting a particular vulnerability of these neural circuits to early caregiving, as well as reductions of brain white matter integrity in the anterior limb of the internal capsule, which have been implicated in various psychiatric disorders such as depression and schizophrenia (Coplan et al., 2010).

A recent study suggests that VFD may have transgenerational effects on the behavior of female offspring never exposed to this condition (Kinnally et al., 2013). Additional research needs to be conducted to determine whether transgenerational effects are also evident in males and the possible mechanisms of transmission, which could range from changes in maternal behavior or observational learning by the infant, to epigenetic modifications in the germ line. Adult macaques exposed to VFD show higher whole-genome and 5HT transporter DNA methylation in blood samples, supporting the possibility of epigenetic modifications (Kinnally et al., 2011).

3.4.4 Infant maltreatment

Childhood maltreatment is not a uniquely human phenomenon but has also been observed in both wild and captive populations of NHPs, including macaques, baboons, and marmosets (Brent et al., 2002; Johnson et al., 1996;

Maestripieri, 1998; Maestripieri et al., 1997; Sanchez, 2006; Troisi et al., 1982). In macaque species, infant maltreatment involves two comorbid behaviors in the mother that result in overt signs of infant distress (screams, tantrums) and happen very early in life: physical abuse, which involves violent behaviors towards the infant that cause pain and distress (e.g., dragging, crushing, throwing the infant); and infant rejection, which consists of pushing the infant away when it solicits contact with the mother (Maestripieri, 1998; McCormack et al., 2006). The majority of infant maltreatment in this animal model occurs in the first 3 months of life when the infant is more dependent on the mother (Maestripieri 1998; McCormack et al., 2006; Sanchez 2006) and, therefore, more vulnerable to trauma.

Infant physical abuse has been more widely studied than rejection and it runs in families, being experientially transmitted from generation to generation (Maestripieri, 2005; Maestripieri & Carroll, 1998; Maestripieri et al., 2000b). Overall, the findings suggest that maltreatment in macaques is a stressful experience that results in elevated activity of the HPA axis and increased emotional reactivity and irritability that persist throughout the juvenile and adolescent periods, comparable to those seen in maltreated children (Cicchetti 1998; Howell et al., 2014b; Koch et al., 2014; McCormack et al., 2006, 2009; Sanchez, 2006; Sanchez & Pollak, 2009; Sanchez et al., 2010). Social deficits, including delayed independence from the mother and less exploration and play, as well as reduced affiliation and increased aggression during the juvenile/adolescent periods, have also been reported in this model (Howell et al., 2013; Maestripieri & Carroll, 1998; Maestripieri et al., 2000a). Additional neuroendocrine evidence supports the conclusion that the experience of abuse during infancy is stressful, as abused infants show increased HPA axis activity and blunted ACTH responses to CRF pharmacological challenge, which confirms an adaptation of the pituitary to stress-induced hypothalamic CRF overactivity (Koch et al., 2014; Sanchez et al., 2010). Recent neuroimaging studies by our group have reported increased amygdala volume associated with abuse rates received by the animals during infancy, as well as reduced cortical white matter integrity in tracts important for behavioral and emotional regulation, and a link between these neural alterations and elevated levels of the stress hormone cortisol found early in life in abused infants (Howell et al., 2014b, 2013). These findings parallel long-term consequences found in maltreated humans, supporting the construct validity of this model and its translational value to understand mechanisms underlying the developmental outcomes associated with this adverse early experience in humans.

Interestingly, infant rejection (which implies an act of omission by depriving the infant of a caregiving behavior, and is close to the neglect construct in humans), more so than physical abuse, is a strong predictor of negative physiological and neurobehavioral outcomes, including reduced brain 5HT and dopamine function, and increased anxiety and activation of pro-inflammatory pathways (Maestripieri et al., 2006a,b; Sanchez et al., 2007; Sanchez & Pollak, 2009). Altogether these findings parallel long-term consequences found in maltreated humans, and highlight the critical role of a sensitive mother (or father) for infant primate development, particularly early in life before animals start exploring – around weaning (Howell & Sanchez, 2011). However, they also bring up important questions not addressed in these studies, such as the potential role of social support from other members of the family or group to explain individual variability to the adverse experiences.

3.4.5 Stress inoculation and the issue of timing of early adversity

In contrast to the evidence presented so far that disruptions in parental care result in alterations in primate neurobehavioral development and physiological impacts, there is an interesting body of literature suggesting that some stressors at specific times of development may actually increase resilience to future challenges. Most of this evidence in NHPs comes from studies in squirrel monkeys showing that mild stress exposure at specific developmental times (weaning, when infants are not as dependent on maternal care) may be protective, instead allowing the animal to better adapt to challenges later in life (Lyons & Parker, 2007; Lyons et al., 2010; Parker et al., 2004). This phenomenon, termed "stress inoculation," involves exposure to mild intermittent stress consisting of separation from the mother and social group for 1 hour/week for 10 weeks. Unlike evidence from rodent studies, the effects don't seem to be mediated by changes in maternal care following reunion, but by the infant's reactivity to the separation (Parker et al., 2006). Several positive behavioral outcomes of this experience have been reported, including increased exploratory behavior in adolescence and inhibitory control of behavior lasting into early adulthood (Parker et al., 2005, 2012). The HPA axis stress response also seems better adapted to handle challenges, as shown by reduced basal levels of stress hormones, but an intact ability to mount a healthy response to a moderate stressor (Parker et al., 2005, 2012). Neurobiological effects of this manipulation include alterations in PFC structure and GR receptor expression in reward circuits, without impact to the hippocampus (Lyons et al., 2002; Lyons & Schatzberg, 2003; Patel et al., 2008). Although seemingly contradictory to everything presented so far, the resilience could be explained by the fact that these infants are in a later developmental stage (weaning) when exposed to stress and, therefore, are less dependent on maternal care. We have to understand the ecological and ethological implications of these experimental separations as, in this species, unlike macaques, mothers periodically leave newly weaned offspring on their own, at 3–6 months of age, to forage for food (Boinski & Fragaszy, 1989; Lyons et al., 1998). Therefore separation stress is built into the normative developmental experiences of this species. These studies highlight the importance of the ecological validity and the timing/age of the experience for our interpretation of the findings in relation to human psychiatric disorders (Parker & Maestripieri, 2011; Howell & Sanchez, 2011).

3.5 Impact of early life stress on prefrontal-limbic brain circuits across species: biological and evolutionary mechanisms

Early traumatic/stressful experiences, including infant/child maltreatment (which, as reviewed earlier in the chapter, rodent and NHP species also experience), happen at a time of drastic and rapid neurodevelopmental changes, when this plasticity becomes a vulnerability factor in which the impact of trauma can be encoded (Andersen, 2003; Knudsen, 2004; Rice & Barone, 2000). These developmental trajectories vary from one brain region to another, explaining why there are region-specific sensitive periods that sometimes last for several years in primates, as in the case of the PFC, due to their protracted development (Andersen, 2003). Thus, cortical maturation occurs first in regions that process visual or somatosensory stimuli, and later on in the association cortices that integrate these sensory inputs, including temporal and frontal cortices, and follows an evolutionary pattern, with phylogenetically older regions maturing earlier than newer regions, such as the PFC (Giedd, 2004; Giedd & Rapoport 2010; Gogtay et al., 2004; Shaw et al., 2008). This evidence suggests that specific brain regions with protracted developmental trajectories, including the PFC, association cortices and temporal lobe structures such as the amygdala and hippocampus, are particularly vulnerable to early postnatal experiences, especially maternal care, explaining why infant/childhood maltreatment is a strong risk factor for later psychopathology, consistently affecting socioemotional and stress regulation functions supported by these cortico-limbic circuits. Indeed, human (Bremner & Randall, 1997; De Bellis, 2005; De Bellis et al., 1999a,b; Drevets et al. 2011; Teicher et al., 2003; Tottenham & Sheridan, 2009) and animal studies (Arabadzisz et al., 2010; Bale et al., 2010; Law et al., 2008, 2009; Coplan et al., 1996, 1998, 2001, 2010; Howell et al., 2014b; Jackowski et al., 2011; Mathew, et al., 2003; O'Connor & Cameron, 2006; Pryce et al., 2005; Sanchez et al., 2001; Spinelli et al., 2009) provide evidence of consistent impact of adverse caregiving on the PFC, amygdala, and hippocampus and their connectivity (see Chapter 12). Because these PFC-limbic circuits play critical roles in emotion regulation and the stress response, including hypothalamic-pituitary-adrenal (HPA) axis function (Herman et al., 2003, 2005; Ulrich-Lai & Herman, 2009), it is not surprising that one of the most consistent effects of adverse caregiving, including childhood maltreatment, in different species is increased emotional and stress reactivity. Recent neuroimaging studies in a NHP model of infant maltreatment demonstrated a positive correlation between abuse rates received by the animals during infancy and amygdala volume during adolescence, as well as reduced white matter integrity in cortico-cortical tracts important for behavioral and emotional regulation, and a link between these brain alterations and elevated cortisol levels in abused infants (Howell et al., 2013,2014b). These findings are similar to those found in maltreated human populations (Dannlowski et al., 2012; McCrory et al., 2012; Teicher et al., 2014).

The high plasticity of these PFC–amygdala circuits and their sensitivity to early experiences probably have an adaptive purpose. In mammals, a main role of the infant brain is to bond to the mother/caregiver at any cost. Elegant studies in rodent models have dissected biological mechanisms by which specific maternal behaviors regulate brain development (Eghbal-Ahmadi et al., 1999; for a review, see Howell & Sanchez, 2011, Korosi & Baram, 2009, and Sanchez et al., 2001). These mechanisms include feeding regulation of the pup's heart rate through milk effects on gastrointestinal receptors; and tactile stimulation through grooming and licking, which stimulates sensory pathways that regulate not only the activity, but the development of limbic systems including PFC–amygdala circuits that control emotional and stress responses. Therefore, somatosensory information derived from the pup's suckling or from maternal licking and grooming can reach amygdala nuclei such as the central nucleus of the amygdala through projections from the laterodorsal tegmental and pedunculopontine nuclei that receive somatosensory inputs from the spinal cord. A third biological mechanism includes maternal behavior-induced epigenetic modifications (e.g., DNA methylation) in the pup's genes like the GR, estrogen receptor, neurotrophic factors (e.g. BDNF) and proteins that regulate brain synaptic development (e.g., protocadherins). These epigenetic modifications collectively produce long-term genomic programming impacts that lead to extensive and coordinated biological responses whose purpose seem to be to adapt to the early environment. These altered responses can get transmitted to future generations through epigenetic modifications in the germ line.

Additional studies in rodents have characterized the major neurobiological attachment systems that allow infants to recognize and bond with their mother/caregiver (Moriceau & Sullivan, 2005; Sullivan & Lasley, 2010) (see Chapter 4) and that are particularly vulnerable to adverse forms of caregiving, such as physical abuse (Rincon et al., 2014). These seminal studies by Sullivan and colleagues have shown that the mammalian infant brains (rodent, NHP or human) are similar in the way they are wired to form and maintain strong bonds with the mother/caregiver, although through different sensory systems (olfactory in the case of rat pups). In fact, the neonatal rat uses a different learning circuit from that used in adults, which involves noradrenergic (NE) projections from the locus coeruleus (LC). During the sensitive period for attachment formation to the mother (PND 1–9), when the pups are confined to the nest, this LC–NE system is overactive and releases high amounts of

NE during dam–pup interactions, which facilitates learning of a robust and rapid preference of the pup for the mother. At the same time, brain circuits that mediate fear/avoidance learning, such as the amygdala, are turned "off" during this period of critical infant dependence on the mother. The activity of attachment/approach systems and inactivity of fear/avoidance learning explain why the attachment to the caregiver is not broken even in painful relationships, when she/he is physically abusive, as shown in humans (Helfer et al., 1997), and animal species (Fisher, 1955; Harlow & Harlow, 1965; Sanchez et al., 2010). Now, when the rat pup starts exploring outside the nest (after PND 10), the fear/avoidance learning system becomes active and the attachment/approach LC automatic system becomes less active, although the mother's presence still has the power to switch the pup's amygdala to a more immature (fear "off") state (Rincon et al., 2014). These developmental brain-behavioral strategies are very adaptive for the survival of infants in altricial species, where the proximity to mother early in life provides protection, nutrition, warmth and physiological regulation, while, when the infant grows older and starts exploring, fear is switched "on" to stir youngsters from danger and towards a secure base (mother and nest). A similar developmental switch characterized by increased fear (gaze aversion, freezing) appears around 1 year of age in humans when we start walking and there is increased risk for exposure to threats in the environment (Sroufe, 1977). These similar developmental switches in approach-avoidance strategies in primate and rodent infants seem supported by neurodevelopmental switches in amygdala function and the nature of its connectivity with the PFC both in humans (Gee et al., 2013) and NHPs (Raper et al., 2014). The plasticity of these neural systems and the complexity of the normative developmental changes they undergo make them very vulnerable to the impact of early traumatic experiences, including childhood maltreatment, leading to a myriad long-term alterations in emotional regulation and stress responses and, therefore, psychopathology.

3.6 Conclusions

Early traumatic experiences, including childhood maltreatment, are major risk factors for psychiatric disorders. Studies in animals offer a unique opportunity to understand the basic neurobiological and developmental mechanisms that translate these adverse experiences into negative outcomes. This includes understanding the underlying cellular/molecular mechanisms involved and the critical sensitive periods. An important, but often overlooked, factor is the need to have a strong understanding of the normative patterns of neurobehavioral development involved not only in children, but also in the animal models being used (Machado & Bachevalier, 2003), which requires the selection and development of models and experiences with strong ecological and ethological validity.

Acknowledgements

We thank the members of the NIMH-funded "Early Experience, Stress and Neurobehavioral Development Center" (P50 MH078105) for the stimulating discussions that influenced some of the views presented here. This work was supported by grants P50 MH078105 and F31 MH086203 from the National Institute of Mental Health (NIMH, grants HD055255 and HD077623 from the National Institute of Child Health & Human Development (NICHD), grant DA038588 from the National Institute of Drug Abuse (NIDA) and grant BCS-1439258 from the National Science Foundation (NSF). The content is solely the responsibility of the authors and does not necessarily represent the official views of the NIMH, NICHD, NIDA or the National Institutes of Health of the NSF. The project was also supported by the Office of Research Infrastructure Programs/OD (ORIP/OD) P51OD11132 (YNPRC Base grant, formerly NCRR P51RR000165). The YNPRC is fully accredited by the Association for the Assessment and Accreditation of Laboratory Care, International.

References

Ainsworth MDS (1969) Object relations, dependency, and attachment: A theoretical review of the infant-mother relationship. *Child Dev* 969–1025.

Ainsworth MS (1979) Infant–mother attachment. *Am Psychol* 34, 932.

Andersen SL (2003) Trajectories of brain development: point of vulnerability or window of opportunity? *Neurosci Biobehav Rev* 27, 3–18.

Andrews MW, Rosenblum LA (1994) The development of affiliative and agonistic social patterns in differentially reared monkeys. *Child Dev* 65, 1398–1404.

Arabadzisz D, Diaz-Heijtz R, Knuesel I et al. (2010) Primate early life stress leads to long-term mild hippocampal decreases in corticosteroid receptor expression. *Biol Psychiatry* 67, 1106–1109.

Bale TL, Baram TZ, Brown AS et al. (2010) Early life programming and neurodevelopmental disorders. *Biol Psychiatry* 68, 314–319.

Baram TZ, Davis EP, Obenaus A et al. (2012) Fragmentation and unpredictability of early-life experience in mental disorders. *Am J Psychiatry* 169, 907–915.

Barbas, H (2000) Connections underlying the synthesis of cognition, memory, and emotion in primate prefrontal cortices. *Brain Res Bull* 52, 319–330.

Barr CS, TK Newman et al. (2003) The utility of the non-human primate; model for studying gene by environment interactions in behavioral research. *Genes Brain Behav* 2, 336–340.

Bauman MD, Lavenex P et al. (2004) The development of social behavior following neonatal amygdala lesions in rhesus monkeys. *J Cogn Neurosci* 16, 1388–1411.

Bayart F, Hayashi KT et al. (1990) Influence of maternal proximity on behavioral and physiological reponses to separation in infant rhesus monkeys (Macaca mulatta). *Behav Neurosci* 104, 98–107.

Bernstein IS (1976) Dominance, aggression and reproduction in primate societies. *J Theor Biol* 60: 459–472.

Bernstein IS, Gordon TP (1974) The function of aggression in primate societies. *Am Sci* 62, 304–311.

Bernstein IS, Gordon TP et al. (1974) Aggression and social controls in rhesus monkey (Macaca mulatta) groups revealed in group formation studies. *Folia Primatol (Basel)* 21, 81–107.

Boinski S, Fragaszy, DM (1989) The ontogeny of foraging in squirrel monkeys, Saimiri oerstedi. *Animal Behaviour* 37, 415–428.

Bowlby J (1965) *Attachment*. New York: Basic Books.

Bremner JD, Randall PR (1997) MRI-based measurement of hippocampal volume in posttraumatic stress disorder related to childhood physical and sexual abuse: A preliminary report. *Biol Psychiatry* 41, 23–32.

Brent L, Koban T et al. (2002) Abnormal, abusive, and stress-related behaviors in baboon mothers. *Biol Psychiatry* 52, 1047–56.

Cicchetti, D (1998) Child abuse and neglect-usefulness of the animal data: comment on Maestripieri and Carroll (1998) *Psychol Bull* 123, 224–230.

Coplan JD, Abdallah CG, Tang CY et al. (2010) The role of early life stress in development of the anterior limb of the internal capsule in nonhuman primates. *Neurosci Lett* 480, 93–96.

Coplan JD, Andrews MW, Rosenblum LA et al. (1996) Persistent elevations of cerebrospinal fluid concentrations of corticotropin-releasing factor in adult nonhuman primates exposed to early-life stressors: implications for the pathophysiology of mood and anxiety disorders. *Proc Natl Acad Sci USA* 93, 1619–1623.

Coplan JD, Smith EL, Altemus M et al. (2001) Variable foraging demand rearing: sustained elevations in cisternal cerebrospinal fluid corticotropin-releasing factor concentrations in adult primates. *Biol Psychiatry* 50, 200–204.

Coplan JD, Trost RC, Owens MJ et al. (1998) Cerebrospinal fluid concentrations of somatostatin and biogenic amines in grown primates reared by mothers exposed to manipulated foraging conditions. *Archiv Gen Psychiatry* 55, 473–477.

Coplan JD, Altemus M et al. (2005) Synchronized maternal-infant elevatons of primate CSF CRF concentrations in response to variable foraging demand. *CNS Spectr* 10, 530–536.

Coplan JD, Mathew SJ et al. (2010) Early-life stress and neurometabolites of the hippocampus. *Brain Res* 1358, 191–199.

Croxson PL, Johansen-Berg H, Behrens TEJ et al. (2005) Quantitative investigation of connections of the prefrontal cortex in the human and macaque using probabilistic diffusion tractography. *J Neurosci* 25, 8854–8866.

Dannlowski U, Stuhrmann A, Beutelmann V et al.(2012) Limbic scars: long-term consequences of childhood maltreatment revealed by functional and structural magnetic resonance imaging. *Biol Psychiatry* 71:286–293.

De Bellis MD (2005) The psychobiology of neglect. *Child Maltreat* 10, 150–172.

De Bellis MD, Baum AS, Birmaher B et al. (1999a). A.E. Bennett Research Award. Developmental traumatology. Part I: Biological stress systems. *Biol Psychiatry* 45, 1259–1270.

De Bellis MD, Keshavan MS, Clark DB et al. (2002a) Early deprivation and behavioral and physiological responses to social separation/novelty in the marmoset. *Pharmacol Biochem Behav* 73, 259–269.

Dettling AC, Feldon J, Pryce CR (2002b). Repeated parental deprivation in the infant common marmoset (*Callithrix jacchus*, primates) and analysis of its effects on early development. *Biol Psychiatry* 52, 1037–1046.

Dettmer AM, Novak MA, Suomi SJ et al. (2012) Physiological and behavioral adaptation to relocation stress in differentially reared rhesus monkeys: hair cortisol as a biomarker for anxiety-related responses. *Psychoneuroendocrinology* 37, 191–199.

Diamond A (1991) Frontal lobe involvement in cognitive changes during the first year of life. Brain maturation and cognitive development: Comparative and cross-cultural perspectives, 127–180.

Drevets WC, Gadde KM, Krishnan KRR (2011) Neuroimaging studies of mood. In: Charney DS, Nestler EJ (eds), *Neurobiology of Mental Illness*. Oxford University Press, New York, pp. 461–490.

Eghbal-Ahmadi M, Avishai-Eliner S, Hatalski CG et al. (1999) Differential regulation of the expression of corticotropin-releasing factor receptor type 2 (CRF2) in hypothalamus and amygdala of the immature rat by sensory input and food intake. *J Neurosci* 19, 3982–3991.

Erickson K, KE Gabry et al. (2005) Social withdrawal behaviors in nonhuman primates and changes in neuroendocrine and monoamine concentrations during a separation paradigm. *Dev Psychobiol* 46: 331–339.

Fisher AE (1955) The effects of differential early treatment on the social and exploratory behavior of puppies. Doctoral Dissertation, Pennsylvania State University.

Gee DG, Humphreys KL, Flannery J et al. (2013) A developmental shift from positive to negative connectivity in human amygdala–prefrontal circuitry. *J Neurosci* 33, 4584–4593.

Gibson KR (1991) Myelination and behavioral development: a comparative perspective on questions of neotony, altriciality, and intelligence. In: Gibson KR, Petersen AC (eds) *Brain Maturation and Cognitive Development: Comparative and Cross-cultural Perspectives*. Aldine de Gruyter, Hawthorne, NY, pp. 29–63.

Giedd JN, Rapoport JL (2010) Structural MRI of pediatric brain development: what have we learned and where are we going? *Neuron* 67:728–34.

Giedd JN (2004) Structural magnetic resonance imaging of the adolescent brain. *Ann NY Acad Sci* 1021, 77–85.

Gogtay N, Giedd JN, Lusk L et al. (2004) Dynamic mapping of human cortical development during childhood through early adulthood. *Proc Natl Acad Sci USA USA* 101, 8174–8179.

Gunnar MR, DM Vazquex (2006) Stress neurobiology and developmental psychopathology. In: Cicchetti D, Cohen D (eds) *Developmental Psychopathology: Developmental Neuroscience*. Wiley Press, New York, NY, pp. 533–577.

Harlow HF (1958) The nature of love. *Am Psychol* 13, 673.

Harlow, HF and Harlow, MK (1965) The affectional systems. In: Shrier AM, Harlow HF, Stollnitz F (eds) *Behavior of Nonhuman Primates* (Vol. 2). Academic Press, New York.

Harlow HF, MK Harlow et al. (1971) From thought to therapy: Lessons from a primate laboratory. *Am Sci* 59, 538–549.

Harlow HF, Dodsworth RO et al. (1965) Total social isolation in monkeys. *Proc Natl Acad Sci USA* 54, 90–97.

Heim C, Ehlert U et al. (2000) The potential role of hypocortisolism in the pathophysiology of stress-related bodily disorders. *Psychoneuroendocrinology* 25, 1–35.

Helfer ME, Kempe RS, Krugman RD (1997) *The Battered Child*. University of Chicago Press, Chicago.

Herman JP, Figueiredo H, Mueller NK et al. (2003) Central mechanisms of stress integration: hierarchical circuitry controlling hypothalamo-pituitary-adrenocortical responsiveness. *Front Neuroendocrinol* 24, 151–180.

Herman JP, Ostrander MM, Mueller NK et al. (2005) Limbic system mechanisms of stress regulation: hypothalamo-pituitary-adrenocortical axis. *Progr Neuropsychopharmacol Biol Psychiatry* 29, 1201–1213.

Higley JD, MF Hasert et al. (1991) Nonhuman primate model of alchol abuse: effects of early experience, personality, and stress on alchol consumption. *Proc Natl Acad Sci USA* 15: 7261–7265.

Howell BR, Grand AP, McCormack KM et al. (2014b) Early adverse experience increases emotional reactivity in juvenile rhesus macaques: Relation to amygdala volume. *Dev Psychobiol* 56, 1735–1746.

Howell BR, McCormack KM, Grand AP et al. (2013) Brain white matter microstructure alterations in adolescent rhesus monkeys exposed to early life stress: associations with high cortisol during infancy. *Biol Mood Anxiety Disord* 3.

Howell BR, Sanchez, MM (2011) Understanding behavioral effects of early life stress using the reactive scope and allostatic load models. *Dev Psychopathol* 23, 1001–16.

Huttenlocher PR, Dabholkar AS (1997) Regional differences in synaptogenesis in human cerebral cortex. *J Comparative Neurol* 387, 167–178.

Ichise M, D Vines C et al. (2006) Effects of early life stress on [11C]DASB positron emission tomography imaging of serotonin transporters in adolescent peer-and mother-reared rhesus monkeys. *J Neurosci* 26, 4638–4643.

Ivy AS, Brunson KL, Sandman C et al. (2008) Dysfunctional nurturing behavior in rat dams with limited access to nesting material: a clinically relevant model for early-life stress. *Neuroscience* 154, 1132–1142.

Jackowski A, Perera TD, Abdallah CG et al. (2011) Early-life stress, corpus callosum development, hippocampal volumetrics, and anxious behavior in male nonhuman primates. *Psychiatry Res* 192, 37–44.

Johnson EO, Kamilaris TC, Calogero AE et al. (1996) Effects of early parenting on growth and development in a small primate. *Pediatr Res* 39, 999–1005.

Kaffman A, Meaney MJ (2007) Neurodevelopmental sequelae of postnatal maternal care in rodents: clinical and research implications of molecular insights. *J Child Psychol Psychiatry* 48, 224–244.

Kinnally EL, Feinberg C et al. (2011) DNA methylation as a risk factor in the effects of early life stress. *Brain Behav Immun* 25, 1548–1553.

Kinnally EL, Feinberg C et al. (2013) Transgenerational effects of variable foraging demand stress in female bonnet macaques. *Am J Primatol* 75, 509–517.

Knudsen EI (2004) Sensitive periods in the development of the brain and behavior. *J Cogn Neurosci* 16, 1412–1425.

Koch H, McCormack K, Sanchez MM et al. (2014) The development of the hypothalamic-pituitary-adrenal axis in rhesus monkeys: Effects of age, sex, and early experience. *Dev Psychobiol* 56, 86–95.

Korosi A, Baram, TZ (2009) The pathways from mother's love to baby's future. *Front Behav Neurosci*, 3, 1–8.

Law AJ, Pei Q, Feldon J et al. (2009) Gene expression in the anterior cingulate cortex and amygdala of adolescent marmoset monkeys following parental separations in infancy. *Int J Neuropsychopharmacol* 12, 761–772.

Law AJ, Pei Q, Walker M et al. (2008) Early parental deprivation in the marmoset monkey produces long-term changes in hippocampal expression of genes involved in synaptic plasticity and implicated in mood disorder. *Neuropsychopharmacology* 34, 1381–1394.

Lyons DM, Parker KJ (2007) Stress inoculation-induced indications of resilience in monkeys. *J Traum Stress* 20, 423–433.

Lyons DM, Schatzberg AF (2003) Early maternal availability and prefrontal correlates of reward-related memory. *Neurobiol Learn Mem* 80, 97–104.

Lyons DM, Afarian H, Schatzberg AF et al. (2002) Experience-dependent asymmetric variation in primate prefrontal morphology. *Behav Brain Res* 136, 51–59.

Lyons DM, Parker KJ, Schatzberg AF (2010) Animal models of early life stress: implications for understanding resilience. *Dev Psychobiol* 52, 616–624.

Lyons DM, Kim S, Schatzberg AF et al. (1998) Postnatal foraging demands alter adrenocortical activity and psychosocial development. *Dev Psychobiol* 32, 285–291.

Lyons DM, S Kim et al. (1998) Postnatal foraging demands alter adrenocortical activity and psychosocial development. *Dev Psychobiol* 32: 285–291.

Machado CJ, Bachevalier, J (2003) Non-human primate models of childhood psychopathology: the promise and the limitations. *J Child Psychol Psychiatry* 44, 64–87.

Maestripieri, D (1998) Parenting styles of abusive mothers in group-living rhesus macaques. *Anim Behav* 55, 1–11.

Maestripieri, D (2005) Early experience affects the intergenerational transmission of infant abuse in rhesus monkeys. *Proc Natl Acad Sci USA USA* 102, 9726–9729.

Maestripieri D, Carroll KA (1998) Risk factors for infant abuse and neglect in group-living rhesus monkeys. *Psychol Sci* 9, 143–145.

Maestripieri D, Jovanovic T, & Gouzoules, H. (2000a). Crying and infant abuse in rhesus monkeys. *Child Dev* 71, 301–309.

Maestripieri D, Wallen K et al. (1997) Genealogical and demographic influences on infant abuse and neglect in group-living sooty mangabeys (*Cercocebus atys*). *Dev Psychobiol* 31: 175–180.

Maestripieri D, Lindell SG, Higley JD et al. (2006a). Early maternal rejection affects the development of monoaminergic systems and adult parenting in rhesus macaques. *Behav Neurosci* 120, 1017–24.

Maestripieri D, McCormack KM, Higley JD, Lindell SG, & Sanchez MM(2006b). Influence of parenting style on the offspring's behavior and CSF monoamine metabolites in cross-fostered and noncrossfostered rhesus macaques. *Behavioural Brain Research* 175, 90–95.

Maestripieri D, Megna NL, Jovanovic T (2000b). Adoption and maltreatment of foster infants by rhesus macaque abusive mothers. *Dev Sci* 3, 287–293.

Marco EM, Macri S, Laviola G (2011) Critical age windows for neurodevelopmental psychiatric disorders: evidence from animal models. *Neurotox Res* 19, 286–307.

Mathew SJ, Shungu DC, Mao X et al. (2003) A magnetic resonance spectroscopic imaging study of adult nonhuman primates exposed to early-life stressors. *Biol Psychiatry* 54, 727–735.

Mathew SJ, Coplan JD et al. (2002) Cerebrospinal fluid concentrations of biogenic amines and corticotropin-releasing factor in adolescent non-human primates as a function of the timing of adverse early rearing. *Stress* 5, 185–193.

McCormack K, Newman TK, Higley JD et al. (2009) Serotonin transporter gene variation, infant abuse, and responsiveness to stress in rhesus macaque mothers and infants. *Horm Behav* 55, 538–547.

McCormack K, Sanchez MM, Bardi M et al. (2006) Maternal care patterns and behavioral development of rhesus macaque abused infants in the first 6 months of life. *Dev Psychobiol* 48, 537–550.

McCrory E, De Brito SA, Viding E (2012) The link between child abuse and psychopathology: a review of neurobiological and genetic research. *J R Soc Med* 105, 151–156.

Molet J, Maras PM, Avishai-Eliner S et al. (2014) Naturalistic rodent models of chronic early-life stress. *Developmental Psychobiology* 56, 1675–1688.

Moriceau S, Sullivan R (2005) Neurobiology of infant attachment. *Dev Psychobiol* 47, 230–242.

Nelson EE, Winslow JT (2008) Non-human primates: model animals for developmental psychopathology. *Neuropsychopharmacology* 34, 90–105.

O'Connor TG, JL Cameron (2006) Translating research findings on early experience to prevention: animal and human evidence on early attachement relationships. *Am J Prev Med* 31:S175-S181.

Parker KJ, Maestripieri, D (2011) Identifying key features of early stressful experiences that produce stress vulnerability and resilience in primates. *Neurosci Biobehav Rev* 35, 1466–1483.

Parker KJ, Maestripieri, D (2011) Identifying key features of early stressful experiences that produce stress vulnerability and resilience in primates. *Neurosci Biobehav Rev* 35, 1466–1483.

Parker KJ, Buckmaster CL, Justus KR et al. (2005) Mild early life stress enhances prefrontal-dependent response inhibition in monkeys. *Biol Psychiatry* 57, 848–855.

Parker KJ, Buckmaster CL, Lindley SE et al. (2012) Hypothalamic-pituitary-adrenal axis physiology and cognitive control of behavior in stress inoculated monkeys. *Int J Behav Dev* 36, 45–52.

Parker KJ, Buckmaster CL, Schatzberg AF et al. (2004) Prospective investigation of stress inoculation in young monkeys. *Archiv Gen Psychiatry* 61, 933–941.

Parker KJ, Buckmaster CL, Sundlass K et al. (2006) Maternal mediation, stress inoculation, and the development of neuroendocrine stress resistance in primates. *Proc Natl Acad Sci USA USA* 103, 3000–3005.

Parker KJ, Rainwater KL et al. (2007) Early life stress and novelty seeking behavior in adolescent monkeys. *Psychoneuroendocrinology* 32, 785–792.

Patel PD, Katz M, Karssen AM et al. (2008) Stress-induced changes in corticosteroid receptor expression in primate hippocampus and prefrontal cortex. *Psychoneuroendocrinology* 33, 360–367. *Pediatric Research* 39: 999–1005.

Provençal N, Suderman MJ, Guillemin C et al. (2012) The signature of maternal rearing in the methylome in rhesus macaque prefrontal cortex and T cells. *J Neurosci* 32, 15626–15642.

Pryce CR (2008) Postnatal ontogeny of expression of the corticosteroid receptor genes in mammalian brains: Inter-species and intra-species differences. *Brain Res Rev* 57, 596–605.

Pryce CR, Dettling AC, Spengler M et al. (2004b) Deprivation of parenting disrupts development of homeostatic and reward systems in marmoset monkey offspring *Biol Psychiatry* 56, 72–79

Pryce CR, Dettling A, Spengler M et al. (2004a) Evidence for altered monoamine activity and emotional and cognitive disturbance in marmoset monkeys exposed to early life stress. *Ann NY Acad Sci* 1032, 245–249

Pryce CR, Rüedi-Bettschen D, Dettling AC et al. (2005) Long-term effects of early-life environmental manipulations in rodents and primates: Potential animal models in depression research. *Neurosci Biobehav Rev* 29, 649–674.

Raper J, Stephens SBZ, Henry A et al. (2014) Neonatal amygdala lesions lead to increased activity of brain CRF systems and hypothalamic-pituitary-adrenal axis of juvenile rhesus monkeys. *J Neurosci* 34, 11452–11460.

Reep, R (1984) Relationship between prefrontal and limbic cortex: a comparative anatomical review. *Brain Behav Evol* 25, 5–80.

Rice D, Barone Jr, S (2000) Critical periods of vulnerability for the developing nervous system: evidence from humans and animal models. *Env Health Perspect* 108(Suppl 3), 511.

Rilling JK, Winslow JT et al. (2001) Neural correlates of maternal separation in rhesus monkeys. *Biol Psychiatry* 49, 146–157.

Rincon-Cortes M, Sullivan RM (2014) Early life trauma and attachment: immediate and enduring effects on neurobehavioral and stress axis development. *Front Endocrinol* 5, 33.

Rincón-Cortés, M., Sullivan, R. M. (2014). Early life trauma and attachment: Immediate and enduring effects on neurobehavioral and stress axis development. *Frontiers in Endocrinology* 5, 1–15.

Rosenblum LA, GS Paully (1984) The effects of varying environmental demands on maternal and infant behavior. *Child Dev* 55, 305–314.

Roth TL, Lubin FD, Funk AJ et al. (2009) Lasting epigenetic influence of early-life adversity on the BDNF gene. *Biol Psychiatry* 57, 823–831.

*Roth TL, Sullivan RM (2005) Memory of early maltreatment: neonatal behavioral and neural correlates of maternal maltreatment within the context of classical conditioning. *Biol Psychiatry* 57, 823–831.

Sade D (1967) Determinants of dominance in a group of free ranging rhesus monkeys. In: Altmann SA (ed.) *Social Communication among Primates*. University of Chicago Press, Chicago, IL, pp. 99–114.

Sanchez MM, Hearn EF et al. (1998) Differential rearing affects corpus callosum size and cognitive fuction of rhesus monekys. *Brain Res* 812, 38–49.

Sanchez MM, Pollak SD (2009) Socio-emotional development following early abuse and neglect: Challenges and insights from translational research. In: de Haan M, Gunnar MR (eds) *Handbook of Developmental Social Neuroscience*. The Guilford Press, New York, pp. 497–520.

Sanchez MM, Alagbe O, Felger JC et al. (2007) Activated p38 MAPK is associated with decreased CSF 5-HIAA and increased maternal rejection during infancy in rhesus monkeys. *Mol Psychiatry* 12, 895–897.

Sanchez MM, McCormack K, Grand AP et al. (2010) Effects of sex and early maternal abuse on adrenocorticotropin hormone and cortisol responses to the corticotropin-releasing hormone challenge during the first 3 years of life in group-living rhesus monkeys. *Dev Psychopathol* 22, 45–53.

Sanchez MM, Young LJ, Plotsky PM et al. (2000) Distribution of corticosteroid receptors in the rhesus brain: relative absence of glucocorticoid receptors in the hippocampal formation. *J Neurosci* 20, 4657–4668.

Sanchez, MM (2006) The impact of early adverse care on HPA axis development: Nonhuman primate models. *Horm Behav* 50, 623–631.

Sanchez MM, Ladd CO et al. (2001) Early adverse experience as a developmental risk factor for later psychopathology: Evidence for rodent and primate models. *Dev Psychopathol* 13, 419–449.

Sanchez MM, McCormack K et al. (2010) Effects of sex and early maternal abuse on adrenocorticotropin hormone and cortisol responses to the corticotropin-releasing hormone challenge during the first 3 years of life in group-living rhesus monkeys. *Dev Psychopathol* 22, 45–53.

Sanchez MM, Noble PM et al. (2005) Alterations in diurnal cortisol rhythms and acoustic startle response in nonhuman primates with adverse rearing. *Biol Psychiatry* 15: 373–381.

Seay B and Gottfried NW (1975) A phylogenetic perspective for social behavior in primates. *J Gen Psychol* 92, 5–17.

Shaw P, Kabani NJ, Lerch JP et al. (2008) Neurodevelopmental trajectories of the human cerebral cortex. *J Neurosci* 28, 3586–3594.

Spinelli S, Chefer S et al. (2009) Early-life stress induces long-term morphologic changes in primate brain. *Arch Gen Psychiatry* 66, 658–665.

Sroufe LA (1977) Wariness of strangers and the study of infant development. *Child Dev* 48, 731–746.

Stevens HE, Leckman JF, Coplan JD et al. (2009) Risk and resilience: early manipulation of macaque social experience and persistent behavioral and neurophysiological outcomes. *Journal of the American Acad Child Adol Psychiatry* 48, 114–127.

Sullivan R, Lasley, EN (2010) *Fear in Love: Attachment, Abuse, and the Developing Brain. Cerebrum,* September 2010. The Dana Foundation.

Suomi SJ, 2005 Mother-infant attachment, peer relationships, and the development of social networks in rhesus monkeys *Hum Dev* 48, 67–79

Suomi SJ Harlow HF et al. (1971) Behavioral effects of prolonged partial social isolation in the rhesus monkey. *Psychol Rep* 29: 1171–1177.

Suomi SJ, Harlow HF, Kimball SD (1971) Behavioral effects of prolonged partial social isolation in the rhesus monkey. *Psychol Reports* 29, 1171–1177.

Teicher MH, Andersen SL, Polcari A et al. (2003) The neurobiological consequences of early stress and childhood maltreatment. *NeurosciBiobehav Rev* 27, 33–44.

Teicher MH, Anderson CM, Ohashi K et al. (2014) Childhood maltreatment: altered network centrality of cingulate, precuneus, temporal pole and insula. *Biol Psychiatry* 76:297–305.

Thiebaut de Schotten M, Dell'Acqua F, Valabregue R et al. (2012) Monkey to human comparative anatomy of the frontal lobe association tracts. *Cortex* 48, 82–96.

Tottenham N, Sheridan MA (2009) A review of adversity, the amygdala and the hippocampus: a consideration of developmental timing. *Front Hum Neurosci* 3, 68.

Troisi, A FRD'Amato et al. (1982) Infant abuse by a wild-born group-living Japanese macaque mother. *J Abnorm Psychol* 91: 451–456.

Ulrich-Lai YM, Herman JP (2009) Neural regulation of endocrine and autonomic stress responses. *Nat Rev Neurosci* 10, 397–409.

Yehuda R, Halligan SL et al. (2001) Childhood trauma and risk for PTSD: relationship to intergeneraltional effects of trauma, parental PTSD, and cortisol excretion. *Dev Psychopathol* 13, 733–753.

CHAPTER 4

Amygdala contributions to fear and safety conditioning: insights into PTSD from an animal model across development

Christopher Cain & Regina Sullivan

Department of Child and Adolescent Psychiatry, New York University School of Medicine, New York, NY, and The Emotional Brain Institute, Nathan S. Kline Institute for Psychiatric Research, Orangeburg, NY, USA,

4.1 Introduction

Posttraumatic stress disorder (PTSD) is a unique anxiety disorder that is largely defined by trauma exposure and dysfunctional emotional memory processes. Most PTSD symptoms relate to associative memory for the traumatic experience. For instance, intrusion symptoms include flashbacks, nightmares, recurrent traumatic memories, and intense or prolonged stress reactions to traumatic reminders. Avoidance of trauma-related cues, thoughts or feelings is also an important symptom of PTSD. Finally, PTSD symptoms must persist for at least 1 month, as most individuals exhibit PTSD-like symptoms post-trauma, but then recover naturally. Given these diagnostic criteria, it is perhaps unsurprising that Pavlovian fear and safety conditioning are leading models for studying neurobiological mechanisms relevant to PTSD.

During fear conditioning (FC), neutral cues rapidly form strong associations with aversive or painful events. Following conditioning, these cues elicit emotional reactions and support avoidance. FC memories are also extremely persistent; in the laboratory, even a single conditioning session leads to lifelong fear of the traumatic cue (Gale et al., 2004). Safety conditioning (extinction and conditioned inhibition) can reduce fear responding post-trauma. We will discuss the neurobiological mechanisms of fear and safety conditioning, focusing first on findings from studies in adult rodents and then the ontogenetic emergence of fear in early life. The amygdala will be featured in this discussion, as this brain region is critical for conditioned fear. Finally, we will discuss the potential role that dysfunctional threat processing plays in PTSD.

Posttraumatic Stress Disorder: From Neurobiology to Treatment, First Edition.
Edited by J. Douglas Bremner.
© 2016 John Wiley & Sons, Inc. Published 2016 by John Wiley & Sons, Inc.

4.2 Stress and defensive responding

All organisms have an innate capacity to respond defensively to stressful or threatening stimuli. Although specific responses vary considerably between organisms, the basic functions of stress response systems are similar: to prevent threat escalation, escape danger, and return the organism to its "preferred activity pattern" (Fanselow & Lester, 1988). Stress responding has both physiological and behavioral components. For instance, in mammals, acute stressors activate the hypothalamic–pituitary–adrenal (HPA) axis and trigger sympathetic responses that alter blood flow and respiration. This diverts bodily resources from non-essential processes (e.g., digestion) to sensory and motor systems important for defense. Stressors also activate brain "survival" circuits, which restrict behavior to innate, species-specific defensive responses such as flight or freezing (LeDoux, 2012).

The exact defensive behavior triggered by a stressor depends on many factors, such as the species, the perceived magnitude and proximity of the threat, response options in the environment and the level of maturation/independence of the organism. However, generally speaking, defensive behaviors fall along a continuum, with more intense stressors eliciting greater survival circuit activation and stronger, more reflexive defensive responses. Distant, ambiguous, or mild stressors activate survival circuits less intensely (or activate different parts of the circuit), causing more sustained, but less urgent, responding. For instance, rats rapidly flee an attacking cat, but only show risk assessment behaviors after encountering cat hair (Litvin et al., 2008). Defensive responses on the high end of this spectrum model human fear responses, whereas responses on the lower end of the spectrum are more akin to anxiety (Figure 4.1).

An adaptive stress response is also transient. Once a threat is removed, the system should decay to its basal state allowing the organism to return to its preferred activity pattern. Although little is known about the behavioral processes operating during the return to baseline after a stressful experience, more

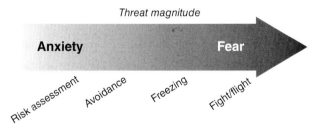

Figure 4.1 Threats trigger survival circuit activation and initiate defensive responding. Defensive responses are organized hierarchically, and greater threats lead to greater survival circuit activation and more intense, reflexive responses. Responses at the high end of the spectrum model human fear (e.g., freezing), whereas those at the low end of the spectrum model anxiety (e.g., risk assessment behaviors).

intense stressors elicit greater deviations from the preferred activity pattern and require more time for recovery. At the physiological level, active feedback mechanisms promote recovery from stress. For example, HPA axis activation leads to release of cortisol/corticosterone (CORT) into the peripheral circulation. CORT is a primary mediator of the global stress response; however, it also provides the key negative feedback signal to halt the stress response by suppressing release of corticotropin-releasing factor (CRF), adrenocorticotropic hormone and norepinephrine in the brain (Vermetten & Bremner, 2002). Not surprisingly, dysfunctions in CORT signaling and feedback are implicated in PTSD (see Chapter 11).

4.3 Fear conditioning

Survival circuits evolved to respond to innate threats and naturally painful or harmful stimuli. This first line of defense is important, as it protects the organism with automatic (unlearned) responses. Plasticity in survival circuits allows animals to adapt to new threats. Pavlovian FC is a simple form of associative learning that leads to plasticity in survival circuits and defensive responding to previously innocuous stimuli. Dysfunction in FC processes can lead to maladaptive or pathological reactions to threats.

4.3.1 Procedure
Fear conditioning involves temporal pairings of a neutral conditioned stimulus (CS; e.g., tone or odor) and an aversive unconditioned stimulus (US; e.g., footshock; Figure 4.2). Any sensory stimulus can be a CS, including complex configural cues such as contexts, and any aversive stimulus can act as a US. After conditioning, CS presentations elicit robust behavioral, autonomic, and endocrine reactions, collectively referred to as conditioned fear responses (CRs; Figure 4.3).

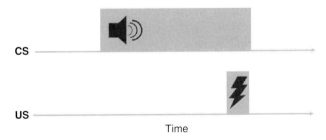

Figure 4.2 Pavlovian fear conditioning. Conditioned stimulus (CS) presentations (e.g., tones) usually precede aversive unconditioned stimulus (US) presentations (e.g., shocks) by seconds or minutes and the stimuli coterminate. Unlike instrumental conditioning, subjects have no control over the delivery of stimuli with a Pavlovian procedure.

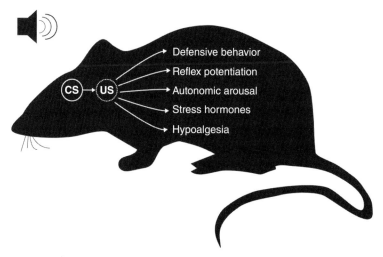

Figure 4.3 Fear conditioning is believed to form a link between conditioned stimulus (CS) and unconditioned stimulus (US) representations in the brain (rather than a direct link between the CS and individual defensive responses). This allows the animal to anticipate the US and emit defensive responses appropriate to the situation. Conditioned responses are typically weaker than unconditioned responses because the CS activates the US representation less intensely than the US itself.

4.3.2 Memory content

Although Pavlovian CRs are sometimes considered to be reflexes, it is unlikely that standard FC procedures produce an associative link between the CS and individual defensive responses (stimulus–response or S–R learning). Instead, FC produces an associative link between CS and US representations (stimulus–stimulus or S–S learning), so the CS predicts the US and allows for defensive responding appropriate to the situation. True Pavlovian CRs depend on the CS–US contingency during the acquisition phase; unpaired or random presentations of the CS and US fail to create an excitatory association and are common control procedures (Rescorla, 1967).

4.3.3 Conditioned responses

Fear conditioning plasticity allows the CS to gain control over innate defensive responses. Although CRs sometimes resemble unconditioned responses to the US, more often they take a different form. For example, rats jump when presented with brief footshocks but primarily freeze when presented with a tone that was previously paired with footshock. Some common CRs include freezing, potentiated startle, suppression of appetitive behavior and hypoalgesia. However, a CR can be any change in CS-elicited responding that depends on the CS–US relationship during conditioning. For animal studies, the term "conditioned fear" is used as shorthand for all defensive CRs that result from conditioning. This should not be confused with explicit memory or consciously experienced emotions and feelings in humans (LeDoux, 2012).

4.3.4 Memory phases

To understand the neurobiological mechanisms of FC, it will be important to appreciate the different phases of memory formation and stabilization. Memory formation begins with the *acquisition* phase (sometimes called *learning* or *conditioning*). This refers to initial behavioral and neural plasticity that occurs during CS–US training trials. Acquisition establishes *short-term memory* (STM) processes that are maintained transiently (~6–12 hours). Following acquisition, separate *consolidation* processes stabilize the memory trace converting STM to *long-term memory* (LTM). If consolidation is disrupted, STM processes decay and the memory is essentially forgotten. For FC, the LTM trace is usually stabilized within 24 hours, and, in the absence of further training, LTM is maintained permanently (never forgotten) (Gale et al., 2004). Following acquisition, CS presentations trigger *retrieval* of the FC memory and *expression* or *performance* of CRs. Aside from triggering CRs, retrieval can also return the memory trace to a labile state that is sensitive to disruption for several hours (*reactivation*). Reactivated LTM undergoes a *reconsolidation* process that restabilizes the memory within 24 hours of retrieval. If reconsolidation is disrupted, post-reactivation STM processes decay and the memory is essentially erased. However, reconsolidation normally allows for memory updating (Schiller et al., 2010).

4.3.5 Neurobiology of FC

Fear conditioning is widely studied for several important reasons: the paradigm is simple, the procedure is quick, experimenters have a high degree of control over experimental stimuli, learning is rapid, memory is robust and long-lasting, and the paradigm is amenable to neurobiological studies (Cain et al., 2013). The neural mechanisms of FC also appear to be highly conserved, which allows for meaningful translational research (Pattwell et al., 2013). We will summarize a large body of research revealing the neurobiology of FC in rodents. These studies overwhelmingly implicate the amygdala in the learning, storage, and expression of Pavlovian FC memories.

4.3.5.1 Amygdala connectivity

The amygdala is a complex of 13 interconnected nuclei in the medial temporal lobe (Pitkänen, 2000). Amygdala nuclei can be differentiated by function, connectivity, cytoarchitecture, and chemoarchitecture. Three amygdala nuclei have received the greatest attention in studies of FC: lateral amygdala (LA), basal amygdala (BA) and central amygdala (CeA).

The LA is the main sensory interface of the amygdala and receives CS inputs from both thalamus and cortex. Auditory inputs synapse in dorsal LA on glutamatergic pyramidal neurons and on GABAergic neurons that provide feed-forward inhibition. The neural pathway(s) providing US information to the LA are less clear (reviewed in Johansen et al., 2010b).

The BA lies ventral to the LA and receives heavy projections from the LA. The BA is the target of the heaviest hippocampal inputs to the amygdala, which may transmit contextual CS information to the fear circuit. BA also receives inputs from the prefrontal cortex (PFC). The BA projects to both the LA and CeA within the amygdala, and sends heavy projections to several extra-amygdala targets, including the PFC, hippocampus, and striatum.

The CeA lies medial to both the LA and BA and receives input from both. The medial division of the CeA (CeM) is a major output of the amygdala and projects to many regions mediating fear responses (reviewed in Cain & LeDoux, 2008). For instance, the CeA projects heavily to the hypothalamus, periacqueductal gray, nucleus reticularis pontis caudalis and brainstem modulatory centers, and most of these regions project back to the CeA. The CeA also receives input from the hippocampus and PFC, as well as sparse sensory inputs from the thalamus and cortex.

4.3.5.2 Role of amygdala nuclei in FC

Pre- or post-training lesions of LA severely disrupt CS-elicited fear in LTM tests (Amorapanth et al., 2000; Campeau & Davis, 1995). Further, temporary inactivation of LA neurons during conditioning or testing prevents acquisition and expression, respectively, of CS-related fear (Maren et al., 2001; Muller et al., 1997). Injections of protein synthesis inhibitors into the LA after conditioning or reactivation impair LTM, but leave STM (and post-reactivation STM) processes intact, indicating that protein synthesis plays a role in memory consolidation and reconsolidation (Nader & LeDoux, 2000; Schafe & LeDoux, 2000). Together, these findings indicate that plasticity critical for the FC memory trace is acquired, consolidated, and reconsolidated in LA. In rodents, lesions of LA impair FC even 18 months after the conditioning session (Gale et al., 2004), which strongly suggests that LA is a permanent site of memory storage.

The CeA is also critical for FC. Lesions of the CeA before or after conditioning abolish conditioned fear (Goosens & Maren, 2001; Hitchcock & Davis, 1991). Initially, the CeA was thought to play a more passive role in the mediation of CRs, receiving CS information from LA and orchestrating conditioned responding via projections to downstream effector regions. This was mainly because agents known to impair synaptic plasticity, such as NMDA-receptor (NMDAR) blockers, impaired FC when infused into the LA, but not when infused into the CeA (Fanselow & Kim, 1994). However, more recent work demonstrates that blocking neural activity or protein synthesis in the CeA impairs LTM (Ciocchi et al., 2010; Wilensky et al., 2006). Thus, like LA, plasticity in the CeA is also important for FC.

The BA has received less attention than the LA and CeA, although interest in this nucleus is increasing. The BA does not appear to be necessary for FC; pre-conditioning lesions produce no significant impairment in acquisition, STM or LTM (e.g., Sotres-Bayon et al., 2004). However, post-conditioning lesions or inactivation impair conditioned responding (Amano et al., 2011; Anglada-Figueroa & Quirk, 2005). This suggests that BA is normally part of the amygdala FC circuit; however, when damaged, other pathways are capable of supporting FC on their own. At present, it is not known whether BA contributes to acquisition, consolidation, or storage of the FC memory, although it clearly contributes to expression.

4.3.5.3 Plasticity in amygdala FC circuits

Sensory afferents carrying CS and US information converge on pyramidal neurons in the dorsal portion of LA (Romanski et al., 1993). This convergence is believed to trigger Hebbian synaptic plasticity in the CS pathway to LA during FC (Bailey et al., 2000; Blair et al., 2001; Humeau et al., 2003; Maren, 2005; Figure 4.4). "Hebbian" refers to plasticity induced by coincident, or nearly coincident, pre- and postsynaptic activity, which Donald Hebb first suggested as a neural mechanism for associative learning (Hebb, 1949). Prior to conditioning, CS inputs elicit weak responses in LA neurons that are insufficient to drive fear responses. During conditioning, coincident pre- and postsynaptic activity,

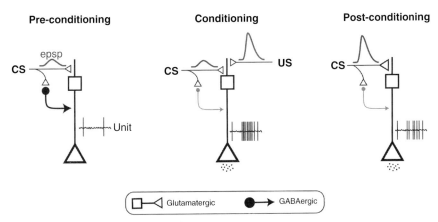

Figure 4.4 Hebbian fear conditioning plasticity in the lateral amygdala (LA). Prior to conditioning, conditioned stimulus (CS) presentations result in weak depolarization of LA neurons and little to no activation of downstream brain areas mediating conditioned fear responses. However, with CS – unconditioned stimulus (US) pairings, neurons are strongly depolarized resulting in initiation of an LTP-like process that strengthens the synapses between CS afferents and LA neurons. Following conditioning, CS presentations strongly depolarize LA neurons, triggering action potentials and neurotransmitter release to activate downstream targets. epsp, excitatory postsynaptic potential. (*See color plate section for the color representation of this figure.*)

induced by the CS and US, respectively, leads to long-term potentiation (LTP) of CS synapses (Fourcaudot et al.,). After conditioning, strengthened CS inputs can drive LA output and fear responses. Several lines of evidence strongly support this model. First, FC strengthens CS-evoked unit responses in LA (e.g., Quirk et al., 1995). Second, FC induces LTP and occludes artificially induced LTP in the LA, suggesting a shared mechanism (McKernan & Shinnick-Gallagher, 1997; Rogan et al., 1997; Tsvetkov et al., 2002). Third, US-induced depolarization of LA pyramidal cells is necessary for LTP of CS inputs during FC (Rosenkranz & Grace, 2002). Fourth, pairing CS presentations with optogenetic depolarization of LA neurons is sufficient to induce FC (Johansen et al., 2010a). Finally, manipulations that block LTP of CS inputs to LA also block behavioral FC (Apergis-Schoute et al., 2005; Rodrigues et al., 2002). Although FC produces plasticity in many brain regions, these findings demonstrate a central role for Hebbian plasticity in LA. Also, FC-related plasticity in regions upstream of LA often depends on LA plasticity (Armony et al., 1998; Maren et al., 2001).

It is not clear if synaptic plasticity in BA is necessary for FC; however, FC leads to the emergence of CS-responsive neurons in BA (e.g., Amano et al., 2011). Although these could simply reflect plasticity upstream, BA units show longer responses that mirror behavioral fear, unlike rapidly adapting LA responses. LTP of hippocampal projections to BA may also contribute to contextual fear (Maren & Fanselow, 1995).

Recent studies have identified an inhibitory microcircuit in CeA that plays a crucial role in fear learning and expression. It consists of two populations of GABAergic neurons in the lateral/capsular division (CeL), and GABAergic projection neurons in the CeM. The CeL neurons have been dubbed "ON" and "OFF" cells because they fire more or less to an aversive CS post-conditioning (Ciocchi et al., 2010; Duvarci et al., 2011). Identification and manipulation of ON and OFF cells is possible because they express distinct molecular markers. Most OFF cells express PKC-δ and oxytocin receptors, whereas ON cells express somatostatin (Gozzi et al., 2010; Haubensak et al., 2010; Li et al., 2013). ON and OFF cells reciprocally inhibit each other (Haubensak et al., 2010), and OFF cells send a more dense projection to CeM (Li et al., 2013).

Selective stimulation of the CeM triggers fear reactions like freezing, consistent with the CeM being the major amygdala output mediating fear reactions (Ciocchi et al., 2010). Interestingly, freezing can be triggered in naïve rodents by inactivating CeL or selectively stimulating ON neurons (Ciocchi et al., 2010; Li et al., 2013). Further, expression of conditioned freezing is enhanced when OFF cells are silenced (Haubensak et al., 2010), and impaired when OFF cells are stimulated (Knobloch et al., 2012). Together, these findings suggest that the CeL gates conditioned fear, with CS inputs to the CeL ultimately generating CRs by disinhibiting CeM projection neurons (Figure 4.5).

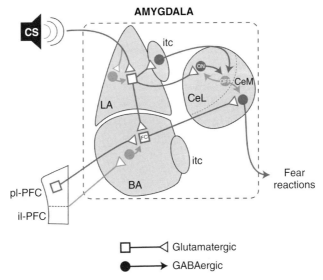

Figure 4.5 Amygdala FC circuitry. After conditioning, conditioned stimulus (CS) presentations activate lateral amygdala (LA) neurons, which project to basal amygdala (BA) "fear cells," intercalated cells (itc), and lateral/capsular division (CeL) of the central amygdala (CeA). CS processing in these regions leads to simultaneous stimulation and disinhibition of the medial division of the CeA (CeM). The CeM projects to downstream effector regions (e.g., periacqueductal gray) that mediate specific fear reactions (e.g., freezing). Prelimbic-prefrontal cortex (pl-PFC) neurons help sustain conditioned responding over longer intervals via projections to the BA. Pathways contributing to expression of conditioned fear responses are highlighted in red. il-PFC, infralimbic-PFC. (*See color plate section for the color representation of this figure.*)

The impressive work above describes how LA plasticity can be translated into CRs; however, it does not describe how learning-related plasticity within the CeA contributes to FC. Available data suggest that plasticity is not required in CeM or CeL OFF cells. Very recent work provides an important piece of the puzzle. Li et al. (2013) show strengthening of synaptic connections between LA neurons and CeL-ON cells as a result of FC. This aligns with work showing the emergence of CS-elicited unit responses (ON cells) with conditioning (Duvarci et al., 2011). Further, hyperpolarization of ON cells during FC blocks this plasticity and impairs LTM, consistent with a Hebbian mechanism. Thus, FC appears to induce associative plasticity at specific synapses in the CeL, leading to CS-evoked disinhibition of CeM and generation of CRs.

4.3.5.4 Molecular mechanisms of FC
The molecular mechanisms of FC have been intensely studied over the past two decades, and comprehensive reviews of this work are available elsewhere

(e.g., Johansen et al., 2011). We will highlight the contributions of several molecular pathways in the LA to FC plasticity and memory.

Acquisition of FC is believed to depend on Hebbian coincidence detection in LA pyramidal neurons and covalent modification of existing synaptic proteins. NMDARs are important for coincidence detection and the initiation of associative, synapse-specific plasticity (Malenka & Nicoll, 1999). NMDARs require two simultaneous events to open their channel and pass calcium into the cell: the binding of glutamate to the receptor site; and postsynaptic depolarization to eject magnesium ions that normally block the channel pore. In relation to FC, afferents carrying CS information to the synapse provide the glutamate. Strong postsynaptic depolarization probably results from activation of AMPA receptors (AMPARs) at synapses receiving US inputs followed by cell-wide depolarization via action potentials. Strong depolarization also opens voltage-dependent calcium channels (VGCCs) that pass additional calcium into the cell. Intracellular calcium activates several protein kinases that are important for acquisition. For instance, calcium activates calcium/calmodulin-dependent kinase-II (CamKII) (Silva, 2003), which can phosphorylate AMPARs, leading to insertion at the synapse and strengthening of synaptic transmission (Nedelescu et al., 2010; Rumpel et al., 2005; Yeh et al., 2006). Thus, glutamate receptors and dendritic kinases translate specific patterns of synaptic activity into LTP-like strengthening of CS synapses in LA.

During acquisition, intracellular signaling cascades are set in motion that ultimately lead to the consolidation of LTM. In brief, consolidation involves synapse to nucleus signaling that initiates gene transcription, protein translation, and structural synaptic changes that maintain the memory trace. Synapse to nucleus signaling mostly involves the activation of kinases, such as protein kinase A (PKA), mitogen-activated protein kinase (MAPK), phosphoinositide-3 (PI3) kinase, and protein kinase C (PKC). Some kinases translocate to the nucleus when activated and phosphorylate transcription factors that initiate gene expression.

One critical transcription factor is cyclic-AMP response-element binding protein (CREB). CREB promotes transcription of genes downstream from cyclic-AMP response elements (CRE sequences), such as immediate early genes like *c-fos*, and genes encoding neurotrophins and neuropeptides, such as brain-derived neurotrophic factor (BDNF) and CRF (Alberini, 2009). In the LA, CREB enhances long-term FC and contributes to competitive processes that determine which neurons are incorporated into the memory trace (Josselyn, 2010). The specific genes and gene products necessary to stabilize long-term FC memories are still being investigated (e.g., Ploski et al., 2010). However, it appears that FC memories are maintained by structural changes at the synapse and specific molecular alterations within the cell. For instance, synapse size increases in LA with FC (Ostroff et al., 2010), which is consistent with the requirement for cytoskeletal rearrangement and synaptic AMPAR insertion during consolidation of FC (Lamprecht & LeDoux, 2004). Recent studies also implicate epigenetic mechanisms in fear memory maintenance (Zovkic & Sweatt, 2013).

Finally, neuromodulatory systems can also powerfully regulate Hebbian learning and consolidation (Bailey et al., 2000). This is certainly true of FC, where monoamines, neurotrophins and neuropeptides all make important contributions. For instance, norepinephrine and dopamine can facilitate Hebbian processes in LA pyramidal neurons, both directly and indirectly (Bissiere et al., 2003; Sears et al., 2013; Tully et al., 2007). Activation of beta-adrenergic receptors (β-ARs) or dopamine receptors on pyramidal neurons can amplify intracellular signaling in PKA and PKC pathways. They can also suppress feed-forward inhibition in CS pathways to the LA, which increases pyramidal cell excitability and lowers the threshold for plasticity induction. Consistent with this, pre-training blockade of β-ARs or D1-dopamine receptors in LA impairs fear acquisition (Bush et al., 2010; Guarraci et al., 1999). Neurotrophins like BDNF are important for consolidation processes in LA (Cowansage et al., 2010). BDNF may facilitate consolidation via activation of TrkB receptors which activate MAPK and PI3-kinase. Neuropeptides in LA also modulate fear learning and consolidation. For instance, CRF appears to promote consolidation at low levels but impairs consolidation at high levels (Isogawa et al., 2013), although the exact mechanism is unclear.

4.4 Safety conditioning

Although plasticity in survival circuits allows animals to adaptively respond to new threats, the threshold for FC is low and the system is prone to errors. Fortunately, there are simple forms of inhibitory (safety) conditioning that can limit or suppress conditioned fear reactions. We refer specifically to fear extinction and conditioned inhibition. Considerably less is known about the precise neurobiological mechanisms of safety conditioning, however, plasticity in the amygdala, and/or regions that regulate the amygdala, appears critical.

4.4.1 Fear extinction

Extinction training involves repeated CS-alone presentations in a safe setting. This contradicts the predictive validity of the CS and creates a new inhibitory CS–no US association (Bouton et al., 2006). Extinction can reduce or eliminate conditioned responding, depending on the amount of training. Extinction doesn't erase the original CS–US association; rather, behavior post-extinction is the net result of competition between excitatory and inhibitory CS memories. Evidence for this comes mainly from behavioral experiments showing that fear relapse occurs with context changes (renewal), passage of time

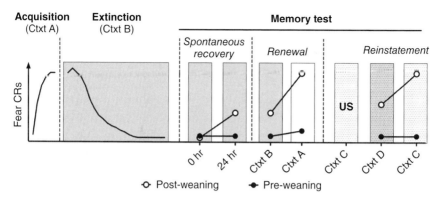

Figure 4.6 Relapse-prone vs. relapse-resistant fear extinction. After acquisition, conditioned stimulus (CS)-alone presentations lead to a gradual and progressive weakening of fear conditioned responses (CRs) (extinction). In adults, extinction creates a new inhibitory memory that suppresses, but does not erase, the fear conditioning (FC) memory. This allows the subject to flexibly respond to threats depending on the context. However, fear relapse is common after adult extinction; fear returns with the passage of time (spontaneous recovery), with context changes (renewal) and with stress (reinstatement). Early in development, fear extinction is relapse-resistant and probably results from erasure or weakening of the original FC memory. Ctxt, context.

(spontaneous recovery), or US exposure (reinstatement) (Figure 4.6). Many forms of cognitive-behavioral therapy rely on fear extinction to alleviate anxiety (Craske et al., 2008; Foa 2011).

We are beginning to understand the neural circuits and cellular mechanisms of fear extinction (Milad & Quirk, 2012; Figure 4.7). For instance, the ventromedial PFC (vmPFC) is essential for rapidly expressing extinction memories. Neural activity in vmPFC increases after extinction training, and electrical or growth factor (BDNF) stimulation of vmPFC can induce extinction. vmPFC projects to inhibitory intercalated cells in the amygdala that can suppress CeA outputs and block fear reactions (Amano et al., 2010; Quirk et al., 2003). The LA and BA also play key roles in extinction learning. Several studies indicate that NMDARs, VGCCs, BDNF, calcineurin, MAPK, cannabinoid receptors, neuromodulators and GABA receptors in these regions participate in fear extinction learning (Davis & Bauer, 2012; Myers & Davis, 2007). BA neurons may contribute by selecting between high and low fear states post-extinction (Herry et al., 2010). Synaptic depression has also been observed in projections from vmPFC to BA principal cells, which shifts the excitation/inhibition balance in amygdala towards inhibition (Cho et al., 2013). GABAergic inhibitory synapses have also been observed to reorganize around previously fear-responsive neurons in BA after extinction (Trouche et al., 2013). Opioid-mediated input from the periacqueductal gray may provide the error signal driving extinction plasticity

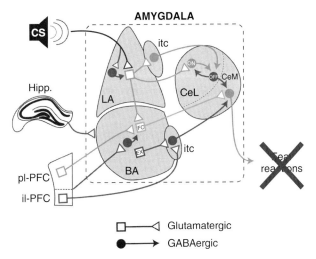

Figure 4.7 Amygdala fear extinction circuitry (adult). Extinction learning counteracts fear responding in a number of ways: (i) by strengthening feed-forward inhibition in the lateral amygdala (LA); (ii) through infralimbic-prefontal cortex (il-PFC) activation of intercalated cells (itc) that inhibit medial division of the central amygdala (CeM); (iii) through a subset of basal amygdala (BA) "extinction cells" that project to GABAergic neurons, possibly itc neurons, which inhibit CeM output; (iv) through synaptic depression of projections from PFC to BA "fear cells" (FC); and (v) through increased inhibition of fear conditioning cells in the BA by local interneurons. The hippocampus plays a critical role in gating extinction according to context via connections to the il-PFC and BA. Pathways contributing to expression of fear extinction are highlighted in blue. (*See color plate section for the color representation of this figure.*)

(McNally et al., 2004). Finally, the hippocampus plays a critical role in the context-dependent expression of fear extinction (Bouton et al., 2006).

4.4.2 Conditioned inhibition

Unlike extinction, where the CS comes to have ambiguous meaning, conditioned inhibition (CI) training produces a stimulus that has purely inhibitory properties. This "safety signal" indicates that no harm will come. There are many variations of the CI procedure, but they all share one important feature: the safety signal is negatively correlated with aversive US presentations. Following training, safety signals can suppress behaviors indicative of anxiety, fear, and even depression in rodents (Pollak et al., 2008). Surprisingly little is known about the neurobiological mechanisms of CI learning. However, some recent studies suggest that CI learning is associated with a reduction of synaptic size and strength in the LA and an increase in synaptic strength in striatum (Ostroff et al., 2010; Rogan et al., 2005). Safety conditioning is also associated with alterations in dopamine and substance P signaling in the basolateral (BA + LA) amygdala (Pollak et al., 2008).

4.5 Ontogeny of fear and safety conditioning

Our understanding of the development of survival circuits lags behind our understanding of the adult system; however, striking developmental differences in stress responding, FC, and safety conditioning have already been documented.

4.5.1 Development of stress and defensive responses

Defensive responding changes dynamically as animals transition from dependence on a caregiver to independence. For instance, early in development rat pups are ill-equipped to evade predators and instead rely on maternal protection. Thus, separation from the mother elicits anxiety-like responses, including ultrasonic distress calls to signal alarm (Winslow & Insel, 1991). Physiological stress responses are also much different early in life. For instance, most stressors fail to elicit significant glucocorticoid release until the second or third week of life (Figure 4.8). This stress hyporesponsive period (SHRP) has been observed in both rodent and human infants (Hostinar et al., 2013), and has profound effects on the outcome of FC.

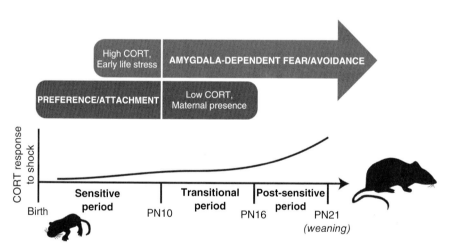

Figure 4.8 Ontogeny of fear conditioning. During the sensitive period, odor-shock conditioning produces an odor preference through an amygdala-independent mechanism. This odor conditioned stimulus (CS) can also support attachment interactions with the mother. As pups age and exit the stress hyporesponsive period, conditioning elicits a greater cortisol/corticosterone (CORT) response, which engages amygdala processes that produce fear/avoidance of the odor CS. Abusive rearing conditions can lead to abnormally high CORT responses in the late sensitive period and precocious fear/avoidance learning. Maternal presence during the transitional period weakens the CORT response and enables preference learning. After postnatal day 16 (PN16), conditioning produces fear/avoidance and CORT only modulates the degree of learning. (*See color plate section for the color representation of this figure.*)

4.5.2 Ontogeny of amygdala-dependent FC

Fear conditioning does not emerge in rodents until the second week of life. Paradoxically, prior to developmental emergence of FC around postnatal day 10 (PN10), an aversive US paired with a novel odor produces an odor-CS that supports approach responses and permits nipple attachment and social interactions with the mother (Landers & Sullivan, 2012), much like the natural maternal odor. This occurs despite the pup's ability to detect and respond to pain. Importantly, prior to PN10, CS and US presentations produce neural and gene expression changes in the basolateral amygdala; however, FC-related plasticity is absent. This initial "sensitive period" is believed to have evolved to suppress accidental fear and avoidance responses to the caregiver, which would probably prove fatal at this stage of development (Figure 4.8).

Interestingly, amygdala-dependent FC is possible in the "transitional sensitive period" (~ PN10–15 in rat pups). Animals at this stage show a preference for a fear-conditioned CS when CORT reactions to the US are low, and fear/avoidance when CORT is high. Thus, unlike the adult, where CORT levels influence the *degree* of FC (Sullivan & Holman, 2010), in this transitional period CORT levels change the *sign* of learning (preference/maternal odor vs. aversion) (Moriceau & Sullivan, 2006). Finally, during the "post-sensitive period" (> PN16), CORT is no longer required for FC, though it can still positively modulate FC as in the adult (Sullivan & Holman, 2010). Thus, the amygdala is capable of supporting FC very early in life, but this is suppressed during the SHRP.

The retrieval/retention of fear memories also differs dramatically across development. In rats, conditioned fear is retained and expressed across the entire adult lifetime (Gale et al., 2004). However, FC conducted at PN16 produces an initially strong memory that rapidly decays (Callaghan & Richardson, 2013). Such *infantile amnesia* has been observed for a variety of learning phenomena and in most altricial species, including humans (Josselyn & Frankland, 2012). However, it is important to note that infantile amnesia for FC is usually observed with a single conditioning session; repeated FC in young pups leads to robust memory that lasts throughout the life span (Raineki et al., 2012).

4.5.3 Ontogeny of fear extinction

In adults, fear extinction induces inhibitory learning and fear is prone to relapse when inhibition fails (Bouton et al., 2006). Interestingly, extinction early in development appears qualitatively different (Nair et al., 2001). Although CS exposure still leads to decreased fear, relapse does not occur (dubbed *relapse-resistant extinction*; Callaghan & Richardson, 2013). These studies suggest that extinction early in development fails to engage PFC and leads to the erasure of the original fear memory.

4.5.4 Ontogeny of conditioned inhibition and implications for safety

In contrast to adults, explicitly unpaired CS and US presentations fail to produce a safety signal during the first few weeks of life (Stanton, 2000). However, pups appear capable of learning a safety signal through associative conditioning as pups learn the maternal odor, but also through FC prior to functional ontogeny of the amygdala (Sullivan et al., 2000). Specifically, there are indications that conditioned maternal odors can function as safety signals and modulate learning during development. For instance, in older pups that have left the SHRP, maternal cues can block CORT responses to aversive stimuli (Stanton, 2000). Such "maternal buffering" also prevents fear learning and reinstates the learning of maternal odor with FC (Moriceau & Sullivan, 2006). This odor remains important into adulthood, where it can reduce FC, depression-like behavior and amygdala activity (Sevelinges et al., 2011), similar to conditioned inhibitors acquired in adulthood (Pollak et al., 2008; Rogan et al., 2005). These data suggest that "safety signals" may be acquired differently in early life compared with adulthood.

4.6 Implications for PTSD

Most researchers agree that FC occurs with traumatic experience and contributes to PTSD phenomenology. However, there continue to be debates regarding which FC processes are dysfunctional in PTSD and how to exploit associative learning to enhance treatment. We will first consider the possible relationship between fear and safety conditioning processes and PTSD in adults. Then we will highlight important developmental considerations.

4.6.1 Adult

There are two major hypotheses regarding dysfunctional FC processes in adult PTSD (resulting from adult trauma): PTSD occurs because the FC memory is excessively strong; and PTSD occurs because safety conditioning processes important for coping are deficient. Although not mutually exclusive, available data are more consistent with the latter option. As mentioned earlier, PTSD may largely be a disorder of recovery, as most traumatized individuals exhibit PTSD-like symptoms acutely but recover without treatment. When subjected to controlled FC procedures measuring implicit fear responses, PTSD cohorts show impaired fear extinction recall, compared with trauma-exposed, non-PTSD controls (Milad et al., 2009). Fear acquisition effects in those with PTSD are less consistent; some studies show facilitated FC, some do not, and still others report normal CRs, but excessive responding to non-threatening cues (generalization) (Grillon & Morgan 1999; Jovanovic et al., 2010; Milad et al., 2009; Orr et al., 2000). Thus, the major deficit appears to involve inhibitory fear learning, and especially retrieval of the extinction memory, as PTSD patients learn extinction normally but fail to remember it. This specific memory pattern points to dysfunctions in PFC and hippocampal processes that gate amygdala-dependent fear during extinction retrieval (Bouton et al., 2006; Quirk et al., 2000), and those with PTSD show abnormal PFC, hippocampal, and amygdalar activation with functional magnetic resonance imaging analyses (Milad et al., 2009).

Another hypothesis suggests that *overconsolidation* and stronger FC memories are the primary problem in PTSD (Pitman & Delahanty, 2005). Although a recent study failed to detect overconsolidation in PTSD patients (Milad et al., 2009), this model also hypothesizes a role for reminder-induced strengthening of the FC memory, to account for the progressive worsening of symptoms in PTSD. This is actually predicted by the impaired-extinction model discussed earlier; retrieval episodes that fail to induce extinction trigger stress responses, such as CRF and norepinephrine release, that enhance reconsolidation leading to incubation (strengthening) of the FC memory (Debiec et al., 2011; Pickens et al., 2009). It remains to be determined whether such a secondary "over-reconsolidation" process contributes to PTSD.

The FC framework has helped to identify dysfunctional learning processes in PTSD and has provided a neurobiological foundation for studies investigating potential cures. For instance, PTSD is commonly treated with extinction-based therapies, which are imperfect, but still effective for many patients (Foa, 2011). As extinction is impaired in PTSD, pharmacological agents that enhance extinction may improve treatment outcomes. Candidate drugs are being selected based on their interaction with neurobiological processes known to be important for extinction. For example, augmentation of NMDAR, norepinephrine, cannabinoid, and BDNF signaling have each been shown to improve long-term extinction, sometimes in humans (Andero & Ressler, 2012; Davis, 2011; Holmes & Quirk, 2010; Kaplan & Moore, 2011). In a similar vein, agents that block reconsolidation or incubation processes (e.g., CRF1 or β-AR antagonists) may also facilitate recovery from fear (Cain et al., 2012). Finally, researchers are using combined knowledge of reconsolidation and extinction processes to design new patterns of CS exposure that may enhance the efficacy of exposure therapy (Schiller et al., 2010). Thus, FC studies in adults represent an evidence-based approach towards identifying dysfunctional learning processes in PTSD and discovering better treatments.

4.6.2 Developmental considerations

The finding that FC procedures fail to produce an aversive CS early in life might suggest that trauma effects are attenuated in infancy. However, a large body of literature shows robust and enduring effects of early life trauma (Yehuda et al., 2010). Indeed, short-term detrimental effects of FC can be found provided pups are stressed. For instance, natural stress, induced through interactions with an abusive caregiver, or exogenous CORT, can produce precocious termination of the SHRP and amygdala-dependent FC even in infancy (Sullivan & Holman, 2010). This very early FC experience is associated with reduced social interactions with the mother and amygdala hyperactivity (Raineki et al., 2010). Enduring amygdala-dependent effects have also been observed as pups develop independence, suggesting delayed developmental emergence of the effects of trauma; at weaning, social interaction deficits with peers emerge, followed by depressive-like behaviors (Raineki et al., 2012; Sevelinges et al., 2011). And unpaired odor-shock conditioning, which does not produce infant FC or depressive-like behaviors later in life, results in adult anxiety-like behaviors (Sarro et al., 2014). Early life stress is also associated with closure of developmental windows and precocious expression of adult fear retrieval and fear extinction phenotypes (Callaghan & Richardson, 2013; Sullivan & Holman, 2010). Together, these findings suggest that trauma or stress during the sensitive period may alter brain programming related to adult anxiety and depression. They also suggest the need for unique criteria for childhood PTSD. Most notably, a failure to show effects of trauma in early life may not be a sufficient cause to prevent or discontinue treatment.

Developmental work also raises an exciting new treatment possibility for PTSD: reopening critical periods to recruit early-life fear expression and extinction mechanisms. This could lead to blunted fear memories and/or relapse-resistant extinction following therapy. Several recent studies suggest that this may be possible. First, researchers found that the emergence of perineuronal nets (PNNs) in the basolateral amygdala coincides with the transition from relapse-resistant to relapse-prone (adult-like) extinction (Gogolla et al., 2009). Degrading basolateral amygdala PNNs prior to extinction in adults led to relapse-resistant fear suppression. Second, systemic or intra-amygdalar infusions of fibroblast growth factor-2 before extinction training produces relapse-resistant extinction (Graham & Richardson, 2011). Finally, a recent study found that chronic administration of the selective serotonin reuptake inhibitor fluoxetine reduced PNNs in basolateral amygdala and led to enhanced extinction that was resistant to fear relapse (Karpova et al., 2011). This last finding is supported by a human study showing that SSRIs combined with prolonged exposure therapy leads to more enduring relief from PTSD symptoms (Schneier et al., 2012).

4.7 Conclusion

Many PTSD symptoms relate to associative memory for the traumatic experience. Fear and safety conditioning paradigms model important aspects of trauma learning and recovery processes, allowing researchers to examine the neurobiology in detail. This work overwhelmingly implicates plasticity in amygdala–PFC circuits, and highlights important developmental differences in the mechanisms of threat processing. Identifying dysfunctional CS processing in these circuits should allow researchers and clinicians to target specific molecular mechanisms and normalize responding through combinations of behavioral and drug therapies. Although it is beyond the scope of this chapter, continued work on the development and mechanisms of innate fear (Rosen & Schulkin, 1998), avoidance (Cain & LeDoux, 2008; McGaugh et al., 2002), generalization (Golub et al., 2009), stress-enhanced fear learning (Poulos et al., 2013), and individual differences (Yehuda & LeDoux, 2007) should enhance our understanding of survival circuits and help to identify factors that contribute to risk vs. resilience post-trauma.

Acknowledgement

Research was funded by MH097125 to C.C., and MH091451 and NIH-DC009910 to R.M.S.

References

Alberini CM (2009) Transcription factors in long-term memory and synaptic plasticity. *Physiol Rev* 89, 121–45.

Amano T, Duvarci S, Popa D, Pare D (2011) The fear circuit revisited: contributions of the basal amygdala nuclei to conditioned fear. *J Neurosci* 31, 15481–9.

Amano T, Unal CT, Pare D (2010) Synaptic correlates of fear extinction in the amygdala. *Nat Neurosci* 13, 489–94.

Amorapanth P, LeDoux JE, Nader K (2000) Different lateral amygdala outputs mediate reactions and actions elicited by a fear-arousing stimulus. *Nat Neurosci* 3, 74–9.

Andero R, Ressler KJ (2012) Fear extinction and BDNF: translating animal models of PTSD to the clinic. *Genes Brain Behav* 11, 503–12.

Anglada-Figueroa D, Quirk GJ (2005) Lesions of the basal amygdala block expression of conditioned fear but not extinction. *J Neurosci* 25, 9680–5.

Apergis-Schoute AM, Debiec J, Doyere V, LeDoux JE, Schafe GE (2005) Auditory fear conditioning and long-term potentiation in the lateral amygdala require ERK/MAP kinase signaling in the auditory thalamus: a role for presynaptic plasticity in the fear system. *J Neurosci* 25, 5730–9.

Armony JL, Quirk GJ, LeDoux JE (1998) Differential effects of amygdala lesions on early and late plastic components of auditory cortex spike trains during fear conditioning. *J Neurosci* 18, 2592–601.

Bailey CH, Giustetto M, Huang YY, Hawkins RD, Kandel ER (2000) Is heterosynaptic modulation essential for stabilizing Hebbian plasticity and memory? *Nat Rev Neurosci* 1, 11–20.

Bissiere S, Humeau Y, Luthi A (2003) Dopamine gates LTP induction in lateral amygdala by suppressing feedforward inhibition. *Nat Neurosci* 6, 587–92.

Blair HT, Schafe GE, Bauer EP, Rodrigues SM, LeDoux JE (2001) Synaptic plasticity in the lateral amygdala: a cellular hypothesis of fear conditioning. *Learn Mem* 8, 229–42.

Bouton ME, Westbrook RF, Corcoran KA, Maren S (2006) Contextual and temporal modulation of extinction: behavioral and biological mechanisms. *Biol Psychiatry* 60, 352–60.

Bush DE, Caparosa EM, Gekker A, Ledoux J (2010) Beta-adrenergic receptors in the lateral nucleus of the amygdala contribute to the acquisition but not the consolidation of auditory fear conditioning. *Front Behav Neurosci* 4, 154.

Cain CK, LeDoux JE (2008) Brain mechanisms of Pavlovian and Instrumental Aversive Conditioning In *Handbook of Anxiety and Fear*, ed. DJ Nutt, RJ Blanchard, DC Blanchard, G Griebel, pp. 103–25. Amsterdam: Elsevier Academic Press.

Cain CK, Maynard GD, Kehne JH (2012) Targeting memory processes with drugs to prevent or cure PTSD. *Expert opinion on investigational drugs* 21, 1323–50.

Cain CK, Sullivan GM, LeDoux JE (2013) The neurobiology of fear and anxiety: contributions of animal models to current understanding. In: Charney DS, Buxbaum JD, Sklar P et al. (eds) *Neurobiology of Mental Illness*. Oxford University Press, New York.

Callaghan BL, Richardson R (2013) Early experiences and the development of emotional learning systems in rats. *Biol Mood Anxiety disord* 3, 8.

Campeau S, Davis M (1995) Involvement of the central nucleus and basolateral complex of the amygdala in fear conditioning measured with fear-potentiated startle in rats trained concurrently with auditory and visual conditioned stimuli. *J Neurosci* 15, 2301–11.

Cho JH, Deisseroth K, Bolshakov VY (2013) Synaptic encoding of fear extinction in mPFC-amygdala circuits. *Neuron* 80, 1491–507.

Ciocchi S, Herry C, Grenier F et al (2010) Encoding of conditioned fear in central amygdala inhibitory circuits. *Nature* 468, 277–82.

Cowansage KK, LeDoux JE, Monfils MH (2010) Brain-derived neurotrophic factor: a dynamic gatekeeper of neural plasticity. *Curr Mol Pharmacol* 3, 12–29.

Craske MG, Kircanski K, Zelikowsky M et al. (2008) Optimizing inhibitory learning during exposure therapy. *Behav Res Ther* 46, 5–27.

Davis M (2011) NMDA receptors and fear extinction: implications for cognitive behavioral therapy. *Dialog Clin Neurosci* 13, 463–74.

Davis SE, Bauer EP (2012) L-type voltage-gated calcium channels in the basolateral amygdala are necessary for fear extinction. *J Neurosci* 32, 13582–6.

Debiec J, Bush DE, LeDoux JE (2011) Noradrenergic enhancement of reconsolidation in the amygdala impairs extinction of conditioned fear in rats--a possible mechanism for the persistence of traumatic memories in PTSD. *Depress Anxiety* 28, 186–93.

Duvarci S, Popa D, Pare D (2011) Central amygdala activity during fear conditioning. *J Neurosci* 31, 289–94.

Fanselow MS, Kim JJ (1994) Acquisition of contextual Pavlovian fear conditioning is blocked by application of an NMDA receptor antagonist D,L-2-amino-5-phosphonovaleric acid to the basolateral amygdala. *Behav Neurosci* 108, 210–12.

Fanselow MS, Lester LS (1988) A functional behavioristic approach to aversively motivated behavior: predatory imminence as a determinant of the topography of defensive behavior. In Bolles RC, Beecher MD (eds) *Evolution and Learning*. Erlbaum, Hillsdale, NJ, pp. 185–211.

Foa EB (2011) Prolonged exposure therapy: past, present, and future. *Depress Anxiety* 28, 1043–7.

*Fourcaudot E, Gambino F, Casassus G et al. (2009) L-type voltage-dependent Ca(2+) channels mediate expression of presynaptic LTP in amygdala. *Nat Neurosci* 12, 1093–5.

Gale GD, Anagnostaras SG, Godsil BP, et al (2004) Role of the basolateral amygdala in the storage of fear memories across the adult lifetime of rats. *J Neurosci* 24, 3810–5.

Gogolla N, Caroni P, Luthi A et al. (2009) Perineuronal nets protect fear memories from erasure. *Science* 325, 1258–61.

Golub Y, Mauch CP, Dahlhoff M, Wotjak CT (2009) Consequences of extinction training on associative and non-associative fear in a mouse model of posttraumatic stress disorder (PTSD). *Behav Brain Res* 205, 544–9.

Goosens KA, Maren S (2001) Contextual and auditory fear conditioning are mediated by the lateral, basal, and central amygdaloid nuclei in rats. *Learn Mem* 8, 148–55.

Gozzi A, Jain A, Giovanelli A, Bertollini C, Crestan V, et al (2010) A neural switch for active and passive fear. *Neuron* 67, 656–66.

Graham BM, Richardson R (2011) Intraamygdala infusion of fibroblast growth factor 2 enhances extinction and reduces renewal and reinstatement in adult rats. *J Neurosci* 31, 14151–7.

Grillon C, Morgan CA, 3rd, (1999) Fear-potentiated startle conditioning to explicit and contextual cues in Gulf War veterans with posttraumatic stress disorder. *J Abnorm Psychol* 108, 134–42.

Guarraci FA, Frohardt RJ, Kapp BS (1999) Amygdaloid D1 dopamine receptor involvement in Pavlovian fear conditioning. *Brain Res* 827, 28–40.

Haubensak W, Kunwar PS, Cai H et al (2010) Genetic dissection of an amygdala microcircuit that gates conditioned fear. *Nature* 468, 270–76.

Hebb DO (1949) *The Organization of Behavior: A neuropsychological theory*. John Wiley and Sons, New York.

Herry C, Ferraguti F, Singewald N et al. (2010) Neuronal circuits of fear extinction. *Eur J Neurosci* 31, 599–612.

Hitchcock JM, Davis M (1991) Efferent pathway of the amygdala involved in conditioned fear as measured with the fear-potentiated startle paradigm. *Behav Neurosci* 105, 826–42.

Holmes A, Quirk GJ (2010) Pharmacological facilitation of fear extinction and the search for adjunct treatments for anxiety disorders – the case of yohimbine. *Trends Pharmacol Sci* 31, 2–7.

Hostinar CE, Sullivan RM, Gunnar MR (2013) Psychobiological mechanisms underlying the social buffering of the hypothalamic-pituitary-adrenocortical axis: a review of animal models and human studies across development. *Psychol Bull* 140, 256–82.

*Humeau Y, Shaban H, Bissiere S et al. (2003) Presynaptic induction of heterosynaptic associative plasticity in the mammalian brain. *Nature* 426, 841–5.

Isogawa K, Bush DE, LeDoux JE (2013) Contrasting effects of pretraining, posttraining, and pretesting infusions of corticotropin-releasing factor into the lateral amygdala: attenuation of fear memory formation but facilitation of its expression. *Biol Psychiatry* 73, 353–9.

Johansen JP, Cain CK, Ostroff LE, LeDoux JE (2011) Molecular mechanisms of fear learning and memory. *Cell* 147, 509–24.

Johansen JP, Hamanaka H, Monfils MH et al. (2010a) Optical activation of lateral amygdala pyramidal cells instructs associative fear learning. *Proc Natl Acad Sci USA* 107, 12692–7.

Johansen JP, Tarpley JW, LeDoux JE, Blair HT. 2010b. Neural substrates for expectation-modulated fear learning in the amygdala and periaqueductal gray. *Nat Neurosci* 13, 979–86.

Josselyn SA (2010) Continuing the search for the engram: examining the mechanism of fear memories. *J Psychiatry Neurosci* 35, 221–8.

Josselyn SA, Frankland PW (2012) Infantile amnesia: a neurogenic hypothesis. *Learn Mem* 19, 423–33.

Jovanovic T, Norrholm SD, Blanding NQ et al (2010) Impaired fear inhibition is a biomarker of PTSD but not depression. *Depress Anxiety* 27, 244–51.

Kaplan GB, Moore KA (2011) The use of cognitive enhancers in animal models of fear extinction. *Pharmacol Biochem Behav* 99, 217–28.

Karpova NN, Pickenhagen A, Lindholm J et al (2011) Fear erasure in mice requires synergy between antidepressant drugs and extinction training. *Science* 334, 1731–4.

Knobloch HS, Charlet A, Hoffmann LC et al (2012) Evoked axonal oxytocin release in the central amygdala attenuates fear response. *Neuron* 73, 553–66.

Lamprecht R, LeDoux J (2004) Structural plasticity and memory. *Nat Rev Neurosci* 5, 45–54.

Landers MS, Sullivan RM (2012) The development and neurobiology of infant attachment and fear. *Dev Neurosci* 34, 101–14.

LeDoux JE (2012) Rethinking the emotional brain. *Neuron* 73, 653–76.

Li H, Penzo MA, Taniguchi H et al. (2013) Experience-dependent modification of a central amygdala fear circuit. *Nat Neurosci* 16, 332–9.

Litvin Y, Pentkowski NS, Pobbe RL et al.(2008) Unconditioned models of fear and anxiety In: Blanchard RJ, Blanchard DC, Griebel G et al. (eds) *Handbood of Anxiety and Fear*. Academic Press, Amsterdam, pp. 81–99.

Malenka RC, Nicoll RA (1999) Long-term potentiation--a decade of progress? *Science* 285, 1870–4.

Maren S (2005) Synaptic mechanisms of associative memory in the amygdala. *Neuron* 47, 783–6.

Maren S, Fanselow MS (1995) Synaptic plasticity in the basolateral amygdala induced by hippocampal formation stimulation *in vivo*. *J Neurosci* 15, 7548–64.

Maren S, Yap SA, Goosens KA (2001) The amygdala is essential for the development of neuronal plasticity in the medial geniculate nucleus during auditory fear conditioning in rats. *J Neurosci* 21, RC135.

McGaugh JL, McIntyre CK, Power AE (2002) Amygdala modulation of memory consolidation: interaction with other brain systems. *Neurobiol Learn Mem* 78, 539–52.

McKernan MG, Shinnick-Gallagher P (1997) Fear conditioning induces a lasting potentiation of synaptic currents in vitro. *Nature* 390, 607–11.

McNally GP, Pigg M, Weidemann G (2004) Opioid receptors in the midbrain periaqueductal gray regulate extinction of pavlovian fear conditioning. *J Neurosci* 24, 6912–9.

Milad MR, Pitman RK, Ellis CB et al (2009) Neurobiological basis of failure to recall extinction memory in posttraumatic stress disorder. *Biol Psychiatry* 66, 1075–82.

Milad MR, Quirk GJ (2012) Fear extinction as a model for translational neuroscience: ten years of progress. *Ann Rev Psychol* 63, 129–51.

Moriceau S, Sullivan RM (2006) Maternal presence serves as a switch between learning fear and attraction in infancy. *Nat Neurosci* 9, 1004–6.

Muller J, Corodimas KP, Fridel Z, LeDoux JE (1997) Functional inactivation of the lateral and basal nuclei of the amygdala by muscimol infusion prevents fear conditioning to an explicit conditioned stimulus and to contextual stimuli. *Behav Neurosci* 111, 683–91.

Myers KM, Davis M (2007) Mechanisms of fear extinction. *Molecular psychiatry* 12, 120–50.

Nader K, Schafe GE, LeDoux JE (2000) Fear memories require protein synthesis in the amygdala for reconsolidation after retrieval. *Nature* 406, 722–6.

Nair HP, Berndt JD, Barrett D, Gonzalez-Lima F (2001) Maturation of extinction behavior in infant rats: large-scale regional interactions with medial prefrontal cortex, orbitofrontal cortex, and anterior cingulate cortex. *J Neurosci* 21, 4400–7.

Nedelescu H, Kelso CM, Lazaro-Munoz G et al (2010) Endogenous GluR1-containing AMPA receptors translocate to asymmetric synapses in the lateral amygdala during the early phase of fear memory formation: an electron microscopic immunocytochemical study. *J Comp Neurol* 518, 4723–39.

Orr SP, Metzger LJ, Lasko NB et al. (2000) De novo conditioning in trauma-exposed individuals with and without posttraumatic stress disorder. *J Abnorm Psychol* 109, 290–8.

Ostroff LE, Cain CK, Bedont J et al. (2010) Fear and safety learning differentially affect synapse size and dendritic translation in the lateral amygdala. *Proc Natl Acad Sci USA* 107, 9418–23.

*Pattwell SS, Mouly AM, Sullivan RM, Lee FS (2013) Developmental Components of Fear and Anxiety in Animal Models. In: Charney DS, Sklar P, Buxbaum JD et al. (eds) *Neurobiology of Mental Illness*. Oxford University Press, New York, pp. 593–605.

Pickens CL, Golden SA, Adams-Deutsch T et al. (2009) Long-lasting incubation of conditioned fear in rats. *Biol Psychiatry* 65, 881–6.

Pitkänen A (2000) Connectivity of the rat amygdaloid complex In: Aggleton JP (ed.) *The Amygdala: A Functional Analysis*. Oxford University Press, Oxford, , pp. 31–115.

Pitman RK, Delahanty DL (2005) Conceptually driven pharmacologic approaches to acute trauma. *CNS Spectr* 10, 99–106.

Ploski JE, Park KW, Ping J, Monsey MS, Schafe GE (2010) Identification of plasticity-associated genes regulated by Pavlovian fear conditioning in the lateral amygdala. *J Neurochem* 112, 636–50.

Pollak DD, Monje FJ, Zuckerman L et al. (2008) An animal model of a behavioral intervention for depression. *Neuron* 60, 149–61.

Poulos AM, Reger M, Mehta N et al (2013) Amnesia for early life stress does not preclude the adult development of posttraumatic stress disorder symptoms in rats. *Biol Psychiatry* 76, 306–14.

Quirk GJ, Likhtik E, Pelletier JG, Pare D (2003) Stimulation of medial prefrontal cortex decreases the responsiveness of central amygdala output neurons. *J Neurosci* 23, 8800–7.

Quirk GJ, Repa C, LeDoux JE (1995) Fear conditioning enhances short-latency auditory responses of lateral amygdala neurons: parallel recordings in the freely behaving rat. *Neuron* 15, 1029–39.

Quirk GJ, Russo GK, Barron JL, Lebron K (2000) The role of ventromedial prefrontal cortex in the recovery of extinguished fear. *J Neurosci* 20, 6225–31.

Raineki C, Cortes MR, Belnoue L, Sullivan RM (2012) Effects of early-life abuse differ across development: infant social behavior deficits are followed by adolescent depressive-like behaviors mediated by the amygdala. *J Neurosci* 32, 7758–65.

Raineki C, Moriceau S, Sullivan RM (2010) Developing a neurobehavioral animal model of infant attachment to an abusive caregiver. *Biol Psychiatry* 67, 1137–45.

Rescorla RA (1967) Pavlovian conditioning and its proper control procedures. *Psychol Rev* 74, 71–80.

Rodrigues SM, Bauer EP, Farb CR et al. (2002) The group I metabotropic glutamate receptor mGluR5 is required for fear memory formation and long-term potentiation in the lateral amygdala. *J Neurosci* 22, 5219–29.

Rogan MT, Leon KS, Perez DL et al. (2005) Distinct neural signatures for safety and danger in the amygdala and striatum of the mouse. *Neuron* 46, 309–20.

Rogan MT, Staubli UV, LeDoux JE (1997) Fear conditioning induces associative long-term potentiation in the amygdala. *Nature* 390, 604–7.

Romanski LM, LeDoux JE, Clugnet MC et al. (1993) Somatosensory and auditory convergence in the lateral nucleus of the amygdala. *Behav Neurosci* 107, 444–50.

Rosen JB, Schulkin J (1998) From normal fear to pathological anxiety. *Psychol Rev* 105, 325–50.

Rosenkranz JA, Grace AA (2002) Dopamine-mediated modulation of odour-evoked amygdala potentials during pavlovian conditioning. *Nature* 417, 282–7.

Rumpel S, LeDoux J, Zador A et al. (2005) Postsynaptic receptor trafficking underlying a form of associative learning. *Science* 308, 83–8.

Sarro EC, Sullivan RM, Barr G (2014) Unpredictable neonatal stress enhances adult anxiety and alters amygdala gene expression related to serotonin and GABA. *Neuroscience* 258, 147–61.

Schafe GE, LeDoux JE (2000) Memory consolidation of auditory pavlovian fear conditioning requires protein synthesis and protein kinase a in the amygdala. *J Neurosci* 20, RC96.

Schiller D, Monfils MH, Raio CM et al. (2010) Preventing the return of fear in humans using reconsolidation update mechanisms. *Nature* 463, 49–53.

Schneier FR, Neria Y, Pavlicova M et al (2012) Combined prolonged exposure therapy and paroxetine for PTSD related to the World Trade Center attack: a randomized controlled trial. *Am J Psychiatry* 169, 80–8.

Sears RM, Fink AE, Wigestrand MB et al.(2013) Orexin/hypocretin system modulates amygdala-dependent threat learning through the locus coeruleus. *Proc Natl Acad Sci USA* 110, 20260–5.

Sevelinges Y, Mouly AM, Raineki C et al.(2011) Adult depression-like behavior, amygdala and olfactory cortex functions are restored by odor previously paired with shock during infant's sensitive period attachment learning. *Dev Cogn Neurosci* 1, 77–87.

Silva AJ (2003) Molecular and cellular cognitive studies of the role of synaptic plasticity in memory. *J Neurobiol* 54, 224–37.

Sotres-Bayon F, Bush DE, LeDoux JE (2004) Emotional perseveration: an update on prefrontal-amygdala interactions in fear extinction. *Learn Mem* 11, 525–35.

Stanton ME (2000) Multiple memory systems, development and conditioning. *Behav Brain Res* 110, 25–37.

Sullivan RM, Holman PJ (2010) Transitions in sensitive period attachment learning in infancy: the role of corticosterone. *Neurosci Biobehav Rev* 34, 835–44.

Sullivan RM, Landers M, Yeaman B et al. (2000) Good memories of bad events in infancy. *Nature* 407, 38–9.

Trouche S, Sasaki JM, Tu T et al. (2013) Fear extinction causes target-specific remodeling of perisomatic inhibitory synapses. *Neuron* 80, 1054–65.

Tsvetkov E, Carlezon WA, Benes FM et al. (2002) Fear conditioning occludes LTP-induced presynaptic enhancement of synaptic transmission in the cortical pathway to the lateral amygdala. *Neuron* 34, 289–300.

Tully K, Li Y, Tsvetkov E, Bolshakov VY (2007) Norepinephrine enables the induction of associative long-term potentiation at thalamo-amygdala synapses. *Proc Natl Acad Sci USA* 104, 14146–50.

Vermetten E, Bremner JD (2002) Circuits and systems in stress. I. Preclinical studies. *Depress Anxiety* 15, 126–47.

Wilensky AE, Schafe GE, Kristensen MP et al. (2006) Rethinking the fear circuit: the central nucleus of the amygdala is required for the acquisition, consolidation, and expression of pavlovian fear conditioning. *J Neurosci* 26, 12387–96.

Winslow JT, Insel TR (1991) The infant rat separation paradigm: a novel test for novel anxiolytics. *Trends Pharmacol Sci* 12, 402–4.

Yeh SH, Mao SC, Lin HC, Gean PW (2006) Synaptic expression of glutamate receptor after encoding of fear memory in the rat amygdala. *Mol Pharmacol* 69, 299–308.

Yehuda R, Flory JD, Pratchett LC et al. (2010) Putative biological mechanisms for the association between early life adversity and the subsequent development of PTSD. *Psychopharmacology (Berl)* 212, 405–17.

Yehuda R, LeDoux J (2007) Response variation following trauma: a translational neuroscience approach to understanding PTSD. *Neuron* 56, 19–32.

Zovkic IB, Sweatt JD (2013) Epigenetic mechanisms in learned fear: implications for PTSD. *Neuropsychopharmacology* 38, 77–93.

CHAPTER 5

Preclinical evidence for benzodiazepine receptor involvement in the pathophysiology of PTSD, comorbid substance abuse, and alcoholism

Robert Drugan, Nathaniel P. Stafford & Timothy A. Warner

Department of Psychology, University of New Hampshire, Durham, NH, USA

5.1 Introduction

Trauma exposure has many physical and psychological sequelae, with the most common psychiatric condition manifested as posttraumatic stress disorder (PTSD; Bremner et al., 1993, 1994; Singer et al., 1995; Yehuda et al., 1995). According to the *Diagnostic and Statistical Manual of Mental Disorders* (DSM-IV-TR; American Psychiatric Association, 2000), the diagnostic criteria for PTSD include the person experiencing or witnessing an event that involved actual or threatened death, or serious injury to that person or others. In addition, the reaction of the person to the event is intense fear, helplessness, or horror. The individual subsequently re-experiences the event in one or more of several ways: symptom cluster B, which includes intrusive recollections, nightmares, flashbacks; symptom cluster C, which includes avoidance and psychic numbing; and symptom cluster D, which includes hyperarousal, and these symptoms last for more than 1 month (American Psychiatric Association, 2000). Importantly, PTSD is often comorbid with a number of other psychiatric disorders, including panic disorder, generalized anxiety disorder, major depressive disorder, and substance abuse (Friedman & Yehuda, 1995). Although great strides have been made in the treatment of those with PTSD, more research needs to be conducted if we are to be able to effectively treat all PTSD patients.

Animal models of PTSD provide great insight into the pathophysiology and treatment of PTSD. Some have briefly noted (van der Kolk, 1985, 1987) that symptoms of PTSD were evident in early neurosis paradigms (Gantt, 1944;

Posttraumatic Stress Disorder: From Neurobiology to Treatment, First Edition.
Edited by J. Douglas Bremner.
© 2016 John Wiley & Sons, Inc. Published 2016 by John Wiley & Sons, Inc.

Masserman, 1943; Pavlov, 1927; Wolpe, 1952) where animals exhibited lethargy or withdrawn action as well as sudden eruptions of agitated behavior (Mineka & Hendersen, 1985; Mineka & Kihlstrom, 1978). Obviously, it is arduous for animal models to mirror all symptoms of PTSD, because it is impossible to assess the emotional components. However, animal models allow researchers to assess most of the prominent features of the disorder – non-verbal cues (Mineka, 1985). There are several animal models of PTSD: behavioral sensitization, time-dependent sensitization, and kindling (Charney et al., 1993; Post et al., 1995; Yehuda & Antelman, 1993). In addition, learned helplessness, although initially conceptualized as an animal model of behavioral depression (Weiss et al., 1981), has more recently been suggested to be an animal model of PTSD, due to the nature of inescapable shock (IS; Petty et al., 1997; Koba et al., 2001; Hammack et al., 2012). In fact, uncontrollability of stressors (i.e., shock) results in coping deficits noted by the failure to escape or terminate shock (Maier, 2001). When rats are exposed to escapable shock (ES; controllability) there are evident signs of an attenuation of contextual fear in comparison to rats that receive IS (Brennan & Riccio, 1975; Mineka et al., 1984; Mowrer & Viek, 1948; Weiss, 1968), as long as there are at least 20 shocks (Rosellini et al., 1987), which suggests that IS elicits greater generalized fear. Stress-induced analgesia, resulting from IS exposure (Maier & Keith, 1987; Moye et al., 1983), seems to parallel the numbing typically expressed in PTSD patients evoked by trauma-related stress, and further contributes to the validity of learned helplessness as an animal model of PTSD.

The endogenous mechanism responsible for the deficits observed after IS exposure includes various neurotransmitter systems, including norepinephrine (Weiss et al., 1970, 1981), serotonin (Maier & Watkins, 1998, 2005), dopamine (Anisman et al., 1980), and the benzodiazepine (BDZ)/GABA$_A$ receptor system (Drugan et al., 1984, 1985a).

5.2 Stress and the Benzodiazepine Receptor

The first clue that BDZ systems may be involved in the etiology of IS-induced deficits came from an anecdotal observation of rats undergoing ES vs. IS stress. During the inter-trial interval of the shock stress session, the respiratory cadence was much faster in rats receiving IS than in those receiving ES (R.C. Drugan, unpublished observations). This difference was hypothesized to be due to higher and lower levels of anxiety for the IS and ES groups, respectively. If high anxiety during the stress session set the stage for the subsequent behavioral depression, then alleviating this anxiety should block the subsequent stress effects. This is exactly what happened. Two well-replicated consequences of exposure to inescapable stress are cognitive deficits, manifested as an inability to escape from a shuttlebox where shock occurs and escape is indeed possible, and the development of long-term analgesia, or insensitivity to pain. Administration of an anxiolytic BDZ, chlordiazepoxide (Librium), prior to IS prevented both the shuttle escape deficit and long-term analgesia typically observed 24 hours later (Drugan et al., 1984). However, a BDZ that is administered only before shuttlebox testing, not prior to IS, reduces fear associated with shuttlebox testing, but has no effect on the escape deficit (Maier, 1990), and thus illustrates the importance of BDZs prior to IS (Deutsch et al., 1988). Concurrent work evaluating fear conditioning to the stress environment verified our observations. Rats exposed to IS showed greater fear of the stress context than rats exposed to ES (Mineka et al., 1984). A subsequent study revealed that anxiety was both necessary and sufficient for producing these effects, in that administration of the anxiogenic compound, β-carboline (FG 7142), which binds as an inverse agonist to the BDZ binding site of the $GABA_A$ receptor complex, given in lieu of IS resulted in the shuttlebox escape deficit. This anxiety-induced depression could be prevented by prior administration of the high-affinity BDZ receptor antagonist flumazenil (Drugan et al., 1985).

Although this clearly demonstrated that the prevention as well as induction of anxiety could produce these effects, it was unknown what was happening in the brains of the ES and IS groups, and whether BDZ receptor changes were concomitant with this stress exposure. Prior to conducting brain receptor analysis, an *in vivo* functional test of changes in the BDZ/$GABA_A$ receptor was conducted using susceptibility to $GABA_A$ receptor antagonist (i.e., bicuculline)-induced seizures. There was a noted bidirectional effect of inescapable vs. escapable stress on subsequent seizure susceptibility. ES protected against bicuculline-induced seizure, while IS exposure rendered the rats hypersusceptible to seizure (Drugan et al., 1985; Figure 5.1).

Research into the neurochemical changes associated with IS exposure indicated a controllability-dependent change in the $GABA_A$ receptor complex, with IS resulting in a distinct pattern compared with ES (Drugan et al., 1985b, 1994). Subsequent *in vitro* and *in vivo* receptor analysis indicated that unique BDZ receptor changes occurred in rats unable to cope with stress and that subsequently developed behavioral depression, whereas these changes were not observed in rats that appeared resilient to the effects of IS (Drugan et al., 1989, 1993). Exposure to IS, and subsequent failure in the shuttlebox escape task, was associated with a significant reduction in the functional component of the BDZ/$GABA_A$ receptor complex, as measured by muscimol-stimulated $^{36}Cl^-$ uptake in cerebral cortex, in comparison to naïve controls (Drugan et al., 1989; Figure 5.2).

In addition, IS-induced deficits in shuttle escape performance were associated with a reduction in *in vivo* binding of [^3H]Ro15-1788, a BDZ receptor antagonist, in the cortex, hippocampus, and striatum in comparison to naïve controls (Drugan et al., 1989; Figure 5.3).

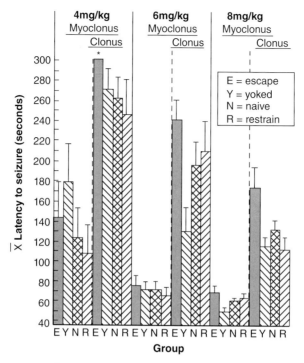

Figure 5.1 Mean (+ SEM) latency to onset of myoclonus and clonus following an intraperitoneal injection of bicuculline (4, 6, or 8 mg/kg) 2 hours after 80 escapable shocks, inescapable shocks, restraint, or no treatment (naïve). Vertical bars represent standard errors. * denotes that all subjects went to the cut-off without a seizure. (From Drugan et al., 1985, with permission.)

5.3 Interaction of Stress, Alcohol Intake and the Benzodiazepine Rector

The functional significance of these changes became apparent in more recent studies that showed a differential response to central nervous system (CNS) depressants following exposure to IS vs. ES.

More specifically, IS exposure resulted in an exaggerated behavioral response to a threshold hypnotic dose of ethanol either immediately or 2 hours post-stress compared with naïve controls (Drugan et al., 1992; Figure 5.4).

The observation of enhanced reactivity to ethanol was extended by subsequent research looking into a more clinically relevant dose of ethanol. More specifically, rather than investigating the hypnotic or sleep-inducing effects of alcohol, the motor ataxic effects of much lower doses were examined to provide greater translational value to the human condition. Again, exposure to IS but not ES resulted in a significant potentiation of the motor ataxic effects of ethanol

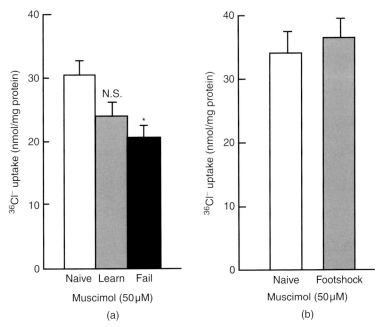

Figure 5.2 The effects of inescapable shock on muscimol-stimulated $^{36}Cl^-$ uptake. (a) Muscimol-stimulated $^{36}Cl^-$ uptake is decreased in cerebral cortical synaptoneurosomes from rats that fail to learn the shuttlebox escape task on day 2 of the learned helplessness paradigm when compared with naïve controls. Each bar represents the mean + SEM of $^{36}Cl^-$ uptake measured in six individual subjects following the shuttle escape task. Muscimol-stimulated $^{36}Cl^-$ uptake was decreased 29% from 30.4 ± 2.2 in naïve controls to 21.6 ± 1.0 nmol/mg protein in subjects that "fail". Subjects from each experimental group were assayed simultaneously. (b) Inescapable footshock alone (comparable to the "fail" condition in a) did not alter muscimol-stimulated $^{36}Cl^-$ uptake. Each bar represents the mean + SEM of $^{36}Cl^-$ uptake measured in quadruplicate in six individual subjects. Control: 34.16 ± 3.6 vs. footshock: 36.66 ± 3.1 nmol/mg protein. *$P < 0.05$, by Newman–Keuls *post hoc* comparison with naïve controls after ANOVA. (From Drugan et al., 1989, with permission.)

at 2 hours post-stress at a threshold dose of 0.6 mg/kg, but not at higher doses such as 0.8 and 1.0 g/kg (Drugan et al., 1996; Figure 5.5).

Importantly, this effect was replicated looking at the same threshold dose (0.6 g/kg), and rather than testing the ataxic effects 5 minutes after ethanol injection, it was also observed when ethanol was injected 12 minutes prior to the rotarod test (Drugan et al., 1996; Figure 5.6).

Subsequent research extended the time course of this IS-induced enhancement of alcohol reactivity demonstrating that this phenomenon occurred both 2 and 24 hours after exposure to IS when compared with non-stressed controls (Drugan et al., 2007; Figure 5.7)

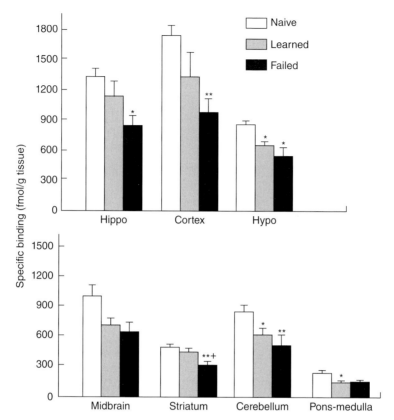

Figure 5.3 *In vivo* [3H]Ro15-1788 binding is decreased in cortex and hippocampus (hippo) of rats that fail to learn the shuttlebox escape task on day 2 of the learned helplessness paradigm. [3H]Ro15-1788 *in vivo* binding is decreased in hypothalamus (hypo), midbrain and cerebellum of both subjects that "learn" and subjects that "fail" the shuttlebox escape task 24 hours after exposure to inescapable shock. Each bar represents the mean + SEM of specific binding in eight to 15 subjects. There was no change in non-specific binding in either "learn" or "fail" subjects compared with controls. *$P < 0.05$, **$P < 0.01$, by Newman–Keuls *post hoc* comparison to naïve control values after ANOVA. (From Drugan et al., 1989, with permission.)

The generality of the IS-induced enhancement of ethanol's effects was tested on other minor tranquillizers including the BDZs. IS but not ES exposure significantly enhanced the motor ataxic effects of midazolam when tested at several doses in comparison to naïve controls (Drugan et al., 1996; Figure 5.8).

These preclinical results demonstrate that an exteroceptive, environmental stressor can markedly influence the subsequent reactivity to both ethanol and midazolam. However, in order to have greater translational value to the human condition, it would be desirable to demonstrate that the intense anxiety/fear caused by the stress is critical and not the physical stressor *per se*. The discovery

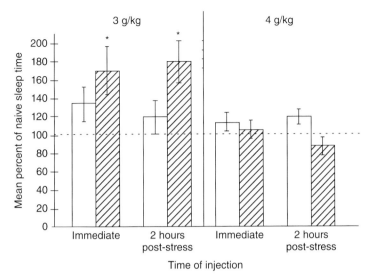

Figure 5.4 Mean percentage of naïve control ethanol-induced sleep time for rats given escapable shock (open bars) or yoked-inescapable shock (hatched bars). The left panel represents the response when the injection was given in a dose of 3 g/kg either immediately or 2 hours after stress, and the right panel represents the response when the drug was given in a dose of 4 g/kg either immediately or 2 hours after stress (n = 8–16 rats per group. Vertical bars represent SEM. * indicates significantly different from naïve control ($P < 0.05$) by Newman–Keuls *post hoc* comparison after ANOVA. (From Drugan et al., 1992, with permission.)

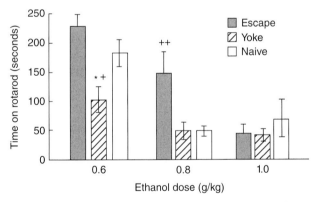

Figure 5.5 Mean time spent on the rotarod for rats 2 hours following exposure to escapable shock, yoked-inescapable shock, or no shock (naïve) and injected with 0.6, 0.8, or 1.0 g/kg of ethanol 5 minutes prior to rotarod testing. Vertical bars represent + SEM (8–10 subjects/group). * (at the 0.6 g/kg dose) indicates a significant difference from the naïve group ($P < 0.05$); + indicates a significant difference from the escape group ($P < 0.01$). For the 0.8 g/kg group, ++ indicates significantly different from both yoked and naïve groups ($P < 0.01$) by Newman–Keuls *post hoc* comparisons after ANOVA. (From Drugan et al., 1996, with permission.)

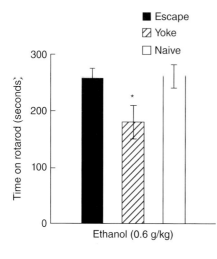

Figure 5.6 Mean time spent on the rotarod 2 hours post-stress for rats exposed to escapable shock, yoked-inescapable shock or no shock (naïve), and injected with 0.6 g/kg ethanol 12 minutes prior to rotarod testing. Vertical bars represent mean ± SEM (10–12 rats per group). * indicates a significant difference from both escapable shock and naïve groups by Newman–Keuls *post hoc* comparisons after ANOVA. (From Drugan et al., 1996, with permission.)

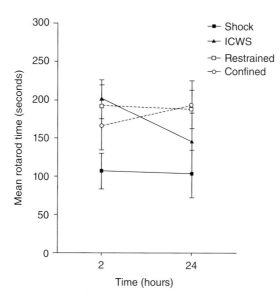

Figure 5.7 Mean (± SEM) time spent on the rotarod 2 or 24 hours after stress exposure. Rotarod performance was assessed 12 minutes after an ataxic dose of ethanol hydroxide. Inescapable shock significantly reduced time on the rotarod compared with all other groups at both 2 and 24 hours post-stress by Newman–Keuls *post hoc* comparisons after ANOVA. (From Drugan et al., 2007, with permission.)

of inverse agonists (e.g., β-carbolines) at the BDZ receptor has served as a pharmacological tool for studying the pathophysiology of anxiety. Contrary to the anxiolytic effects of BDZs, β-carbolines induce intense anxiety as confirmed in both animal (Skolnick et al., 1984) and human studies (Dorow et al., 1983). Thus, demonstration of intense anxiety by an interoceptive stressor (i.e.,

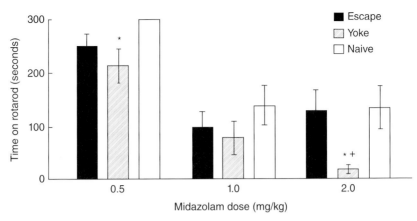

Figure 5.8 Mean time spent on rotarod 2 hours following stress for rats receiving escapable shock, yoked-inescapable shock, or no shock (naïve). Rats were injected with 0.5, 1.0 or 2.0 mg/kg midazolam (intraperitoneally) 10 minutes before the rotarod test. Vertical bars represent mean ± SEM (8–10 rats per group). * indicates a significant difference from the naïve group ($P < 0.01$); + indicates a significant difference from the escapable shock group ($P < 0.05$) by Newman–Keuls *post hoc* comparisons after ANOVA. (From Drugan et al., 1996, with permission.)

drug-induced) would provide key evidence that the enhanced anxiety resulting from stress is both necessary and sufficient to alter subsequent reactivity to these minor tranquillizers. More recent reports from our laboratory have shown that β-carboline-induced anxiety (either alone or in combination with restraint stress) result in an exaggerated motor ataxic response to both ethanol and midazolam. This effect is observed 24 hours after injection for ethanol as well as midazolam (Austin et al., 1999; Figures 5.9 and 5.10)

This evidence clearly demonstrates that traumatic, inescapable stress exposure alters BDZ receptor binding and the functional, transducing mechanism of this receptor complex (i.e. $^{36}CL^-$ ion flux). Furthermore, the behavioral functional significance of these changes is revealed by exaggerated hypnotic and ataxic properties of several classes of minor tranquillizers, including alcohol and BDZs.

5.4 Stress, Drug Abuse and the Benzodiazepine Receptor

This enhanced drug reactivity increases the reinforcing value of these drugs and may set the stage for subsequent stress-induced abuse and addiction. This may explain the mechanism responsible for the high comorbidity of PTSD with alcohol/substance abuse/addiction (Brady & Sinha, 2005).

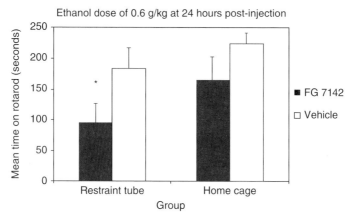

Figure 5.9 Mean time spent on the rotarod for subjects 24 hours after an injection of either FG7142 or equivolume vehicle solution, and subsequent placement in a restraining tube of a Plexiglas home cage. Ten minutes prior to the rotarod test all subjects received an intraperitoneal injection of ethanol (0.6 g/kg). The histograms indicate means ($n = 8$–10 per group), and vertical bars represent SEMs. * indicates significantly different from vehicle-home cage controls as determined by Newman–Keuls *post hoc* comparisons ($P < 0.05$) after ANOVA. (From Austin et al., 1999, with permission.)

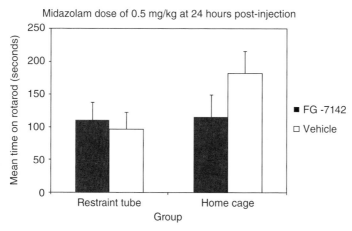

Figure 5.10 Mean time spent on the rotarod for subjects 24 hours following an injection of either FG 7142 or vehicle, and subsequent placement in either restraint tubes or a Plexiglas home cage. Ten minutes prior to the rotarod test, all subjects were injected (intraperitoneally) with 0.5 mg/kg midazolam. Histograms represent means ($n = 12$–14 per group), and vertical bars indicate SEMs. (From Austin et al., 1999, with permission.)

Additional preclinical data demonstrate that prior exposure to inescapable traumatic stress such as uncontrollable shock increases the behavioral and physiological reactivity to a number of classes of drugs of abuse, including psychomotor stimulants and opioids (Logrip et al., 2012). Amphetamine- and cocaine-induced stereotypy are enhanced following IS (MacLennan & Maier, 1983). However, IS appears only to affect the rewarding properties of cocaine, but not those of amphetamine, in a conditioned place preference paradigm (CPP; Will et al., 1998, 2002).

The effects of IS on an opiate such as morphine are more stable. With regard to shuttlebox testing following IS exposure, morphine has no impact on escape latencies (Drugan et al., 1981), whereas an opioid antagonist, naltrexone, extinguishes the escape learning deficit (Maier, 1990). Exposure to uncontrollable shock potentiates the analgesic response to morphine; this effect also occurs in lieu of shock from administration of the BDZ inverse agonist methyl-6,7-dimethoxy-4-ethyl-beta-carboline-3-carboxylate (DMCM), and this effect is subsequently blocked by administration of diazepam (Sutton et al., 1997). IS also increases CPP for morphine, and DMCM administration in the absence of shock similarly enhances the rewarding properties of morphine (Will et al., 1998). Furthermore, opiate antagonist-precipitated withdrawal is potentiated following IS but not ES (Williams et al., 1984). In addition, IS reinstates previously conditioned preference of both cocaine and morphine chambers in a CPP task, which is consistent with clinical populations of addiction/abuse and trauma-related relapse (Logrip et al., 2012).

There are also other drugs of abuse to be discussed, such as cannabinoids and alcohol. There are mixed viewpoints on the anxiolytic and anxiogenic effects of cannabinoids. Recent work has suggested cannabinoids might be able to mitigate the effects of anxiety (Rodgers et al., 2003; Haller et al., 2004; Marco et al., 2004), which could help to extinguish IS-induced anxiogenic effects (Christianson et al., 2008, 2009, 2010). However, the efficacy of cannabinoids is an area of concern, as the results are dependent on the dosage, environmental conditions, and history of the animal subjects (Haller et al., 2004; Marco et al., 2004; Rodgers et al., 2003). For the assessment of the effects of cannabinoids on anxiety, most reports have studied anxiety using exploratory conflict tests such as the open field or elevated plus maze. For instance, the CB1 inverse agonist AM251 produced similar anxiogenic effects to the BDZ inverse agonist FG-7142 in the open field and elevated plus maze (Sink et al., 2010). Another study evaluated the anxiogenic effects of cannabinoids following IS via ultrasonic vocalizations (Arnold et al., 2010), which have been suggested to serve as an indicator of emotions in rodents (Miczek et al., 1995; Rodgers, 1997). In looking solely at the effects of cannabinoids, Arnold et al. (2010) determined that a cannabinoid receptor agonist produced anxiety-like behavior in Wistar (but not Lewis) rats, indicating strain specificity for the drug. The same laboratory noted a similar cannabinoid-induced anxiogenic outcome indicated by more c-Fos expression (a marker of neural activation) in the anxiety-related region of the central nucleus of the amygdala for Wistar, but not Lewis, rats (Arnold et al. 2001). In terms of IS-induced deficits, the cannabinoid receptor agonist, which may have targeted CB1 receptors, heightened IS-induced contextual fear for rats regardless of strain (Arnold et al., 2010).

Uncontrollable shock also has been associated with mixed outcomes in response to alcohol. Numerous studies have reported an increase in alcohol consumption (Anisman & Waller 1974; Füllgrabe et al., 2007; Kinney & Schmidt 1979; Mills et al., 1977; Siegmund et al., 2005; Volpicelli et al., 1990; Vengeliene et al., 2003), while others have noted a decrease in alcohol intake (Bond 1978; Champagne & Kirouac 1987; Darnaudery et al., 2007) following IS. There are even some who have found no noticeable shock-related changes with regard to the consumption of alcohol (Brunell & Spear 2005; Fidler & LoLordo 1996; Myers & Holman 1967; Powell et al., 1966). Interestingly, Meyer et al. (2012) noted that rats significantly consumed more alcohol after exposure to IS, but this effect was not relevant if there was a prior drinking history for the rats that later received IS.

Inescapable shock also induces physiological changes in response to drugs of abuse. Opiates are of particular interest when comes to IS, because IS yields long-term neurochemical alterations for the endogenous opiate systems; specifically, in the μ-receptors (Stuckey et al., 1989) Enkephalin agonists acting on δ-receptors reverse IS-induced shuttlebox escape deficits (Tejedor-Real et al., 1998).

5.5 Translation from Neurobiology to PTSD

These preclinical observations concerning the importance of BDZ systems in the pathophysiology and treatment of PTSD have been validated in human studies. Brain BDZ receptor binding is significantly reduced in PTSD patients compared with controls (Bremner et al., 2000). Although recent recommendations have steered clinicians away from the use of BDZs in the treatment of PTSD, they are still used with some frequency, especially among veterans (Hermos et al., 2007; Lund et al., 2013). Also, BDZs (e.g., clonazepam) can be an effective treatment for certain symptom clusters of PTSD, such as prevailing anxiety, intrusive thoughts, and hyperarousal, although it also appears to have effects on the serotonergic system (Hermos et al., 2007; Hageman et al., 2001).

Clinical observations also confirm the above preclinical work indicating that traumatic stress exposure changes the behavioral reactivity to drugs of abuse. There is a high comorbidity of PTSD symptomology with substance abuse (Bonin et al., 2000; Brady et al., 1994; Deykin et al., 1997; LaCoursiere et al., 1980), with prevalence rates of substance abuse disorders in PTSD patients ranging from 19% to 35%, and an even higher prevalence rate (36–52%) focusing specifically on the comorbidity between PTSD and alcohol (Breslau & Davis, 1992; Kessler et al., 1995) The substance abuse is quite varied and includes various drug of abuse (e.g., alcohol, cannabinoids, and opiates). Additionally, substance abuse is used to relieve distressing psychological symptoms that parallel the development of PTSD, and signs of abuse increase with the severity of the symptoms (Bremner et al., 1996; Khantzian, 1985). The self-medication hypothesis holds that individuals typically attempt to diminish initial trauma-induced anxiety with alcohol or BDZs in an effort to forget painful, traumatic memories (Stewart et al 1998).

Hermos et al. (2007) recently reported that veterans within the New England Veterans Integrated Service Network (VISN 1) are typically prescribed low, stable long-term dosages of BDZs for PTSD-related anxiety. However, those prescribed high, increasing dosages of long-term BDZs reported greater substance abuse prevalence. Specifically, younger patients reporting comorbid PTSD and alcoholism as well as concurrent opiate (oxycodone/acetaminophen) prescriptions required higher-dose BDZs (Hermos et al., 2007). These data suggest dual dependencies, as opioid prescription or alcohol is needed to supplement tolerance to BDZs.

It is clear from the aforementioned literature that the BDZ/GABA$_A$ receptor complex is an important component of stress responsivity in the learned helplessness model of PTSD. However, since recent clinical administration of BDZs has waned in the treatment of PTSD symptoms (Lund et al., 2013), and comorbid substance abuse is quite prevalent (Norman et al., 2012), endogenous GABA$_A$ receptor ligands may serve as an alternative treatment option. Preclinical observations have indicated several putative endogenous ligands as allosteric modulators. These include, diazepam binding inhibitor (Costa et al., 1994), the brain-derived steroid pregnenolone (Jung-Testas et al., 1989), and neuroactive 3-alpha reduced hydroxy steroids. One such steroid, 3-alpha, 5 alpha-tetrahydrodeoxycorticosterone (THDOC), prolongs GABA$_A$ receptor recovery from desensitization to augment inhibitory postsynaptic GABAergic signaling (Mellon & Griffin, 2002). The A-ring-reduced metabolite of progesterone, 3-alpha-hydroxy-5 alpha-pregnan-20-one (allopregnanolone) also has important anxiolytic properties (Crawley et al., 1986). This substance augments GABA-activated chloride channels analogous to the most efficacious BDZs (Purdy et al., 1991), and inhibits [35s]TBPS binding (Gee et al., 1987), which is associated with resilience to IS-induced deficits (Drugan et al., 1993). Furthermore, certain drugs of abuse affect brain allopregnanolone levels. Interestingly, administration of Δ9-tetrahydrocannabinol elevates cortical levels of the neurosteroid to a greater extent than morphine, while cocaine has no effect (Grobin et al., 2005).

5.6 Conclusions

In sum, we have demonstrated changes in the BDZ/GABA$_A$ receptor complex associated with traumatic, uncontrollable stress. The functional significance of these changes in this animal model of PTSD are revealed, in that there is a subsequent hypersensitivity to the pharmacological and psychoactive actions of a number of drugs of abuse, including BDZs, alcohol, opiates, and cocaine. This change may reflect the etiology of the high comorbidity of PTSD with substance abuse and alcoholism. We have developed a hybrid animal model of depression called the intermittent swim stress (ISS) paradigm (Brown et al., 2001; Christianson & Drugan, 2005). It is a hybrid model because it draws from both the learned helplessness model (i.e., intermittent stress) as well as the behavioral despair model (the use of cold water swim as the stressor). We initially demonstrated ISS-induced behavioral depression using several endpoints such as the forced swim test and instrumental learning tests. Recent data have revealed that ISS produces a long-term increase in anxiety as measured by the juvenile social exploration test 24 hours post-ISS (Christianson et al., 2008; Warner et al., 2013; Stafford et al., 2015). Therefore, the ISS paradigm may have additional utility as an animal model of PTSD. We plan on testing the reactivity to a number of minor tranquillizers following ISS to test the generality of the IS-induced changes described here.

References

American Psychiatric Association (2000) *Diagnostic and Statistical Manual DSM-IV*, text revision (TR). American Psychiatric Press, Washington, DC.

Anisman H, Waller TG (1974) Effects of inescapable shock and shock-produced conflict on self selection of alcohol in rats. *Pharmacol Biochem Behav* 2, 27–33.

Anisman H, A Suissa, LS Sklar (1980) Escape deficits induced by uncontrollable stress: Antagonism by dopamine and norepinephrine agonists. *Behavioral and Neural Biology* 28, 34–37.

Arnold J C, Dielenberg RA, McGregor IS (2010) Cannabinoids increase conditioned ultrasonic vocalisations and cat odour avoidance in rats: strain differences in drug-induced anxiety. *Life Sci* 87, 572–578.

Arnold JC, Topple AN, Mallet PE et al. (2001) The distribution of cannabinoid-induced Fos expression in rat brain: differences between the Lewis and Wistar strain. *Brain Res* 921, 240–255.

Austin M, Myles V, Brown PL et al. (1999) FG 7142- and restraint-induced alterations in the ataxic effects of alcohol and midazolam in rats are time dependent. *Pharmacol Biochem Behav* 62, 45–51.

Bond NW (1978) Shock induced alcohol consumption in rats: role of initial preference. *Pharmacol Biochem Behav* 9, 39–42.

Bonin MF, Norton GR, Asmundson JG et al. (2000) Drinking away the hurt: the nature and prevalence of PTSD in substance abuse patients attending a community-based treatment program. *J Behav Ther* 31, 55–66.

Brady KT, Sinha, R. (2007) Co-occurring mental and substance use disorders: the neurobiological effects of chronic stress. *Am J Psychiatry* 162, 1483–1493.

Brady KT, Killeen T, Saladin ME et al. (1994) Comorbid substance abuse and post traumatic stress disorder. *Am J Addict* 3, 160–164.

Bremner JD, Innis RB, Southwick SM et al. (2000) Decreased benzodiazepine receptor binding in prefrontal cortex in combat-related posttraumatic stress disorder. *Am J Psychiatry* 157, 1120–1126.

Bremner JD, Southwick SM, Charney DS. (1994) Etiologic factors in the development of post-traumatic stress disorder. In Mazure CM (ed) *Stress and Psychiatric Disorders*, American Psychiatric Press, Washington DC, pp. 149–186.

Bremner JD, Southwick SM, Darnell A et al. (1996) Chronic PTSD in Vietnam combat veterans: course of illness and substance abuse. *Am J Psychiatry* 153, 369–375.

Bremner JD, Steinberg M, Southwick SM et al. (1993) Use of the Structured Clinical Interview for DSM-IV dissociative disorders for systematic assessment of dissociative symptoms in posttraumatic stress disorder. *Am J Psychiatry* 150, 1011–1014.

Brennan, J. F, Riccio DC (1975) Stimulus generalization of suppression in rats following aversively motivated instrumental or Pavlovian training. *J Comp Physiol Psychol* 88, 570–579.

Breslau N, Davis GC, 1992. Post-traumatic stress disorder in an urban population of young adults: risk factors for chronicity. *Am J Psychiatr* 149, 671–675.

Brown PL, Hurley C, Repucci, N et al. (2001) Behavioral characterization of stress controllability effects in a new swim stress paradigm. *Pharmacol Biochem Behav* 68, 263–272.

Brunell SC, Spear LP (2006) Effect of stress on the voluntary intake of a sweetened ethanol solution in pair-housed adolescent and adult rats. *Alcohol Clin Exp Res* 29, 1641–1653.

Champagne F, Kirouac G. (1987) Effects of unavoidable electric shocks on voluntary alcohol consumption in the rat. *Percept Motor Skills* 64, 335–338.

Charney DS, Deutch AY, Krystal JH et al. (1993) Psychobiologic mechanisms of post-traumatic stress disorder. *Archiv Gen Psychiatry* 50, 294–305.

Christianson JP, Drugan RC (2005) Intermittent cold-water swim stress increases immobility and interferes with escape performance in rat. *Behavioural Brain Res* 165, 58–62.

Christianson JP, Paul ED, Irani M et al. (2008) The role of prior stressor controllability and the dorsal raphe nucleus in sucrose preference and social exploration. *Behavioural Brain Res* 193, 87–93.

Christianson JP, Ragole T, Amat J et al. (2010) 5-hydroxytryptamine 2C receptors in the basolateral amygdala are involved in the expression of anxiety after uncontrollable traumatic stress. *Biol Psychiatry* 67, 339–345.

Christianson JP, Thompson BM, Watkins LR et al. (2009) Medial prefrontal cortical activation modulates the impact of controllable and uncontrollable stressor exposure on a social exploration test of anxiety in the rat. *Stress* 12, 445–450.

Darnaudery M, Louvart H, Defrance L et al. (2007) Impact of an intense stress on ethanol consumption in female rats characterized by their pre-stress preference: modulation by prenatal stress. *Brain Res* 1131, 181–186.

*Deutsch SI, Drugan RC, Vocci FJ et al. (1988) The benzodiazepine/GABA receptor complex in experimental stress, anxiety and depression. In: Brilley M, Filon G (eds) *New Concepts in Depression*. MacMillan Publishers, London, pp. 351–362.

Deykin EY, Buka SL. (1997) Prevalence and risk factors for posttraumatic stress disorder among chemically dependent adolescents. *Am J Psychiatry* 154, 752–757.

Dorow, R, Horowski, R, Paschelke, G, Amin, M, & Braestrup, C. (1983). Severe anxiety induced by FG7142, a -carboline ligand for benzodiazepine receptors. *The Lancet* 2, 98–99.

Drugan RC (1999) Coping with traumatic stress interferes with memory of the event: A new conceptual mechanism for the protective effect of stress control. In: Williams L, Banyard V (eds) *Trauma and Memory*. Sage Publications, Thousand Oaks, CA, pp. 245–256.

Drugan RC (2000) The neurochemistry of stress resilience and coping: A quest for nature's own antidote to illness. In: Gillham JE (ed.) *The Science of Optimism and Hope*. Templeton Foundation Press, Radnor, PA, pp. 57–71.

Drugan RC, Grau JW, Maier SF et al. (1981) Cross tolerance between morphine and the long-term analgesic reaction to inescapable shock. *Pharmacol Biochem Behav* 14, 677–682.

Drugan RC, Basile AS, Ha JH et al. (1994) The protective effects of stress control may be mediated by increased brain levels of benzodiazepine receptor agonists. *Brain Res* 661, 127–136.

Drugan RC, Coyle TS, Healy DJ et al. (1996) Stress controllability modulates both midazolam and ethanol-induced ataxia in the rat. *Behav Neurosci* 110, 360–367.

Drugan RC, Deutsch SI, Weizman A et al. (1989) Molecular mechanisms of stress and anxiety: Alterations in the benzodiazepine/GABA receptor complex. In: *Frontiers of Stress Research: Control of Bodily Function: Basic and Clinical Aspects* (H. Weiner, I Florin and D. Hellhammer, eds) Vol 3, Hans Huber Publishers, Toronto, pp. 148–159.

Drugan RC, Maier SF, Skolnick P, Paul SM, Crawley JN (1985a) An anxiogenic benzodiazepine receptor ligand induces learned helplessness. *Eur J Pharmacol* 113, 453–457.

Drugan RC, McIntyre TD, Alpern HP et al. (1985b) Coping and seizure susceptibility: control over shock protects against bicuculline-induced seizures in rats. *Brain Res* 342: 9–17.

Drugan RC, Morrow AL, Weizman R et al. (1989) Stress-induced behavioral depression in the rat is associated with a decrease in GABA receptor-mediated chloride ion flux and brain benzodiazepine receptor occupancy. *Brain Res* 487, 45–51.

Drugan RC, Paul SM, Crawley JN (1993) Decreased forebrain [35S]TBPS binding and increased [3H]muscimol binding in rats that do not develop stress-induced behavioral depression. *Brain Res* 631, 270–276.

Drugan RC, Ryan SM, Minor TR et al. (1984) Librium prevents the analgesia and shuttlebox escape deficit typically observed following inescapable shock. *Pharmacol Biochem Behav* 21, 749–754.

Drugan RC, Scher DM, Sarabanchong V et al. (1992) Controllability and duration of stress alter central nervous system depressant-induced sleep time in rats. *Behav Neurosci* 106, 682–689.

Drugan RC, Skolnick P, Paul SM et al. (1989) A pretest procedure reliably predicts performance in two animal models of inescapable stress. *Pharmacol Biochem Behav* 33, 649–654.

Drugan RC, Wiedholz LM, Holt A et al. (2007) Environmental and immune stressors enhance alcohol-induced motor ataxia in rat. *Pharmacol Biochem Behav* 86, 125–131.

Fidler TL, LoLordo VM (2006) Failure to find postshock increases in ethanol preference. *Alcohol Clin Exp Res* 20, 110–121.

Friedman MJ, and Yehuda R (1995) Post-Traumatic stress disorder and comorbidity: Psychobiological approaches to differential diagnosis In: Friedman MJ, Charney DS, Deutsch AY (eds) *Neurobiological and Clinical Consequences of Stress: From Normal Adaptation to PTSD.* Lippincott-Raven Publishers, Philadelphia, pp. 429–445.

Füllgrabe MW, Vengeliene V, Spanagel, R. (2007) Influence of age at drinking onset on the alcohol deprivation effect and stress-induced drinking in female rats. *Pharmacol Biochem Behav* 86, 320–326.

Gantt, W H. (1944) *Experimental Basis for Neurotic Behavior: Origin and Development of Artificially Produced Disturbances of Behavior in Dogs.* Hoeber, New York.

Gee, KW, Chang, WC, Brinton, RE, & McEwen, BS (1987). GABA-dependent modulation of the Cl- ionophore by steroids in rat brain. *European journal of pharmacology* 136, 419–423.

Grobin AC, VanDoren MJ, Porrino LJ et al. (2005) Cortical 3α-hydroxy-5α-pregnan-20-one levels after acute administration of Δ9-tetrahydrocannabinol, cocaine and morphine. *Psychopharmacology,* 179, 544–550.

Hageman I, Andersen HS, Jørgensen MB (2001) Post-traumatic stress disorder: a review of psychobiology and pharmacotherapy. *Acta Psychiatr Scand* 104, 411–422.

Haller J, Varga B, Ledent C et al. (2004) Context-dependent effects of CB1 cannabinoid gene disruption on anxiety-like and social behaviour in mice. *Eur J Neurosci* 19, 1906–1912.

Hammack SE, Cooper MA, Lezak KR (2012) Overlapping neurobiology of learned helplessness and conditioned defeat: implications for PTSD and Mood disorders. *Neuropharmacology* 62, 565–75.

Jung-Testas, I, Hu, ZY, Baulieu, EE, & Robel, P. (1989) Steroid synthesis in rat brain cell cultures. *Journal of steroid biochemistry* 34, 511–519.

Kessler RC, Sonnega A, Bromet E et al. (1995) Post-traumatic stress disorder in the national co-morbidity survey. *Arch. Gen. Psychiatr.* 52, 1048–1060.

Khantzian EJ (1985) The self-medication hypothesis of addictive disorders: focus on heroin and cocaine dependence. *Am J Psychiatry* 142, 1259–1264.

Kinney L, Schmidt, H. (1979) Effect of cued and uncued inescapable shock on voluntary alcohol consumption in rats. *Pharmacol Biochem Behav* 11, 601–604.

*Koba T, Kodama Y, Shimizu K et al. (2001) Persistent behavioral changes in rats following inescapable shock stress: a potential model of posttraumatic stress disorder. *World J Biol Psychiatry* 2, 34–37.

LaCoursiere RB, Godfrey KE, Ruby LM. (1980) Traumatic neurosis in the etiology of alcoholism: Vietnam and other trauma. *Am J Psychiatry* 137, 966–968.

Logrip ML, Zorrilla EP, Koob GF (2012) *Stress modulation of drug self-administration: implications for addiction comorbidity with post traumatic stress disorder Neuropharmacology* 62, 552–564.

Lund BC, Abrams TE, Bernardy NC et al. (2013) Benzodiazepine Prescribing Variation and Clinical Uncertainty in Treating Posttraumatic Stress Disorder. *Psychiatr Serv* 64, 21–27.

MacLennan AJ, Maier SF (1983) Coping and the stress-induced potentiation of stimulant stereotypy in the rat. *Science* 219, 1091–1093.

Maier SF (1990) Role of fear in mediating shuttle escape learning deficit produced by inescapable shock. *J Exp Psychol* 16, 137–149.

Maier SF (2001) Exposure to the stressor environment prevents the temporal dissipation of behavioral depression/learned helplessness. *Biol Psychiatry* 49, 763–773

Maier, S. F, Keith JR (1987) Shock signals and the development of stress-induced analgesia. *J Exp Psychol* 13, 226–238.

Maier SF, Watkins LR (1998) Stressor controllability, anxiety, and serotonin. *Cogn Ther Res* 22, 595–613.

Maier SF, Watkins LR (2005) Stressor controllability and learned helplessness: the roles of the dorsal raphe nucleus, serotonin, and corticotropin-releasing factor. *Neurosci Biobehav Rev* 29, 829–842.

Marco EM, Perez-Alvarez L, Borcel E et al. (2004) Involvement of 5-HT1A receptors in behavioural effects of the cannabinoid receptor agonist CP 55,940 in male rats. *Behav Pharmacol* 15, 21–27.

Masserman JH (1943) *Behavior and neurosis: An experimental psychoanalytic approach to psychobiologic principles.* University of Chicago Press, Chicago.

Mellon SH, Griffin LD (2002) Neurosteroids: biochemistry and clinical significance. *Trends Endocrinol Metab* 13, 35–43.

Meyer EM, Long V, Fanselow MS et al. (2012) Stress increases voluntary alcohol intake, but does not alter established drinking habits in a rat model of posttraumatic stress disorder. *Alcohol Clin Exp Res* 37, 566–574.

Miczek KA, Weerts EM, Vivian JA et al. (1995) Aggression, anxiety and vocalizations in animals: GABA A and 5-HT anxiolytics. *Psychopharmacology* 121, 38–56.

Mills KC, Bean JW, Hutcheson JS (1977) Shock induced ethanol consumption in rats. *Pharmacol Biochem Behav* 6, 107–115.

Mineka, S. (1985) Animal models of anxiety based disorders. In: Tuma R, Maser J (eds) *Anxiety and Anxiety Disorders.* Erlbaum, Hillsdale, NJ, pp. 199–244.

Mineka S, Cook M, and Miller S. (1984) Fear conditioned with escapable and inescapable shock: the effects of a feedback stimulus. *J Exper Psychol Anim Behav Proc* 10, 307–323.

Mineka S, Hendersen RW (1985) Controllability and predictability in acquired motivation. *Ann Rev Psychol* 36, 495–529.

Mineka S, Kihlstrom JF (1978) Unpredictable and uncontrollable events: A new perspective on experimental neurosis. *J Abnormal Psychol* 2, 256–271.

Mowrer H, Viek, P. (1948) An experimental analogue of fear from a sense of helplessness. *J Abnormal Soc Psychol* 43, 193–200.

Moye TB, Hyson RL, Grau, JW et al. (1983) Immunization of opioid analgesia: Effects of prior escapable shock on subsequentshock-induced and morphine-induced antinociception. *Learning Motiv* 14, 238–251.

Myers RD, Holman RB (1967) Failure of stress of electric shock to increase ethanol intake in rats. *Quart J Studies Alcohol* 28, 132–137.

Norman SB, Myers US, Wilkins KC et al. (2012) Review of biological mechanisms and pharmacological treatments of comorbid PTSD and substance use disorder. *Neuropharmacology* 62, 542–551.

Pavlov IP (1927) *Conditioned Reflexes.* London: Oxford University Press.

Petty F, Kramer GL, Wu JH et al. (1997) Posttraumatic stress and depression: A neurochemical anatomy of the learned helplessness animal model. In: Yehuda R, McFarlane AC (eds) Psychobiology of PTSD. *Anals NY Acad Sci* 822, 529–532.

Post RM, Weiss SRB, Smith MA (1995) Sensitization and kindling: Implications for the evolving neural substrate of PTSD. In: Friedman MJ, Charney DS, Deutsch AY (eds) *Neurobiological and Clinical Consequences of Stress: From Normal Adaptation to PTSD.* Lippincott-Raven Publishers, Philadelphia, pp. 209–229.

Powell BJ, Kamano DK, Martin LK (1966) Multiple factors affecting volitional consumption of alcohol in the Abrams Wistar rat. *Quart J Studies Alcohol* 27, 7–15.

Purdy, RH, Morrow, AL, Moore, PH, & Paul, SM. (1991) Stress-induced elevations of gamma-aminobutyric acid type A receptor-active steroids in the rat brain. *Proceedings of the National Academy of Sciences* 88, 4553–4557.

Rodgers RJ (1997) Animal models of "anxiety": Where next? *Behav Pharmacol* 8, 477–496.

Rodgers RJ, Haller J, Halasz J et al. (2003) 'One-trial sensitization' to the anxiolytic-like effects of cannabinoid receptor antagonist SR141716A in the mouse elevated plus maze. *Eur J Neurosci* 17, 1279–1286.

Rosellini R, Warren D, DeCola J (1987) Predictability and controllability: Differential effects upon contextual fear. *Learning Motivation* 18, 392–420.

Siegmund S, Vengeliene V, Singer MV et al. (2006) Influence of age at drinking onset on long-term ethanol self-administration with deprivation and stress phases. *Alcohol Clin Exp Res* 29, 1139–1145.

Singer MI, Anglin TM, Song LY et al. (1995) Adolescents' exposure to violence and associated symptoms of psychological trauma. *JAMA* 273, 477–482.

Sink KS, Segovia KN, Sink J et al. (2010) Potential anxiogenic effects of cannabinoid CB1 receptor antagonists/inverse agonists in rats: comparisons between AM4113, AM251, and the benzodiazepine inverse agonist FG-7142. *Eur Neuropsychopharmacol* 20, 112–122.

Skolnick P, Crawley JN, Glowa JR, Paul SM (1984) B-carboline-induced anxiety states. *Psychopathology* 17, 52–60.

Stafford NP, Jones AM, Drugan RC (2015) Ultrasonic vocalizations during intermittent swim stress forecasts resilience in a subsequent juvenile social exploration test of anxiety. *Behav Brain Res* 287, 196–199.

Stewart SH (1996) Alcohol abuse in individuals exposed to trauma: A critical review. *Psychol Bull* 120, 83–112.

Stuckey J, Marra S, Minor T et al. (1989) Changes in mu opiate receptors following inescapable shock. *Brain Res* 476, 167–169.

Sutton LC, Grahn RE, Wiertelak EP et al. (1997) Inescapable shock-induced potentiation of morphine analgesia in rats: involvement of opioid, GABAergic, and serotonergic mechanisms in the dorsal raphe nucleus. *Behav Neurosci* 111, 816.

Tejedor-Real P, Micó JA, Smadja C et al. (1998) Involvement of δ-opioid receptors in the effects induced by endogenous enkephalins on learned helplessness model. *Eur J Pharmacol* 354, 1–7.

van der Kolk BA (1987) *Psychological Trauma*. American Psychiatric Press, Washington, DC.

van der Kolk B, Greenberg M, Boyd H et al. (1985) Inescapable shock, neurotransmitters, and addiction to trauma: toward a psychobiology of post-traumatic stress. *Biol Psychiatry* 20, 314–325.

Vengeliene V, Siegmund S, Singer MV et al. (2003) A Comparative Study on Alcohol-Preferring Rat Lines: Effects of Deprivation and Stress Phases on Voluntary Alcohol Intake. *Alcohol Clin Exp Res* 27, 1048–1054.

Volpicelli JR, Ulm RR, Hopson N. (1990) The bidirectional effects of shock on alcohol preference in rats. *Alcohol Clin Exp Res* 14, 913–916.

Warner TA, Lowry CA, Stafford NP, Drugan, RC. Intermittent swim stress effects on anxiety behavior. Program No. 128.18. 2013 Neuroscience Meeting Planner Society for Neuroscience, 2013, San Diego, CA. Online.

Weiss JM (1968) Effects of coping responses on stress. *J Comp Physiol Psychol* 65, 251–260.

Weiss JM, Goodman PA, Losito BG et al. (1981) Behavioral depression produced by an uncontrollable stressor: relationship to norepinephrine, dopamine, and serotonin levels in various regions of rat brain. *Brain Res Rev* 3, 167–205.

Weiss JM, Stone EA, Harrell, N. (1970) Coping behavior and brain norepinephrine level in rats. *J Comp Physiol Psychol* 72, 153–160.

Will MJ, Der-Avakian A, Pepin JL et al. (2002) Modulation of the locomotor properties of morphine and amphetamine by uncontrollable stress. *Pharmacol Biochem Behav* 71, 345–351.

Will MJ, Watkins LR, Maier SF (1998) Uncontrollable stress potentiates morphine's rewarding properties. *Pharmacol Biochem Behav* 60, 655–664.

Williams JL, Drugan RC, Maier SF (1984) Exposure to uncontrollable stress alters withdrawal from morphine. *Behav Neurosci* 98, 836–846.

Wolpe, J, Experimental neuroses as learned behaviour (1952) *British Journal of Psychology* 43, 243–268.

Yehuda R, Antelman SM (1993) Criteria for rationally evaluating animal models of post-traumatic stress disorder *Biol Psychiatry* 33, 479–486.

Yehuda R, Kahana B, Schmeidler J et al. (1995) Impact of cumulative lifetime trauma and recent stress on current posttraumatic stress disorder symptoms in Holocaust survivors. *Am J Psychiatry* 152, 1815–1818.

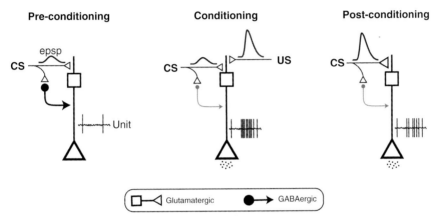

Figure 4.4 Hebbian fear conditioning plasticity in the lateral amygdala (LA). Prior to conditioning, conditioned stimulus (CS) presentations result in weak depolarization of LA neurons and little to no activation of downstream brain areas mediating conditioned fear responses. However, with CS–unconditioned stimulus (US) pairings, neurons are strongly depolarized resulting in initiation of an LTP-like process that strengthens the synapses between CS afferents and LA neurons. Following conditioning, CS presentations strongly depolarize LA neurons, triggering action potentials and neurotransmitter release to activate downstream targets. epsp, excitatory postsynaptic potential.

Posttraumatic Stress Disorder: From Neurobiology to Treatment, First Edition.
Edited by J. Douglas Bremner.
© 2016 John Wiley & Sons, Inc. Published 2016 by John Wiley & Sons, Inc.

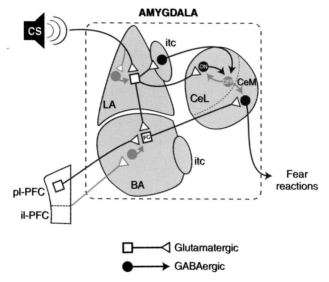

Figure 4.5 Amygdala FC circuitry. After conditioning, conditioned stimulus (CS) presentations activate lateral amygdala (LA) neurons, which project to basal amygdala (BA) "fear cells," intercalated cells (itc), and lateral/capsular division (CeL) of the central amygdala (CeA). CS processing in these regions leads to simultaneous stimulation and disinhibition of the medial division of the CeA (CeM). The CeM projects to downstream effector regions (e.g., periacqueductal gray) that mediate specific fear reactions (e.g., freezing). Prelimbic-prefrontal cortex (pl-PFC) neurons help sustain conditioned responding over longer intervals via projections to the BA. Pathways contributing to expression of conditioned fear responses are highlighted in red. il-PFC, infralimbic-PFC.

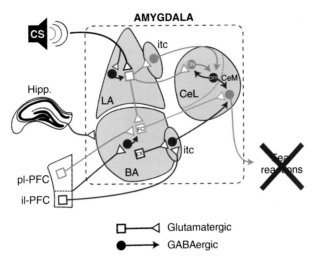

Figure 4.7 Amygdala fear extinction circuitry (adult). Extinction learning counteracts fear responding in a number of ways: (i) by strengthening feed-forward inhibition in the lateral amygdala (LA); (ii) through infralimbic-prefontal cortex (il-PFC) activation of intercalated cells (itc) that inhibit medial division of the central amygdala (CeM); (iii) through a subset of basal amygdala (BA) "extinction cells" that project to GABAergic neurons, possibly itc neurons, which inhibit CeM output; (iv) through synaptic depression of projections from PFC to BA "fear cells" (FC); and (v) through increased inhibition of fear conditioning cells in the BA by local interneurons. The hippocampus plays a critical role in gating extinction according to context via connections to the il-PFC and BA. Pathways contributing to expression of fear extinction are highlighted in blue.

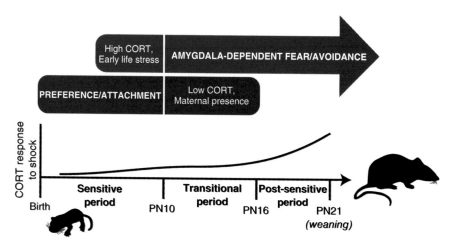

Figure 4.8 Ontogeny of fear conditioning. During the sensitive period, odor-shock conditioning produces an odor preference through an amygdala-independent mechanism. This odor conditioned stimulus (CS) can also support attachment interactions with the mother. As pups age and exit the stress hyporesponsive period, conditioning elicits a greater cortisol/corticosterone (CORT) response, which engages amygdala processes that produce fear/avoidance of the odor CS. Abusive rearing conditions can lead to abnormally high CORT responses in the late sensitive period and precocious fear/avoidance learning. Maternal presence during the transitional period weakens the CORT response and enables preference learning. After postnatal day 16 (PN16), conditioning produces fear/avoidance and CORT only modulates the degree of learning.

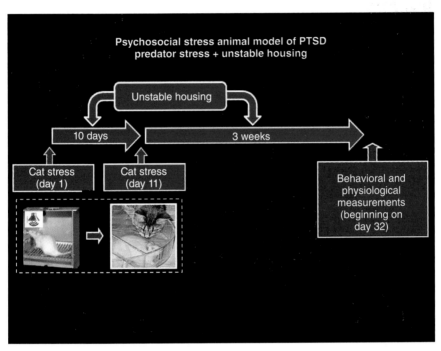

Figure 6.1 General description of the timeline of events in the psychosocial predator stress model of posttraumatic stress disorder (PTSD). Rats were exposed to a fear-conditioning chamber and tone followed by immobilization and cat exposure on days 1 and 11; unstable housing occurring daily from the first day of cat exposure through day 31. Beginning on day 32, fear conditioning memory testing, as well as all behavioral and physiological assessments took place.

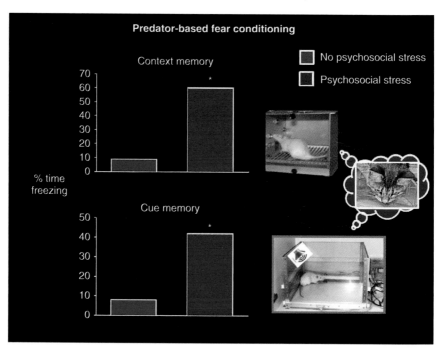

Figure 6.2 Rats exhibited strong fear memory for the context and cue associated with cat exposure. On days 1 and 11, rats were exposed to the fear conditioning chamber for 3 minutes, which terminated with a 20-second tone, followed by immobilization of the rats, followed by cat exposure, which took place in another room. On day 32, rats were re-exposed to the original chamber (context memory) and tone (cue memory) in a different chamber, with an assessment of their conditioning fear (freezing). The group exposed to the chamber/tone followed by cat exhibited significantly greater freezing in response to re-exposure to the context (top) and cue (bottom) compared with the control group, which had not been exposed to the cat. (Data adapted from Zoladz et al., 2008, 2012.)

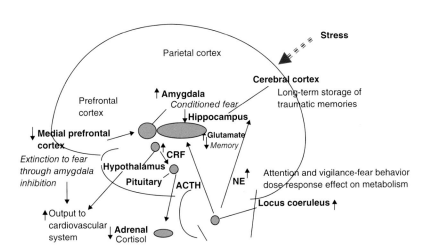

Figure 9.1 Neurotransmitters in posttraumatic stress disorder (PTSD). Neurotransmitters involved in the stress response and PTSD symptoms include norepinephrine (NE), with cell bodies in the locus coeruleus and projections to the amygdala, hippocampus, prefrontal cortex, and hypothalamus, and the hypothalamic–pituitary–adrenal (HPA) axis, with corticotropin-releasing factor (CRF) release from the hypothalamus, which stimulates adrenocorticotropic hormone (ACTH) release from the pituitary, and cortisol from the adrenal.

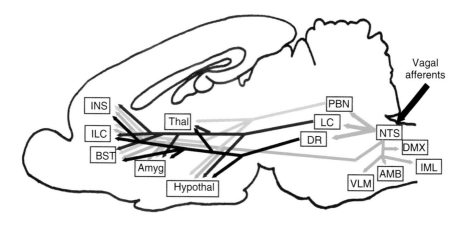

Figure 9.2 Afferents from the vagal nerve to central areas of the brain. AMB = nucleus ambiguous; DMX = dorsal motor nucleus of the vagus, IML = intermediolateral column of spinal cord (symp pregang); VLM = ventrolateral medulla; Amyg = amygdala; INS = insular cortex; ILC - infralimbic cortex; PBN = parabrachial nucleus; DR = dorsal Raphe; LC = locus coeruleus; Thal = thalamus; Hypothal = hypothalamus. (Used with permission from Thomas Cunningham PhD, University of North Texas Health Sciences Center.)

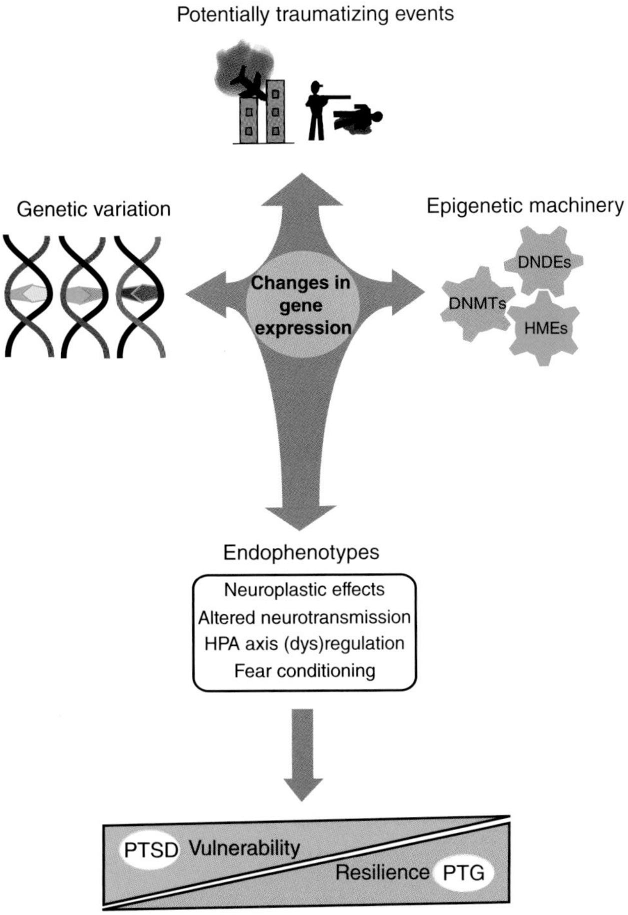

Figure 10.1 Simplified heuristic representation of the mechanisms leading to the development of posttraumatic stress disorder (PTSD) and posttraumatic growth (PTG). A complex interplay among potentially traumatizing events, multiple gene variants, and epigenetic mechanisms results in changes in the expression of genes that are involved in the regulation of neurotransmission, hypothalamic–pituitary–adrenal (HPA) axis activity, emotion and cognition. This shapes endophenotypes and, ultimately, vulnerability or resilience phenotypes. DNDEs, DNA demthylating enzymes; DNMTs, DNA methyltransferases; HMEs, histone-modifying enzymes.

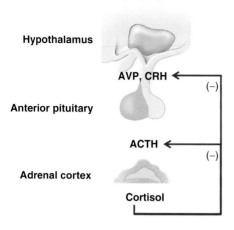

Figure 11.1 Normal functioning of the hypothalamic–pituitary–adrenal axis. The normal reaction to acute or brief stress or threat involves increases in cortisol and corticotropin-releasing hormone (CRH) and arginine vasopressin (AVP). CRH stimulates the release of adrenocorticotropic hormone (ACTH) from the pituitary, which in turn stimulates the production of cortisol in the adrenal cortex. Cortisol provides negative feedback and inhibits the further release of CRH, AVP and ACTH, leading to the containment of the stress response and return to homeostasis.

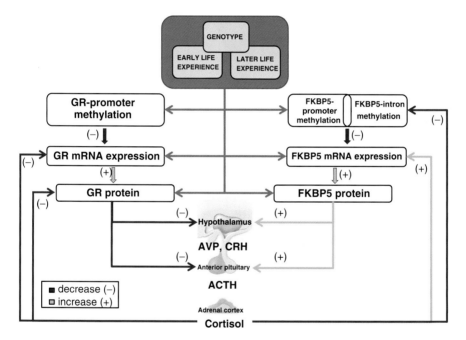

Figure 11.2 Conceptual model of hypothalamic–pituitary–adrenal axis regulation by glucocorticoid receptor (GR) and FK506 binding protein 5 (FKBP5). Early life experience (e.g., adversity) and later life stressors (e.g., trauma) may influence GR and FKBP5 methylation; these influences may interact with genotype to increase risk. Higher GR responsiveness and lower cortisol in PTSD may result from lower GR methylation and expression. Low cortisol levels probably contribute to higher *FKBP5* methylation and lower *FKBP5* gene expression, corresponding to lower FKBP5 protein expression, and ultimately more GR responsiveness (glucocorticoid negative feedback) at the hypothalamus and pituitary. Green arrows indicate a positive influence (+) and red arrows a negative influence (−). Blue arrows depict a relationship. GR encoded by the *NR3C1* gene, FKBP5 FK506 binding protein 5 encoded by the *FKBP5* gene. CRH, corticotropin-releasing hormone; AVP, arginine vasopressin; ACTH, adrenocorticotropic hormone.

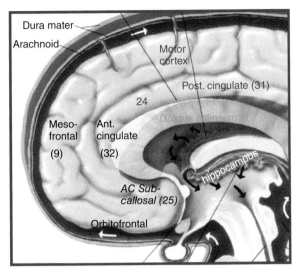

Figure 12.1 Brain regions involved stress and emotion. The medial prefrontal cortex includes parts of the prefrontal cortex, including mesofrontal cortex (Brodmann's area (BA 9), anterior cingulate (AC, BA 32), subcallosal gyrus (BA 25), and orbitofrontal cortex. Other areas shown include the motor cortex, posterior cingulate (BA 31), and hippocampus.

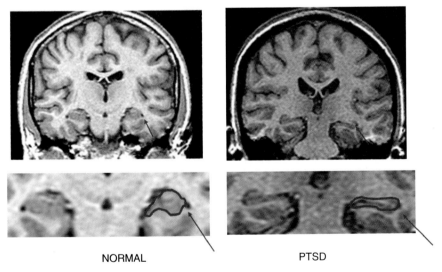

NORMAL   PTSD

Figure 12.2 Hippocampal volume on magnetic resonance imaging in posttraumatic stress disorder (PTSD). There is smaller hippocampal volume in this patient with PTSD compared with a control (from Bremner, 2005).

Medial PFC
(BA 25)

AC
(BA32)

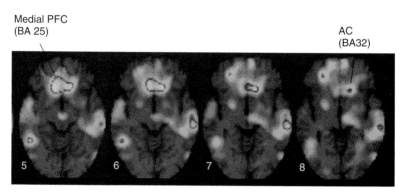

Figure 12.3 Medial prefrontal cortex (PFC) dysfunction in PTSD. There was a failure of medial prefrontal activation in a group of combat veterans with PTSD compared with combat veterans without PTSD during exposure to traumatic combat-related slides and sounds. The yellow areas represent decreased function in the medial PFC, which includes both Brodmann's rea (BA) 25 and anterior cingulate (AC) BA 32. Each image represents an adjacent slice of the brain, with the yellow areas representing a composite of areas of relative decrease in blood flow in PTSD patients compared with controls (from Bremner, 2005).

CHAPTER 6

Psychosocial predator stress model of PTSD based on clinically relevant risk factors for trauma-induced psychopathology

Phillip R. Zoladz[1] & David Diamond[2]

[1] Department of Psychology, Sociology, & Criminal Justice, Ohio Northern University, Ada, OH, USA
[2] Departments of Psychology and Molecular Pharmacology & Physiology, University of South Florida, Tampa, FL, USA

6.1 Introduction

Posttraumatic stress disorder (PTSD) is a psychiatric disorder which is unique in that it has a known etiological feature composed of a single trauma or repeated life-threatening experiences, such as wartime combat, a motor vehicle accident, rape or other assault to an individual or to a loved one (*Diagnostic and Statistical Manual of Mental Disorders-V* [DSM-V]). The horrific triggering experience(s) can transform a healthy individual into one with a cluster of debilitating symptoms, including hypervigilance, cognitive deficits and pathologically intense and intrusive memories of the trauma, which can persist for a lifetime. PTSD is not a modern disorder, as the symptoms of traumatized individuals have been described throughout recorded human history. For example, the biographer Plutarch wrote of PTSD-like symptoms involving chronic anxiety, sleep disturbances, and alcohol abuse of Gaius Marius, a Roman General in the first century BC, who was (Plutarch, 1920):

> … tortured by his reflections and bringing into review his long wandering, his flights, and his perils, as he was driven over land and sea, he fell into a state of dreadful despair, and was prey to nightly terrors and harassing dreams … since above all things he dreaded the sleepless nights, he gave himself up to drinking-bouts and drunkenness at unseasonable hours and in a manner unsuited to his years, trying thus to induce sleep as a way of escape from his anxious thoughts" (p. 594).

Posttraumatic Stress Disorder: From Neurobiology to Treatment, First Edition.
Edited by J. Douglas Bremner.
© 2016 John Wiley & Sons, Inc. Published 2016 by John Wiley & Sons, Inc.

In the 19th century, the emotional and physical toll of combat on soldiers in the US Civil War was referred to as "soldier's heart," and following World War I, trauma symptoms were referred to as "shell shock," because of the presumed relationship of the heightened anxiety and startle reactivity to the intense sounds and stress of combat. In 1952, the persistent effects of psychological trauma were formally termed "gross stress reaction" in DSM-I, and in 1980 the syndrome was given its contemporary nomenclature, "post-traumatic stress disorder," with the publication of the DSM-III (Andreasen, 2010).

Logistical challenges and ethical restrictions limit the study of the biology of PTSD under controlled conditions in human subjects. Therefore, insight into the neurobiology and neuroendocrinology of the persistent effects of trauma on brain and behavior may be achieved indirectly through translational approaches involving the study of traumatic stress in animals. This approach has spawned a vast amount of research on the effects of exposing animals, primarily rodents, to strong stressful experiences followed by behavioral and physiological testing, which, in theory, provides insight into PTSD in traumatized people. However, we assert that there remain conceptual limitations to linking the study of stress in animals to generating a syndrome which resembles clinical features of PTSD. For example, people who experience a horrific event, as well as rats exposed to a painful shock, can have a strong memory of the trauma, but an emotional memory of an experience alone does not sufficiently represent the cluster of symptoms that define PTSD. PTSD develops from the inability to cope with the memory of the trauma; the memory itself is only one component of the entire syndrome. A multifaceted goal for any animal model of PTSD, therefore, is to administer a strong stressful (traumatic) experience to an animal, and then to demonstrate that the animal has a conditioned fear memory for that experience, and that the trauma produces a cluster of behavioral and biological abnormalities that resemble those found in people diagnosed with PTSD.

This chapter reviews a subset of research studies that have addressed this goal. First, we provide a description of the basic features of PTSD, followed by a global review of diverse preclinical approaches that have modeled PTSD. We then discuss our animal model of PTSD, which is based on predator exposure administered in the context of clinically relevant risk factors, including social instability. The pathological outcomes generated in our model may provide insight into behavioral and biological abnormalities that develop in the subset of traumatized people that develop PTSD, as well as to provide a model that optimizes the development of novel pharmacotherapies for PTSD.

6.2 General characteristics of PTSD

Individuals exposed to life-threatening trauma, such as wartime combat, motor vehicle accidents, or natural disasters, are at risk for developing PTSD. People who develop PTSD respond to a traumatic event with intense feelings of fear, helplessness, or horror and subsequently endure chronic psychological distress by repeatedly re-living their trauma through intrusive, flashback memories (Ehlers et al., 2004; Hackmann et al., 2004; Reynolds et al., 1999; Speckens et al., 2007). These characteristics of the disorder foster the development of other debilitating symptoms, including persistent anxiety, exaggerated startle and cognitive impairments, as well as a predisposition toward substance abuse and comorbid psychiatric disorders, such as major depressive disorder (Nemeroff et al., 2006; Stam et al., 2007).

Posttraumatic stress disorder is also characterized by a complex aberrant biological profile involving several physiological systems, including the hypothalamus–pituitary–adrenal (HPA) axis and the sympathetic nervous system (SNS; Krystal & Neumeister, 2009; Pervanidou et al., 2010; Vidovic et al., 2011; Zoladz & Diamond, 2013). For instance, although findings have been mixed, extensive work has reported abnormally low baseline levels of cortisol in PTSD, which has been associated with the presence of enhanced negative feedback of the HPA axis and an elevated density of glucocorticoid receptors in these individuals (Yehuda, 2005, 2009). The reduced basal cortisol levels with PTSD do not appear to reflect adrenal insufficiency, as PTSD patients display robust HPA axis responsiveness, as evidenced by greater cortisol levels in response to, and in anticipation of, acute laboratory stressors, compared with control subjects (Bremner et al., 2003; Liberzon et al., 1999; Elzinga et al., 2003). People with PTSD also demonstrate greater baseline and stress-induced elevations of SNS activity (Buckley & Kaloupek, 2001), as measured by elevated baseline heart rate (HR), systolic blood pressure (BP) and diastolic BP, findings that resonate with research reporting an association between PTSD and increased risk for cardiovascular disease (Boscarino & Chang, 1999; Kubzansky et al., 2007).

In response to traumatic reminders and standard laboratory stressors, people with PTSD display significantly greater increases in HR, BP, skin conductance, epinephrine, and norepinephrine than do control subjects. Another indication of accentuated SNS activity in PTSD patients is the exaggerated responsiveness (i.e., greater increases in HR, greater increases in BP, greater expression of anxiety-like behavior) they exhibit following administration of yohimbine, an α_2-adrenergic receptor antagonist that leads to increased central norepinephrine activity (Bremner et al., 1996, 1997; Southwick et al., 1993, 1999). These findings, as well as evidence of greater norepinephrine levels in PTSD patients (Krystal & Neumeister, 2009; Amihaesei & Mungiu, 2012; Strawn & Geracioti,

2008), have suggested a major role for exaggerated noradrenergic activity in the hyperarousal component of PTSD (Strawn & Geracioti, 2008).

Whereas numerous brain regions contribute to the behavioral and physiological manifestations of PTSD, much of the research has focused on the involvement of three primary structures, the amygdala, prefrontal cortex (PFC) and hippocampus (Bremner, 2007; Pitman et al., 2012; Zoladz & Diamond, 2013). People with PTSD exhibit abnormal fear responses and diminished extinction of conditioned fear, which is suggestive of amygdala hyperactivity (Elzinga & Bremner, 2002; Koenigs & Grafman, 2009; Orr et al., 2000; Peri et al., 2000). Studies have also shown that PTSD patients have decreased PFC volume (Carrion et al., 2001; De Bellis et al., 2002; Fennema-Notestine et al., 2002; Rauch et al., 2003; Woodward et al., 2006; Yamasue et al., 2003) and reduced activation of the PFC in response to the presentation of trauma-related, or fear-eliciting, stimuli (Bremner et al., 1999; Britton et al., 2005; Lanius et al., 2001; Lindauer et al., 2004; Shin et al., 2004). PTSD patients are also impaired in tasks involving executive functioning, indicating impaired PFC functioning. Given the importance of the PFC in inhibiting amygdala-modulated emotional responses, reduced PFC activity in PTSD patients could promote amygdala hyperactivity, as well as the hypervigilance component of the disorder. Moreover, repeated activation of the traumatic memory, which would involve activation of the amygdala in conjunction with impaired PFC functioning, would contribute to traumatic memories becoming even more intrusive and debilitating over time.

Extensive work has also shown that people with PTSD have cognitive deficits that are suggestive of hippocampal dysfunction. This has been documented by reports of smaller hippocampal volume (Grossman et al., 2002; Liberzon et al., 2008; Nutt & Malizia, 2004; Shin et al., 2006) and impaired hippocampus-dependent learning and memory in PTSD patients (Bremner et al., 1995; Gilbertson et al., 2001). However, close scrutiny of the literature suggests that severe deficits in hippocampal functioning with PTSD are relatively uncommon, with numerous studies that have not provided evidence of a global hippocampal impairment of hippocampal functioning in PTSD (Zoladz & Diamond, 2013). Moreover, impaired hippocampal functioning may actually be a risk factor for, rather than an outcome of, PTSD (Gilbertson et al., 2002; Pitman et al., 2006).

In summary, clinical research has provided strong evidence of increased sympathetic activation which underlies the hypervigilance component of PTSD, as well as PFC and amygdala abnormalities. Thus, symptoms including impaired attention, working memory, and executive functioning all point to impaired PFC functioning in conjunction with hyper-responsiveness, and perhaps hypertrophy, of the amygdala in PTSD. However, whether there are hippocampus-specific deficits in PTSD remains to be determined.

6.3 Preclinical models of PTSD

Whereas clinical research is vital for the implementation of novel treatments, animal models of PTSD provide a crucial complementary component in this process. In addition to their key role in establishing the safety and initial efficacy of novel compounds, animal models are valuable in three key areas of treatment development. First, they allow the rapid, cost-effective development of proof of concept studies to identify the most promising pharmacological candidates that can block trauma-induced behavioral and physiological abnormalities. This approach, with direct molecular assays of neural tissue, can improve our understanding of the mechanism of action of these compounds. Second, animal research provides for the assessment of the effects of interventions initiated prior to, or soon after, trauma occurs, which provides the opportunity to develop preventive strategies that would be high risk, expensive and potentially unethical to undertake in people. Finally, animal studies provide for the study of direct tests for different PTSD comorbidities and risk factors that might influence treatment responses in people, such as early life abuse, gender, and traumatic brain injury.

The development of valid and informative animal models of psychiatric disorders, in general, and PTSD in particular, has been a challenge. The human response to trauma can be considered to be composed of two distinct components, both of which should be included in animal models of PTSD. First, the person with PTSD typically has a pathologically intense and intrusive memory for the traumatic experience. Hence, the person commonly avoids any cues associated with the traumatic experience. Therefore, an animal model should include a component in which the traumatized animal exhibits a powerful fear-provoking memory for the stressful experience. Second, in patients with PTSD there are numerous abnormalities in their physiology and behavior. That is, a person with PTSD not only exhibits an intense memory for the traumatic event which may last for a lifetime, he or she also experiences significant post-trauma changes in physiology and behavior, including comorbid psychiatric disorders such as depression. Therefore, a clinically relevant animal model of PTSD should generate a powerful memory of the traumatic experience, as well as persistent changes in physiology and behavior in common with people with PTSD.

Preclinical researchers have used several types of stressors to model aspects of PTSD in animals (Stam, 2007). Such stressors have included electric shock (Garrick et al., 2001; Li et al., 2006; Milde et al., 2003; Pynoos et al., 1996; Rau et al., 2005; Sawamura et al., 2004; Servatius et al., 1995; Shimizu et al., 2004, 2006; Siegmund & Wotjak, 2007a,b; Wakizono et al., 2007), underwater trauma (Cohen & Zohar, 2005; Richter-Levin, 1998), stress–restress and single prolonged stress paradigms (Harvey et al. , 2003; Khan & Liberzon, 2004; Kohda et al., 2007; Liberzon et al., 1997; Takahashi et al., 2006) and exposure to predators (Adamec & Shallow, 1993; Adamec et al., 1997, 1999a,b; 2006, 2007) or predator-related cues (Cohen & Zohar, 2005; Cohen et al., 2000, 2006; Goswami et al., 2013). The stressors employed in these studies typically produce behavioral signs of anxiety that persist beyond the time of the stress experience, and in some cases, exaggerated startle, cognitive impairments, enhanced fear conditioning, resistance to fear extinction, and reduced social interaction.

Although these studies have reported physiological and behavioral changes resembling those observed in people with PTSD, most have utilized only a small set of assessments, such as stress-induced changes in anxiety, without assessing the extensive abnormalities that make up routine symptoms of PTSD. Moreover, many of these studies have evaluated stress-induced changes in responses for a relatively short period of time. Finally, it is quite rare to find animal models of PTSD that assess the animal's memory for the traumatic experience; typically the stress exposure is used only to disturb post-stress brain and behavior, instead of assessing the memory for the trauma experience itself.

We consider all of the aforementioned approaches to have contributed toward our understanding of how traumatic stress changes aspects of behavior and physiology, in general, and how a subset have enhanced our understanding of the neurobiology and endocrinology of PTSD. In the following section, we discuss our psychosocial predator-based animal model of PTSD and how our findings may shed light on the development of novel pharmacotherapies for trauma, as well as neurobiological and endocrine abnormalities observed in people diagnosed with PTSD.

6.4 Psychosocial predator stress model of PTSD

Pioneering research by Caroline and Robert Blanchard described how rats exhibit a strong fear of a predator, such as a cat (Blanchard et al., 1975). Their work also contributed to the development of studies examining predator scent, provided, for example, by cat or fox urine, as a stress-provoking stimulus which can substitute for the live animal (Apfelbach et al., 2005; Rosen, 2004). Further evidence of the effectiveness of predator exposure as a means with which to generate a fear response are findings in which cat exposure or predator scent activates the HPA axis (Morrow et al., 2000). At a functional level, extensive research demonstrates that predator exposure exerts a profound impairment of spatial memory and a suppression of synaptic plasticity in the hippocampus (Diamond et al., 1999; Mesches et al., 1999; Park et al., 2008; Vanelzakker et al., 2011; Woodson et al., 2003 ; Zoladz et al., 2012). It has also been reported that live predator exposure can enhance synaptic plasticity in the amygdala (Vouimba et al., 2006). Therefore, the ethological relevance and potency of predator exposure provides a highly relevant approach toward producing an intense, purely psychological, fear response in rodent models of PTSD.

Based on these observations of the instinctual fear generated in rats by cat exposure, our group has published a series of studies based on a predator-exposure animal model of PTSD (Roth et al., 2011; Zoladz et al., 2008, 2012, 2013). The primary components of the PTSD model were based on trauma-induction features that are known to be associated with a greater susceptibility of a subset of traumatized people to develop PTSD. Specifically, a subset of the DSM-V criteria for the diagnosis of PTSD includes the following three conditions: PTSD can be triggered by an event that involves threatened death or a threat to one's physical integrity; a person's response to the event involves intense fear, helplessness, or horror; and in the aftermath of the trauma, the person feels as if the traumatic event were recurring, including a sense of re-living the experience. Therefore, in our work, rats are immobilized and placed in close proximity to a cat. As noted, rats have an instinctual and intense fear of cats (Blanchard et al., 1990, 2003, 2005; Hubbard et al., 2004), which, in theory, would be intensified by their inability to escape (Amat et al., 2005; Bland et al., 2006, 2007; Maier & Watkins, 2005). Although there is no physical contact between the rats and cat, the experience produces a profound physiological stress response in the rats, including elevated HR, BP and corticosterone levels.

A core symptom of PTSD is the repeated "re-experiencing" of the traumatic event that people with PTSD suffer in response to activation of intense and intrusive memories of their trauma. For this reason, we included a "re-experiencing" component in our animal model of PTSD by giving rats the second cat exposure 10 days after the first. Moreover, the first predator exposure occurs during the light cycle, and the second predator exposure occurs during the dark cycle, thereby adding an element of unpredictability as to when the rats might re-experience the traumatic event. A lack of predictability in one's environment is a major factor in the development of PTSD, as a means with which to increase the susceptibility of a subset of people to develop PTSD in response to trauma, as well as to influence the later expression of PTSD symptoms (Orr et al., 1990; Regehr et al., 2007; Solomon et al., 1988, 1989).

The second cat exposure occurred 10 days after the first, based on findings of Chattarji's group, who observed increased dendritic arborization of amygdala neurons 10 days after a single immobilization experience (Mitra et al., 2005). In theory, therefore, the second cat exposure on day 11 activated a sensitized amygdala with hypertrophied neurons, thereby reinforcing stress-induced changes in brain and behavior that would have been initiated by the first cat exposure. The second exposure of rats to the cat also relates to work showing that PTSD develops in some people only after they have repeated traumatic experiences and work revealing that prolonged exposure to trauma increases the likelihood of developing symptoms of PTSD (Gurvits et al., 1996; Resnick et al., 1995; Taylor & Cahill, 2002). Thus, the repeated inescapable cat exposure served as a powerful reminder of the stress experience, as well as a manipulation that potentially increased the likelihood of the rats to exhibit physiological and behavioral seque-lae that can be broadly applied to people who develop PTSD as a result of multiple traumatic experiences.

An additional risk factor for PTSD is insufficient social support and an unstable social life (Andrews et al., 2003; Boscarino, 1995; Brewin et al., 2000; Ullman & Filipas, 2001). Therefore, we included daily social instability in the model to increase the likelihood of producing long-lasting sequelae in the rats. Beginning with the day of the first cat exposure, the stressed rats are exposed to unstable housing conditions for the next 31 days. The rats are pair-housed, and every day, their cohort pair combination is randomly changed, which results in the stressed rats having different cage mates on a daily basis during the 31-day stress period. Following this 31-day stress period, the rats are given a battery of physiological and behavioral assessments to examine the development of PTSD-like seque-lae in the animals. The social instability component is an integral component of the model, as predator exposure alone does not produce persistent PTSD-like changes in the behavior of the rats (Zoladz et al., 2008).

We have found that exposing rats to our psychosocial predator-based animal model of PTSD results in a number of physiological and behavioral abnormali-ties, all of which are remarkably similar to those observed in people with PTSD. For instance, 3 weeks after the second predator exposure, rats exposed to our animal model of PTSD exhibit reduced growth rate, reduced thymus weight, greater adrenal gland weight, increased anxiety, exaggerated startle, impaired memory, greater cardiovascular and hormonal reactivity to an acute stressor and an exaggerated physiological and behavioral response to the α_2-adrenergic receptor antagonist, yohimbine (Zoladz et al., 2008). Importantly, these effects depended on the combination of both cat exposures and daily social instability. Thus two cat exposures in conjunction with social instability produced greater anxiogenic effects on rat behavior than either cat exposure or social instability alone (Zoladz et al., 2008).

As we mentioned earlier in this chapter, a pathologically intense memory of the trauma is a hallmark feature of PTSD. Therefore, it was important to include a method with which to measure the rat's memory for the cat exposure experi-ences. To accomplish this goal, in recent work we measured the rat's memory for trauma indirectly by placing the rat in a fear conditioning chamber immediately prior to each of the two cat exposures (Zoladz et al., 2012). It is notable that the rats were not exposed to any aversive stimuli while they were in the chamber. The rats were in the chamber for 3 minutes, and during the last 30 seconds of each exposure, they were presented with a tone. Then, they were removed from the chamber and immediately immobilized and given the 1-hour cat exposure. The strategy behind this manipulation was to use a form of classical conditioning, which traditionally involves the pairing of a neutral stimulus, such as a tone, with a strong stimulus, such as shock to the tail. An illustration of the entire sequence

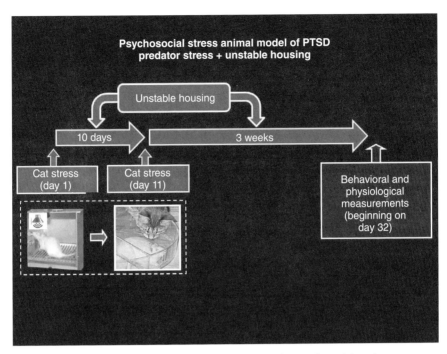

Figure 6.1 General description of the timeline of events in the psychosocial predator stress model of posttraumatic stress disorder (PTSD). Rats were exposed to a fear-conditioning chamber and tone followed by immobilization and cat exposure on days 1 and 11; unstable housing occurring daily from the first day of cat exposure through day 31. Beginning on day 32, fear conditioning memory testing, as well as all behavioral and physiological assessments took place. (*See color plate section for the color representation of this figure.*)

of events in the psychosocial predator stress model, including the predator-based fear conditioning component, is depicted in Figure 6.1.

As a result of the pairing of the two stimuli, cat-exposed rats exhibit evidence of memory by displaying fear when later exposed only to the tone. In our case, rats associated the chamber and the tone with the fear-provoking cat experience. The association that rats form between the chamber and cue with the cat is analogous to the panic response people with PTSD exhibit when they experience a cue, such as an odor or a sound, that reminds them of their traumatic experience. Our test of the rat's memory of the cat was confirmed with the finding that psychosocially stressed rats exhibited significant immobility (fear memory-induced freezing) in response to being returned to the chamber, as well as the tone, paired with the cat exposures. These findings are illustrated in Figure 6.2. Thus, our animal model of PTSD is unique in that the rats stressed in this paradigm display a powerful memory for the context and cue associated with the predator stress experiences, and they exhibit physiological and behavioral symptoms that occur in people with PTSD.

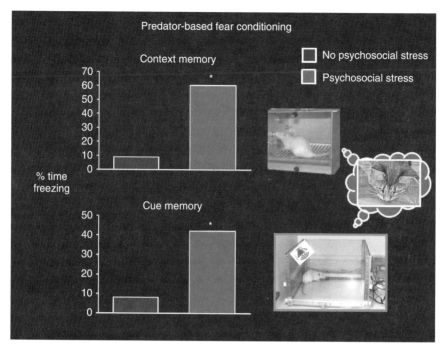

Figure 6.2 Rats exhibited strong fear memory for the context and cue associated with cat exposure. On days 1 and 11, rats were exposed to the fear conditioning chamber for 3 minutes, which terminated with a 20-second tone, followed by immobilization of the rats, followed by cat exposure, which took place in another room. On day 32, rats were re-exposed to the original chamber (context memory) and tone (cue memory) in a different chamber, with an assessment of their conditioning fear (freezing). The group exposed to the chamber/tone followed by cat exhibited significantly greater freezing in response to re-exposure to the context (top) and cue (bottom) compared with the control group, which had not been exposed to the cat. (Data adapted from Zoladz et al., 2008, 2012.) (*See color plate section for the color representation of this figure.*)

As discussed, PTSD is characterized by an aberrant biological profile in multiple physiological systems. One of the most extensively researched physiological systems in people with PTSD is the HPA axis. Empirical investigations of the adrenal hormone, cortisol, have often reported abnormally low baseline levels of cortisol in PTSD patients. One explanation for the presence of low baseline cortisol levels in people with PTSD is that the disorder is associated with enhanced negative feedback inhibition of the HPA axis. Indeed, studies have reported that people with PTSD display an increased number and sensitivity of glucocorticoid receptors and an increased suppression of cortisol and adrenocorticotropic hormone (ACTH) following the administration of dexamethasone, a synthetic glucocorticoid (Duval et al., 2004; Goenjian et al., 1996; Grossman et al., 2003; Stein et al., 1997; Yehuda et al., 1995, 2002, 2004) . Studies have also employed the dexamethasone-corticotropin-releasing hormone (CRH) challenge paradigm to study abnormal HPA axis functioning in people with PTSD. An advantage of this paradigm is that the subjects are treated with dexamethasone prior to CRH administration, thereby activating negative feedback mechanisms before acute HPA axis stimulation. Studies employing this paradigm have generally reported reduced ACTH levels in dexamethasone-treated PTSD patients who were subsequently administered CRH (de Kloet et al., 2006; Rinne et al., 2002; Strohle et al., 2008).

Based on the clinical findings of abnormal HPA activity in PTSD, we examined the effects of our animal model on rat corticosterone levels at baseline and following dexamethasone administration. We found that, at baseline, psychosocially stressed animals exhibited significantly lower corticosterone levels than non-stressed rats. Following dexamethasone administration, psychosocially stressed rats displayed a blunted increase in corticosterone levels and a more rapid post-stressor recovery of those levels, relative to non-stressed control animals, following administration of an acute stressor (Zoladz et al., 2012). These findings bear resemblance to those from human studies employing the dexamethasone–CRH challenge paradigm and suggest that our PTSD regimen might result in enhanced negative feedback of the HPA axis.

One of the most promising areas of PTSD research is the study of the interaction of genetic and epigenetic factors with environmental stressors (Zoladz & Diamond, 2013). Epigenetic alterations of the brain-derived neurotrophic factor (BDNF) gene have been linked to brain functioning, memory, stress, and neuropsychiatric disorders (Domschke, 2012; Zovkic & Sweatt, 2013). Therefore, we examined whether there was a link between our model and BDNF DNA methylation. We found that psychosocially stressed rats exhibited increased BDNF DNA methylation in the dorsal hippocampus, with the most robust hypermethylation detected in the dorsal CA1 subregion (Roth et al., 2011). On the other hand, psychosocially stressed rats also displayed decreased methylation in the ventral hippocampus (CA3). No changes in BDNF DNA methylation were detected in the medial prefrontal cortex or basolateral amygdala. Finally, we also observed decreased levels of BDNF mRNA in both the dorsal and ventral CA1 regions of psychosocially stressed animals. These results provide evidence that traumatic stress occurring in adulthood can induce CNS gene methylation and, specifically, support the hypothesis that epigenetic marking of the BDNF gene may underlie hippocampal dysfunction in response to traumatic stress. Furthermore, this work provides support for the speculative notion that altered hippocampal BDNF DNA methylation is a cellular mechanism underlying the persistent cognitive deficits which are prominent features of the pathophysiology of PTSD.

One goal of our animal model of PTSD was to assess whether pharmacotherapeutic agents can block the stress-induced abnormalities. We recently examined the differential effectiveness of amitriptyline (tricyclic antidepressant), clonidine (noradrenergic antagonist), and tianeptine (glutamate modulator) in blocking the physiological and behavioral sequelae manifested by our psychosocial predator stress model (Zoladz et al., 2013). We found that while each of the drugs had some sort of therapeutic effects, tianeptine was the only agent to prevent the effects of chronic psychosocial stress on our entire battery of physiological and behavioral end-points. Specifically, tianeptine blocked the expression of fear-conditioned memory in psychosocially stressed rats when they were re-exposed to the context and cue that were paired with the two cat exposures, and also prevented the effects of psychosocial stress on anxiety, startle, cardiovascular reactivity, growth rate, adrenal gland weight and thymus weight. Importantly, these salutary effects of tianeptine occurred in the absence of any adverse side-effects. To emphasize that the design of our experiment had clinical relevance, we did not begin the administration of pharmacological agents until the day after the stress paradigm commenced (i.e., 1 day after the first cat exposure). Treatment beginning 24 hours after exposing rats to an intense stressor is potentially relevant to treatment applications begun in people within 24 hours of a traumatic experience. This strategy may also highlight the importance of beginning a treatment regimen as soon as possible after a person experiences trauma.

6.5 Summary: the challenge of modeling PTSD in animals

In this chapter we have addressed the challenge of translating stress research in animals to clinically relevant factors involved in PTSD. Too often, research on animals focuses on either the stress response alone or the memory of the stress procedure, as measured by fear conditioning, which we have suggested addresses only fragments of the broad spectrum of PTSD symptoms. We emphasized the importance of appreciating the range of clinically relevant features of PTSD, which includes the intrusive memory of the traumatic experience, in conjunction with risk factors, such as social support, and the chronic anxiety following trauma, because all components interact to influence whether or not a traumatized individual will develop PTSD. Hence, PTSD results from the impaired ability to cope with the traumatic experience and the memory it generated, rather than PTSD being composed of a strong memory of the trauma alone. We therefore developed an animal model of PTSD which is based on clinically relevant features of susceptibility of an individual to develop stress-induced psychopathology. Specifically, we administered predator exposure to immobilized rats to provide them with a life-threatening experience in conjunction with an inability to escape. In theory, this experience to the rat is analogous to the PTSD induction feature involving a condition that evokes fear and horror in conjunction with a life-threatening experience. However, despite the fact that this experience provokes a powerful stress response in rats, cat exposure alone does not produce persistent PTSD-like abnormalities in behavior. It was only when we combined predator exposure with social instability that we observed persistent behavioral and physiological abnormalities in the rats, which are remarkably similar to those found in people diagnosed with PTSD, including a strong memory of the trauma, increased anxiety, exaggerated startle, impaired memory for new information, increased cardiovascular and hormonal reactivity to an acute stressor, abnormally low corticosterone levels, increased sensitivity to dexamethasone, and an exaggerated physiological and behavioral response to the α_2-adrenergic receptor antagonist, yohimbine. Moreover, we have provided guidance for clinical research on PTSD with the finding of epigenetic modifications (methylation) of the BDNF gene in the hippocampus, which may provide the basis for impaired cognitive functioning in traumatized people. Finally, our work has identified the antidepressant tianeptine as a potentially useful pharmacological approach toward treatment of the cluster of symptoms found in PTSD.

Acknowledgements

The authors were supported by Career Scientist and Merit Review Awards from the Veterans Affairs Department during the production of this review. The opinions expressed in this chapter are those of the authors and not of the Department of Veterans Affairs or the US Government.

References

Adamec R, Muir C, Grimes M et al. (2007) Involvement of noradrenergic and corticoid receptors in the consolidation of the lasting anxiogenic effects of predator stress. *Behav Brain Res* 179, 192–207.

Adamec RE, Blundell J, Burton P (2006) Relationship of the predatory attack experience to neural plasticity, pCREB expression and neuroendocrine response. *Neurosci Biobehav Rev* 30, 356–375.

Adamec RE, Burton P, Shallow T et al. (1999a) NMDA receptors mediate lasting increases in anxiety-like behavior produced by the stress of predator exposure--implications for anxiety associated with posttraumatic stress disorder. *Physiol Behav* 65, 723–737.

Adamec RE, Burton P, Shallow T et al. (1999b) Unilateral block of NMDA receptors in the amygdala prevents predator stress-induced lasting increases in anxiety-like behavior and unconditioned startle--effective hemisphere depends on the behavior. *Physiol Behav* 65, 739–751.

Adamec RE, Shallow T, Budgell J (1997) Blockade of CCK(B) but not CCK(A) receptors before and after the stress of predator exposure prevents lasting increases in anxiety-like behavior: implications for anxiety associated with posttraumatic stress disorder. *Behav Neurosci* 111, 435–449.

Adamec RE, Shallow T (1993) Lasting effects on rodent anxiety of a single exposure to a cat. *Physiol Behav* 54, 101–109.

Amat J, Baratta MV, Paul E et al. (2005) Medial prefrontal cortex determines how stressor controllability affects behavior and dorsal raphe nucleus. *Nat Neurosci* 8, 365–371.

Amihaesei IC, Mungiu OC (2012) Posttraumatic stress disorder: neuroendocrine and pharmacotherapeutic approach. *Rev Med Chir Soc Med Nat Iasi* 116, 563–566.

Andreasen NC (2010) Posttraumatic stress disorder: a history and a critique. *Ann NY Acad Sci* 1208, 67–71.

Andrews B, Brewin CR, Rose S (2003) Gender, social support, and PTSD in victims of violent crime. *J Trauma Stress* 16, 421–427.

Apfelbach R, Blanchard CD, Blanchard RJ et al. (2005) The effects of predator odors in mammalian prey species: a review of field and laboratory studies. *Neurosci Biobehav Rev* 29, 1123–1144.

Blanchard DC, Canteras NS, Markham CM et al. (2005) Lesions of structures showing FOS expression to cat presentation: effects on responsivity to a Cat, Cat odor, and nonpredator threat. *Neurosci Biobehav Rev* 29, 1243–1253.

Blanchard DC, Griebel G, Blanchard RJ (2003) Conditioning and residual emotionality effects of predator stimuli: some reflections on stress and emotion. *Prog Neuro-Psychopharmacol Biol Psychiatry* 27, 1177–1185.

Blanchard RJ, Blanchard DC, Rodgers J et al. (1990) The characterization and modelling of antipredator defensive behavior. [Review]. *Neurosci Biobehav Rev* 14, 463–472.

Blanchard RJ, Mast M, Blanchard DC (1975) Stimulus control of defensive reactions in the albino rat. *J Comp Physiol Psychol* 88, 81–88.

Bland ST, Schmid MJ, Greenwood BN et al. (2006) Behavioral control of the stressor modulates stress-induced changes in neurogenesis and fibroblast growth factor-2. *NeuroReport* 17, 593–597.

Bland ST, Tamlyn JP, Barrientos RM et al. (2007) Expression of fibroblast growth factor-2 and brain-derived neurotrophic factor mRNA in the medial prefrontal cortex and hippocampus after uncontrollable or controllable stress. *Neuroscience* 144, 1219–1228.

Boscarino JA (1995) Post-traumatic stress and associated disorders among Vietnam veterans: the significance of combat exposure and social support. *J Trauma Stress* 8, 317–336.

Boscarino JA, Chang J (1999) Electrocardiogram abnormalities among men with stress-related psychiatric disorders: implications for coronary heart disease and clinical research. *Ann Behav Med* 21, 227–234.

Bremner JD (2007) Functional neuroimaging in post-traumatic stress disorder. *Expert Rev Neurother* 7, 393–405.

Bremner JD, Innis RB, Ng CK et al. (1997) Positron emission tomography measurement of cerebral metabolic correlates of yohimbine administration in combat-related posttraumatic stress disorder. *Archiv Gen Psychiatry* 54, 246–254.

Bremner JD, Krystal JH, Southwick SM et al. (1996) Noradrenergic mechanisms in stress and anxiety: II. *Clinical studies. Synapse* 23, 39–51.

Bremner JD, Randall P, Scott TM et al. (1995) Deficits in short-term memory in adult survivors of childhood abuse. *Psychiatry Res* 59, 97–107.

Bremner JD, Staib LH, Kaloupek D et al. (1999) Neural correlates of exposure to traumatic pictures and sound in Vietnam combat veterans with and without posttraumatic stress disorder: A positron emission tomography study. *Biol Psychiatry* 45, 806–816.

Bremner JD, Vythilingam M, Vermetten E et al. (2003) Cortisol response to a cognitive stress challenge in posttraumatic stress disorder (PTSD) related to childhood abuse. *Psychoneuroendocrinol* 28, 733–750.

Brewin CR, Andrews B, Valentine JD (2000) Meta-analysis of risk factors for posttraumatic stress disorder in trauma-exposed adults. *J Consult Clin Psychol* 68, 748–766.

Britton JC, Phan KL, Taylor SF et al. (2005) Corticolimbic blood flow in posttraumatic stress disorder during script-driven imagery. *Biol Psychiatry* 57, 832–840.

Buckley TC, Kaloupek DG (2001) A meta-analytic examination of basal cardiovascular activity in posttraumatic stress disorder. *Psychosom Med* 63, 585–594.

Carrion VG, Weems CF, Eliez S et al. (2001) Attenuation of frontal asymmetry in pediatric posttraumatic stress disorder. *Biol Psychiatry* 50, 943–951.

Cohen H, Benjamin J, Kaplan Z et al. (2000) Administration of high-dose ketoconazole, an inhibitor of steroid synthesis, prevents posttraumatic anxiety in an animal model. *Eur Neuropsychopharmacol* 10, 429–435.

Cohen H, Kaplan Z, Matar MA et al. (2006) Anisomycin, a protein synthesis inhibitor, disrupts traumatic memory consolidation and attenuates posttraumatic stress response in rats. *Biol Psychiatry* 60, 767–776.

Cohen H, Zohar J (2004) An animal model of posttraumatic stress disorder: the use of cut-off behavioral criteria. *Ann N Y Acad Sci* 1032, 167–178.

De Bellis MD, Keshavan MS, Shifflett H et al. (2002) Brain structures in pediatric maltreatment-related posttraumatic stress disorder: a sociodemographically matched study. *Biol Psychiatry* 52, 1066–1078.

de Kloet CS, Vermetten E, Geuze E et al. (2006) Assessment of HPA-axis function in posttraumatic stress disorder: pharmacological and non-pharmacological challenge tests, a review. *J Psychiatr Res* 40, 550–567.

Diamond DM, Park CR, Heman KL et al. (1999) Exposing rats to a predator impairs spatial working memory in the radial arm water maze. *Hippocampus* 9, 542–552.

Domschke K (2012) Patho-genetics of posttraumatic stress disorder. *Psychiatr Danub* 24, 267–273.

Duval F, Crocq MA, Guillon MS et al. (2004) Increased adrenocorticotropin suppression after dexamethasone administration in sexually abused adolescents with posttraumatic stress disorder. *Ann N Y Acad Sci* 1032, 273–275.

Ehlers A, Hackmann A, Michael T (2004) Intrusive re-experiencing in post-traumatic stress disorder: phenomenology, theory, and therapy. *Memory* 12, 403–415.

Elzinga BM, Bremner JD (2002) Are the neural substrates of memory the final common pathway in posttraumatic stress disorder (PTSD)? *J Affect Disord* 70, 1–17.

Elzinga BM, Schmahl CG, Vermetten E et al. (2003) Higher cortisol levels following exposure to traumatic reminders in abuse-related PTSD. *Neuropsychopharmacology* 28, 1656–1665.

Fennema-Notestine C, Stein MB, Kennedy CM et al. (2002) Brain morphometry in female victims of intimate partner violence with and without posttraumatic stress disorder. *Biol Psychiatry* 52, 1089–1101.

Garrick T, Morrow N, Shalev AY et al. (2001) Stress-induced enhancement of auditory startle: an animal model of posttraumatic stress disorder. *Psychiatry* 64, 346–354.

Gilbertson MW, Gurvits TV, Lasko NB et al. (2001) Multivariate assessment of explicit memory function in combat veterans with posttraumatic stress disorder. *J Trauma Stress* 14, 413–432.

Gilbertson MW, Shenton ME, Ciszewski A et al. (2002) Smaller hippocampal volume predicts pathologic vulnerability to psychological trauma. *Nat Neurosci* 5, 1242–1247.

Goenjian AK, Yehuda R, Pynoos RS et al. (1996) Basal cortisol, dexamethasone suppression of cortisol, and MHPG in adolescents after the 1988 earthquake in Armenia. *Am J Psychiatry* 153, 929–934.

Goswami S, Rodriguez-Sierra O, Cascardi M et al. (2013) Animal models of post-traumatic stress disorder: face validity. *Front Neurosci* 7, 89.

Grossman R, Buchsbaum MS, Yehuda R (2002) Neuroimaging studies in post-traumatic stress disorder. Psychiatr Clin North Am 25, 317.

Grossman R, Yehuda R, New A et al. (2003) Dexamethasone suppression test findings in subjects with personality disorders: associations with posttraumatic stress disorder and major depression. *Am J Psychiatry* 160, 1291–1298.

Gurvits TV, Shenton ME, Hokama H et al. (1996) Magnetic resonance imaging study of hippocampal volume in chronic, combat-related posttraumatic stress disorder. *Biol Psychiatry* 40, 1091–1099.

Hackmann A, Ehlers A, Speckens A et al. (2004) Characteristics and content of intrusive memories in PTSD and their changes with treatment. *J Trauma Stress* 17, 231–240.

Harvey BH, Naciti C, Brand L et al. (2003) Endocrine, cognitive and hippocampal/cortical 5HT 1A/2A receptor changes evoked by a time-dependent sensitisation (TDS) stress model in rats. *Brain Res* 983, 97–107.

Hubbard DT, Blanchard DC, Yang M et al. (2004) Development of defensive behavior and conditioning to cat odor in the rat. *Physiol Behav* 80, 525–530.

Khan S, Liberzon I (2004) Topiramate attenuates exaggerated acoustic startle in an animal model of PTSD. *Psychopharmacology (Berl)* 172, 225–229.

Koenigs M, Grafman J (2009) Posttraumatic stress disorder: the role of medial prefrontal cortex and amygdala. *Neuroscientist* 15, 540–548.

Kohda K, Harada K, Kato K et al. (2007) Glucocorticoid receptor activation is involved in producing abnormal phenotypes of single-prolonged stress rats: A putative post-traumatic stress disorder model. *Neuroscience* 148, 22–33.

Krystal JH, Neumeister A (2009) Noradrenergic and serotonergic mechanisms in the neurobiology of posttraumatic stress disorder and resilience. *Brain Res* 1293, 13–23.

Kubzansky LD, Koenen KC, Spiro A, III et al. (2007) Prospective study of posttraumatic stress disorder symptoms and coronary heart disease in the Normative Aging Study. *Arch Gen Psychiatry* 64, 109–116.

Kubzansky LD, Koenen KC (2007) Is post-traumatic stress disorder related to development of heart disease? *Future Cardiol* 3, 153–156.

Lanius RA, Williamson PC, Densmore M et al. (2001) Neural correlates of traumatic memories in posttraumatic stress disorder: a functional MRI investigation. *Am J Psychiatry* 158, 1920–1922.

Li S, Murakami Y, Wang M et al. (2006) The effects of chronic valproate and diazepam in a mouse model of posttraumatic stress disorder. *Pharmacol Biochem Behav* 85, 324–331.

Liberzon I, Abelson JL, Flagel SB et al. (1999) Neuroendocrine and psychophysiologic responses in PTSD: a symptom provocation study. *Neuropsychopharmacology* 21, 40–50.

Liberzon I, Krstov M, Young EA (1997) Stress-restress: effects on ACTH and fast feedback. *Psychoneuroendocrinol* 22, 443–453.

Liberzon I, Sripada CS (2008) The functional neuroanatomy of PTSD: a critical review. *Prog Brain Res* 167, 151–169.

Lindauer RJ, Booij J, Habraken JB et al. (2004) Cerebral blood flow changes during script-driven imagery in police officers with posttraumatic stress disorder. *Biol Psychiatry* 56, 853–861.

Maier SF, Watkins LR (2005) Stressor controllability and learned helplessness: the roles of the dorsal raphe nucleus, serotonin, and corticotropin-releasing factor. *Neurosci Biobehav Rev* 29, 829–841.

Mesches MH, Fleshner M, Heman KL et al. (1999) Exposing rats to a predator blocks primed burst potentiation in the hippocampus in vitro. *J Neurosci* 19:RC18.

Milde AM, Sundberg H, Roseth AG et al. (2003) Proactive sensitizing effects of acute stress on acoustic startle responses and experimentally induced colitis in rats: relationship to corticosterone. *Stress* 6, 49–57.

Mitra R, Jadhav S, McEwen BS et al. (2005) Stress duration modulates the spatiotemporal patterns of spine formation in the basolateral amygdala. *Proc Natl Acad Sci U S A* 102, 9371–9376.

Morrow BA, Redmond AJ, Roth RH et al. (2000) The predator odor, TMT, displays a unique, stress-like pattern of dopaminergic and endocrinological activation in the rat. *Brain Res* 864, 146–151.

Nemeroff CB, Bremner JD, Foa EB et al. (2006) Posttraumatic stress disorder: A state-of-the-science review. *J Psychiatr Res* 40, 1–21.

Nutt DJ, Malizia AL (2004) Structural and functional brain changes in posttraumatic stress disorder. *J Clin Psychiatry* 65 Suppl 1, 11–17.

Orr SP, Claiborn JM, Altman B et al. (1990) Psychometric profile of posttraumatic stress disorder, anxious, and healthy Vietnam veterans: correlations with psychophysiologic responses. *J Consult Clin Psychol* 58, 329–335.

Orr SP, Metzger LJ, Lasko NB et al. (2000) De novo conditioning in trauma-exposed individuals with and without posttraumatic stress disorder. *J Abnorm Psychol* 109, 290–298.

Park CR, Zoladz PR, Conrad CD et al. (2008) Acute predator stress impairs the consolidation and retrieval of hippocampus-dependent memory in male and female rats. *Learn Mem* 15, 271–280.

Peri T, Ben Shakhar G, Orr SP et al. (2000) Psychophysiologic assessment of aversive conditioning in posttraumatic stress disorder. *Biol Psychiatry* 47, 512–519.

Pervanidou P, Chrousos GP (2010) Neuroendocrinology of post-traumatic stress disorder. *Prog Brain Res* 182, 149–160.

Pitman RK, Gilbertson MW, Gurvits TV et al. (2006) Clarifying the origin of biological abnormalities in PTSD through the study of identical twins discordant for combat exposure. *Ann N Y Acad Sci* 1071, 242–254.

Pitman RK, Rasmusson AM, Koenen KC et al. (2012) Biological studies of post-traumatic stress disorder. *Nat Rev Neurosci* 13, 769–787.

Plutarch (1920) *The Life of Marius*, 9 edn. Chicago: Loeb Classical Library edition.

Pynoos RS, Ritzmann RF, Steinberg AM et al. (1996) A behavioral animal model of posttraumatic stress disorder featuring repeated exposure to situational reminders. *Biol Psychiatry* 39, 129–134.

Rau V, DeCola JP, Fanselow MS (2005) Stress-induced enhancement of fear learning: an animal model of posttraumatic stress disorder. *Neurosci Biobehav Rev* 29, 1207–1223.

Rauch SL, Shin LM, Segal E et al. (2003) Selectively reduced regional cortical volumes in post-traumatic stress disorder. *NeuroReport* 14, 913–916.

Regehr C, LeBlanc V, Jelley RB et al. (2007) Previous trauma exposure and PTSD symptoms as predictors of subjective and biological response to stress. *Can J Psychiatry* 52, 675–683.

Resnick HS, Yehuda R, Pitman RK et al. (1995) Effect of previous trauma on acute plasma cortisol level following rape. *Am J Psychiatry* 152, 1675–1677.

Reynolds M, Brewin CR (1999) Intrusive memories in depression and posttraumatic stress disorder. *Behav Res Ther* 37, 201–215.

Richter-Levin G (1998) Acute and long-term behavioral correlates of underwater trauma—potential relevance to stress and post-stress syndromes. *Psychiatry Res* 79, 73–83.

Rinne T, de Kloet ER, Wouters L et al. (2002) Hyperresponsiveness of hypothalamic-pituitary-adrenal axis to combined dexamethasone/corticotropin-releasing hormone challenge in female borderline personality disorder subjects with a history of sustained childhood abuse. *Biol Psychiatry* 52, 1102–1112.

Rosen JB (2004) The neurobiology of conditioned and unconditioned fear: a neurobehavioral system analysis of the amygdala. *Behav Cogn Neurosci Rev* 3, 23–41.

Roth TL, Zoladz PR, Sweatt JD et al. (2011) Epigenetic modification of hippocampal Bdnf DNA in adult rats in an animal model of post-traumatic stress disorder. *J Psychiatr Res* 45, 919–926.

Sawamura T, Shimizu K, Nibuya M et al. (2004) Effect of paroxetine on a model of posttraumatic stress disorder in rats. *Neurosci Lett* 357, 37–40.

Sawchuk CN, Roy-Byrne P, Goldberg J et al. (2005) The relationship between post-traumatic stress disorder, depression and cardiovascular disease in an American Indian tribe. *Psychol Med* 35, 1785–1794.

Servatius RJ, Ottenweller JE, Natelson BH (1995) Delayed startle sensitization distinguishes rats exposed to one or three stress sessions: further evidence toward an animal model of PTSD. *Biol Psychiatry* 38, 539–546.

Shimizu K, Kikuchi A, Wakizono T et al. (2006) [An animal model of posttraumatic stress disorder in rats using a shuttle box]. *Nihon Shinkei Seishin Yakurigaku Zasshi* 26, 93–99.

Shimizu K, Sawamura T, Nibuya M et al. (2004) [An animal model of posttraumatic stress disorder and its validity: effect of paroxetine on a PTSD model in rats]. *Nihon Shinkei Seishin Yakurigaku Zasshi* 24, 283–290.

Shin LM, Orr SP, Carson MA et al. (2004) Regional cerebral blood flow in the amygdala and medial prefrontal cortex during traumatic imagery in male and female Vietnam veterans with PTSD. *Arch Gen Psychiatry* 61, 168–176.

Shin LM, Rauch SL, Pitman RK (2006) Amygdala, medial prefrontal cortex, and hippocampal function in PTSD. *Ann NY Acad Sci* 1071, 67–79.

Siegmund A, Wotjak CT (2007a) Hyperarousal does not depend on trauma-related contextual memory in an animal model of Posttraumatic Stress Disorder. *Physiol Behav* 90, 103–107.

Siegmund A, Wotjak CT (2007b) A mouse model of posttraumatic stress disorder that distinguishes between conditioned and sensitised fear. *J Psychiatr Res* 41, 848–860.

Solomon Z, Mikulincer M, Avitzur E (1988) Coping, locus of control, social support, and combat-related posttraumatic stress disorder: a prospective study. *Journal of Personality & Social Psychology* 55, 279–285.

Solomon Z, Mikulincer M, Benbenishty R (1989) Locus of control and combat-related post-traumatic stress disorder: the intervening role of battle intensity, threat appraisal and coping. *Br J Clin Psychol* 28 (Pt 2):131–144.

Southwick SM, Krystal JH, Morgan CA et al. (1993) Abnormal noradrenergic function in post-traumatic stress disorder. *Arch Gen Psychiatry* 50, 266–274.

Southwick SM, Morgan CA, III, Charney DS et al. (1999) Yohimbine use in a natural setting: effects on posttraumatic stress disorder. *Biol Psychiatry* 46, 442–444.

Speckens AE, Ehlers A, Hackmann A et al. (2007) Intrusive memories and rumination in patients with post-traumatic stress disorder: a phenomenological comparison. *Memory* 15, 249–257.

Stam R (2007) PTSD and stress sensitisation: a tale of brain and body Part 1: human studies. *Neurosci Biobehav Rev* 31, 530–557.

Stam R (2007) PTSD and stress sensitisation: a tale of brain and body Part 2: animal models. *Neurosci Biobehav Rev* 31, 558–584.

Stein MB, Yehuda R, Koverola C et al. (1997) Enhanced dexamethasone suppression of plasma cortisol in adult women traumatized by childhood sexual abuse. *Biol Psychiatry* 42, 680–686.

Strawn JR, Geracioti TD, Jr (2008) Noradrenergic dysfunction and the psychopharmacology of posttraumatic stress disorder. *Depress Anxiety* 25, 260–271.

Strohle A, Scheel M, Modell S et al. (2008) Blunted ACTH response to dexamethasone suppression-CRH stimulation in posttraumatic stress disorder. *J Psychiatr Res* 42, 1185–1188.

Takahashi T, Morinobu S, Iwamoto Y et al. (2006) Effect of paroxetine on enhanced contextual fear induced by single prolonged stress in rats. *Psychopharmacology (Berl)* 189, 165–173.

Taylor F, Cahill L (2002) Propranolol for reemergent posttraumatic stress disorder following an event of retraumatization: a case study. *J Trauma Stress* 15, 433–437.

Ullman SE, Filipas HH (2001) Predictors of PTSD symptom severity and social reactions in sexual assault victims. *J Trauma Stress* 14, 369–389.

Vanelzakker MB, Zoladz PR, Thompson VM et al. (2011) Influence of Pre-Training Predator Stress on the Expression of c-fos mRNA in the Hippocampus, Amygdala, and Striatum Following Long-Term Spatial Memory Retrieval. *Front Behav Neurosci* 5, 30.

Vidovic A, Gotovac K, Vilibic M et al. (2011) Repeated assessments of endocrine- and immune-related changes in posttraumatic stress disorder. *Neuroimmunomodulation* 18, 199–211.

Vouimba RM, Munoz C, Diamond DM (2006) Differential effects of predator stress and the antidepressant tianeptine on physiological plasticity in the hippocampus and basolateral amygdala. *Stress* 9, 29–40.

Wakizono T, Sawamura T, Shimizu K et al. (2007) Stress vulnerabilities in an animal model of post-traumatic stress disorder. *Physiol Behav* 90, 687–695.

Woodson JC, Macintosh D, Fleshner M et al. (2003) Emotion-induced amnesia in rats: working memory-specific impairment, corticosterone-memory correlation, and fear versus arousal effects on memory. *Learn Mem* 10, 326–336.

Woodward SH, Kaloupek DG, Streeter CC et al. (2006) Decreased anterior cingulate volume in combat-related PTSD. *Biol Psychiatry* 59, 582–587.

Yamasue H, Kasai K, Iwanami A et al. (2003) Voxel-based analysis of MRI reveals anterior cingulate gray-matter volume reduction in posttraumatic stress disorder due to terrorism. *Proc Natl Acad Sci USA* 100, 9039–9043.

Yehuda R (2005) Neuroendocrine aspects of PTSD. *Handb Exp Pharmacol* 371–403.

Yehuda R (2009) Status of glucocorticoid alterations in post-traumatic stress disorder. *Ann NY Acad Sci* 1179, 56–69.

Yehuda R, Boisoneau D, Lowy MT et al. (1995) Dose-response changes in plasma cortisol and lymphocyte glucocorticoid receptors following dexamethasone administration in combat veterans with and without posttraumatic stress disorder. *Arch Gen Psychiatry* 52, 583–593.

Yehuda R, Golier JA, Halligan SL et al. (2004) The ACTH response to dexamethasone in PTSD. *Am J Psychiatry* 161, 1397–1403.

Yehuda R, Halligan S, Grossman R et al. (2002) The cortisol and glucocorticoid receptor response to low dose dexamethasone administration in aging combat veterans and holocaust survivors with and without posttraumatic stress disorder. *Biol Psychiatry* 52, 393.

Zoladz PR, Conrad CD, Fleshner M et al. (2008) Acute episodes of predator exposure in conjunction with chronic social instability as an animal model of post-traumatic stress disorder. *Stress* 11, 259–281.

Zoladz PR, Conrad CD, Fleshner M et al. (2008) Acute episodes of predator exposure in conjunction with chronic social instability as an animal model of post-traumatic stress disorder. *Stress* 11, 259–281.

Zoladz PR, Diamond DM (2013) Current status on behavioral and biological markers of PTSD: A search for clarity in a conflicting literature. *Neurosci Biobehav Rev* 37, 860–895.

Zoladz PR, Fleshner M, Diamond DM (2013) Differential effectiveness of tianeptine, clonidine and amitriptyline in blocking traumatic memory expression, anxiety and hypertension in an animal model of PTSD. *Prog Neuropsychopharmacol Biol Psychiatry* 44C, 1–16.

Zoladz PR, Fleshner M, Diamond DM (2012) Psychosocial animal model of PTSD produces a long-lasting traumatic memory, an increase in general anxiety and PTSD-like glucocorticoid abnormalities. *Psychoneuroendocrinol* 37, 1531–1545.

Zoladz PR, Park CR, Halonen JD et al. (2012) Differential expression of molecular markers of synaptic plasticity in the hippocampus, prefrontal cortex, and amygdala in response to spatial learning, predator exposure, and stress-induced amnesia. *Hippocampus* 22, 577–589.

Zovkic IB, Sweatt JD (2013) Epigenetic mechanisms in learned fear: implications for PTSD. *Neuropsychopharmacology* 38, 77–93.

CHAPTER 7

Coping with stress in wild birds – the evolutionary foundations of stress responses

Molly J. Dickens[1] & Michael Romero[2]

[1] Department of Integrative Biology, University of California, Berkeley, Berkeley, CA, USA
[2] Department of Biology, Tufts University, Medford, MA, USA

7.1 Introduction

Often, when we think of *stress in the wild,* we picture a classic predator/prey scenario – a gazelle being chased across the savanna by a lion or something similar. At this basic level, the physiological and behavioral responses that are initiated when that gazelle perceives that lion are generally thought to be *adaptive* – helping the animal survive when faced with a life-threatening scenario. Although modern humans rarely face this type of predation risk, the range of stressors (from extreme to mild) that humans may encounter in their lifetime also initiate this basic, evolutionarily conserved suite of physiological and behavioral responses that we classify as the *acute stress response*.

We consider this scenario – a single incident, mounting a single response to a single stressor with adequate time to recover and return to baseline functioning – as the "good" side of stress. The negative side of stress, in both wild animals and humans, occurs when this system is pushed beyond its normal functional capacity to respond and recover; this can occur following exposure to extreme, sustained, and/or repeated stressors. To emphasize this distinction between "good stress" and "bad stress," we will define these scenarios with two categories:

- Acute stress – beneficial, adaptive, important for survival
- Chronic stress – detrimental, maladaptive, decreasing survival.

In chronic stress, the beneficial response elements of the acute stress response are pushed beyond their adaptive capacity and into a state of dysregulation

Posttraumatic Stress Disorder: From Neurobiology to Treatment, First Edition.
Edited by J. Douglas Bremner.
© 2016 John Wiley & Sons, Inc. Published 2016 by John Wiley & Sons, Inc.

(Romero et al., 2009). A chronically stressed animal no longer responds appropriately to life-threatening stimuli and maintenance of basal output of the stress pathways (e.g., circadian rhythm of glucocorticoids) is dysregulated.

The dysregulation of physiological and behavioral systems resulting from chronic stress has been the subject of decades of human clinical and preclinical research. Much of what we've learned has been discovered using laboratory rodents as surrogates for human responses. However, the clean, regimented, controlled, and fairly constant environment (i.e., cages) that laboratory rodents experience during their lifetimes has little in common with the chaotic, messy, ever-changing environments experienced by most humans. Consequently, wild animals (i.e., those animals also experiencing chaotic, messy, and ever-changing environments) might provide better models for how humans respond to stress.

Recently, there has been an increased focus on using free-living and wild-caught birds to investigate the adaptive stress response and the effects of chronic stress. Most wild birds are diurnal and conspicuous, making them more tractable for study than the mostly nocturnal and secretive wild rodents. There is mounting evidence that the mechanisms and pathways underlying the physiological stress response system are very similar across species, including avian species. For example, the fight-or-flight response is initiated immediately following stressor exposure (Nephew et al., 2003) and, as in mammals, is driven by the sympathetic nervous system (SNS) and epinephrine release (Cyr et al., 2009). On a slower timescale, the hypothalamic–pituitary–adrenal (HPA) axis, and the resulting secretion of glucocorticoids (corticosterone [CORT] being the predominant glucocorticoid in birds), is initiated with concentrations peaking 15–30 minutes after stressor exposure (Wingfield & Romero, 2001). Although higher brain regions regulating stressor perception and HPA regulation are not as well mapped or characterized in the avian brain as in the mammalian brain, early studies suggest a high homology between regions involved in the neural stress response pathways; for example, the avian hippocampus (Atoji & Wild, 2006) and amygdala (Atoji et al., 2006; Saint-Dizier et al., 2009) appear to have neural connections that suggest similar regulatory roles during stress as the mammalian hippocampus and amygdala. And when wild birds encounter multiple or sustained stressors in a manner they cannot cope appropriately with (either behaviorally or physiologically), the physiological stress response can be pushed into a state of dysregulation at multiple levels (as discussed below). Research on the effects of acute and chronic stress in wild avian species highlight the consequences of the maladaptive response while also emphasizing the basics of the adaptive response that may make individuals more or less susceptible to the effects of chronic stress. The fundamentally conserved nature of the underlying physiological and behavioral stress mechanisms indicates that what we learn from wild birds will have relevance to human conditions, and perhaps better relevance than the highly artificial conditions of laboratory rodent studies.

7.2 Physiological changes associated with chronic stress in wild birds

7.2.1 Fight-or-flight response

In the scenario discussed earlier with the gazelle and the lion, the gazelle's initial response is to initiate a fight-or-flight response. This classic response is mediated via the SNS and epinephrine release. Although the behavioral aspects of this response are fairly easy to measure in free-living birds, sympathetic activation is more difficult to demonstrate. The primary solution has been to monitor SNS activity through heart rate (HR) and heart rate variability (HRV).

Early studies clearly indicate that measurements of HR as indicators of the fight-or-flight system in free-living birds demonstrate responses to acute stressors as we would expect. For example, female ptarmigans incubating eggs on their nests increase HR in response to approaching predators (Steen et al., 1988) and approaching tourists induce marked bradycardia in penguins (Nimon et al., 1996).

Analysis of HRV has been applied much more recently to avian species. HRV is used as a measurement of the balance between SNS drive and parasympathetic nervous system (PNS) drive, such that decreased HRV indicates an increase in sympathetic drive while an increase in HRV indicates the opposite (Billman, 2011). For example, when birds are exposed to restraint stress, HR increases immediately while HRV decreases (Cyr et al., 2009). When birds are exposed experimentally to different stimuli that induce chronic stress, there are marked changes in both baseline function and the stress responsiveness of HR and HRV.

In a study by Cyr et al. (2009), European starlings (*Sturnus vulgaris*) were subjected to a chronic stress protocol utilizing rotating acute stressors given four times/day for 21 days. During this period of chronic stress, the birds showed a delayed increase in daytime HR but no change in HRV (Figure 7.1). The increase in baseline HR during chronic stress appears to indicate that chronic stress results in an over-active sympathetic drive. However, the lack of change in HRV suggests exactly the opposite – that increased SNS activity is not driving the increased HR. Instead, the data suggest that both sympathetic drive and parasympathetic inhibition are down-regulated. The ratio of SNS and PNS input remains the same, resulting in no change in HRV, while decreased inhibition from the PNS allows HR to elevate. This situation is often referred to as parasympathetic withdrawal. Humans subjected to psychological stress (Delaney & Brodie, 2000) and patients suffering from cardiomyopathy (Binkley et al., 1991) show signs of parasympathetic withdrawal, and parasympathetic withdrawal has been suggested as the

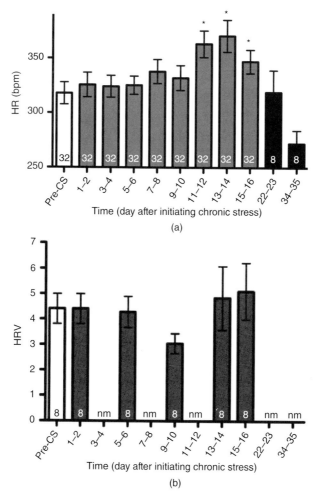

Figure 7.1 Daytime measurements of baseline heart rate (HR) (a) and HR variability (HRV) (b) before (pre-chronic stress [CS]; white bars), during (days 1–16; gray bars), and after (after day 22; black bars) chronic stress treatment. Because measurements were taken every other day, with half of the birds measured on one day and the other half measured the next, means are grouped in 2-day increments. Sample sizes are indicated within bars. Asterisks indicate significant differences from pre-CS values. Spaces (labeled "nm" for "not measured") were added in (b) so that the graphs line up. (From Cyr et al., 2009; reprinted with permission.)

cause of increased risk of sudden cardiac death after exercise (Billman & Hoskins, 1989; Cole et al., 1999, 2000). This suggests that chronic stress has induced incipient cardiac disease in the starlings.

Cyr et al. (2009) also showed that chronically stressed birds have a decreased HR response to an acute stressor (Figure 7.2). Cyr et al. suggest that this finding indicates an insufficient signal operating through the SNS (e.g., potential

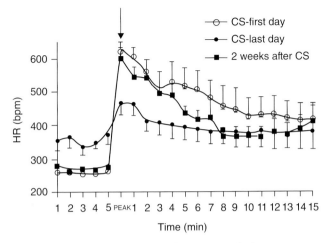

Figure 7.2 Mean heart rate (HR) taken before and 15 minutes during an acute stressor (restraint) on the first day (open circles) and the last day (filled circles) of the chronic stress (CS) period, as well as days 34–35 (dashed line, black squares; i.e., 18–19 days after the completion of the CS period). The arrow denotes the initiation of restraint. Note the increased baseline HR at the end of chronic stress that is repeated from Figure 7.1, but the relative lack of response to restraint. bpm, beats/minute. (From Cyr et al., 2009; reprinted with permission.)

down-regulation of epinephrine/norepinephrine receptors) combined with the acute decrease in parasympathetic inhibition indicated in Figure 7.1.

Using a different model of chronic stress – introduction to captivity – we found both similarities and differences in HR and HRV response in starlings (Dickens & Romero, 2009). Moving wild-caught birds into captivity results in a series of stressor exposures: capture and human handling, confinement and transport, and release to a novel, captive environment. Not surprisingly, this scenario resulted in an increase in HR and a decrease in HRV in the recently captured birds as compared with control birds. A massive increase in sympathetic drive is exactly what would be predicted. Interestingly, however, the increase in HR returned to control levels within 24 hours of capture from the wild, yet the decrease in HRV remained lower for another 24 hours. We speculated that this decrease in HRV indicated a sustained drive of the SNS for 48 hours after the introduction to captivity, but with SNS desensitization such that the relative balance between the SNS and the PNS is reflected in a normal HR despite underlying continuous exposure to elevated catecholamine concentrations.

Perhaps most surprising, we found a profound long-term disruption in their capacity to respond to a startle stressor. When newly captive birds were exposed to a brief loud noise, their HR response remained blunted, as compared with control birds, for at least 10 days (Figure 7.3). These data suggest that despite recovery of baseline regulation of HR within 48 hours, there are lasting changes in the fight-or-flight response to a mild acute stressor.

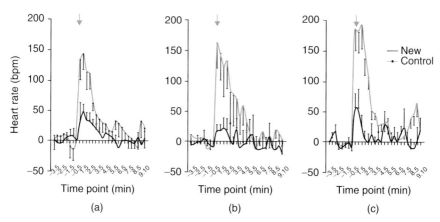

Figure 7.3 Heart rate responses to a startle stressor. Startle response for wild-caught, newly captive starlings (new) and long-term captivity controls (controls) at 36 hours (a), 88 hours (b), or 228 hours (c) after surgery, which occurred < 6 hours after initial trapping. The arrow indicates the time period at which the startle was given. (From Dickens & Romero, 2009; reprinted with permission.)

All of these studies were done on captive birds. There are numerous commercially available systems for collecting HR data in animals restricted to small cages, and the systems designed for laboratory rodents have proven amenable for use in birds as well. Monitoring changes in HR in free-living birds is difficult and requires using either HR loggers or transmitters. These devices are custom-made and require capturing the bird for implantation and/or affixing to the feathers. Transmitters send HR data to receivers and have the advantage of collecting data immediately. The disadvantage, however, is that they require a researcher to be nearby to collect the data, which can often be quite challenging in an animal that can fly wherever it wants. Transmitters are also limited by the size of the battery required to send the signal. Until very recently, transmitters were quite large and therefore required a large bird as a subject. Improvements in battery design and receiver technology are currently opening these techniques to smaller species. Loggers avoid many of these problems by collecting the HR data and storing them in the device. Their disadvantage, however, is that the data are unavailable until the animal is trapped a second time, something that can often be very difficult. Notwithstanding these technical challenges, measuring stress-induced changes in HR in free-living birds is a growing area of research.

7.2.2 Hypothalamic–pituitary–adrenal axis

Our studies of chronic stress in either free-living or wild-caught birds have shown a number of consistent changes across the HPA axis. Most of these changes parallel preclinical and clinical findings.

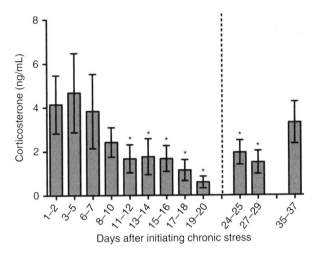

Figure 7.4 Baseline corticosterone concentrations during and after the chronic stress period. Because measurements were taken every other day, with half of the birds measured on one day and the other half measured the next, means are grouped in 2-day increments. Asterisks represent significant difference from controls. (From Rich & Romero, 2005; reprinted with permission.)

The protocol detailed earlier (21 days of rotating acute stressors – see Figure 7.1) was first utilized by Rich and Romero (2005). Their study demonstrated that chronically stressed starlings exhibited a decrease in baseline CORT (Figure 7.4), a decrease in stress-induced CORT, and a blunted pituitary response as indicated with an adrenocorticotropin hormone (ACTH) challenge. Cyr et al. (2007) repeated the study. These data seem counterintuitive because chronic stress is generally thought to result in elevated CORT. However, there are numerous preclinical studies showing chronically stressed animals with HPA inhibition (e.g., Blanchard, 1995) and some human clinical studies suggest cortisol levels are lower in people suffering from posttraumatic stress disorder (PTSD) following chronic stress (Rohleder et al., 2004; Roth et al., 2006). An increase in CORT during chronic stress is not a universal response (Dickens & Romero, 2013) and the wild birds seem to match some human clinical data.

Figure 7.4 comes from laboratory data. To ascertain whether similar responses occur in free-living chronically stressed birds, female starlings that were incubating eggs (females were thus invested in their nests and did not simply leave the area when harassed) were exposed to four rotating acute stressors per day to induce chronic stress. These birds showed similar decreases in baseline CORT (Cyr & Romero, 2007). Furthermore, these starlings also showed an increase in fecal glucocorticoid metabolites (Cyr & Romero, 2008). CORT metabolites are thought to be deposited fairly constantly in the feces, making fecal metabolites an integrated measure of plasma concentrations during the period between defecations. The increases in fecal CORT metabolites suggest reduced efficiency of the CORT negative feedback signal, which would normally result in a rapid shut-off of stress-induced CORT release. Without a functional negative feedback signal, stress-induced CORT will remain elevated, albeit at a lower level than non-chronically stressed birds, for an extended period of time. The result would be extended CORT release into the circulation and thus more metabolites appearing in the fecal material.

Similar results were obtained using a different model of chronic stress. Translocation is a conservation procedure where animals are taken from an area where they are common and moved to an area where they have been extirpated. The idea is to "seed" a new population and thus forestall extinction. We studied the effects of translocation in terms of the four component stressors; animals are (1) captured from the wild, (2) confined and (3) transported to a captive facility for a short period of time, and then (4) released back into the wild but at a novel site (Dickens et al., 2009b). The combination of these four stressors is a potent inducer of chronic stress (Dickens et al., 2010). In translocated wild chukar partridge (*Alectoris chukar*), as compared with non-translocated controls, we also found a decrease in baseline CORT and a decrease in stress-induced CORT (Figure 7.5). These results closely match the data from starlings discussed earlier.

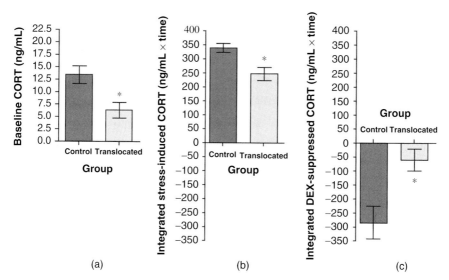

Figure 7.5 Corticosterone (CORT) responses following translocation stress. Birds recaptured after the translocation procedure were compared with control individuals that were not exposed to human interference prior to sampling. (a) Baseline plasma concentrations (mean ± SE). (b) Total CORT released after 15 minutes of restraint stress as mean ± SE of individual integrated stress-induced CORT concentrations. (c) Total CORT decrease 30 minutes after dexamethasone (DEX) suppression test as mean ± SE of individual integrated DEX-suppressed CORT concentrations. Asterisk indicates significance at $P < 0.05$. (Adapted from Dickens et al., 2009; reprinted with permission.)

In addition, these birds had an attenuated CORT suppression using a dexamethasone (DEX) suppression test (DST). The DST was designed to ascertain the efficacy of glucocorticoid negative feedback in humans (Carroll et al., 1981) and has been adapted for use in wild animals (Sapolsky et al., 1995) The resistance to DEX in the translocated chukar (Figure 7.5c) suggests that HPA negative feedback is blunted in these chronically stressed individuals. When these birds were tested during the captivity phase of the experiment, we also noted a decrease in stress responsiveness and a complete elimination of DEX suppression (Dickens et al., 2009c). However, at the time of release (10 days of captivity), the DEX suppression response had returned, suggesting that this aspect of HPA regulation was returning to pre-captivity levels. Stress-induced CORT remained suppressed at time of release, however, suggesting that the chronic stress of translocation results in lasting effects on this component of the HPA response.

Interestingly, in all of the studies in which we noted physiological changes in HPA physiology, regardless of differences in species and models of chronic stress, we also found decreases in body weight. This factor appears to be the one consistent measure of chronic stress effects in models across species and techniques (Dickens & Romero, 2013).

7.2.3 Neural changes

In chronically stressed starlings, we have shown that there are neural changes associated with the HPA changes. We focused on changes in expression of two glucocorticoid binding receptors – type 1, mineralocorticoid receptors (MRs); and type 2, glucocorticoid receptors (GRs). We found evidence for down-regulation of receptor expression in the avian hippocampus (Dickens et al., 2009a). In the hippocampus, chronically stressed birds showed a decrease in MR expression as determined from both cell counts and relative expression levels. As GR expression did not change in this brain region, the data suggest that chronic stress is causing the hippocampal MR : GR ratio to shift. A shift in the balance between the two receptors has been suggested to result in decreased HPA axis sensitivity (De Kloet, 1991), which may underlie the decreased baseline and stress-induced CORT demonstrated in these individuals.

We also demonstrated receptor changes in the paraventricular nucleus of the hypothalamus (PVN). The PVN contains the cell bodies of neurons producing corticotropin-releasing factor (CRF) that are primarily involved with the HPA activation. There was a decrease in the relative expression of GR in the PVN. The CRF neurons in this brain area are key sites of negative feedback acting to rapidly return stress-induced CORT concentrations to baseline. With a decrease in the negative feedback signal, stress-induced CORT will remain elevated for an extended period of time. This result was suggested in the fecal glucocorticoid metabolites measured in these birds (Cyr & Romero, 2008).

7.3 Lessons from wild birds

7.3.1 Not all stressors are created equal

The acute stress response is not an all or nothing response. It is graded depending on the perception of the severity of the stressor. This has long been shown to be the case for HPA responses (e.g., Hennessy & Levine, 1978), but is also true for fight-or-flight responses. For example, Nephew and Romero (2003) exposed birds to a mild stressor that progressively increased in intensity and found evidence of a graded sympathetic response (increase in HR). Furthermore, Nephew et al. (2003) showed that mild stressors could evoke strong HR responses, but with a smaller CORT response when birds were exposed to these mild stressors as compared with more severe stressors such as restraint stress (Remage-Healey & Romero, 2000). This provided evidence that the HPA and SNS responses to stress could be uncoupled.

Perception of severity may also change depending on individual context. For example, European starlings are seasonal breeders. In the breeding season, males and females pair and defend a nest – pairs are isolated and males are highly territorial. In the non-breeding season, males and females form large flocks – they feed, fly, and roost in close proximity with other starlings. Using males in the conditions representative of these two seasons, we compared individual responses to the introduction of intruders into an individual's home cage. We found that the birds in breeding condition mounted a sympathetic response (increased HR) to having a single intruder introduced into their cage. Birds in the non-breeding season did not respond to a single intruder and only showed evidence of mounting a sympathetic response when the number of intruders reached a point of crowding (five additional birds in a 34 × 38 × 45 cm cage). In both seasons, however, CORT did not increase with any number of intruders.

Considering these findings, it appears that a sympathetic response can occur without stimulation of the HPA axis and perception of a "stressor" may shift depending on individual circumstances.

7.3.2 Not all individuals are created equal

Although examining responses on an individual level in wild birds can be quite difficult, there is evidence for marked differences in how stimuli are interpreted between related species.

For example, two vireo species – the endangered black-capped vireo (*Vireo atricapilla*) and the common white-eyed vireo (*Vireo griseus*) – show very different sympathetic responses to humans. For each species, individuals were equipped with HR transmitters and then chased by the researchers for several hours. The intent was to monitor the responses of the birds to human activities. Black-capped vireos increased HR in response to chasing (Bisson et al., 2011) whereas the white-eyed vireos did not (Bisson et al., 2009). Therefore, it appears that the endangered species was much more sensitive to disturbance than the common species. Although the difficult nature of these studies has so far precluded examining individual differences in fight-or-flight responses, this difference in sensitivity between closely related species suggests that the different sensitivities in individual humans is likely to be reflected in individual free-living birds as well. Furthermore, the species-specific sensitivity resulting in hyper-responsiveness in more sensitive species (e.g., black-capped vireos) as compared with less sensitive species (e.g., white-eyed vireos) may make an animal more vulnerable to chronic stress effects (and may provide a partial explanation for why black-capped vireos are endangered). In addition, such differences in sensitivity may be amplified when encountering extreme stressors such as anthropogenic stressors associated with human encroachment.

An indication of the effects of differences in sensitivity can be seen in a laboratory-bred species, the Japanese quail, which were bred to show higher or lower "emotionality" (utilizing a quantifiable behavioral characteristic similar to the helplessness model in rodents). When exposed to chronic stress, individuals bred for higher emotionality exhibited changes in the HPA axis (reduced baseline CORT), whereas the birds bred for lower emotionality did not show any physiological changes (Calandreau et al., 2011). In this way, sensitivity may result in susceptibility, as physically responding to more stressors can result in a dysregulated state.

7.3.3 Lack of control can exacerbate chronic stress effects

Using similar chronic stress protocols, two studies investigated physiological dysregulation resulting from chronic stress in different species of free-living birds and obtained very different results. As discussed, exposing incubating female starlings to a series of nest-directed stressors resulted in decreased baseline plasma CORT and elevated fecal glucocorticoid metabolites (Cyr et al., 2007). These data suggested that despite reduced baseline CORT in the circulation, there may be dysregulation of HPA responsiveness and CORT negative feedback such that exposure to subsequent stressors results in sustained elevation of CORT.

Despite the evident HPA dysregulation in the European starlings, studies in two species of vireo by Butler et al. (2009) did not find the same result. Using similar nest-directed stressors with black-capped vireos and white-eyed vireos, neither baseline CORT nor stress-induced CORT differed from control birds that were not exposed to chronic stress. As posited by the authors, the lack of change in these species may be attributed to nesting strategy. European starlings are cavity nesters – incubating adults have one small entrance and exit to the nest such that a predation attempt (e.g., a snake) will most likely result in the death of the parent as well as the offspring. Vireos, on the other hand are open cup nesters. Parents sitting on the nest have a 360° view and, therefore, do not face the same predation risk as cavity nesters. These contrasting results suggest that situational control (perceived escape potential) plays a role in how birds respond to individual stressors and, therefore, the likelihood that such stressors in series will push an animal into a state of chronic stress.

7.4 Conclusions

Linking what we have observed and theorized about wild animals to stress-induced pathology in humans generally, and PTSD specifically, may be far from a stretch. Already we can see a fascinating potential parallel: the data from translocated chukar match data in some studies from translocated humans. Serum cortisol levels were lower in war refugees from Kosovo (Roth et al., 2006) and Bosnia (Rohleder et al., 2004). However, lower cortisol is not universal in human refugees (Sondergaard & Theorell, 2003) and the specific response may result from differences in stressors (Meewise et al., 2007) or in how well individual refugees are coping (Almedom et al., 2005).

Evidence from our research and others suggests that exposure to a series of relatively severe anthropogenic stressors can push a wild bird into a state of chronic stress as demonstrated by the dysregulated physiology. We theorize that this shift may be caused by physically responding to an extreme or sustained stressor or a series of acute stressors in a manner that does not allow full recovery of the physiological pathways (Romero et al., 2009). Responsiveness to single stressors may be the key to understanding why some individuals are pushed into a state of chronic stress while others are not, despite similar stress exposure.

Humans show the same physiological responses as wild animals, and all species studied to date, including humans, respond to both mild stress and severe stress using similar physiological pathways. Humans also show a capacity for the system to be dysregulated similar to wild animals pushed beyond their adaptive capacity, resulting in vulnerability to stress-induced pathology. Furthermore, both the stressors that humans encounter in the modern "wild" and the anthropogenic stressors affecting wild animals are, from an evolutionary perspective, quite recent. Therefore, we propose that the fields of PTSD research and the ecophysiology of stress can learn and build off each other to further understand the underlying basis for stress pathologies and the roles played by the differences in sensitivity, context-dependent responsiveness, and perception of stress severity due to changes in sense of control.

Acknowledgements

Funding was provided by NIH grant F32HD072732 to M.J.D. and NSF grant IOS-1048529 to L.M.R.

References

Almedom AM, Teclemichael T, Romero LM et al. (2005) Postnatal salivary cortisol and sense of coherence (SOC) in eritrean mothers. *Am J Hum Biol* 17, 376–379.

Atoji Y, Saito S, Wild JM (2006) Fiber connections of the compact division of the posterior pallial amygdala and lateral part of the bed nucleus of the stria terminalis in the pigeon (Columba livia). *J Comp Neurol* 499, 161–182.

Atoji Y, Wild JM (2006) Anatomy of the avian hippocampal formation. *Rev Neurosci* 17, 3–15.

Billman GE (2011) Heart rate variability – a historical perspective. *Frontiers Physiol* 2, 1–13.

Billman GE, Hoskins RS (1989) Time-series analysis of heart rate variability during submaximal exercise. Evidence for reduced cardiac vagal tone in animals susceptible to venticular fibrillation. *Circulation* 80, 146–157.

Binkley PF, Nunziata E, Haas GJ et al. (1991) Parasympathetic withdrawal is an integral component of autonomic imbalance in congestive heart failure: Demonstration in human subjects and verification in a paced canine model of ventricular failure. *J Am Coll Cardiol* 18, 464–472.

Bisson IA, Butler LK, Hayden TJ et al. (2011) Energetic response to human disturbance in an endangered songbird. *Anim Conserv* 14, 484–491.

Bisson IA, Butler LK, Hayden TJ et al. (2009) No energetic cost of anthropogenic disturbance in a songbird. *Proc R Soc B-Biol Sci* 276, 961–969.

Blanchard DC (1995) Visible burrow system as a model of chronic social stress: Behavioral and neuroendocrine correlates. *Psychoneuroendocrinology* 20, 117–134.

Butler LK, Bisson IA, Hayden TJ et al. (2009) Adrenocortical responses to offspring-directed threats in two open-nesting birds. *Gen Comp Endocrinol* 162, 313–318.

Calandreau L, Favreau-Peigne A, Bertin A et al. (2011) Higher inherent fearfulness potentiates the effects of chronic stress in the Japanese quail. *Behav Brain Res* 225, 505–510.

Carroll BJ, Feinberg M, Greden JF (1981) A specific laboratory test for the diagnosis of melancholia. Standardization, validation, and clinical utility. *Archives of General Psychiatry* 38, 15–22.

Cole CR, Blackstone EH, Pashkow FJ et al. (1999) Heart-rate recovery immediately after exercise as a predictor of mortality. *New Engl J Med* 341, 1351–1357.

Cole CR, Foody JM, Blackstone EH et al. (2000) Heart rate recovery after submaximal exercise testing as a predictor of mortality in a cardiovascularly healthy cohort. *Ann Intern Med* 132, 552–555.

Cyr NE, Dickens MJ, Romero LM (2009) Heart rate and heart rate variability responses to acute and chronic stress in a wild-caught passerine bird. *Physiol Biochem Zool* 82, 332–344.

Cyr NE, Earle K, Tam C et al. (2007) The effect of chronic psychological stress on corticosterone, plasma metabolites, and immune responsiveness in European starlings. *Gen Comp Endocrinol* 154, 59–66.

Cyr NE, Romero LM (2007) Chronic stress in free-living European starlings reduces corticosterone concentrations and reproductive success. *Gen Comp Endocrinol* 151, 82–89.

Cyr NE, Romero LM (2008) Fecal glucocorticoid metabolites of experimentally stressed captive and free-living starlings: Implications for conservation research. *Gen Comp Endocrinol* 158, 20–28.

De Kloet ER (1991) Brain corticosteroid receptor balance and homeostatic control. *Frontiers in Neuroendocrinology* 12, 95–164.

Delaney JPA, Brodie DA (2000) Effects of short-term psychological stress on the time and frequency domains of heart-rate variability. *Percept Motor Skills* 91, 515–524.

Dickens M, Romero LM, Cyr NE et al. (2009a) Chronic stress alters glucocorticoid receptor and mineralocorticoid receptor mRNA expression in the European starling (*Sturnus vulgaris*) brain. *J Neuroendocrinol* 21, 832–840.

Dickens MJ, Delehanty DJ, Romero LM (2009b) Stress and translocation: alterations in the stress physiology of translocated birds. *Proceedings of the Royal Society B: Biological Sciences* 276, 2051–2056.

Dickens MJ, Delehanty DJ, Romero LM (2010) Stress: An inevitable component of animal translocation. *Biol Conserv* 143, 1329–1341.

Dickens MJ, Earle KA, Romero LM (2009c) Initial transference of wild birds to captivity alters stress physiology. *Gen Comp Endocrinol* 160, 76–83.

Dickens MJ, Romero LM (2009) Wild European starlings (Sturnus vulgaris) adjust to captivity with sustained sympathetic nervous system drive and a reduced fight-or-flight response. *Physiol Biochem Zool* 82, 603–610.

Dickens MJ, Romero LM (2013) A consensus endocrine profile for chronically stressed wild animals does not exist. *Gen Comp Endocrinol* 191, 177–189.

Hennessy MB, Levine S (1978) Sensitive pituitary-adrenal responsiveness to varying intensities of psychological stimulation. *Physiology and Behavior* 21, 295–297.

Meewise ML, Reitsma JB, De Vries GJ et al. (2007) Cortisol and post-traumatic stress disorder in adults – Systemic review and meta-analysis. *Br J Psychiatry* 191, 387–392.

Nephew BC, Kahn SA, Romero LM (2003) Heart rate and behavior are regulated independently of corticosterone following diverse acute stressors. *Gen Comp Endocrinol* 133, 173–180.

Nephew BC, Romero LM (2003) Behavioral, physiological, and endocrine responses of starlings to acute increases in density. *Horm Behav* 44, 222–232.

Nimon AJ, Schroter RC, Oxenham RK (1996) Artificial eggs: measuring heart rate and effects of disturbance in nesting penguins. *Physiol Behav* 60, 1019–1022.

Remage-Healey L, Romero LM (2000) Daily and seasonal variation in response to stress in captive starlings (Sturnus vulgaris): glucose. *Gen Comp Endocrinol* 119, 60–68.

Rich EL, Romero LM (2005) Exposure to chronic stress downregulates corticosterone responses to acute stressors. *Am J Physiol Regul Integr Comp Physiol* 288, R1628–1636.

Rohleder N, Joksimovic L, Wolf JM et al. (2004) Hypocortisolism and increased glucocorticoid sensitivity of proinflammatory cytokine production in Bosnian war refugees with posttraumatic stress disorder. *Biological Psychiatry* 55, 745–751.

Romero LM, Dickens MJ, Cyr NE (2009) The reactive scope model - A new model integrating homeostasis, allostasis, and stress. *Horm Behav* 55, 375–389.

Roth G, Ekbad S, Agren H (2006) A longitudinal study of PTSD in a sample of adult mass-evacuated Kosovars, some of whom returned to their home country. *Eur Psychiatry* 21, 152–159.

Saint-Dizier H, Constantin P, Davies DC et al. (2009) Subdivisions of the arcopallium/posterior pallial amygdala complex are differentially involved in the control of fear behaviour in the Japanese quail. *Brain Res Bull* 79, 288–295.

Sapolsky R, Brooke S, Stein-Behrens B (1995) Methodologic issues in studying glucocorticoid-induced damage to neurons. *J Neurosci Methods* 58, 1–15.

Sondergaard HP, Theorell T (2003) A longitudinal study of hormonal reactions accopanying life events in recently resettled refugees. *Psychotherapy and Psychosomatics* 72, 49–58.

Steen JB, Gabrielsen GW, Kanwisher JW (1988) Physiological aspects of freezing behavior in willow ptarmigan hens. *Acta Physiol Scand* 134, 299–304.

Wingfield JC, Romero LM (2001) Adrenocortical responses to stress and their modulation in free-living vertebrates. In: McEwen BS, Goodman HM (eds) *Handbook of Physiology; Section 7: The Endocrine System; Volume IV: Coping with the Environment: Neural and Endocrine Mechanisms*. Oxford University Press, New York, pp. 211–234.

CHAPTER 8

Stress, fear, and memory in healthy individuals

Christian J. Merz[1], Bernet M. Elzinga[2] & Lars Schwabe[3]

[1] Institute of Cognitive Neuroscience, Cognitive Psychology, Ruhr-University, Bochum, Germany
[2] Institute for Psychological Research, Section Clinical Psychology, Leiden University, The Netherlands
[3] Institute for Psychology, Department of Cognitive Psychology, University of Hamburg, Hamburg, Germany

8.1 Introduction

Life-threatening experiences such as car accidents, assaults, or natural disasters usually produce powerful and intrusive memories. In vulnerable individuals, these overly strong memories may persist and lead to the debilitating condition of posttraumatic stress disorder (PTSD). In addition to strongly encoded emotional memories, impoverished memory functioning or disruptions in memory have been associated with exposure to stress. These two, apparently opposing, memory processes have also been identified as key memory impairments in PTSD patients, in the form of highly emotional traumatic memories that are easily triggered and general memory impairments (American Psychiatric Association, 2013).

In this chapter, we summarize the research findings on the impact of acute stress on memory functioning in healthy individuals, which may shed light on the underlying neurobiological processes related to these two apparently distinct memory processes.

The strength of traumatic memories has been related to the action of hormones and neurotransmitters that are released during the traumatic event (Pitman, 1989; Pitman et al., 2012). Although such extreme experiences are relatively rare, we all experience stress in varying degrees and forms every day, with work-related stress, financial problems, relationship distress, or chronic illness being only a few examples. Albeit less intense, it is assumed that the biological responses to everyday stress are highly similar to the physiological responses to life-threatening stress experiences. The stress response begins when the prefrontal cortex (PFC) and limbic structures, in particular the amygdala and the hippocampus, appraise a situation or a stimulus as a potential threat (i.e., a stressor) to the organism. These brain areas are intimately

Posttraumatic Stress Disorder: From Neurobiology to Treatment, First Edition.
Edited by J. Douglas Bremner.
© 2016 John Wiley & Sons, Inc. Published 2016 by John Wiley & Sons, Inc.

linked to the hypothalamus, the control center of two major stress response systems of the body: the rapidly acting sympathetic nervous system and the hypothalamus–pituitary–adrenal (HPA) axis (Joëls & Baram, 2009; see Figure 8.1 and Chapters 9 and 11). When prefrontal and limbic structures signal that a situation is threatening, the hypothalamus rapidly activates the sympathetic nervous system, which triggers, within seconds, the release of epinephrine and norepinephrine from the adrenal medulla. Although these catecholamines

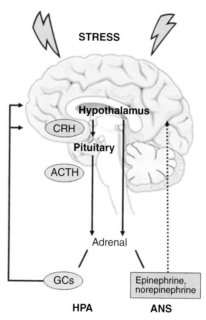

Figure 8.1 Circuits activated by stress. If a situation is perceived as a threat for the physiological or psychological integrity of the organism, the brain activates two lines of defense mechanisms that serve to adapt to the demand and to restore balance: the rapidly acting autonomic nervous system (ANS) and the slower hypothalamic–pituitary–adrenal (HPA) axis. The first line of defense sets in immediately after the stressor occurs when the amygdala activates the hypothalamus. Activation of the hypothalamus in turn stimulates the sympathetic arm of the ANS, which secretes norepinephrine at its postganglionic nerve endings. Among the effector organs of the ANS is the adrenal medulla, which releases epinephrine and norepinephrine. Autonomic activation can indirectly (via the vagal nerve, solitary tract nucleus, and locus coeruleus) lead to the release of norepinephrine in the brain. The second line of defense is initiated by the secretion of corticotropin-releasing hormone (CRH) from the paraventricular nucleus of the hypothalamus. CRH causes the secretion of β-endorphin and adrenocorticotropic hormone (ACTH) from the anterior pituitary, which is transported in the bloodstream to the cortex of the adrenal glands, inducing the secretion of glucocorticoids. Glucocorticoids exert negative feedback via receptors at the pituitary and hypothalamus, thereby reducing the enhanced activity of the HPA axis. (Reproduced from Schwabe et al., 2010b.)

cannot cross the blood–brain barrier, they exert indirect effects on the brain via the vagus nerve, which then further activates central noradrenergic systems, particularly the locus coeruleus and the nucleus tractus solitarius (Williams & Clayton, 2001). In addition to the activation of the sympathetic nervous system, the hypothalamus also triggers the HPA axis by releasing corticotropin-releasing hormone (CRH). CRH provokes the secretion of another hormone, adreno-corticotropic hormone (ACTH), from the pituitary. ACTH, in turn, stimulates the release of glucocorticoids (mainly cortisol in humans and corticosterone in rodents) from the adrenal cortex. Glucocorticoids are steroid hormones that can cross the blood–brain barrier. Through binding to glucocorticoid receptors (GRs) and mineralocorticoid receptors (MRs) in the brain, glucocorticoids modulate, in concert with norepinephrine and other hormones and neurotransmitters that are released in response to stressors, learning and memory processes by acting on various brain areas, including the hippocampus, amygdala, and PFC. Understanding how stress, through these stress mediators, may yield strongly consolidated emotional memories and impaired memory functioning could enhance our understanding of the pathogenesis of PTSD and potentially open the door to novel treatment approaches.

In this chapter, we first focus on the impact of stress and stress hormones on human episodic memory, i.e., memory for events that can be explicitly stated and tested, such as the memory for your last birthday party. Next, we review stress effects on human fear conditioning, an important model of PTSD, where fear memories can be established without explicit awareness of the learning process. In the third part of this chapter, we will summarize recent findings showing that stress may alter the contributions of multiple memory systems to learning, thus promoting a shift from flexible, "cognitive" to rather rigid, "habit" learning and memory. Finally, we discuss the implications of these findings on stress and memory in healthy humans for trauma memory, the core feature of PTSD. Findings related to neuropsychological studies of memory function in PTSD patients are covered elsewhere in this book (see Chapter 12).

8.2 Time-dependent effects of stress on episodic memory in healthy humans

When learning, storing, and retrieving new information, the hippocampus and adjacent medial temporal lobe regions are the key locus of episodic memory in the brain (Dickerson & Eichenbaum, 2010; Tulving & Markowitsch, 1998). At the same time, the hippocampus is one of the brain areas with the highest density of GRs and MRs (de Kloet et al., 1998; McEwen et al., 1986), suggesting that it is particularly sensitive to stress and glucocorticoid effects. Indeed, there is converging evidence from neurophysiological, neuroimaging, and behavioral studies showing that stress and stress hormones affect hippocampal activity and functionality (Diamond et al., 2007; Kim et al., 2001; Pruessner et al., 2008; de Quervain et al., 2003; Schwabe et al., 2009a). Hippocampus-dependent learning and memory processes may be enhanced or impaired by stress, depending on whether or not stress occurs around the time and within the context of a learning episode (Joëls et al., 2006). In a stressful situation, the hippocampus turns to a 'memory formation mode' during which strong memories are created for everything that is related to the stressor. When the stress situation is over, the hippocampus appears to shift to a "memory storage mode" that is dedicated to the consolidation of the memories of the stressful event (Schwabe et al., 2012a). The prioritized encoding and storage of memories of stressful experiences is obviously adaptive; our survival may depend on remembering these stressful episodes from our past. However, the superior memory for information related to a stressor may come at the cost or detriment of stressor-unrelated memory processes. In the following sections, we discuss the effect of stress on every stage of a memory – encoding, consolidation, retrieval, and post-retrieval reconsolidation – in more detail (see also Figure 8.2).

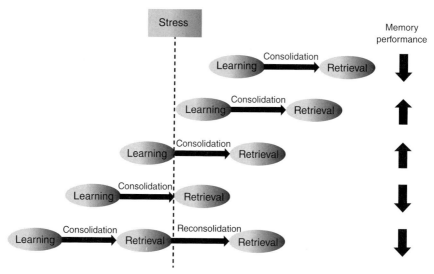

Figure 8.2 Time-dependent effects of stress on hippocampus-dependent episodic memory. Stress before learning may enhance memory when it occurs within the context of a learning experience (e.g., shortly before or during learning), whereas stress out of the learning context (e.g., relatively long before learning) impairs memory. Stress shortly after learning strengthens subsequent memory, particularly for emotionally arousing information. Conversely, stress before retention testing typically reduces retrieval performance, again particularly for emotionally arousing information. In addition, stress may also interfere with the re-stabilization ("reconsolidation") of memories after retrieval. (Reproduced from Schwabe & Wolf, 2013.)

8.2.1 Stress and memory encoding

One of the challenges in investigating the specific effects of stress on memory encoding is that stress effects on encoding can hardly be disentangled from those on memory consolidation, and in some studies the stress effects may influence encoding, consolidation, and retrieval. Studies in which participants were exposed to a (unrelated) stressor before encoding yielded heterogeneous results, with some studies reporting enhanced (Henckens et al., 2009; Nater et al., 2007; Schwabe et al., 2008; Van Stegeren et al., 2010), and others impaired, subsequent memory performance (Elzinga et al., 2005; Kirschbaum et al., 1996; Lupien et al., 1997). Several factors have been proposed to account for these discrepant findings. For example, it has been suggested that stress has different effects on the encoding of neutral and emotional material (Payne et al., 2006; Tops et al., 2003) or that the direction of the stress effects depends on the stressor intensity and the associated glucocorticoid level (Abercrombie et al., 2003). Based on models derived from neurophysiological studies in rodents (Diamond et al., 2007; Joëls et al., 2006), it has recently been argued that the time of the stress exposure relative to the learning episode might be the critical factor that determines whether stress before learning enhances or impairs memory. It is assumed that catecholamines and rapid, non-genomic glucocorticoid actions enhance the memory for currently ongoing events, whereas the slowly developing genomic glucocorticoid actions impair memory formation (Joëls et al., 2006, 2011). Such a biphasic effect of glucocorticoids on the hippocampus was recently confirmed in the human brain (Lovallo et al., 2010). Moreover, a recent behavioral study reported that memory was impaired when healthy subjects were stressed 30 minutes before learning, but enhanced when subjects were exposed to the stressor shortly before learning (Zoladz et al., 2011). In line with these findings, other studies showed that psychosocial stress shortly before or during learning enhanced the retention of material that is conceptually related to the stress situation, such as stressor-related, high-arousal words (Smeets et al., 2007, 2009). However, stress around the time of learning may not necessarily boost memory. If stress is not related to the learning experience, it may act as a distractor and result in severely impaired memory (Schwabe & Wolf, 2010a). In sum, many factors determine how exactly stress affects memory encoding, and the details are still not fully understood.

8.2.2 Stress and memory consolidation

Compared with neutral events, emotionally arousing experiences are typically very well remembered (Christianson, 1992; McGaugh, 2000; Winograd & Neisser, 1992). Understanding how the superior memory for emotional material is created has important implications for the intrusive traumatic memories that typically develop in PTSD. The emotional memory enhancement is thought to be a result of the influence of adrenal hormones on amygdala activity, which in turn promotes consolidation processes in other brain regions such as the hippocampus. For instance, amygdala activity during encoding correlates significantly with the strength of emotional memories (Cahill et al., 1996) and amygdala dysfunction abolishes the superior memory for emotional material (Cahill et al., 1995). Adrenergic activity is critical for the superior memory for an emotionally arousing event. For instance, studies showed a correlation between the level of the plasma metabolite of norepinephrine, 3-methoxy-4-hydroxyphenylglycol (MHPG), and the strength of emotional memory formation in the context of a pharmacological challenge (Southwick et al., 2002). Blocking the activity of norepinephrine by means of the β-adrenergic antagonist propranolol eliminates both the emotional memory enhancement and the associated increase in amygdala activity (Cahill et al., 1994; Strange & Dolan, 2004), and hence is theoretically an interesting treatment for direct use after exposure to a traumatic event. In line with the idea that hormones and neurotransmitters that are released in response to stress facilitate memory consolidation, stress and elevated glucocorticoid or epinephrine levels shortly after training also enhance subsequent memory (Andreano & Cahill, 2006; Beckner et al., 2006; Cahill & Alkire, 2003; Cahill et al., 2003). The enhancing effects of stress on memory consolidation are particularly pronounced for emotionally arousing material (Cahill et al., 2003). Moreover, glucocorticoids appear to be most effective in individuals who are emotionally aroused (Abercrombie et al., 2006). These latter findings corroborate the view that glucocorticoids interact with emotional arousal-induced noradrenergic activation to boost memory consolidation, which has been convincingly shown in rodents (Roozendaal et al., 2006a,b).

8.2.3 Stress and memory retrieval

Stress or the administration of glucocorticoids shortly before retention testing is often associated with reduced memory performance (de Quervain et al., 2000; Kuhlmann et al., 2005; Schwabe & Wolf, 2009a, 2014; Tollenaar et al., 2008, 2009; but for indications of enhanced retrieval during or after stress, see Hupbach & Fieman, 2012; Schilling et al., 2013; Schönfeld et al., 2014; Schwabe et al., 2009b), suggesting that memory retrieval is, in contrast to memory consolidation, impaired by stress. The disruptive effect of stress or glucocorticoids on retrieval performance is paralleled by reduced activity in the PFC and the hippocampus during retention testing (Kukolja et al., 2008; Oei et al., 2007). Emotionally arousing memories are, again, particularly sensitive to the influence of stress and stress hormones (Buchanan et al., 2006; Kuhlmann et al., 2005). Blocking the arousal-related noradrenergic activity pharmacologically with a β-adrenergic antagonist prevents the impact of stress on memory retrieval (de Quervain et al., 2007; Schwabe et al., 2009b), whereas it does not affect retrieval *per se* (Tollenaar et al., 2009). Thus, there is strong evidence that the impairing effect of stress on memory retrieval requires, as with the enhancing effect on memory consolidation, concurrent glucocorticoid and noradrenergic activation.

8.2.4 Stress and memory reconsolidation

The past 15 years have seen renewed interest in the idea that the reactivation of a consolidated memory during retrieval returns this memory to an unstable state again from which it needs to be stabilized anew during a process of "reconsolidation" (Dudai, 2006; Nader & Hardt, 2009). Recent evidence suggests that stress may affect memory also when administered after retrieval, i.e., during reconsolidation. The direction of these effects, however, is not yet fully clear. One study reported that stress during reconsolidation enhances subsequent memory (Coccoz et al., 2011), similar to stress during initial consolidation. Other studies, however, showed that stress after retrieval impairs updating of memory traces (Schmidt et al., 2014) and disrupts the re-stabilization of memories during reconsolidation, resulting in impaired subsequent recall (Schwabe & Wolf, 2010c; Zhao et al., 2009). Given the potential opportunity to modify unwanted memories after their reactivation, stress hormone effects on memory reconsolidation might be particularly interesting in the context of PTSD and are therefore an important avenue for future research.

8.3 Stress and fear conditioning in humans

In addition to the episodic memory of the traumatic event, conditioned fear is an important part of the trauma memory (see Chapter 4). Fear conditioning processes are thought to play a major role in the development of anxiety disorders in general (Mineka & Oehlberg, 2008; Mineka & Zinbarg, 2006) and fear conditioning is one of the most important models of fear learning relevant to PTSD (Graham & Milad, 2011; Mineka & Oehlberg, 2008). During fear conditioning, an individual learns that a neutral stimulus is reliably paired with an aversive event (unconditioned stimulus, UCS) leading to a fear response (unconditioned response). As a result of these pairings, the initially neutral stimulus alone can trigger the fear response and is now referred to as a conditioned stimulus (CS). The CS can be a cue (cue-dependent conditioning) or a context (context-dependent conditioning). Because human fear conditioning studies have used mainly cue-dependent conditioning, we will focus mainly on this form of conditioning (for context-dependent conditioning in animals, see Maren et al., 2013; for the effects of development on fear learning, see Chapter 4).

Repeated presentations of the CS without the UCS result in fear extinction during which fear memories are suppressed. Exposure to phobic stimuli and situations, or trauma-related memories in the case of PTSD, is based on fear extinction and represents the most effective therapeutic strategy to treat anxiety disorders (Foa & Kozak, 1986; Vervliet et al., 2013). However, after extinction, the fear is not gone, it is just not expressed. Return of fear is often observed when individuals are exposed to the CS after a delay (spontaneous recovery), after a change in context (renewal), or after unsignalled presentations of the UCS (reinstatement; see Bouton, 2004).

It is well established that the amygdala is the central structure for fear conditioning in the brain, both in humans and other animals (LeDoux, 2000). Moreover, the anterior cingulate cortex, the insula, the ventromedial PFC (vmPFC), and the hippocampus are important parts of the fear and extinction network (Mechias et al., 2010; Sehlmeyer et al., 2009). Interestingly, abnormalities in this fear circuitry have been repeatedly found in PTSD patients (Elzinga & Bremner, 2003; Etkin & Wager, 2007). In the following sections, we review the findings regarding the impact of stress and stress hormones on fear memory formation, extinction, and the return of fear.

8.3.1 Stress and fear memory formation

How stress affects fear acquisition in healthy individuals remains controversial; some studies reported enhanced, others reduced, conditioned fear memory after stress. Part of these discrepancies is the result of differences in the timing of the stress experience. For instance, autonomic activity setting in rapidly after stressor onset appears to be associated with enhanced conditioned fear (Antov et al., 2013). In line with these findings, pharmacological elevations in noradrenergic stimulation by the α_2-adrenoreceptor antagonist yohimbine strengthens subsequent fear memory, as indicated by slower extinction learning, heightened fear retrieval after reinstatement, and increased fear reacquisition (Soeter & Kindt, 2011). In contrast to the influence of autonomic arousal, the delayed cortisol response to a stressor appears to be negatively correlated with fear memory formation (Antov et al., 2013). This is in line with findings that the cortisol response 30 minutes after stress exposure is negatively associated with amygdala activation (Oei et al., 2012). However, it is important to note that there is accumulating evidence for significant sex differences in stress effects on fear conditioning, in line with animal data (Dalla & Shors, 2009; Shors, 2004). For instance, stress induction 1 hour before fear conditioning enhanced fear responses in men but appeared to inhibit fear memory in women (Jackson et al., 2006). Similarly, stress-induced cortisol elevations after fear conditioning strengthen fear memory consolidation in men but not in women (Zorawski et al., 2005, 2006). Exposure to psychosocial stress led to the same pattern of results: stress attenuated conditioned fear responses in men, but enhanced fear responses in women taking oral contraceptives (Merz et al., 2013).

Pharmacological studies suggest that glucocorticoids may further modulate fear conditioning processes differently in men and women sex-dependently.

Cortisol attenuated fear contextualization and increased fear generalization in women taking oral contraceptives, whereas the opposite pattern was observed in men (Van Ast et al., 2012). More specifically, in women, cortisol enhanced fear towards cues signaling danger in threatening and safe contexts, as well as towards safety signals in a threatening context. Such deficits in fear contextualization may constitute a vulnerability factor in the development of anxiety and trauma-related disorders such as PTSD. Moreover, it has been consistently shown that pharmacological elevations of cortisol diminish fear responses in men and free-cycling women, but increase fear in women taking oral contraceptives (Merz et al., 2010, 2012; Stark et al., 2006; Tabbert et al., 2010). Neuroimaging revealed that glucocorticoid administration and stress affected the fear network, including the amygdala and the hippocampus (Henckens et al., 2010, 2012; de Quervain et al., 2003), which are critical for the formation of emotional memories (Cahill & McGaugh, 1998; McGaugh, 2000). Cortisol also exerted sex hormone status-related effects in areas involved in fear expression and regulation, such as the anterior cingulate or the orbitofrontal cortex. Further evidence points to sex-dependent effects of stress hormones, particularly on amygdala activity. For example, noradrenergic stimulation led to increased amygdala activity in response to fearful faces in women but to decreased amygdala responses in men (Schwabe et al., 2013a). In line with these findings, rapid cortisol effects reduced amygdala responsivity to fearful faces (Henckens et al., 2010) and also impaired resting state functional connectivity of the amygdala to the hippocampus in men (Henckens et al., 2012).

Taken together, autonomic activity and rapid, non-genomic glucocorticoid actions appear to enhance fear memory formation. However, when stress hormone concentrations peak shortly before or during acquisition they inhibit transiently the fear circuit surrounding the amygdala and the hippocampus in general, but increase fear in women taking oral contraceptives. Slowly developing, genomic glucocorticoid effects, on the other hand, seem to enhance fear acquisition again. How exactly stress hormones evoke these opposite fear response patterns is still not fully understood.

8.3.2 Stress, extinction, and the return of fear

The majority of human studies on the influence of stress on fear conditioning processes have focused on fear acquisition, yet over the past few years also fear extinction and the subsequent return of fear received increasing attention. For example, cortisol administration before fear learning has been shown to reduce activation of the amygdala or the hippocampus during subsequent extinction learning in women taking oral contraceptives (Tabbert et al., 2010). However, here, cortisol effects on fear acquisition and extinction could not be separated. To overcome this problem, in a recent functional magnetic resonance imaging experiment, cortisol was given directly after fear learning, 45 minutes before fear extinction took place (Merz et al., 2014). The results showed that cortisol increased electrodermal fear responses during extinction in men, which was paralleled by attenuated activation of the amygdala, medial PFC, and nucleus accumbens. These findings suggest that cortisol disrupted the interplay between these structures, which may have delayed fear extinction. Whereas this study used a 1-day design in which fear acquisition und extinction were separated only by a short delay, another recent study in healthy humans tested how stress alters extinction of a conditioned fear memory that was acquired 1 day before (Bentz et al., 2013). Here, stress reduced fear retrieval expressed as UCS expectancy in men, but not in women. However, this effect was evident only at the first CS presentation in the extinction session as well as in another test on a third day, indicating that stress inhibited fear retrieval rather than that it affected extinction learning. These findings parallel experiments in phobic patients, who benefit from cortisol intake prior to exposure sessions, which are based on the principle of extinction learning (de Quervain et al., 2011; Soravia et al., 2006; see below).

Several further attempts have been made to enhance extinction learning and to prevent the return of fear mainly by pharmacological alterations of noradrenergic activity (see Holmes & Quirk, 2010, for an overview of the animal literature). Pharmacologically increased noradrenergic activity before exposure therapy attenuates fear at a 1-week follow-up in acrophobic patients (Powers et al., 2009). In line with findings in episodic memory (discussed earlier), it is tempting to speculate that yohimbine made extinction memories more arousing and thus better consolidated.

Building on the proposed lability of memories after their reactivation (Nader & Hardt, 2009), several recent studies aimed to tackle fear memories during reconsolidation. Administration of the β-adrenergic antagonist propranolol given either before or after fear memory reactivation by a single CS presentation reduced the return of fear in subsequent reinstatement and renewal protocols, even 1 month later (Soeter & Kindt, 2010, 2012a,b).

Taken together, augmentation of (nor)adrenergic transmission seems to promote consolidation of fear extinction. Neuroimaging studies exploring the neural underpinnings of the effects of norepinephrine are still largely missing. The animal literature, however, suggests an enhancement of the excitability of neurons in the vmPFC (Mueller & Cahill, 2010).

8.4 Stress-induced modulation of multiple memory systems

The previous two sections dealt with stress effects on single memory systems, mainly the hippocampus and the amygdala. Stress may affect the performance of these systems and thus alter quantitative memory parameters such as the number of remembered items or the strength of the fear memory. Over the past few years, evidence has accumulated suggesting that stress affects not only how much we learn or remember in a given situation but also how we learn and which strategies we use during learning (Schwabe et al., 2010b).

Many tasks can be solved in different ways; they can be acquired by distinct memory systems that differ in the mode of operation and the type of information that is processed (Squire, 2004). Stress may have a critical impact on which of these systems is engaged during learning. Route learning, for example, may be supported by a hippocampus-dependent spatial memory system that learns the relationship between multiple cues in the environment and by a dorsal striatum-dependent stimulus–response (S–R) memory system that associates a single stimulus with a certain response (McDonald & White, 1993; Packard et al., 1989). In line with earlier rodent data (Kim et al., 2001; Packard & Wingard, 2004), stress before learning promotes in humans S–R learning at the expense of spatial learning (Schwabe et al., 2007). Glucocorticoids seem to play an important role in the switch between flexible, "cognitive" spatial learning and rather rigid, "habitual" S–R learning (Bohbot et al., 2011; Schwabe et al., 2009c). Probabilistic classification learning may also be subserved by a hippocampal and a striatal system (Foerde et al., 2006; Knowlton et al., 1996) and which memory controls learning can also be influenced by stress. Stress before classification learning favors striatum-dependent "procedural" learning over hippocampus-dependent "declarative" learning (Schwabe & Wolf, 2012). Neuroimaging data confirmed that stress shifted classification learning from hippocampal to striatal control and suggested that this shift may be due to an impairment of the hippocampus-dependent system (Schwabe & Wolf, 2012). The shift from hippocampus-dependent to striatum-dependent memory is orchestrated by the amygdala, as indicated by findings showing that stress increases amygdala connectivity with the dorsal striatum, whereas amygdala connectivity with the hippocampus decreases after stress (Schwabe et al., 2013b).

Instrumental learning can also be controlled by two separate memory systems: a PFC-based "goal-directed" system that encodes the association between an action and the outcome that is engendered by the action; and a dorsolateral striatum-based "habit" system that associates a response with preceding stimuli (Balleine & O'Doherty, 2010; Dickinson, 1985). Stress promotes habit learning (Schwabe & Wolf, 2009b, 2010b). This stress-induced bias towards habits is correlated with the cortisol increase in response to stress and can be prevented by a β-adrenergic antagonist (Schwabe et al., 2011), suggesting that stress effects on the engagement of goal-directed and habit systems necessitate, in same way as stress effects on hippocampal memory (Roozendaal et al., 2006a), simultaneous glucocorticoid and noradrenergic activation. Corroborating this conclusion, pharmacological elevations of both glucocorticoid and noradrenergic activity resulted in habitual learning, whereas behavior remained goal-directed when only one of the two stress response systems was stimulated (Schwabe et al., 2010a, 2012b). At the neural level, habit learning after concurrent glucocorticoid and noradrenergic activity is associated with sensitivity of prefrontal areas to changes in the motivational value of an outcome (Schwabe et al., 2012b).

In sum, stress may modulate the engagement of multiple memory systems in a manner that favors "habit" over "cognitive" memory and this appears to be due to an impairment of "cognitive" memory systems, thus allowing "habit" systems to dominate behavior (Schwabe & Wolf, 2013).

8.5 Stress and memory in healthy subjects: implications for PTSD

Stress affects how much we learn and remember. Emotionally arousing events are typically remembered much better than neutral events. Moreover, stress during or shortly after a learning experience may enhance episodic or fear memory, particularly when the content is related to the stressor, whereas memory retrieval appears to be impaired by stress (Roozendaal et al., 2006a; Schwabe et al., 2012a). In addition to these stress effects on quantitative memory performance, stress may also modulate the engagement of multiple memory systems in a manner that facilitates rather rigid, inflexible memory processes at the expense of flexible but cognitively demanding memory processes (Schwabe & Wolf, 2013). These different stress effects on memory may help to explain the apparently opposing memory processes in PTSD patients, who suffer from strong intrusive, trauma-related memories on the one hand, but show general memory impairments or distortions for information that is unrelated to the traumatic event, on the other.

The extreme stress during a traumatic experience leads to a strong release of glucocorticoids and catecholamines. As described earlier, these stress mediators promote the formation of lasting memories, in particular if stress occurs in the context of the learning episode, as is the case during a traumatic experience. Thus, the action of stress hormones during the trauma may result in an "overconsolidation" of the traumatic event, through episodic memory processes and fear conditioning (Elzinga & Bremner, 2003; Pitman, 1989; Pitman et al., 2012), resulting in memories that are easily triggered by a wide range of reminders. In addition, the extreme stress during a traumatic experience may alter the recruitment of multiple memory systems in memory formation. Based on research in healthy individuals (Schwabe, 2013), it can be predicted that the stressful experience favors the engagement of habit or S–R memory that is subserved by the striatum over PFC- or hippocampus-dependent cognitive memory. In addition to the fear conditioning processes, the aberrant engagement of habit or S–R memory processes may be reflected in the strong emotional responding to single trauma-related cues (e.g., odors or sounds) that is often observed in PTSD patients (Liberzon et al., 1999; Pissiota et al., 2002). Furthermore, the predominance of striatum-based habit memory under stress, at the expense of hippocampal learning, could also account for the disorganization of trauma memory and why it is often difficult for PTSD patients to integrate the traumatic experience into autobiographical memory (Ehlers & Clark, 2000), which is part of hippocampus-dependent memory. Moreover, stress alters the neurocircuitry of fear, which might explain the aberrant fear response in PTSD. Interestingly, the stress-induced alterations in fear memory appear to be more pronounced in women, who also show a higher prevalence of PTSD than men (Kilpatrick et al., 2013). These examples show that the research on stress effects on memory may enhance our understanding of the neurobiological basis of stress-related disorders such as PTSD.

In addition, however, the findings regarding the impact of stress on memory might also open the door to novel treatment approaches for PTSD. For instance, based on evidence indicating that stress and glucocorticoids impair memory retrieval (Buchanan et al., 2006; de Quervain et al., 2000), it has been hypothesized that stress hormones could also reduce trauma memory retrieval (de Quervain & Margraf, 2008).

It has been shown that glucocorticoids may attenuate phobic fear (Mouthaan et al., 2014; Soravia et al., 2006; de Quervain et al., 2011). There is also some evidence that glucocorticoids may indeed reduce memory-related PTSD symptoms, such as intrusive re-experiencing or nightmares (Aerni et al., 2004). Another strategy makes use of the fact that stress or glucocorticoid effects on memory necessitate noradrenergic arousal (McGaugh, 2000; Roozendaal et al., 2006a), suggesting that blockade of noradrenergic activity might prevent the "overconsolidation" of memory. Indeed, there is some evidence that pharmacological blockade of norepinephrine action by the β-adrenergic antagonist propranolol shortly after a potentially traumatic event reduces PTSD symptoms 3 months later (Pitman et al., 2002; Vaiva et al., 2003). However, trauma memory formation can only be interfered with in a short time window after the traumatic event when clinical treatment is often not available, which limits the practical utility of modifications of initial trauma memory formation. An alternative strategy to circumvent this problem could be the modification of traumatic memories after their reactivation, i.e., during reconsolidation. Memory modification during reconsolidation provides an opportunity to change consolidated, seemingly robust, memories (Nader & Hardt, 2009). In line with evidence from healthy subjects showing that propranolol during fear reactivation can erase subsequent fear (Kindt et al., 2009), propranolol during or after trauma reactivation has been shown to reduce subsequent intrusions (Brunet et al., 2008, 2011), a pathological hallmark of PTSD.

These results are certainly preliminary and much more research is needed to determine the potential use of stress hormone manipulations in the treatment of traumatic memories. Only the first steps have been taken on the long road to the development of novel treatment strategies for PTSD and it is unclear whether it will be successful. However, in light of the suffering associated with PTSD, these efforts are worthwhile.

References

Abercrombie HC, Kalin NH, Thurow ME et al. (2003) Cortisol variation in humans affects memory for emotionally laden and neutral information. *Behav Neurosci* 117, 505–516.

Abercrombie HC, Speck NS, Monticelli RM (2006) Endogenous cortisol elevations are related to memory facilitation only in individuals who are emotionally aroused. *Psychoneuroendocrinology* 31, 187–196.

Aerni A, Traber R, Hock C et al. (2004) Low-dose cortisol for symptoms of post-traumatic stress disorder. *Am J Psychiatry* 161, 1488–1490.

American Psychiatric Association (2013) *Diagnostic and Statistical Manual of Mental Disorders: DSM-V*. American Psychiatric Press, Washington, DC.

Andreano JM, Cahill L (2006) Glucocorticoid release and memory consolidation in men and women. *Psychological Sci* 17, 466–470.

Antov MI, Wölk C, Stockhorst U (2013) Differential impact of the first and second wave of a stress response subsequent fear conditioning in healthy men. *Biol Psychol* 94, 456–468.

Balleine BW, O'Doherty JP (2010) Human and rodent homologies in action control: corticostriatal determinants of goal-directed and habitual action. *Neuropsychopharmacology* 35, 48–69.

Beckner VE, Tucker DM, Delville Y et al. (2006) Stress facilitates consolidation of verbal memory for a film but does not affect memory retrieval. *Behavioral Neurosci* 120, 518–527.

Bentz D, Michael T, Wilhelm FH et al. (2013) Influence of stress on fear memory processes in an aversive differential conditioning paradigm in humans *Psychoneuroendocrinology* 38, 1186–1197.

Bohbot VD, Gupta M, Banner H et al. (2011) Caudate nucleus-dependent response strategies in a virtual navigation task are associated with lower basal cortisol and impaired episodic memory. *Neurobiol Learn Mem* 96, 173–180.

Bouton ME (2004) Context and behavioral processes in extinction. *Learn Mem* 11, 485–494.

Brunet A, Orr SP, Tremblay J et al. (2008) Effect of post-retrieval propranolol on psychophysiologic responding during subsequent script-driven traumatic imagery in post-traumatic stress disorder. *J Psychiatr Res* 42, 503–506.

Brunet A, Poundja J, Tremblay J et al. (2011) Trauma reactivation under the influence of propranolol decreases posttraumatic stress symptoms and disorder: 3 open-label trials. *J Clin Psychopharmacol* 31, 547–550.

Buchanan TW, Tranel D, Adolphs R (2006) Impaired memory retrieval correlates with individual differences in cortisol response but not autonomic response. *Learn Mem* 13, 382–387.

Cahill L, Alkire MT (2003) Epinephrine enhancement of human memory consolidation: interaction with arousal at encoding. *Neurobiol Learn Mem* 79, 194–198.

Cahill L, Babinsky R, Markowitsch HJ et al. (1995) The amygdala and emotional memory. *Nature* 377, 295–296.

Cahill L, Gorski L, Le K (2003) Enhanced human memory consolidation with post-learning stress: interaction with the degree of arousal at encoding. *Learn Mem* 10, 270–274.

Cahill L, Haier RJ, Fallon J et al. (1996) Amygdala activity at encoding correlated with long-term, free recall of emotional information. *Proc Natl Acad Sci USA* 93, 8016–8021.

Cahill L, McGaugh JL (1998) Mechanisms of emotional arousal and lasting declarative memory. *Trends Neurosci* 21, 294–299.

Cahill L, Prins B, Weber M et al. (1994) Beta-adrenergic activation and memory for emotional events. *Nature* 371, 702–704.

Christianson SA (1992) *The Handbook of Emotion and Memory.* L. Erlbaum Associates, Hillsdale, NJ.

Coccoz V, Maldonado H, Delorenzi A (2011) The enhancement of reconsolidation with a naturalistic mild stressor improves the expression of a declarative memory in humans. *Neuroscience* 185, 61–72.

Dalla C, Shors TJ (2009) Sex differences in learning processes of classical and operant conditioning. *Physiol Behav* 97, 229–238.

de Kloet ER, Vreugdenhil E, Oitzl MS et al. (1998) Brain corticosteroid receptor balance in health and disease. *Endocrine Rev* 19, 269–301.

de Quervain DJ, Aerni A, Roozendaal B (2007) Preventive effect of ß-adrenoceptor blockade on glucocorticoid-induced memory retrieval deficits. *Am J Psychiatry* 164, 967–969.

de Quervain DJ, Bentz D, Michael T et al. (2011) Glucocorticoids enhance extinction-based psychotherapy. *Proc Natl Acad Sci USA* 108, 6621–6625.

de Quervain DJ, Henke K, Aerni A et al. (2003) Glucocorticoid-induced impairment of declarative memory retrieval is associated with reduced blood flow in the medial temporal lobe. *Eur J Neurosci* 17, 1296–1302.

de Quervain DJ, Margraf J (2008) Glucocorticoids for the treatment of post-traumatic stress disorder and phobias: a novel therapeutic approach. *Eur J of Pharmacol* 583, 365–371.

de Quervain DJ, Roozendaal B, Nitsch RM et al. (2000) Acute cortisone administration impairs retrieval of long-term declarative memory in humans. *Nature Neurosc* 3, 313–314.

Diamond DM, Campbell AM, Park CR et al. (2007) The temporal dynamics model of emotional memory processing: a synthesis on the neurobiological basis of stress-induced amnesia, flashbulb and traumatic memories, and the Yerkes-Dodson law. *Neural Plasticity* 2007, 60803.

Dickerson BC, Eichenbaum H (2010) The episodic memory system: neurocircuitry and disorders. *Neuropsychopharmacology* 35, 86–104.

Dickinson A (1985) Actions and habits: the development of behavioral autonomy. *Phil Trans R Soc Lond B: Biological Sciences* 308, 67–78.

Dudai Y (2006) Reconsolidation: the advantage of being refocused. *Current Opin Neurobiol* 16, 174–178.

Ehlers A, Clark DM (2000) A cognitive model of posttraumatic stress disorder. *Behav Res Therapy* 38, 319–345.

Elzinga BM, Bakker A, Bremner JD (2005) Stress-induced cortisol elevations are associated with impaired delayed, but not immediate recall. *Psychiatry Res* 134, 211–223.

Elzinga BM, Bremner JD (2003) Are the neural substrates of memory the final common pathway in PTSD? *J Affect Disord* 70, 1–17.

Etkin A, Wager TD (2007) Functional neuroimaging of anxiety: A meta-analysis of emotional processing in PTSD, social anxiety disorder, and specific phobia. *Am J Psychiatry* 164, 1476–1488.

Foa EB, Kozak MJ (1986) Emotional processing of fear: exposure to corrective information. *Psychol Bull* 99, 20–35.

Foerde K, Knowlton BJ, Poldrack RA (2006) Modulation of competing memory systems by distraction. *Proc Natl Acad Sci USA* 103, 11778–11783.

Graham BM, Milad MR (2011) The study of fear extinction: implications for anxiety disorders. *Am J Psychiatry* 168, 1255–1265.

Henckens MJ, van Wingen GA, Joëls M et al. (2012) Corticosteroid induced decoupling of the amygdala in men. *Cerebral Cortex* 22, 2336–2345.

Henckens MJAG, Hermans EJ, Pu Z et al. (2009) Stressed memories: How acute stress affects memory formation in humans. *J Neurosci* 29, 10 111–10 119.

Henckens MJAG, van Wingen GA, Joels M et al. (2010) Time-dependent effects of corticosteroids on human amygdala processing. *J Neurosci* 30, 12 725–12 732.

Holmes A, Quirk GJ (2010) Pharmacological facilitation of fear extinction and the search for adjunct treatments for anxiety disorders – the case of yohimbine. *Trends Pharmacol Sci* 31, 2–7.

Hupbach A, Fieman R (2012) Moderate stress enhances immediate and delayed retrieval of educationally relevant material in healthy young men. *Behav Neurosci* 126:819–825.

Jackson ED, Payne JD, Nadel L et al. (2006) Stress differentially modulates fear conditioning in healthy men and women. *Biol Psychiatry* 59, 516–522.

Joëls M, Baram TZ (2009) The neuro-symphony of stress. *Nat Rev Neurosci* 10, 459–466.

Joëls M, Fernandez G, Roozendaal B (2011) Stress and emotional memory: a matter of timing. *Trends Cogn Sci* 15, 56–65.

Joëls M, Pu Z, Wiegert O et al. (2006) Learning under stress: how does it work? *Trends Cogn Sci* 10, 152–158.

Kilpatrick DG, Resnick HS, Milanak ME et al. (2013) National estimates of exposure to traumatic events and PTSD prevalence using DSM-IV and DSM-5 criteria. *J Traum Stress* 26, 537–547.

Kim J, Lee H, Han J et al. (2001) Amygdala is critical for stress-induced modulation of hippocampal long-term potentiation and learning. *J Neurosci* 21, 5222–5228.

Kindt M, Soeter M, Vervliet B (2009) Beyond extinction: erasing human fear responses and preventing the return of fear. *Nat Neurosci* 12, 256–258.

Kirschbaum C, Wolf OT, May M et al. (1996) Stress- and treatment-induced elevations of cortisol levels associated with impaired declarative memory in healthy adults. *Life Sci* 58, 1475–1483.

Knowlton BJ, Mangels JA, Squire LR (1996) A neostriatal habit learning system in humans. *Science* 273, 1399–1402.

Kuhlmann S, Piel M, Wolf OT (2005) Impaired memory retrieval after psychosocial stress in healthy young men. *J Neurosci* 25, 2977–2982.

Kukolja J, Thiel CM, Wolf OT et al. (2008) Increased cortisol levels in cognitively challenging situations are beneficial in young but not older subjects. *Psychopharmacology* 201, 293–304.

LeDoux JE (2000) Emotion circuits in the brain. *Ann Rev Neurosci* 23, 155–184.

Liberzon I, Taylor SF, Amdur R et al. (1999) Brain activation in PTSD in response to trauma-related stimuli. *Biol Psychiatry* 45, 817–826.

Lovallo WR, Robinson JL, Glahn DC et al. (2010) Acute effects of hydrocortisone on the human brain: an fMRI study. *Psychoneuroendocrinology* 35, 15–20.

Lupien SJ, Gaudreau S, Tchiteya BM et al. (1997) Stress-induced declarative memory impairment in healthy elderly subjects: relationship to cortisol reactivity. *J Clin Endocrinol Metab* 82, 2070–2075.

Maren S, Phan KL, Liberzon I (2013) The contextual brain: implications for fear conditioning, extinction, and psychopathology. *Nature Reviews Neuroscience* 14, 417–428.

McDonald RJ, White NM (1993) A triple dissociation of memory systems: hippocampus, amygdala, and dorsal striatum. *Behav Neurosci* 107, 3–22.

McEwen BS, de Kloet ER, Rostene W (1986) Adrenal steroid receptors and actions in the nervous system. *Physiol Rev* 66, 1121–1188.

McGaugh JL (2000) Memory-a century of consolidation. *Science* 287, 248–251.

Mechias M-L, Etkin A, Kalisch R (2010) A meta-analysis of instructed fear studies: Implications for conscious appraisal of threat. *NeuroImage* 49, 1760–1768.

Merz CJ, Hermann A, Stark R et al. (2014) Cortisol modifies extinction learning of recently acquired fear in men. *Soc Cogn Affect Neurosci* 9, 1426–1434.

Merz CJ, Tabbert K, Schweckendiek J et al. (2010) Investigating the impact of sex and cortisol on implicit fear conditioning with fMRI. *Psychoneuroendocrinology* 35, 33–46.

Merz CJ, Tabbert K, Schweckendiek J et al. (2012) Oral contraceptive usage alters the effects of cortisol on implicit fear learning. *Hormon Behav* 62, 531–538.

Merz CJ, Wolf OT, Schweckendiek J et al. (2013) Stress differentially affects fear conditioning in men and women. *Psychoneuroendocrinology* 11, 2529–2541.

Mineka S, Oehlberg K (2008) The relevance of recent developments in classical conditioning to understanding the etiology and maintenance of anxiety disorders. *Acta Psychol* 127, 567–580.

Mineka S, Zinbarg R (2006) A contemporary learning theory perspective on the etiology of anxiety disorders - It's not what you thought it was. *Am Psychol* 61, 10–26.

Mouthaan J, Sijbrandij M, Luitse JS et al. (2014) The role of acute cortisol and DHEAS in predicting acute and chronic PTSD symptoms. *Psychoneuroendocrinology* 45, 179–186.

Mueller D, Cahill SP (2010) Neuroadrenergic modulation of extinction learning and exposure therapy. *Behav Brain Res* 208, 1–11.

Nader K, Hardt O (2009) A single standard for memory: the case for reconsolidation. *Nat Rev Neurosci* 10, 224–234.

Nater UM, Moor C, Okere U et al. (2007) Performance on a declarative memory task is better in high than low cortisol responders to psychosocial stress. *Psychoneuroendocrinology* 32, 758–763.

Oei NY, Elzinga BM, Wolf OT et al. (2007) Glucocorticoids decrease hippocampal and prefrontal activation during declarative memory retrieval in young men. *Brain Imaging Behav* 1, 31–41.

Oei NY, Veer IM, Wolf OT et al. (2012) Stress shifts brain activation towards ventral 'affective' areas during emotional distraction. *Soc Cogn Affect Neurosci* 7, 403–412.

Packard M, Hirsh R, White NM (1989) Differantial effects of fornix and caudate nucleus lesions on two radial maze tasks: evidence for multiple memory systems. *J Neurosci* 9, 1465–1472.

Packard M, Wingard JC (2004) Amygdala and "emotional" modulation of the relative use of multiple memory systems. *Neurobiol Learn Mem* 82, 243–252.

Payne JD, Jackson ED, Ryan L et al. (2006) The impact of stress on neutral and emotional aspects of episodic memory. *Memory* 14, 1–16.

Pissiota A, Frans O, Fernandez M et al. (2002) Neurofunctional correlates of posttraumatic stress disorder: a PET symptom provocation study. *Eur Archiv Psychiatr Clin Neurosci* 252, 68–75.

Pitman RK (1989) Post-traumatic stress disorder, hormones, and memory. *Biol Psychiatry* 26, 221–223.

Pitman RK, Rasmusson AM, Koenen KC et al. (2012) Biological studies of post-traumatic stress disorder. *Nat Reviews Neuroscience* 13, 769–787.

Pitman RK, Sanders KM, Zusman RM et al. (2002) Pilot study of secondary prevention of post-traumatic stress disorder with propranolol. *Biol Psychiatry* 51, 189–142.

Powers MB, Smits JAJ, Otto MW et al. (2009) Facilitation of fear extinction in phobic participants with a novel cognitive enhancer: A randomized placebo controlled trial of yohimbine augmentation. *J Anxiety Disord* 23, 350–356.

Pruessner JC, Dedovic K, Khalili-Mahani N et al. (2008) Deactivation of the limbic system during acute psychosocial stress: evidence from positron emission tomography and functional magnetic resonance imaging studies. *Biol Psychiatry* 63, 234–240.

Roozendaal B, Okuda S, De Quervain DJ et al. (2006a) Glucocorticoids interact with emotion-induced noradrenergic activation in influencing different memory functions. *Neuroscience* 138, 901–910.

Roozendaal B, Okuda S, Van der Zee EA et al. (2006b) Glucocorticoid enhancement of memory requires arousal-induced noradrenergic activation in the basolateral amygdala. *Proc Natl Acad Sci USA* 103, 6741–6746.

Schilling TM, Kölsch M, Larra MF et al. (2013) For whom the bell (curve) tolls: cortisol rapidly affects memory retrieval by an inverted u-shaped dose-response relationship. *Psychoneuroendocrinolgy* 38, 1565–1572.

Schmidt PI, Rosga K, Schatto C et al. (2014) Stress reduces the incorporation of misinformation into an established memory. *Learn Mem* 21, 744–747.

Schönfeld P, Ackermann K, Schwabe L (2014) Remembering under stress: different roles of autonomic arousal and glucocorticoids in memory retrieval. *Psychoneuroendocrinology* 39, 249–256.

Schwabe L (2013) Stress and the engagement of multiple memory systems: integration of animal and human studies. *Hippocampus* 23, 1035–1043.

Schwabe L, Bohringer A, Chatterjee M et al. (2008) Effects of pre-learning stress on memory for neutral, positive and negative words: Different roles of cortisol and autonomic arousal. *Neurobiol Learn Mem* 90, 44–53.

Schwabe L, Bohringer A, Wolf OT (2009a) Stress disrupts context-dependent memory. *Learn Mem* 16, 110–113.

Schwabe L, Höffken O, Tegenthoff M et al. (2011) Preventing the stress-induced shift from goal-directed to habit action with a beta-adrenergic antagonist. *J Neurosci* 31, 17317–17325.

Schwabe L, Höffken O, Tegenthoff M et al. (2013a) Opposite effects of noradrenergic arousal on amygdala processing of fearful faces in men and women. *Neuroimage* 73, 1–7.

Schwabe L, Joëls M, Roozendaal B et al. (2012a) Stress effects on memory: an update and integration. *Neurosci Biobehav Rev* 36, 1740–1749.

Schwabe L, Oitzl MS, Philippsen C et al. (2007) Stress modulates the use of spatial and stimulus-response learning strategies in humans. *Lear Mem* 14, 109–116.

Schwabe L, Oitzl MS, Richter S et al. (2009c) Modulation of spatial and stimulus-response learning strategies by exogenous cortisol in healthy young women. *Psychoneuroendocrinology* 34, 358–366.

Schwabe L, Römer S, Richter S et al. (2009b) Stress effects on declarative memory retrieval are blocked by a β-adrenoceptor antagonist in humans. *Psychoneuroendocrinology* 34, 446–454.

Schwabe L, Tegenthoff M, Höffken O et al. (2010a) Concurrent glucocorticoid and noradrenergic activity shifts instrumental behavior from goal-directed to habitual control. *J Neurosci* 30, 8190–8196.

Schwabe L, Tegenthoff M, Höffken O et al. (2012b) Simultaneous glucocorticoid and noradrenergic activity disrupts the neural basis of goal-directed action in the human brain. *J Neurosci* 32, 10146–10155.

Schwabe L, Tegenthoff M, Höffken O et al. (2013b) Mineralocorticoid receptor blockade prevents stress-induced modulation of multiple memory systems in the human brain. *Biol Psychiatry* 74, 801–808.

Schwabe L, Wolf OT (2009a) The context counts: Congruent learning and testing environments prevent memory retrieval impairment following stress. *Cogn Affect, and Behav Neurosci* 9, 229–236.

Schwabe L, Wolf OT (2009b) Stress prompts habit behavior in humans. *J Neurosci* 29, 7191–7198.

Schwabe L, Wolf OT (2010a) Learning under stress impairs memory formation. *Neurobiol Learn Mem* 93, 183–188.

Schwabe L, Wolf OT (2010b) Socially evaluated cold pressor stress after instrumental learning favors habits over goal-directed action. *Psychoneuroendocrinology* 35, 977–986.

Schwabe L, Wolf OT (2010c) Stress impairs the reconsolidation of autobiographical memories. *Neurobiol Learn Mem* 94, 153–157.

Schwabe L, Wolf OT (2012) Stress modulates the engagement of multiple memory systems in classification learning. *J Neurosci* 32, 11042–11049.

Schwabe L, Wolf OT (2013) Stress and multiple memory systems: from 'thinking' to 'doing'. *Trends Cogn Sci* 17, 60–68.

Schwabe L, Wolf OT (2014) Timing matters: temporal dynamics of stress effects on memory retrieval. *Cogn Affect & Behav Neurosci* 14, 1041–1048.

Schwabe L, Wolf OT, Oitzl MS (2010b) Memory formation under stress: Quantity and quality. *Neurosci Biobehav Rev* 34, 584–591.

Sehlmeyer C, Schöning S, Zwitserlood P et al. (2009) Human fear conditioning and extinction in neuroimaging: A systematic review. *PLoS ONE* 4, e5865.

Shors TJ (2004) Learning during stressful times. *Learn Mem* 11, 137–144.

Smeets T, Giesbrecht T, Jelicic M et al. (2007) Context-dependent enhancement of declarative memory performance following acute psychosocial stress. *Biol Psychol* 76, 116.123.

Smeets T, Wolf OT, Giesbrecht T et al. (2009) Stress selectively and lastingly promotes learning of context-related high arousing information. *Psychoneuroendocrinolgy* 34, 1152–1161.

Soeter M, Kindt M (2010) Dissociating response systems: Erasing fear from memory. *Neurobiol Learn Mem* 96, 30–41.

Soeter M, Kindt M (2011) Noradrenergic enhancement of associative fear memory in humans. *Neurobiol Learn Mem* 96, 263–271.

Soeter M, Kindt M (2012a) Erasing fear for an imagined threat event. *Psychoneuroendocrinology* 37, 1769–1779.

Soeter M, Kindt M (2012b) Stimulation of the noradrenergic system during memory formation impairs extinction learning but not the disruption of reconsolidation. *Neuropsychopharmacology* 37, 1204–1215.

Soravia LM, Heinrichs M, Aerni A et al. (2006) Glucocorticoids reduce phobic fear in humans. *Proc Natl Acad Sci USA* 103, 5585–5590.

Southwick SM, Horner B, Morgan CA et al. (2002) Relationship of enhanced norepinephrine activity during memory consolidation to enhanced long-term memory in humans. *Am J Psychiatr* 159, 1420–1422.

Squire LR (2004) Memory systems of the brain: a brief history and current perspective. *Neurobiol Learn Mem* 82, 171–177.

Stark R, Wolf OT, Tabbert K et al. (2006) Influence of the stress hormone cortisol on fear conditioning in humans: Evidence for sex differences in the response of the prefrontal cortex. *NeuroImage* 32, 1290–1298.

Strange BA, Dolan RJ (2004) β-adrenergic modulation of emotional memory-evoked human amygdala and hippocampus responses. *Proc Natl Acad Sci USA* 101, 11454–11458.

Tabbert K, Merz CJ, Klucken T et al. (2010) Cortisol enhances neural differentiation during fear acquisition and extinction in contingency aware young women. *Neurobiol Learn Mem* 94, 392–401.

Tollenaar MS, Elzinga BM, Spinhoven P et al. (2008) Long-term outcomes of memory retrieval under stress. *Behavioral Neurosci* 122, 697–703.

Tollenaar MS, Elzinga BM, Spinhoven P et al. (2009) Immediate and prolonged effects of cortisol, but not propranolol, on memory retrieval in healthy young men. *Neurobiol Learn Mem* 91, 23–31.

Tops M, van der Pompe GA, Baas D et al. (2003) Acute cortisol effects on immediate free recall and recognition of nouns depend on stimulus-valence. *Psychophysiology* 40, 167–173.

Tulving E, Markowitsch HJ (1998) Episodic and declarative memory: role of the hippocampus. *Hippocampus* 8, 198–204.

Vaiva G, Ducroca F, Jezequel K et al. (2003) Immediate treatment with propranolol decreases posttraumatic stress disorder two months after trauma. *Biol Psychiatry* 54, 947–949.

Van Ast VA, Vervliet B, Kindt M (2012) Contextual control over expression of fear is affected by cortisol. *Frontiers Behav Neurosci* 6, 67.

Van Stegeren AH, Roozendaal B, Kindt M et al. (2010) Interacting noradrenergic and corticosteroid systems shift human brain activation patterns during encoding. *Neurobiol Learn Mem* 93, 56–65.

Vervliet B, Craske MG, Hermanns D (2013) Fear extinction and relapse: state of the art. *Ann Rev Clin Psychol* 9, 215–248.

Williams CL, Clayton EC (2001) Contribution of brainstem structures in modulating memory storage processes. In: Gold PE, Greenough WT (eds) *Memory Consolidation: Essays in Honor of James L McGaugh*. American Psychological Association, Washington DC, pp. 141–163.

Winograd E, Neisser U (1992) *Affect and Accuracy in Recall: Studies in "Flashbulb Memories"*. Cambridge University Press, New York.

Zhao LY, Zhang XL, Shi J et al. (2009) Psychosocial stress after reactivation of drug-related memory impairs later recall in abstinent heroin addicts. *Psychopharmacology* 203, 599–608.

Zoladz PR, Clark B, Warnecke A et al. (2011) Pre-learning stress differentially affects long-term memory for emotional words, depending on temporal proximity to the learning experience. *Physiol Behav* 103, 467–476.

Zorawski M, Banding NQ, Kuhn CM et al. (2006) Effects of stress and sex on acquisition and consolidation of human fear conditioning. *Learn Mem* 13, 441–450.

Zorawski M, Cook CA, Kuhn CM et al. (2005) Sex, stress and fear: Individual differences in conditioned learning. *Cogn Affect Behav Neurosci* 5, 191–201.

SECTION II
Neurobiology of PTSD

CHAPTER 9

Neurotransmitter, neurohormonal, and neuropeptidal function in stress and PTSD

J. Douglas Bremner[1] & Brad Pearce[2]

[1] *Departments of Psychiatry & Behavioral Sciences and Radiology, Emory University School of Medicine, and the Atlanta VA Medical Center, Atlanta, GA, USA*

[2] *Department of Epidemiology, Rollins School of Public Health, Atlanta, GA, USA*

9.1 Introduction

A wide array of neurotransmitters, neurohormones, and neuropeptides are involved in the stress response. These chemical messenger systems act centrally in the brain as well as in the periphery and are essential for the survival response, resulting in increases in heart rate and blood pressure, respiration, alerting and vigilance behaviors, and shunting energy to the parts of the body that need it most for survival, i.e., the brain and muscles, when the organism is threatened or attacked. These systems include cortisol, norepinephrine, serotonin, dopamine, endogenous benzodiazepines and opiates, and other neuropeptides. Activation of the hypothalamic–pituitary–adrenal (HPA) axis results in release of corticotropin-releasing factor (CRF) from the hypothalamus, with stimulation of adrenocorticotropic hormone (ACTH) release from the pituitary and subsequent release of cortisol from the adrenal (see Figure 9.1). Neuropeptides involved in the stress response or behaviors related to the stress response include neurotensin, somatostatin, substance P, cholecystokinin (CCK), neuropeptide Y (NPY), ghrelin, vasopressin and oxytocin. The excitatory neurotransmitters, including glutamate and gamma-aminobutyric acid (GABA), are also involved. Other peripheral hormones, including testosterone, thyroid hormone, retinoids, estrogen, and adrenal steroids, are affected by the stress response, as well as their regulatory systems.

These hormonal, neurotransmitter, and neuropeptidal systems interact with each other to regulate the stress response. Chronic stress exposure, however, or other factors such as pre-existing vulnerabilities, can cause these systems to develop maladaptive responses. Symptoms of PTSD represent the behavioral

Posttraumatic Stress Disorder: From Neurobiology to Treatment, First Edition.
Edited by J. Douglas Bremner.
© 2016 John Wiley & Sons, Inc. Published 2016 by John Wiley & Sons, Inc.

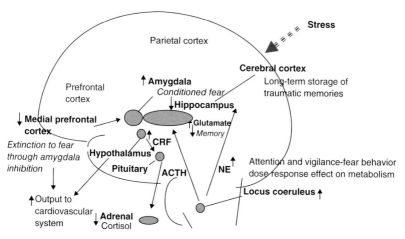

Figure 9.1 Neurotransmitters in posttraumatic stress disorder (PTSD). Neurotransmitters involved in the stress response and PTSD symptoms include norepinephrine (NE), with cell bodies in the locus coeruleus and projections to the amygdala, hippocampus, prefrontal cortex, and hypothalamus, and the hypothalamic–pituitary–adrenal (HPA) axis, with corticotropin-releasing factor (CRF) release from the hypothalamus, which stimulates adrenocorticotropic hormone (ACTH) release from the pituitary, and cortisol from the adrenal. (*See color plate section for the color representation of this figure.*)

manifestation of stress-induced changes in these neurochemical, neurohormonal, and neuropeptidal systems, interacting with specific brain areas involved in the stress response, including the hippocampus, amygdala, and medial prefrontal cortex (mPFC; Bremner, 2003, 2007, 2011; Bremner & Charney, 2010; Elzinga & Bremner, 2002; Garakani et al., 2011; Vermetten & Bremner, 2002a,b). This chapter reviews the effects of stress on neurotransmitter, neurohormonal, and neuropeptide function in animal models as well as in patients with posttraumatic stress disorder (PTSD). Neural circuits, the impact of development, and basic behavioral mechanisms are covered in other chapters of this book.

9.2 Noradrenergic system

Norepinephrine release in the brain is an important part of the behavioral response to stress. Activation of noradrenergic systems centrally in the brain as well as in the peripheral sympathetic system readies the body to prepare to deal with the threat (Bremner et al., 1996a,b). The majority of norepinephrine cell bodies are located in the brain stem, in the locus coeruleus region of the pons, with axons that extend throughout the rest of the brain. Stress activates neurons in the locus coeruleus with subsequent release of norepinephrine in the brain, leading to fear and anxiety behaviors (Abercrombie & Jacobs, 1987a,b; Aston-Jones & Shipley, 1991; Foote et al., 1983; Jedema et al., 2001; Levine et al., 1990; Nisenbaum & Abercrombie, 1993; Redmond & Huang, 1979). Exposure to prior stressors leads to a potentiation of norepinephrine release with subsequent stressors in the hippocampus and mPFC (Finlay et al., 1995; Nisenbaum et al., 1991; Tanaka et al., 2000). Neurons in the mPFC increase the synthetic potential of norepinephrine by increasing the synthetic enzyme tyrosine hydroxylase and cell membrane norepinephrine transporters in response to stress (Miner et al., 2006). Animal models showed that exposure to repeated stressors from which the animal could not escape led to the development of what are called learned helplessness behaviors, where the animal stops trying to avoid the stress, which is associated with a depletion of brain norepinephrine when synthesis does not keep up with demand (Petty et al., 1993; Weiss et al., 1981).

Pharmacological stimulation of the norepinephrine system provokes anxiety and fear-related behaviors in animals. α_2-norepinephrine receptors on norepinephrine neuron cell bodies in the locus coeruleus have an inhibitory effect on locus coeruleus firing (Aston-Jones & Shipley, 1991). Stress exposure results in decreased density of α_2 receptors in the hippocampus and amygdala (Torda et al., 1984) and an increase in yohimbine-induced norepinephrine release in the hippocampus (Nisenbaum & Abercrombie, 1993), which is in part mediated by α_2-adrenoreceptors . Animals deficient in the α_2-adrenoreceptors show increased autonomic activity, startle response, sensitivity to amphetamine, and anxiety-related behaviors (Lahdesmaki & Sallinen, 2002; Lähdesmäki et al., 2004).

Pharmacological agents that are associated with a reduction in anxiety, including benzodiazepines, opiates, alcohol, and antidepressants, are associated with a reduction in firing of neurons in the locus coeruleus (Bremner et al., 1996a). PTSD patients report a decrease in symptoms in the intrusion and hyperarousal categories with these drugs that decrease locus coeruleus firing, while cocaine, which has the opposite effect, increases symptoms (Bremner et al., 1996c). Opiate withdrawal symptoms of anxiety, increased heart rate, and sweating are related to a rebound increased firing of the locus coeruleus as the inhibition is withdrawn. Treatments of opiate withdrawal include agents that decrease locus coeruleus firing, including the α_2-norepinephrine agonist, clonidine, as well as benzodiazepines such as Librium.

Norepinephrine helps the organism prepare for the fight-or-flight response to stress. Norepinephrine sharpens the senses, focuses attention, raises the level of fear, and quickens the heart rate and blood pressure. The norepinephrine system is like a fire alarm that alerts all areas of the brain simultaneously. PTSD symptoms are hypothesized to be related in part to an increase in sensitivity of noradrenergic neurons (Bremner & Charney, 2010; Garakani et al., 2011).

Table 9.1 Evidence for altered catecholaminergic function in PTSD.

Increased resting heart rate and blood pressure	+/−
Increased heart rate and blood pressure in response to traumatic reminders	+++
Increased resting urinary NE and E	+
Increased resting urinary dopamine	+++
Increased resting plasma NE or MHPG	−
Increased plasma NE or MHPG with traumatic reminders	++
Increased plasma NE or MHPG with exercise	+
Increased orthostatic heart rate response to exercise	+
Decreased binding to platelet α_2 receptors	+
Decrease in basal and stimulated activity of cAMP	+
Decrease in platelet MAO activity	+
Increased symptoms, heart rate and plasma MHPG with yohimbine NE challenge	+
Differential brain metabolic response 1 to yohimbine	+

PTSD, posttraumatic stress disorder; NE, norepinephrine; E, epinephrine; MHPG, 3-methoxy-4-hydroxyphenylglycol; cAMP, cyclic adenosine 39,59-monophosphate; MAO, monoamine oxidase.

There is considerable evidence that alterations in noradrenergic and peripheral sympathetic function play a role in the maintenance of symptoms of PTSD (see Table 9.1) (Bremner et al., 1996a, 1996b). A number of symptoms are characteristic of increased noradrenergic function, including irritability, increased startle, hyperarousal and sleep disturbance (Bremner et al., 1996b). Several studies found increased baseline concentrations of norepinephrine and its metabolites in plasma and urine in both children and adults with PTSD (De Bellis et al., 1994b, 1999; Lemieux & Coe, 1995; Mason et al., 1988; Yehuda et al., 1998), although some studies showed no baseline differences (Blanchard et al., 1991; McFall et al., 1992; Mellman et al., 1995; Pitman & Orr, 1990; Southwick et al., 1993). Increased concentrations of baseline norepinephrine and its metabolites were also found in cerebrospinal fluid of PTSD patients (Geracioti et al., 2001). A correlation between cerebrospinal fluid (CSF) norepinephrine and blood pressure was seen in healthy controls, but not PTSD patients, suggesting an uncoupling of central and peripheral sympathetic nervous system function in PTSD (Strawn et al., 2004).

Studies have consistently shown increased noradrenergic reactivity to traumatic reminders and pharmacological stimulation of the noradrenergic system in PTSD. Exposure of PTSD patients to traumatic reminders in the form of combat-related slides and sounds or personalized scripts of the traumatic event are associated with an increase in heart rate, blood pressure, and skin conductance, all markers of sympathetic function (Blanchard et al., 1982, 1986; Malloy et al., 1983; McFall et al., 1990; Orr et al., 1993, 1995, 1998; Orr & Roth, 2000). This is seen in comparison to traumatized individuals without PTSD and is seen in

PTSD related to both combat and civilian traumas or childhood abuse (Bremner et al., 1996b). Exposure to traumatic reminders is also associated with an increase in plasma norepinephrine and epinephrine (Blanchard et al., 1991; McFall et al., 1992). Increased baseline heart rate soon after the trauma was also found to be a predictor of the subsequent development of chronic PTSD (Shalev et al., 1998).

Alterations in other markers of noradrenergic function are also associated with PTSD. PTSD patients have decreased binding to platelet α_2 receptors (Perry et al., 1991), decreased activity of the second messenger, cyclic adenosine monophosphate (cAMP) (Lerer et al., 1987, 1990), and decreased platelet monoamine oxidase activity (Davidson et al., 1985). These findings are consistent with chronic increases in norepinephrine leading to compensatory changes in receptors and other parts of the pathways linked to noradrenergic function. Administration of the α_2-adrenergic receptor, yohimbine, which increases firing of noradrenergic neurons in the locus coeruleus, was associated with an increase in PTSD symptoms and anxiety, as well as an increase in plasma concentrations of the norepinephrine metabolite, 3-methoxy-4-hydroxyphenylglycol, in patients with combat-related PTSD compared to healthy controls (Southwick et al., 1993, 1997). Furthermore, PTSD patients had a decrease in brain function in the mPFC with yohimbine not seen in healthy controls, while increased panic anxiety was correlated with decreased hippocampal function (Bremner et al., 1997a). Overall, these findings show increased central and peripheral noradrenergic function with compensatory changes in receptor and messaging systems.

9.3 HPA axis

The HPA axis plays an important role in the stress response. CRF released from the hypothalamus causes release of ACTH from the pituitary, which causes release of cortisol from the adrenal gland. Cortisol functions to shift energy toward parts of the body that are needed for survival, like the brain and the muscles of the limbs, and away from areas that are not immediately needed, like digestion and reproductive function. Cortisol mobilizes energy stores which facilitates increased arousal, vigilance, and attention. Cortisol and CRF also act centrally to modulate brain areas involved in memory, anxiety, and the fear response, including the hippocampus, amygdala, and PFC (Makino et al., 1995b). Cortisol and similar glucocorticoids have a biphasic effect on memory through actions on the hippocampus (see Chapter 6).

The transient rise of cortisol in response to acute stress induces complex alterations in immune cell trafficking and causes short-term enhancement of innate immunity and inflammatory processes (Dhabhar, 2014). While the enhancement of immune function by cortisol seems to contrast with its well-established immunosuppressive effects (e.g., when given in pharmacological doses), the timing and duration of the stressor and the ability of the HPA axis to re-establish homeostasis are important determinants of cortisol's effect on immune cells. As a stress hormone, cortisol plays a biologically adaptive role in preparing the immune system for physical injury that often accompanies exposure to a traumatic event. However, prolonged or excessive activation of the HPA axis can have deleterious effects on the immune system.

Chronic stress leads to long-term changes in HPA axis function. In animals, chronic stress leads to a sensitization of the HPA axis and increases in central CRF synthesis (Levine et al., 1993; Makino et al., 1995a,b; Stanton et al., 1988). Exposure to early stressors result in long-term alterations in hormonal systems (Yehuda et al., 1995), including sustained increases in plasma glucocorticoid concentrations, potentiation of glucocorticoid responsiveness to subsequent stressors (Ottenweller et al., 1989), resistance to suppression of dexamethasone, increased neuronal secretion of CRF, a compensatory blunting of ACTH responses to CRF (Plotsky & Meaney, 1993; Smith et al., 1997), and alterations in the hippocampus (Sapolsky, 1996). Other studies, however, suggest that chronic stress is associated with a decrease in glucocorticoid response to subsequent stressors (Katz et al., 1981; Rivier & Vale, 1987; Young & Akil, 1985). Early life stress events lead to lasting changes in glucocorticoid receptors and stress-induced CRF and glucocorticoid release (Coplan et al., 1996; Makino et al., 1995b; Plotsky & Meaney, 1993). High levels of glucocorticoids seen during stress, as well as other factors such as elevated levels of brain-derived neurotrophic factor (BDNF) and excitatory amino acids, are associated with damage to neurons in the CA3 region of the hippocampus, a brain area that plays a critical role in learning and memory (Gould et al., 1998; Magarinos et al., 1996; McEwen et al., 1992; Nibuya et al., 1995; Sapolsky et al., 1990; Sapolsky, 1996), as well as deficits in new learning (Diamond et al., 1996; Luine et al., 1994) (see Chapter 6). CRF also has direct effects on the hippocampus, especially during early development (Brunson et al., 2001a,b).

Corticotropin-releasing factor and glucocorticoid (cortisol) receptors (GRs) are located in multiple brain areas including those involved in fear and anxiety, such as the hippocampus, amygdala, and mPFC. In addition to stimulating the HPA axis during stress, CRF also plays a role centrally in the brain to mediate fear-related behaviors. There are two types of CRF receptor, CRF-1 and CRF-2, that are present in all of these areas; however, CRF-1 is uniquely located in the locus coeruleus, nucleus of the solitary tract, thalamus, and striatum, while CRF-2 (but not CRF-1) receptors are in the choroid plexus, certain hypothalamic nuclei, and the nucleus prepositus (Sanchez, 1999). Animals deficient in CRF-1 receptors have decreased fear-related behaviors and impaired response to stress, while animals deficient in CRF-2 have increased fear-related behaviors (Bale et al., 2000, 2002). The HPA axis response to stress is coordinated through an interaction of GRs and mineralocorticoid (MR) receptors (de Kloet et al., 1999).

Studies are consistent with alterations in HPA function in PTSD, although not always in the generalized hypercortisolism seen in many animal studies (Yehuda, 2006). Baseline cortisol levels have been found to be normal or low, with increased cortisol responsiveness to traumatic memories, and other elements of dysregulation. Sexually abused girls in one study were found to have normal baseline cortisol and blunted ACTH response to CRF (De Bellis et al., 1994a), while other studies in abused and neglected children with PTSD showed increased cortisol when measured over a 24-hour period (Cicchetti & Rogosch, 2001; De Bellis et al., 1999; Gunnar et al., 2001; Hart et al., 1996). Depressed pre-school children showed increased cortisol response to separation stress (Luby et al., 2003).

Adults with PTSD both from childhood abuse and combat also show alterations in HPA axis function (Yehuda, 2006). Most studies have shown decreases in cortisol measured over a 24-hour period in plasma or urine (Anisman et al., 2001; Delahanty et al., 2003, 2004; Goenjian et al., 1996; Kanter et al., 2001; Mason et al., 1986, 2002; Oquendo et al., 2003; Seedat et al., 2003; Wessa et al., 2006; Yehuda et al., 1991b, 1994, 1995, 1996b, 2005; Young & Breslau, 2004a,b; Young et al., 2004), although some showed no differences between PTSD patients and controls (Maes et al., 1998; Mason et al., 2002; Pitman & Orr, 1990). The normal cortisol rise after awakening has also has been shown to be blunted in PTSD patients (de Kloet et al., 2007b; Neylan et al., 2005; Wessa et al., 2006), while pre-deployment cortisol response to awakening was not predictive of the development of PTSD (van Zuiden et al., 2011b). Male patients with combat-related PTSD in whom cortisol was measured at multiple time points showed a blunting of the normal diurnal variation and decreased cortisol concentrations in the afternoon (Yehuda et al., 1994, 1996b). Women with PTSD related to childhood sexual abuse where cortisol was measured in plasma at multiple time points over a 24-hour period showed lower cortisol levels in the afternoon, a flattening of the normal diurnal curve, and an increase in pulsatility suggesting dysregulation of CRF release from the hypothalamus (Bremner, 2005, 2007, 2008). Lower cortisol at baseline correlated with increased symptoms of PTSD in the PTSD group (Bremner et al., 2007). Women with PTSD compared with abused controls also had an exaggerated cortisol response to stressors (traumatic stressors involving the reading of a personalized script of the childhood abuse) (Elzinga et al., 2003). Another study of men and women with childhood abuse showed increased cortisol response to cognitive stressors (mental stress challenge involving mental arithmetic and problem-solving with negative feedback), although the magnitude of response was not as great in women with PTSD following traumatic reminder stress (Bremner et al., 2003a). Another study showed that adult women with depression and a history of early childhood abuse had an increased cortisol response to a stressful cognitive challenge relative to controls (Heim et al., 2000) and a blunted ACTH response to CRF challenge (Heim et al., 2001).

Changes in GR function are also associated with PTSD (Vermetten, 2008). Cortisol acts through GRs in the pituitary and hypothalamus to regulate feedback on the HPA axis. GR function cannot be easily measured in the brain, but it can be measured indirectly by assessing cortisol levels following administration of glucocorticoids (e.g., dexamethasone) or through measurement of GR in lymphocytes in the peripheral circulation. Studies show that PTSD is associated with increased suppression of cortisol with low-dose (0.5 mg) dexamethasone, suggesting increased sensitivity of GRs (Goenjian et al., 1996; Stein et al., 1997b; Yehuda et al., 1993; Yehuda & Boisoneau, 1995), although one study found this effect in traumatized non-PTSD subjects as well (de Kloet et al., 2007b). Other studies in PTSD showed increased GR in peripheral lymphocytes (Yehuda et al., 1991a) and hypersensitivity of pituitary response to metyrapone (Yehuda et al., 1996a; although see Kanter et al., 2001), both findings consistent with increased feedback sensitivity in PTSD. Elevated GR was shown to be predictive of the development of PTSD after combat deployment (van Zuiden et al., 2011a). Another study showed that PTSD was associated with a blunted effect of glucocorticoids (dexamethasone) on declarative memory function, suggesting decreased sensitivity of GRs in the hippocampus (Bremner et al., 2004b). One study showed a decrease, however, in GR in leukocytes in both traumatized PTSD and non-PTSD subjects in comparison to healthy controls, and a blunted suppression response of T-cell proliferation in leukocytes to dexamethasone that was specific to PTSD (de Kloet et al., 2007a).

Genetic variability may explain some of the discrepancies. The risk for developing PTSD is modified by genetic polymorphism in the FKBP5, which is a regulator of GR sensitivity (Binder et al., 2008).

Several studies have also found increased concentrations of CRF in the CSF (Baker et al., 1999, 2005; Bremner et al., 1997b; Sautter et al., 2003) and plasma (de Kloet et al., 2008b) in male patients with combat-related PTSD, although one study of civilian PTSD with low levels of comorbid psychiatric diagnoses found no difference in CSF CRF (Bonne et al., 2011). In one study, PTSD patients had a blunted ACTH response to CRF challenge (consistent with decreased pituitary sensitivity to CRF) (Smith et al., 1989), although another showed no difference with controls in ACTH or cortisol after CRF challenge preceded by administration of dexamethasone (de Kloet et al., 2008a). Efforts are under way to develop CRF receptor antagonists as a treatment for PTSD or preventative after exposure to trauma. Some studies have also shown efficacy for cortisol in the treatment of PTSD (Aerni & Traber, 2004). The mechanism for efficacy is unclear.

Overall, these studies suggest that PTSD is associated with long-term changes in function of the HPA axis.

9.4 PTSD and inflammation

Alterations in function of the inflammatory system are associated with chronic stress and PTSD. As described earlier, the ligand-mediated activation of the GR by cortisol mediates the short-term adaptive responses to stress and also restrains the over-production of pro-inflammatory cytokines, regulating the homeostatic tone of the HPA axis (Silverman et al., 2002). For example, cortisol inhibits pro-inflammatory cytokine secretion, while inflammatory cytokines activate the HPA axis, increasing corticotropin-releasing hormone (CRH) and ultimately restraining overproduction of inflammatory mediators by stimulating cortisol release.

Posttraumatic stress disorder is associated with immunoregulatory abnormalities and activation of inflammatory pathways (Pace & Heim, 2011). While these immune changes are complex, the available literature suggests that there is a shift toward inflammation in PTSD, as indicated by elevated C-reactive protein, tumor necrosis factor-alpha (TNFα), interleukin-1 (IL-1) and IL-6 (Eraly et al., 2014; Gill et al., 2009). The vagus nerve plays a key role in the regulation of cytokine responses to stress.

9.5 Acetylcholine and vagal nerve function

In addition to activating stress-responsive brain areas including the amygdala and hippocampus, the vagus regulates communication between immune mediators (e.g., cytokines) and the HPA axis via its neurotransmitter acetylcholine (Figure 9.2). Cytokines present in the circulation signal the brain through intermediates without entering the central nervous system (CNS) parenchyma (Watkins et al., 1995). The local (peripheral) production of pro-inflammatory cytokines can stimulate visceral afferents which in turn communicate with the brain through the vagus. Thus the vagus serves as an afferent route for signaling that up-regulates CRF secretion, altering HPA axis tone through interconnected neuronal circuits involving ascending catecholaminergic fibers of the nucleus of the solitary tract (NTS) projecting to the parvocellular division of the paraventricular nucleus (PVN) of the hypothalamus (Schobitz et al., 1994; Turnbull & Rivier, 1999; Watkins et al., 1995).

The efferent component of vagus nerve stimulation is anti-inflammatory, mainly mediated by activation of the alpha-7 nicotinic receptor by Ach on peripheral immune cells. Numerous studies have demonstrated that diminished vagal tone and increased sympathetic activity are associated with a hyper-inflammatory state characterized by elevated TNFα, IL-6, and high-mobility group box 1 protein (HGMB1) (Bernik et al., 2002; Das, 2007; Li & Olshansky, 2011; Pavlov & Tracey, 2006), while vagus nerve stimulation

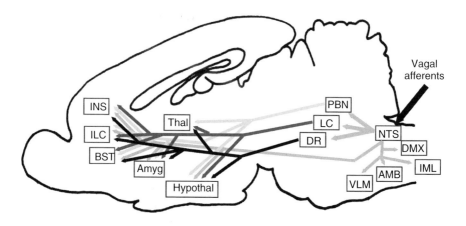

Figure 9.2 Afferents from the vagal nerve to central areas of the brain. AMB = nucleus ambiguous; DMX = dorsal motor nucleus of the vagus, IML = intermediolateral column of spinal cord (symp pregang); VLM = ventrolateral medulla; Amyg = amygdala; INS = insular cortex; ILC - infralimbic cortex; PBN = parabrachial nucleus; DR = dorsal Raphe; LC = locus coeruleus; Thal = thalamus; Hypothal = hypothalamus. (Used with permission from Thomas Cunningham PhD, University of North Texas Health Sciences Center.) (*See color plate section for the color representation of this figure.*)

(VNS) results in an attenuation of endotoxin-induced release of TNFα, IL-1, IL-6 and IL-18, but not the anti-inflammatory cytokine IL-10 (Borovikova et al., 2000). VNS appears to mediate some facets of its anti-inflammatory effects through ghrelin (Bansal et al., 2012).

The vagus nerve also has important interactions with the norepinephrine systems. Vagus activation in animals is associated with an increase in norepinephrine concentration in the hippocampus and cortex (Roosevelt et al., 2006). Lesions of the locus coeruleus interrupt the seizure-reducing properties of VNS (Krahl et al., 1998).

The vagal nerve system also plays an important role in learning and memory. VNS in animals enhances memory in a learning paradigm and is associated with long-term potentiation in the hippocampus (Zuo et al., 2007).

While most of the studies of the so-called cholinergic inflammatory reflex have been performed in experimental animals, a few human studies also support the idea that vagus nerve tone can have profound effects on inflammatory pathways. For example, one study of cardiovascular risk factors in young adults found an inverse correlation between heart rate variability (HRV) and pro-inflammatory cytokines, suggesting that diminished descending vagal signals are linked to inflammation in humans (Sloan et al., 2007). HRV is also diminished in rheumatoid arthritis (Bruchfeld et al., 2010). There are also emerging findings in studies of humans with epilepsy and major depression to support an immunomodulatory effect of VNS (Corcoran et al., 2004; De Herdt et al., 2009; Majoie et al., 2011), but data are lacking in PTSD.

9.6 Dopaminergic system

The majority of dopaminergic neurons have their cell bodies in the ventral tegmental area of the midbrain and release neurotransmitter in several regions of the brain. Dopamine is involved in a number of functions, including the control of locomotion, cognition, affect, neuroendocrine secretion, and the stress response. The three major dopaminergic pathways are the nigrostriatal (projecting from substantia nigra to striatum), mesolimbic (projection from midbrain to nucleus accumbens), and mesocortical/mesoprefrontal (projection from midbrain to the PFC) systems.

The dopaminergic innervation of the mPFC is particularly sensitive to stress. Stress-induced dopamine release occurs in the mPFC preferentially over other areas of the brain with dopaminergic projections (Deutch & Roth, 1990; Roth et al., 1988). Chronic stress results in an increase in turnover of dopamine (evidence by increased dopamine metabolites) in the PFC and nucleus accumbens (Kalivas & Duffy, 1989). Although high enough levels of stress result in activation of several dopaminergic pathways, the mesofrontal pathway is preferentially affected by stress (Deutch et al., 1985; Deutch & Roth, 1990; Roth et al., 1988). Uncontrollable stress activates mPFC dopamine release and inhibits release of dopamine in the nucleus accumbens (Cabib et al., 2002; Ventura et al., 2002).

Multiple neurotransmitter systems modulate dopaminergic neurons as part of the regulatory feedback of the stress response (Kalivas & Abhold, 1987). Dopaminergic innervation of the nucleus accumbens, the mesolimbic pathway, regulates feelings of pleasure, and deficits in this system could underlie feelings of lack of pleasure or anhedonia in patients with stress-related psychiatric disorders (Kalivas & Abhold, 1987). Dopamine release in the PFC, in conjunction with other stress-related neurotransmitters such as norepinephrine, underlies the cognitive impairment that can be associated with the stress response (Arnsten, 2000). Dopaminergic function is also involved in the mediation of extinction to fear responses, and therefore dysfunction of this system could underlie the failure to extinguish traumatic memories, leading to repetitive intrusive thoughts, which are a hallmark of PTSD (Garakani et al., 2011).

Studies in patients with PTSD are consistent with abnormalities of dopaminergic function. Several clinical investigations have reported increased urinary and plasma dopamine concentrations in PTSD patients (Hamner & Diamond, 1993; Lemieux & Coe, 1995). One study found an increase in activity of dopamine beta hydroxylase, an enzyme that converts dopamine to norepinephrine, in PTSD patients (Hamner & Gold, 1998). Candidate genes in the dopamine system studied to date in PTSD include the dopamine receptor D2 gene (DRD2) and the dopamine transporter gene (DAT) (Broekman et al., 2007). Some studies showed an association between the DRD2 A1 allelele and PTSD (Comings et al., 1996; Young et al., 2002), while others did not (Gelernter et al., 1999). In summary, dopamine plays an important role in the stress response, and PTSD is associated with lasting alterations in dopaminergic function.

9.7 NMDA

The excitatory amino acid glutamate and N-methyl-D-aspartate (NMDA) receptors are highly concentrated in the hippocampus and amygdala. In the hippocampus they are involved in new learning and memory, while in the amygdala they play an important role in fear learning and extinction (Bauer et al., 2002; Davis, 1992). Stress is associated with increased release of glutamate in the brain, which is potentially toxic to hippocampal neurons if released in large enough amounts (Chambers et al., 1999; Moghaddam et al., 1997). The NMDA receptor antagonist, ketamine, is associated with an increase in symptoms of dissociation, which are seen in traumatized patients, even when given to healthy human subjects (Krystal et al., 1994). Smaller hippocampal volume is associated with PTSD, and correlates with increased dissociative symptoms in these patients (Bremner et al., 2003b; Stein et al., 1997a).

The epilepsy medication, phenytoin, modulates the glutamatergic system and blocks the effects of stress on the hippocampus (Watanabe et al., 1992b). Phenytoin treatment of PTSD patients results in both an improvement in PTSD symptoms and an increase in right hippocampal and right cerebral volumes (Bremner et al., 2004a, 2005b). The NMDA receptor partial agonist, D-cycloserine (DCS), has been shown to facilitate extinction in animal studies, and was thus proposed as a treatment for PTSD (Davis et al., 2006). Initial studies, however, have not shown efficacy of DCS in the treatment of PTSD (Heresco-Levy et al., 2002).

N-methyl-D-aspartate receptors also interface with the immune system through several mechanisms. For example, the cytokine, interferon gamma, regulates biochemical pathways in numerous cell types, including glia, and shunts tryptophan metabolism toward the kynurenine (KYN) pathway. This has the beneficial effect of depriving invading microorganisms of tryptophan, but it also causes the elevation of KYN and kynurenic acid (KYNA) in the extracellular milieu (Stone et al., 2013). KYNA, in turn, acts as an antagonist of both NMDA and a7NicACh receptors (Stone et al., 2013). The ultimate effect of KYNA on inflammation is thought to be determined by specific characteristics of the receptors on immune cells and glia, but this has not been well studied in PTSD.

9.8 Serotonin

Serotonin regulates a wide variety of behaviors and physiological functions that are relevant to stress-related mental disorders like PTSD. Serotonin is involved in the regulation of anxiety, arousal, vigilance, aggression, mood, impulsivity, food intake, and sleep. It is also involved in controlling physical functions that are a part of the stress response, including cardiovascular function, respiratory activity, motor output, neuroendocrine secretion, and analgesia (Charney & Bremner, 1999; Vermetten & Bremner, 2002a). Serotonin acts on distinct receptors in the brain, including 5-hydroxytryptamine 1A (5-HT_{1A}), 5-HT_{1B}, 5-HT_{1D}, 5-HT_{2A}, 5-HT_{2B}, 5-HT_{2C}, 5-HT_3, and 5-HT_7 receptors. Reuptake of serotonin from the synapse into the neuron is facilitated by the serotonin transporter, which is the target of treatment with the selective serotonin reuptake inhibitors (SSRIs) (Davis et al., 1997).

Stress-induced activation of serotonin stimulates a system that has both anxiogenic and anxiolytic pathways within the forebrain (Charney & Bremner, 1999; Graeff, 1993). Different behaviors related to stress, anxiety, and depression are regulated via different serotonergic pathways with projections to different parts of the brain, or via different serotonin receptor subtypes (Van Praag et al., 1990). The serotonergic innervations of the amygdala and the hippocampus by the dorsal raphe are believed to mediate anxiogenic effects via 5-HT_2 receptors (Charney et al., 2000). In contrast, the median raphe innervation of hippocampal, amygdala, and medial prefrontal 5-HT_{1A} receptors has been hypothesized to facilitate the disconnection of previously learned associations with aversive events, or suppression of the formation of new associations, thus providing a resilience to aversive events (Garakani et al., 2011; Graeff, 1993). Genetically modified mice lacking the 5-HT_{1A} receptor show an increase in anxiety-like behaviors (Klemenhagen et al., 2006). Thus, serotonin plays a role in regulating behavioral responses to stress.

Serotonin also regulates neurohormonal responses to stress through actions on the important stress responsive systems, the HPA axis and the locus coeruleus–noradrenergic systems. Serotonin modifies HPA axis activity both centrally (Dinan, 1996; Phelix et al., 1992) and through regulation of cortisol release at the level of the adrenal gland (Bagdy et al., 1989). Serotonin also has an inhibitory effect on the noradrenergic system, which like the HPA–cortisol system, is activated during stress (Segal, 1979).

Stress affects serotonergic function. Animals exposed to a variety of stressors respond with increased serotonin turnover (Heinsbroek et al., 1991) in brain areas, including the mPFC (Adell et al., 1988; Inoue et al., 1994; Pei et al., 1990; Petty & Sherman, 1983), nucleus accumbens, amygdala, lateral hypothalamus, and locus coeruleus (Kaehler et al., 2000), with preferential release during conditioned fear in mPFC (Inoue et al., 1994). Widespread activation of the serotonergic system after severe stress is associated with the behavioral response termed "learned helplessness," when animals give up trying to escape from the stressful situation. The behavioral deficit of learned helplessness, which is used as a model of stress-induced behavioral disorders like PTSD, is associated with reduced *in vivo* release of serotonin in the frontal cortex (Petty et al., 1992, 1997), probably reflecting a situation where synthesis is not able to keep pace with demand. Adaptation to stress resulted in an increase in hippocampal 5-HT_{1A} binding (Mendelson & McEwen, 1991), while some studies (Watanabe et al., 1993) but not others (Wu et al., 1999) found decreased 5-HT_{1A} receptor binding in the hippocampus with chronic stress. High levels of glucocorticoids, which are seen with chronic stress, also resulted in a decrease in hippocampal 5-HT_{1A} receptor binding (Watanabe et al., 1993). Since glucocorticoids modulate 5-HT_{1A} receptor function, this could represent, at least in part, the mechanism of stress-induced atrophy of the CA3 region of the hippocampus. Other studies showed a reduction in 5-HT_{2A} binding in the amygdala and hypothalamus (Petty et al., 1997; Wu et al., 1999), and decreased serotonin transporter binding in the frontal cortex, with stress (Petty et al., 1997; Wu et al., 1999). Social stress was associated with reduced 5-HT_{1A} binding in the hippocampus and reduced 5-HT_{2A} binding in the parietal cortex (McKittrick et al., 1995).

Preclinical studies have provided evidence of the important role that serotonin plays in behaviors related to stress and anxiety. The capability to increase serotonin metabolism during exposure to inescapable stress prevented the development of learned helplessness (Ronan et al., 2000). Animals with a genetic lack of the serotonin transporter (serotonin transporter knockout mice) had an increase in anxiety behaviors and stress reactivity (Adamec et al., 2006; Holmes et al., 2003b). Serotonin antagonists produced behavioral deficits resembling those seen following inescapable shock (Martin et al., 1990; Sherman & Petty, 1980). Blockade of serotonin transporters during early life resulted in an increase in anxiety in adulthood (Ansorge & Zhou, 2004). Stress-induced learned helplessness was reversed by drugs that enhance serotonin neurotransmission (e.g., SSRIs) (Martin et al., 1990; Sherman & Petty, 1980), and serotonin 5-HT_{1A} receptor agonists, similar to buspirone (Drugan et al., 1987; Przegalinski et al., 1995), which is used in clinical populations for the treatment of anxiety. Learned helplessness in response to stress was also prevented by the injection of serotonin into the frontal cortex (Sherman & Petty, 1982). Pre-administration of benzodiazepines or tricyclic antidepressants prevented stress-induced decreases in serotonin and the acquisition of behavioral deficits (Petty et al., 1992). A natural increase in the level of the serotonin metabolite, 5-hydroxyindoleacetic acid (5-HIAA), in the lateral septum appeared to have a protective effect on the development of adverse behavioral consequences of stress (Petty et al., 1992).

A number of lines of evidence support a role for altered serotonergic function in PTSD (see Table 9.2) (Charney & Bremner, 1999; Davis et al., 1997; Maes

Table 9.2 Evidence for alterations in other neurotransmitter systems in PTSD.

Benzodiazepine	
Increased symptomatologywith benzodiazepine antagonist	+
Decreased number of benzodiazepine receptors on platelets	+
Opiate	
Naloxone-reversible analgesia	++
Increased plasma β-endorphins at rest	+/–
Increased plasma β-endorphin response to exercise	++
Elevated levels of CSF β-endorphin	++
Serotonin	
Decreased serotonin reuptake site binding in platelets	++
Decreased serotonin transmitter in platelets	–
Decreased adenylate cyclase activity in platelets	++
Blunted prolactin response to 5-HT$_{1A}$ probe	–
Altered serotonin effect on cAMP in platelets (5-HT$_{1A}$ probe)	+
Increased anxiogenic responses to 5-HT agonists	+
Decreased serotonin metabolite 5-HIAA in CSF	–
Somatostatin	
Increased somatostatin levels at baseline in CSF	+/–
Cholecystokinin	
Increased anxiogenic responses to CCK agonists	+
Differential effect of CCK on HPA axis function	+
Neuropeptide Y (NPY)	
Decreased baseline plasma NPY	+/–
Reduced NPY with yohimbine challenge	+
Recovery of NPY with successful treatment	+
Substance P	
Increased baseline CSF Substance P	+/–
Reduction in Substance P with treatment	–
Vasopressin	
Increased electrophysiological response to traumatic imagery	+
Oxytocin	
Decreased electrophysiological response to traumatic imagery	+
Estradiol	
Increased baseline plasma estradiol	
Thyroid	
Increased baseline indices of thyroid function	+
Increased TSH response to TRH	+
***Dehydroepiandrosterone* sulfate (DHEA-S)**	
Increased baseline plasma DHEA-S	+/–
Increased diurnal DHEA-S	–/+
***Allopregnanolone* (progesterone metabolite)**	
Decreased baseline CSF allopregnanolone	+
Estradiol	
Reduced baseline plasma estradiol	+/–

cAMP, cyclic adenosine 39,59-monophosphate; CCK, cholecystokinin; CSF, cerebrospinal fluid; 5-HT, serotonin; NS, not studied; PTSD, posttraumatic stress disorder; SPECT, single photon emission computed tomography; TSH, thyroid-stimulating hormone; TRH, thyrotropin-releasing hormone.

et al., 1999; Southwick et al., 1997, 1999; Vermetten & Bremner, 2002b). As mentioned earlier, one of the best lines of evidence is the efficacy of SSRIs and other medications that have actions on the serotonin system in the treatment of PTSD. In addition, studies in human subjects show an association between behaviors seen in PTSD patients, including impulsivity (Brown & Linnoila, 1990; De Cuyper, 1987; Wu et al., 1999), aggression (Brown & Linnoila, 1990), depression and suicide (Mann et al., 1989; Stanly & Stanley, 1990), and decreased serotonergic function. Consistent with this, an increase in 5-HT_2 receptor binding was found in the frontal cortex of suicide victims, suggesting up-regulation of the receptor (Arango et al., 1990; Mann et al., 1986; Stanley & Mann, 1983).

Medications with actions on the serotonin system act on the brain to modify the effects of stress on brain function and behavior. Antidepressant treatments, including SSRIs and other medications acting on the serotonin system, promote nerve growth (neurogenesis) in the hippocampus and/or block the effects of stress on the hippocampus (Czeh et al., 2001; D'Sa & Duman, 2002; Duman, 2004; Duman et al., 1997, 2001; Garcia, 2002; Lucassen et al., 2004; Malberg et al., 2000; McEwen & Chattarji, 2004; Nibuya et al., 1995; Santarelli et al., 2003b; Watanabe et al., 1992b) while stress inhibits neurogenesis (Czeh et al., 2001; D'Sa & Duman, 2002; Duman et al., 2001; Lee et al., 2001; Lucassen et al., 2004; Malberg et al., 2000; Watanabe et al., 1992a). There is also some evidence that neurogenesis is necessary for the positive behavioral effects of antidepressants (Santarelli et al., 2003a; Watanabe et al., 1992a), although this continues to be a source of debate.(Duman, 2004; Henn & Vollmayr, 2004).

Studies in clinical populations of PTSD patients support a role for altered serotonergic function (Southwick et al., 1999). Adenylate cyclase activity in human platelets has been used as a marker of serotonin function. Decreased adenylate cyclase activity at baseline, and decreased forskolin-induced activation of adenylate cyclase activity have been shown in PTSD (Lerer et al., 1990). Victims of Scud missile attacks in Israel with PTSD were also shown to have decreased adenylate cyclase activity at baseline and with forskolin stimulation (Weizmann et al., 1994a). There was no effect of serotonin on forskolin-induced adenylate cyclase activity (a putative probe of the 5-HT_{1A} receptor) (Weizmann et al., 1994a). Patients with PTSD were found to have decreased binding of the SSRI, paroxetine, which binds to the serotonin transporter, as measured with both B_{max} (maximum number of 3H-paroxetine binding sites) and K_D (an inverse measure of affinity of 3H-paroxeting binding to uptake sites), compared with controls (Arora et al., 1993), with decreases in K_D specifically associated with the severity of symptoms of PTSD, anxiety, and depression (Fichtner et al., 1995). Lower baseline K_D predicted a positive response to treatment with the SSRI fluoxetine in PTSD patients (Fichtner et al., 1994). Another study found no difference in platelet serotonin levels or uptake between PTSD patients and controls (Mellman & Kumar, 1994). A study of women with sexual assault-related PTSD found no difference in prolactin response to the 5-HT$_{1A}$ agonist, buspirone (a probe of serotonergic function), between patients and controls (Dinan et al., 1990). Another study found no change in the serotonin metabolite, 5-HIAA, in the CSF, at baseline between PTSD and controls or with trauma-related stimuli (Geracioti et al., 2013). Overall, these studies, albeit representing only peripheral and indirect measures, are consistent with alterations in serotonergic function in clinical populations of PTSD.

The serotonin agonist, meta-chlorophenylpiperazine (mCPP), was used in a pharmacological challenge study to assess serotonergic function in 26 PTSD patients and 14 healthy normal human controls (Southwick et al., 1997). mCPP has agonist properties for the 5-HT$_{1A}$, 5-HT$_{1B}$, 5-HT$_{1D}$, 5-HT$_{2A}$, 5-HT$_{2B}$, 5-HT$_{2C}$, 5-HT$_3$, and 5-HT$_7$ receptors, as well as the serotonin transporter (SERT), with primary effects at 5-HT$_{2B}$ and 5-HT$_{2C}$ receptors (Pettibone & Williams, 1984). It causes mild serotonin uptake inhibition as well as stimulation of release of serotonin in the brain, and is associated with side-effects in normal humans of anxiety, headache, and appetite loss (Pettibone & Williams, 1984). Intravenous infusion of m-CPP resulted in a significant increase in blood pressure as well as symptoms of anxiety, panic, and PTSD in the PTSD patients compared with healthy controls. In all, 31% of the PTSD patients had a panic attack with mCPP and no PTSD patients had a panic attack with a saline placebo infusion. None of the healthy controls had a panic attack with either mCPP or placebo (Southwick et al., 1997). This study provided further evidence that altered central serotonergic function and responsivity is associated with symptoms of PTSD.

Genetic studies are also consistent with altered serotonergic function in PTSD. PTSD patients were found to have altered genotype patterns for genes coding for the serotonin transporter and other serotonin receptors (Kuzelova et al., 2010; Pietrzak et al., 2012). The genotype for the serotonin transporter (5HTTLPR) includes both S and L allele types. The SS allele genotype has been associated with PTSD (Kenna et al., 2012; Koenen et al., 2009; Kuzelova et al., 2010; Lee et al., 2005; Wang et al., 2011). Serotonin transporter 5HTTLPR S allele genotype predicted vulnerability to development of PTSD after natural disaster (Pietrzak et al., 2012) or exposure to childhood adversity.(Xie et al., 2009). Increased PTSD risk was assessed with the L-S and G-A alleles of the serotonin transporter, and increased risk for PTSD was found with L (A) (Grabe et al., 2009). In a study of African-Americans, the G allele of the 5-HT$_{2A}$ receptor genotype (but not the serotonin transporter) was associated with PTSD (Mellman et al., 2009). PTSD patients with the LL allele of the serotonin transporter gene showed enhanced response to SSRIs, and non-responsiveness was associated with the SS allele (Kenna et al., 2012; Mushtaq et al., 2012). The SS allele of 5HTTLPR also predicted poor response to cognitive-behavioral treatment in PTSD (Bryant et al., 2010). These studies show that genes coding for serotonin receptors and the serotonin transporter are predictive of the risk of PTSD as well as response to treatment. Overall, there is considerable evidence that serotonin dysfunction plays a role in PTSD.

9.9 GABA/benzodiazepine system

The GABA-benzodiazepine receptor complex plays an important role in stress and anxiety. GABA is ubiquitous in the CNS and is a major inhibitory neurotransmitter (Roy-Byrne, 2005). The three GABA receptor subtypes are GABA-A, GABA-B, and GABA-C. GABA-A and GABA-C mediate rapid effects through a ligand gated chloride ion channel, while GABA-B mediates slower effects via G protein-coupled effects on calcium and potassium channels. The GABA-benzodiazepine receptor (GABA-A or benzodiazepine receptor) is composed of five glycoprotein subunits that bind benzodiazepine type compounds with an ion channel at the center. Activation of the receptor causes an influx of calcium and membrane hyperpolarization. Binding of benzodiazepines to the benzodiazepine receptor facilitates the actions of GABA by increasing the frequency of ion channel opening. Other compounds acting at this receptor include barbiturates, anesthetics, and alcohol at different sites, but with similar enhancement of the action of GABA. Subunits of the receptor complex include alpha with six isoforms, beta with three isoforms, gamma with three isoforms, theta, epsilon and delta with one isoform each, and rho with three isoforms. The majority of GABA complexes consist of α-1. Each receptor complex has two GABA binding sites and one benzodiazepine binding site. Although endogenous benzodiazepines that bind to the receptor have been hypothesized, they have never been identified. Benzodiazepines do occur naturally in nature, however, and are found in some forms of plants. The evolutionary purpose of benzodiazepine receptors has been hypothesized to be related to the regulation of attention, arousal, and relaxation, and hence its relevance to the anxiety disorders (Nutt & Malizia, 2001; Roy-Byrne, 2005).

Stress is associated with changes in benzodiazepine receptors. Exposure to inescapable stressors such as footshock or forced swim results in a 20–30% decrease in benzodiazepine receptor binding in the frontal cortex (Lippa et al., 1987; Weizman et al., 1989) and cerebral cortex (Drugan et al., 1986, 1989; Medina et al., 1983a,1983b; Weizman et al., 1990), with some studies (Drugan et al., 1989; Medina et al., 1983a,b; Weizman et al., 1990) but not others (Drugan et al., 1986; Havoundjian et al., 1986; Skerritt et al., 1981; Weizman et al., 1989) showing a decrease in the hippocampus. Exposure to stress has no effects on benzodiazepine receptor binding in the pons, striatum, thalamus, cerebellum, midbrain, or occipital cortex (Drugan et al., 1986; Lippa et al., 1987; Medina et al., 1983a,b). One study that used a different model of stressor, defeat stress, showed an increase in benzodiazepine receptor binding in the cortex (Miller et al., 1987). Exposure to prenatal stress results in a decrease in benzodiazepine receptors in the central nucleus of the amygdala and the hippocampus, which is associated with increased anxiety behaviors (Barros & Rodriguez, 2006). A decrease in benzodiazepine receptor binding (B_{max}) was also demonstrated in the Maudsley genetically fearful strain of rat in comparison to non-fearful rats in several brain structures including the hippocampus (Robertson et al., 1978). Inverse agonists to the benzodiazepine receptor promote anxiety reactions in non-human primates (Ninan et al., 1982). These studies are consistent with a role for alterations in benzodiazepine binding in anxiety, with findings showing a specific decrease in the frontal cortex and, although not as consistently, a decrease in the hippocampus. The findings suggest that decreased benzodiazepine receptor binding in the frontal cortex may play a role in the symptoms of PTSD.

Studies in human subjects are also consistent with a relationship between stress and alterations in benzodiazepine receptor binding (Table 9.2) (Dorow et al., 1983; Roy-Byrne, 2005; Weizmann et al., 1987, 1994b). FG7142, a benzodiazepine receptor inverse agonist, induced severe anxiety that resembled panic attacks and biological characteristics of anxiety in healthy subjects (Dorow et al., 1983).

Benzodiazepine function has been investigated in patients with PTSD. A decrease in binding of peripheral benzodiazepine receptors on platelets was found in patients with PTSD (Gavish et al., 1996). Patients with combat-related PTSD did not exhibit a greater behavioral response (i.e., anxiety) with the benzodiazepine receptor antagonist flumazenil than did healthy subjects (Randall et al., 1995); however, flumazenil has no pharmacological effect on the receptor per se.

Brain imaging studies have found alterations in benzodiazepine receptor binding in PTSD. Single photon emission tomography with [I-123]iomazenil, which binds to the benzodiazepine receptor in the human brain, showed decreased frontal binding in Vietnam combat veterans with PTSD compared with controls (Bremner et al., 2000). Another study in veterans of the first Gulf War with PTSD showed no difference in binding with SPECT [I-123]iomazenil from controls (Fujita et al., 2004). PTSD patients in this study did show a significant negative correlation between binding in right superior temporal gyrus and severity of childhood trauma.

The effects of benzodiazepines on anxiety demonstrate a role for the GABA/benzodiazepine system in symptoms of anxiety; however, it is not clear that long-term treatment is useful for PTSD. Benzodiazepine administration has been shown to be efficacious in the treatment of symptoms of chronic anxiety in PTSD patients (Bremner et al., 1996c), although it has not been shown to prevent the development of chronic PTSD (Gelpin et al., 1996) and may not help some of the primary symptoms of PTSD (Braun et al., 1990).

Treatment with the GABA agonist, baclofen, was efficacious in an open-label trial in PTSD (Drake et al., 2003). Other medications that act as GABA agonists or reuptake inhibitors, including gabapentin (Brannon et al., 2000; Pande et al., 2000; Pollack et al., 1998) and tiagabine (Berigan, 2002; Taylor, 2003), were also efficacious for PTSD. These studies suggest that understanding the GABA/benzodiazepine system and how it is affected by stress could lead to the development of newer medications with fewer side-effects and less potential for addiction. Also, as GABA agonists and benzodiazepine receptors bind to the same complex, understanding changes in this complex will be useful to develop new treatments.

9.10 Opioid peptides

An important part of the stress response is opioid-mediated analgesia. This has survival value in allowing the organism not to be disabled by pain while under attack. Stress is associated with release of endogenous opioids, including beta-endorphin, enkephalin, and dynorphin. The beta-endorphins are secreted by the pituitary gland and reach all tissues present in the body by diffusion. There are four major opioid receptor types: delta, kappa, mu, and nociceptin (Loh & Smith, 1990). Opiate systems project from the periaquaeductal gray (PAG) in the midbrain to the nucleus raphe magnus in the medulla, which in turn has noradrenergic and serotonergic projections to the spinal cord (Vaccarino et al., 1999). The opiate system is also involved in regulation of the CRF-HPA and noradrenergic responses to stress (Vythilingam et al., 2000). Medications used in the treatment of opiate overdose, such as naloxone or naltrexone, are selective mu-receptor antagonists.

Stress-induced analgesia mediated by the opiate system occurs with a variety of different kinds of stressful stimuli (Terman et al., 1984). Stress is associated with an increase in endogenous opiate release (Grau et al., 1981) with decreased density of mu-opiate receptors (Stuckey et al., 1989) which may mediate the analgesia associated with stress. Stress-induced analgesia occurs with uncontrollable but not controllable stress (Fanselow, 1986). Sensitization to the analgesic effects of stress also occurs, as evidenced by the re-occurrence of stress-induced analgesia in previously stressed animals upon re-exposure to stress (Maier, 1986). Opioid receptor antagonists such as naloxone block fear learning, suggesting that the opioid system plays a role in the learning of conditioned fear responses (McNally & Cole, 2006). Opioid receptor antagonists also activate CRF and the peripheral hormonal stress response.

Clinical evidence supports a role for alterations in the opiate system in patients with PTSD (Table 9.2). Opiate usage was correlated with an increase in PTSD symptoms in soldiers returning from the war in Vietnam, and PTSD patients endorsed opiates as being efficacious in reducing symptoms, especially in the hyperarousal and intrusive memory categories (Bremner et al., 1996c). This is consistent with the fact that opiates decrease firing of noradrenergic neurons originating in the locus coeruleus, and withdrawal of opiates causes a rebound increase, as is seen in opiate addicts going through withdrawal. The presence of stress-induced analgesia in battered women was correlated with the development of PTSD hyperarousal symptoms 3 months after the initial trauma (Nishith & Griffin, 2002). Studies showed either reduced beta-endorphins in plasma (Hoffman et al., 1989) or no change (Baker et al., 1997), while beta-endorphins were increased in CSF in PTSD with a negative correlation between intrusive and avoidant PTSD symptoms and levels (Baker et al., 1997). Plasma beta-endorphin increased after exercise in PTSD patients to a greater degree than in controls (Hamner & Hitri, 1992). No differences were found in plasma levels of methionine-enkephalin between PTSD patients and controls, although the degradation half-life was significantly higher in the PTSD group (Wolf, 1991). Brain imaging showed decreased mu opiate receptor binding in PTSD in anterior cingulate, while decreases were seen in combat veterans both with and without PTSD in the amygdala, insular and PFC, and nucleus accumbens (Liberzon et al., 2007).

Studies of opioid receptor antagonists in PTSD patients also support a role for this system in the symptoms of PTSD. Administration of morphine in child burn victims had a protective effect on the development of PTSD (Saxe et al., 2001, 2005). A decrease in pain sensitivity following exposure to combat-related materials was blocked by administration of naloxone in patients with PTSD (Pitman et al., 1990; van der Kolk et al., 1989). PTSD was not associated with changes in pain sensitivity at baseline or following mental stress, although another condition commonly associated with early trauma, borderline personality disorder (BPD), was associated with decreased baseline and stress-related pain sensitivity (Schmahl et al., 2010). Open-label studies showed efficacy of opiate antagonists, including naltrexone, in the treatment of PTSD, especially for symptoms of flashbacks (Bills & Kreisler, 1993; Glover, 1993) and in dissociative symptoms in patients with BPD (Schmahl et al., 2012). These studies suggest that endogenous opiate release has a protective effect on the development of PTSD, and that alterations in opioid function are associated with PTSD and pain sensitivity in PTSD.

9.11 Neurotensin

Neurotensin acts as a neurotransmitter in the brain, and its receptors are located in the hypothalamus, septum amygdala, and hippocampus. Centrally administered neurotensin attenuates the development of stress-induced gastric ulcers

(Nemeroff et al., 1982), modulates body temperature and sensory functions relevant to the stress response (Kalivas et al., 1982), and activates stress-responsive systems including dopamine and the HPA axis (Gudelsky et al., 1989). Neurotensin is also functionally and anatomically linked to mesolimbic dopaminergic systems, and these systems function in tandem as part of the stress response (Deutch et al., 1987). To our knowledge, no studies of neurotensin have been conducted in patients with PTSD.

9.12 Somatostatin

Somatostatin (somatotropin release-inhibiting factor) is the major inhibitor of growth hormone secretion in the brain. Somatostatin is located in the PVN of the hypothalamus, the amygdala, hippocampus, cerebral cortex, median preoptic area, nucleus accumbens, and other areas of the b rain (Krisch, 1981). Somatostatin inhibits extinction, and modulates sleep, food intake, locomotor activity, and memory function (Vecsei et al., 1984). Somatostatin levels increase in response to both CRF administration and stress (Benyassi et al., 1993). Chronic stress increases both baseline and stress-induced release of somatostatin with an associated decrease in growth hormone and growth hormone-releasing factor (Armario et al., 1993; Benyassi et al., 1993). One study showed an increase in baseline somatostatin levels in the CSF of patients with PTSD (Bremner et al., 1997b), although another study showed no differences between PTSD patients and controls (Sautter et al., 2003).

9.13 Cholecystokinin

Cholecystokinin (CCK) is a peptide synthesized in the gastrointestinal tract that is similar to gastrin. In addition to mediating effects in the GI tract, such as stimulation of gall bladder secretion, it has central effects in the brain, primarily the stimulation of anxiety. CCK exists in the brain as an octapeptide (CCK-8) and as a tetrapeptide (CCK-4). CCK is co-localized in neurons with opioid peptides and dopamine and modulates their activity. The octapeptide form, CCK-8, is concentrated in the cerebral cortex, amygdala, and hippocampus. CCK receptors, which include CCKA and CCKB, are also located in the periaqueductal gray and substantia nigra regions of the midbrain. CCKB predominates in the brain. Agonists of the CCKB receptor have anxiogenic effects as well as effects on attention and memory, while antagonists are anxiolytic (Bastaki & Hasan, 2003; Cohen et al., 1999). Blockade of CCK receptors in the periaqueductal gray blocks the anxiogenic effects of CCK (Bertoglio & Zangrossi Jr., 2005; Bertoglio et al., 2007).

CCK activation of hippocampal neurons is inhibited by administration of benzo-diazepines (Bouthillier & De Montigny, 1988). CCK-4 administration has been shown to result in an increase in anxiety in PTSD patients compared to healthy subjects, as well as a more blunted ACTH response and more rapid return of cortisol to baseline (Table 9.2) (Kellner et al., 2000). These studies support a role for CCK in anxiety and PTSD.

9.14 Neuropeptide Y

Neuropeptide Y (NPY) is a neuropeptide with anxiolytic properties that is highly concentrated in several brain areas involved in the stress response. Brain areas expressing NPY include the locus coeruleus, PVN of the hypothalamus, brain stem (nucleus of solitary tract and ventrolateral medulla), amygdala, hippocampus, cerebral cortex, basal ganglia, and thalamus (Adrian et al., 1983). There are five NPY receptors, Y1–Y5 (Makino & Baker, 2000; Wahlestedt et al., 1990). Chronic stress results in increased levels of NPY in the amygdala, which may represent an adaptive response to stress exposure (Thorsell et al., 2000). NPY is also involved in the consolidation of fear memories and has a counter-regulatory effect on CRF and noradrenergic systems. Injection of NPY into the amygdala has anxiolytic effects (Heilig et al., 1993) and is protective against the development of stress-induced gastric ulcers (Penner et al., 1993). NPY-transgenic rats show decreased fear responses and insensitivity to the behavioral consequences of stress; impairment of spatial memory acquisition was associated with decreased NPY-Y1 binding in the hippocampus (Thorsell et al., 2000). Patients with combat-related PTSD had reduced baseline and post-pharmacological challenge (yohimbine) plasma levels of NPY (Rasmusson et al., 2000), although another study of intimate partner violence-related PTSD showed no differences in baseline plasma NPY levels (Seedat et al., 2003). Another study found that baseline decreases in NPY corrected following recovery from PTSD (Table 9.2) (Yehuda et al., 2006). These studies support the role of NPY as part of the stress response.

9.15 Galanin

Galanin is a peptide involved in a number of physiological and behavioral functions, including learning and cognition, pain control, food intake, neuroen-docrine control, and cardiovascular regulation, as well as depression and anxiety (Karlsson & Holmes, 2006; Weiss et al., 1998). About 80% of noradrenergic cells in the locus coeruleus co-express galanin. Galanin-containing neural pathways project from the locus coeruleus to the hippocampus, hypothalamus, amygdala, and PFC (Weiss et al., 1998). There are three known galanin receptor subtypes, Gal-R1, Gal-R2, and Gal-R3. The Gal-R1 receptor, in addition to other functions, plays a role in the fear response, and is highly concentrated in the amygdala, hypothalamus, and bed nucleus of the stria terminalis (Gustafson et al., 1996). Galanin reduces locus coeruleus firing, possibly through Gal-R1 (Sevcik et al., 1993), as well as norepinephrine release in the amygdala, hypothalamus, and PFC, possibly through a direct effect on these brain regions via galanin-synthesizing neurons or local galanin receptors (Khoshbouei et al., 2002a).

Galanin plays an important role in stress and fear responses. Administration of galanin is anxiolytic (Kuteeva & Wardi, 2007). Galanin administered into the central nucleus of the amygdala blocks the anxiogenic effects of stress, including a block of release of norepinephrine in the central nucleus of the amygdala; yohimbine administration increases galanin release in the amygdala (Barrera & Hernandez, 2006; Khoshbouei et al., 2002a). Administration of galanin in the brain can have effects on behavior that involve either induction or reduction of fear, depending on the brain region (Bing & Moller, 1993; Karlsson & Holmes, 2005, 2006; Khoshbouei et al., 2002a; Khoshbouei & Cecchi, 2002; Moller & Sommer, 1999). Animals deficient in Gal-R1 receptors demonstrate increased fear and anxiety (Holmes et al., 2003a), while some anxiety-like behaviors (but not all) are associated with Gal-R2 receptor deficiency (Bailey et al., 2007; Gottsch & Zeng, 2005). Galanin-overexpressing transgenic mice are unresponsive to the anxiogenic effects of the α_2-receptor antagonist, yohimbine (Holmes et al., 2002). Galanin administration and galanin overexpression in the hippocampus both result in deficits in conditioned fear learning (Kinney & Starosta, 2002). The galanin receptor agonist, galnon, has anxiolytic-like properties that are reversible when M35, a galanin receptor antagonist, is injected (Rajarao et al., 2007). These studies suggest a possible efficacy of galanin analogs for the treatment of stress-related disorders, although the role of this neuropeptide in PTSD has not been investigated.

9.16 Ghrelin

Ghrelin is a peptide synthesized in the stomach and pancreas that is involved in the regulation of appetite and food digestion. Ghrelin levels rise before meals and stimulate food intake, and alterations in ghrelin function have been linked to obesity (Yildiz et al., 2004). Ghrelin receptors are located in a number of organs of the body as well as the pituitary and the hypothalamus (Stengel et al., 2011). Psychological stress increases ghrelin levels in the plasma (Spencer et al., 2012; Stengel et al., 2011), and ghrelin mediates the stress-induced increase in food intake associated with exposure to chronic stress (Chuang et al., 2011) as well as behavioral responses to stress (Spencer et al., 2012). Ghrelin crosses the blood–brain barrier where it acts through ghrelin receptors in the basolateral nuclear of the hypothalamus to stimulate release of growth hormone. Acting through growth hormone in the amygdala, ghrelin enhances the learning of fear behaviors in animals exposed to an environment of chronic stress. Agonists of ghrelin enhance this effect, while antagonists have the opposite effect (Meyer et al., 2014). These studies suggest that ghrelin plays an important role in fear learning, which is relevant to PTSD, although studies have not yet investigated the clinical role of this neuropeptide.

9.17 Substance P

The neurokinin substance P plays a role in the stress response. The substance P receptor is concentrated in limbic and cortical areas involved in anxiety and stress as well as areas involved in motivation such as the nucleus accumbens. Substance P inhibits baseline HPA axis activity (Donnerer et al., 1991) as well as the duration of the HPA axis response to stress by acting through neurokinin-1 receptors, suggesting that substance P may be an important central agent controlling the transition between acute and chronic stress (Jessop et al., 2000). Substance P is also involved in stress-induced changes in pain sensitivity and immune reactivity (Fehder et al., 1997). Some studies showed increased CSF concentrations of substance P in the CSF of PTSD patients at baseline (Geracioti et al., 2006; Mathew et al., 2011), although one study showed no differences in CSF substance P concentrations between PTSD patients and controls at baseline and no change with antidepressant treatment (Table 9.2) (Bonne et al., 2011). Treatment of PTSD with a neurokinin-1 receptor antagonist showed no difference from placebo in PTSD symptoms (Mathew et al., 2011).

9.18 Vasoactive intestinal peptide

Vasoactive intestinal peptide (VIP) is a peptide originally identified in the intestine which is distributed in multiple organs in the body as well as in the brain. VIP regulates a number of physiological processes that are in general affected by stress, including lipolysis, glycogenolysis, and hormone release from the anterior pituitary gland. Stress stimulates release of VIP, and VIP was shown to prevent stress-induced gastric ulcers (Tuncel et al., 1998).

9.19 Vasopressin and oxytocin

Vasopressin and oxytocin are peptides that play a role in attachment behaviors and are therefore relevant to early stress and PTSD symptoms of avoidance. Vasopressin is released from nerve terminals in the pituitary together with CRF and has a major role in fluid and electrolyte balance in response to dehydration. It is also involved in regulation of the stress response through effects on the HPA axis and other systems, as well as diverse other properties including memory and REM sleep (Aguilera & Rabadan-Diehl, 2000). Vasopressin binds to V1A and V1B receptors in the brain. Animals lacking the V1A receptor have reduced anxiety behaviors (Bielsky et al., 2004; Egashira et al., 2007; Egashira & Tanoue, 2007) while overexpression of V1A is associated with increased anxiety behaviors (Bielsky & Hu, 2005). Vasopressin V1B receptor antagonists have been shown to exhibit anxiolytic and antidepressant effects (Hodgson & Higgins, 2007).

Systemic effects of oxytocin include release of milk and uterine contractility at the time of labor and delivery. It also contributes to HPA axis regulation, potentiating the effect of CRF on ACTH release. Additionally, oxytocin stimulates prolactin secretion and potentiates CRF-stimulated ACTH release (Gibbs, 1986). Increased licking and grooming of rat pups results in increased oxytocin receptor binding in the central nucleus in females, and increased vasopressin receptor binding in males (Francis et al., 2002).

Intranasal administration of vasopressin to PTSD patients resulted in an increase in electrophysiological responses to combat imagery, while oxytocin led to a decrease relative to placebo (Pitman et al., 1993).

9.20 Neurosteroids and neurohormones

Steroids that can cross the blood–brain barrier and have an effect on neurofunction are called neurosteroids (Rupprecht, 2003). Some neurosteroids modulate $GABA_A$ receptors and thus have anxiolytic effects (Rupprecht, 2003). Steroids and hormones that have receptors in the nucleus of cells are part of the nuclear receptor superfamily. These include the receptors for retinoic acid (the active form of vitamin A, RAR), estrogen (ER), androgen (AR), mineralocorticoids (MRs), glucocorticoids (GRs) and thyroid hormone (THR) (Bremner & McCaffery, 2008; McCaffery et al., 2006; Rupprecht, 2003). The receptor is either present in the nucleus or moves from the cytoplasm into the nucleus in the presence of the hormone, and then binds to a response element in the promoter of responsive genes (Bastien & Rochette-Egly, 2004). The binding of the hormone leads to a switch in the conformation of the receptor, followed by a release of co-repressors that removes repression of gene transcription. A chromatin remodeling complex is then recruited that decompacts the chromatin, allowing the transcription to proceed. This leads to genomic modification and protein transcription (Baulieu & Robel, 1998). The members of the nuclear receptor superfamily share in common the fact that they affect behavior and mood.

Some neurosteroids, including 3α-reduced metabolites of progesterone and deoxycorticosterone, modulate ligand-gated channels via nongenomic mechanisms (Strömberg & Haage, 2006). These compounds have anxiolytic effects through positive modulation of $GABA_A$ receptors in the central nucleus of the amygdala (Vanover & Rosenzweig-Lipson, 2000; Wang & Marx, 2007).

Thyroid hormone and thyroid-stimulating hormone (TSH) have a range of actions, including facilitation of energy within the cell, which are relevant to the stress response. Stress results in long-term increases in thyroid hormone (Mason et al., 1968) as well as increased TSH release (Armario & Jolin, 1989) and a blunting of the normal thyroid hormone release to TSH (Armario et al., 1993). Dr. Robert Graves reported the first series of patients with classic symptoms of what would later be determined was due to excessive thyroid hormone production, including increased heart rate and perspiration, anxiety, fatigue, and heat intolerance. He noted that many of the patients developed the condition after exposure to extreme stress. Psychiatric disturbances such as anxiety, depression, mania, and sometimes psychosis occur at an increased rate in patients with hyperthyroidism (Bunevicius & Prange, 2006; Stern et al., 1996). Patients with PTSD have increases in baseline plasma levels of thyroid hormone, both total thyroxine (T4) and free and total triiodothyronine (T3) (Mason et al., 1994) and an increased TSH response to thyrotropin-releasing hormone TRH challenge (Kosten et al., 1990).

Adrenal androgens such as dehydroepiandrosterone (DHEA) and DHEA-sulfate 7 (DHEA-S) are sensitive to stress. Chronic stress increases DHEA and DHEA-S (Fuller et al., 1984). DHEA also has anti-stress effects, blocking the effects of glucocorticoids on peripheral tissues as well as the hippocampus (Kaminska et al., 2000; Kimonides et al., 1998) and decreasing anxiety (Prasad et al., 1997). Studies of DHEA in PTSD based on a single plasma sample have shown decreases (Kanter et al., 2001), increases (Spivak et al., 2000), or no difference between PTSD patients and controls (Rasmusson et al., 2004), although a study involving multiple measurements over a 24-hour period showed elevations in DHEA-S in women with early childhood abuse-related PTSD (Bremner et al., 2007).

Progesterone has anxiolytic effects, largely through its metabolite allopregnanolone acting on GABA-A receptors in the amygdala and other brain areas (Reddy & O'Malley, 2005). One study showed decreased CSF concentrations of allopregnanolone in women with PTSD (Rasmusson & Pinna, 2006).

Stress has inhibitory effects on reproductive function that are mediated through reproductive hormonal systems. Gonadotropin-releasing hormone from the hypothalamus causes release of luteinizing hormone (LH) and follicle-stimulating hormone (FSH) from the pituitary. This in turn stimulates production and release of the sex hormones testosterone and estradiol from the gonads. Stress resulted in decreased estrogen levels in plasma in some studies (Goncharov et al., 1979; Osadchuka et al., 2000) but not others (Anderson et al., 1996; Goldman & Vogel, 1985). Stress results in an inhibition of growth hormone release (Armario et al., 1993) and LH release from the pituitary (Dobson et al., 1999; Kam et al., 2000, 2002; Tilbrook et al., 1999). Some women, during the peri-menopausal period (Schmidt et al., 1997) or post-oophorectomy (Sherwin & Gelfand, 1985), when estradiol levels are low, develop symptoms of depression that reverse with estradiol treatment (Almeida & Barclay, 2001; Carlson et al., 2000; Schmidt et al., 2000; Soares et al., 2001; Steffen et al., 1999). Chronic work stress resulted in a decrease in plasma estradiol levels (Hertting & Theorell, 2002). Women with a history of violent victimization had lower estradiol levels only in the age range 41–45 years, while early abuse was related to increased levels of FSH (Allsworth et al., 2001). Plasma estrogen levels measured at multiple time points over a 24-hour period showed no differences between women with early childhood abuse-related PTSD and controls (Bremner et al., 2007).

Retinoids are the biological family of compounds derived from retinol or vitamin A, which plays an important role in the regulation of vision and other bodily functions. Retinoids also play a role in the regulation of genetic transcription during *in utero* development, which accounts for their potential for teratogenicity if administered to pregnant women. Retinoids can lead to neurological side-effects, and they have recently been shown to act as neurotransmitters in the brain, regulating neurogenesis in the hippocampus and other functions relevant to stress-related mental disorders (Bremner et al., 2012). Vitamin A is obtained in the diet in the form of retinyl esters or beta-carotene from various meats and vegetables (especially those that are orange in color) and is converted in the body to the active form of vitamin A, retinoic acid (13-*trans*-retinoic acid) (Bremner & McCaffery, 2008; Mey & McCaffery, 2004).

The RARs are widely distributed in the adult brain, although there is a more restricted range for retinoic acid (Krezel et al., 1999; Mey & McCaffery, 2004; Zetterstrom et al., 1994, 1999). Retinoid receptors in the brain include RAR α, β, and γ subtypes and retinoid X receptors (RXR) α, β, and γ subtypes (Lane & Bailey, 2005; Zetterstrom et al., 1994,1999). RAR and RXR receptors function as RAR-RXR heterodimers and play a critical role in the regulation of embryonic development (Bastien & Rochette-Egly, 2004; Chambon, 1996; Colbert et al., 1993; Idres et al., 2002; Krezel et al., 1999; Luo et al., 2004; Mendelsohn et al., 1994; Toresson et al., 1999; Waclaw et al., 2004; Zhang et al., 2003). The response element for retinoic acid in the nucleus of cells is called retinoic acid response element (Chambon, 1996). Retinoic acid signaling occurs in the limbic system, including the hippocampus (Krezel et al., 1999; Luo et al., 2004; Misner et al.,

2001; Sakai et al., 2004; Zetterstrom et al., 1999), as well as the mPFC, thalamus and hypothalamus (Luo et al., 2004).

Retinoids have a number of effects on brain areas involved in the stress response. They regulate neurogenesis in the hippocampus, which suggested a possible role in stress-related mental disorders (Crandall et al., 2004; Misner et al., 2001; Sakai et al., 2004). Animals deficient in RAR (Chiang et al., 1998) or suffering from vitamin A deficiency (Misner et al., 2001) show deficits in new learning and memory (Cocco et al., 2002) consistent with an effect on hippocampal function. High levels of the enzyme responsible for conversion of retinol to retinoic acid in the cells, class-1 aldehyde dehydrogenase, are found in brain areas involved in the stress response. These include the basal forebrain, and axons and terminals of the dopaminergic neurons of the mesostriatal and mesolimbic system (McCaffery & Drager, 1994a,b). The distribution of retinoid receptors in the brain corresponds to limbic brain areas that have been implicated in stress-related mental disorders, including hippocampus, hypothalamus, mPFC, bed nucleus of the stria terminalis, olfactory bulb, amygdala and thalamus (Krezel et al., 1999). These brain areas are responsive to retinoids during development as well as in the adult brain (Thompson Haskell et al., 2002). Retinoids modulate gene expression in the brain in a very broad spectrum and have effects on several stress-responsive neurochemical systems, including dopamine, serotonin and norepinephrine (Goodman, 1998). Retinoic acid administration results in increases in D2 receptor mRNA expression (Farooqui, 1994). Mice with double mutations for RARβ-/- RXRβ-/-, RARβ-/- RXRγ-/-, and RXRβ-/- RXRγ-/- show behaviors consistent with deficits in mesolimbic dopamine function, including deficits in rearing and locomotion (Krezel et al., 1998). Retinoid receptor-deficient mice also show reduced expression of D1 and D2 receptors in the ventral striatum, and blunted behavioral responses to cocaine, which acts by blocking dopamine reuptake into striatal neurons (Goodman, 1995, 1998; LaMantia, 1999).

Another key brain area involved in regulation of the stress response that is also endogenously regulated by retinoic acid is the hypothalamus (Shearer et al., 2010). Retinol is converted to retinoic acid by RALDH enzymes in the processes of tanycytes, the specialized ependymal cells that provide a gateway between the CSF in the third ventricle and neural cells of the hypothalamus where there are RARs. Retinoic acid is released into the hypothalamus via the long processes of the tanycytes that reach into the hypothalamus where it can regulate genes including the RAR as well as ACTH (Shearer et al., 2010) and CRH (Kasckow et al., 1994). Studies have found increased density of cells expressing RARα in the PVN of the hypothalamus in post-mortem brains of patients with affective disorders (Chen et al., 2009) and this receptor co-localized with those neurons expressing CRH. Similarly, in a rat model of depression, RARα levels were raised in the PVN (Chen et al., 2009). Thus, retinoic acid plays an important role in the hypothalamus, suggesting a role in the stress response and stress-related mental disorders.

Retinoids also have effects on behavior. Several studies showed that isotretinoin administered to animals resulted in depression-like behaviors (Ferguson et al., 2005b; Ferguson & Berry, 2007; O'Reilly et al., 2006). Studies also found changes in metabolites of serotonin and dopamine in the striatum and dopamine in the hippocampus with isotretinoin (Ferguson et al., 2005a). Another study found that isotretinoin increased serotonin 5-HT_{1A} protein and serotonin transporter protein, which could potentially lead to decreased serotonin in the synapse (O'Reilly et al., 2007).

The retinoid, isotretinoin (13-*cis*-retinoic acid), an isomer of retinoic acid, is used as a pharmaceutical treatment of acne. Isotretinoin has been associated with depression, psychosis, and suicide (Bremner et al., 2012; Bremner & McCaffery, 2008), as well as a decrease in function of the orbitofrontal cortex, which plays an important role in the regulation of mood, behavior and the stress response (Bremner et al., 2005a). These studies show that members of the nuclear receptor superfamily, including the retinoids, play a role in mood responses and stress.

9.21 Conclusions

This chapter has reviewed neurochemical and neurohormonal responses to stress. There are a number of different messaging systems that help the organism prepare to cope with attack or other stressors, and these systems also interact and mutually regulate each other. Neurotransmitters involved include cortisol, norepinephrine, serotonin, and dopamine. GABA and the benzodiazepine system regulate anxiety, and opiates are involved in stress-induced changes in pain sensitivity. The HPA axis regulates both the peripheral stress response and the centrally mediated behavioral responses to stress. Neuropeptides involved in the stress response or behaviors related to the stress response include neurotensin, somatostatin, substance P, CCK, NPY, somatostatin, ghrelin, vasopressin and oxytocin. Other systems include excitatory neurotransmitters and hormones, including testosterone, thyroid hormone, retinoids, estrogen, and adrenal steroids.

Although these systems are needed for survival, chronic stress or particular vulnerabilities can lead to long-term dysregulation of these systems. This, in turn, can manifest as stress-related mental disorders such as PTSD, mediated by changes in these systems interacting with brain areas involved in the stress response, e.g., the hippocampus, amygdala, and mPFC. Targeting these systems in the development of new medications may help to advance the treatment of PTSD patients for whom there are currently limited therapeutic alternatives.

References

Abercrombie ED, Jacobs BL (1987a) Single-unit response of noradrenergic neurons in the locus coeruleus of freely moving cats. *I. Acutely presented stressful and non-stressful stimuli. J Neurosci* 7, 2837–2847.

Abercrombie ED, Jacobs BL (1987b) Single-unit response of noradrenergic neurons in the locus coeruleus of freely moving cats. *II. Adaptation to chronically presented stressful stimuli. J Neurosci* 7, 2844–2848.

Adamec R, Burton P, Blundell J et al. (2006) Vulnerability to mild predator stress in serotonin transporter knockout mice. *Behav Brain Res* 170, 126–140.

Adell A, Garcia-Marquez C, Armario A et al. (1988) Chronic stress increases serotonin and noradrenaline in rat brain and sensitizes their responses to a further acute stress. *J Neurochem* 50, 1678–1681.

Adrian TE, Allen JM, Bloom SR et al. (1983) Neuropeptide Y distribution in human brain. *Nature* 306, 584–686.

Aerni A, Traber R, Hock C et al.(2004) Low-dose cortisol for symptoms of posttraumatic stress disorder. *Am J Psychiatry* 161, 1488–1490.

Aguilera G, Rabadan-Diehl CV (2000) Vasopressinergic regulation of the hypothalamic-pituitary-adrenal axis: implications for stress adaptation. *Regul Peptides* 96, 23–29.

Allsworth JE, Zierler S, Krieger N et al. (2001) Ovarian function in late reproductive years in relation to lifetime experiences of abuse. *Epidemiology* 12, 676–681.

Almeida OP, Barclay L (2001) Sex hormones and their impact on dementia and depression: a clinical perspective. *Expert Opin Pharmacother* 2, 527–535.

Anderson SM, Saviolakis GA, Bauman RA et al. (1996) Effects of chronic stress on food acquisition, plasma hormones, and the estrous cycle of female rats. *Physiol Behav* 60, 325–329.

Anisman H, Griffiths J, Matheson K et al. (2001) Posttraumatic stress symptoms and salivary cortisol levels. *Am J Psychiatry* 158, 1509–1511.

Ansorge MS, Zhou M Lira A et al. (2004) Early-life blockade of the 5-HT transporter alters emotional behavior in adult mice. *Science* 306, 879–881.

Arango V, Ernsberger P, Marzuk PM et al. (1990) Autoradiographic demonstration of increased serotonin 5-HT-2 and alpha-adrenergic receptor binding sites in the brain of suicide victims. *Arch Gen Psychiatry* 47, 1038–1047.

Armario A, Jolin T (1989) Influence of intensity and duration of exposure to various stressors on serum TSH and GH levels in adult male rats. *Life Sci* 44, 215–221.

Armario A, Marti O, Gavalda A et al. (1993) Effects of chronic immobilization stress on GH and TSH secretion in the rat: response to hypothalamic regulatory factors. *Psychoneuroendocrinology* 18, 405–413.

Arnsten AF (2000) Stress impairs prefrontal cortical function in rats and monkeys: role of dopamine D1 and norepinephrine alpha-1 receptor mechanisms. *Prog Brain Res* 126, 183–192.

Arora RC, Fichtner CG, O'Connor F et al. (1993) Paroxetine binding in the blood platelets of posttraumatic stress disorder patients. *Life Sci* 53, 919–928.

Aston-Jones G, Shipley MT, Chouvet G et al. (1991) Afferent regulation of locus coeruleus neurons: anatomy, physiology and pharmacology. *Progr Brain Res* 88, 47–75.

Bagdy G, Calogero AE, Murphy DL et al. (1989) Serotonin agonists cause parallel activation of the sympathoadrenomedullary system and the hypothalamo-pituitary-adrenocortical axis in conscious rats. *Endocrinology* 125, 2664–2669.

Bailey KR, Pavlova MN, Rohde AD et al. (2007) Galanin receptor subtype 2 (GalR2) null mutant mice display an anxiogenic-like phenotype specific to the elevated plus-maze. *Pharmacol Biochem Behav* 86, 8–20.

Baker DG, Ekhator NN, Kasckow JW et al. (2005) Higher levels of basal serial CSF cortisol in combat veterans with posttraumatic stress disorder. *Am J Psychiatry* 162, 992–994.

Baker DG, West SA, Nicholson WE et al. (1999) Serial CSF corticotropin-releasing hormone levels and adrenocortical activity in combat veterans with posttraumatic stress disorder. *Am J Psychiatry* 156, 585–588.

Baker DG, West SA, Orth DN et al. (1997) Cerebrospinal fluid and plasma π-endorphin in combat veterans with post-traumatic stress disorder. *Psychoneuroendocrinology* 22, 517–529.

Bale TL, Contarino A, Smith GW et al. (2000) Mice deficient for corticotrophin-releasing hormone receptor-2 display anxiety-like behavior and are hypersensitive to stress. *Nat Genet* 24, 410–414.

Bale TL, Picetti R, Contarino A et al. (2002) Mice deficient for both corticotrophin-releasing factor receptor 1 (CRFR1) and CRFR2 have an impaired stress response and display sexually dichotomous anxiety-like behavior. *J Neurosci* 22, 193–199.

Bansal V, Ryu SY, Lopez N et al. (2012) Vagal stimulation modulates inflammation through a ghrelin mediated mechanism in traumatic brain injury. *Inflammation* 35, 214–220.

Barrera G, Hernandez A, Poulin JF et al. (2006) Galanin-mediated anxiolytic effect in rat central amygdala is not a result of corelease from noradrenergic terminals. *Synapse* 59, 27–40.

Barros VG, Rodriguez P, Martijena ID et al. (2006) Prenatal stress and early adoption effects on benzodiazepine receptors and anxiogenic behavior in the adult rat brain. *Synapse* 60, 609–618.

Bastaki SM, Hasan MY, Chandranath, S.I., Schmassmann, A.,Garner, A. (2003a). PD -136,450: a CCK2 (gastrin) receptor antagonist with antisecretory, anxiolytic and antiulcer activity. *Mol. Cell Biochem.* 252:83–90. (2003)

Bastaki, S.M., Hasan, M.Y., Chandranath, S.I., Schmassmann, A., Garner, A. (2003b). PD -136,450: a CCK2 (gastrin) receptor antagonist with antisecretory, anxiolytic and antiulcer activity. Mol. Cell Biochem. 252:83–90. *Molecular & Cellular Biology* 252, 83–90.

Bastien J, Rochette-Egly C (2004) Nuclear retinoid receptors and the transcription of retinoid-target genes. *Gene* 328, 1–16.

Bauer EP, Schafe GE, LeDoux JE (2002) NMDA receptors and L-type voltage-gated calcium channels contribute to long-term potentiation and different components of fear memory formation in the lateral amygdala. *J Neurosci* 22, 5239–5249.

Baulieu EE, Robel P (1998) Dehydroepiandrosterone (DHEA) and dehydroepiandrosterone sulfate (DHEAS) as neuroactive neurosteroids. *Proc Natl Acad Sci USA* 95, 4089–4091.

Benyassi A, Gavalda A, Armario A et al. (1993) Role of somatostatin in the acute immobilization stress-induced GH decrease in rat. *Life Sci* 52, 361–370.

Berigan T (2002) Treatment of posttraumatic stress disorder with tiagabine [letter]. *Can J Psychiat* 47, 788.

Bernik TR, Friedman SG, Ochani M et al. (2002) Pharmacological stimulation of the cholinergic antiinflammatory pathway. *The Journal of experimental medicine* 195, 781–788.

Bertoglio, L.J., de Bortoli, V.C., Zangrossi, H. Jr., (2007) Cholecystokinin-2 receptors modulate freezing and escape behaviors evoked by the electrical stimulation of the rat dorsolateral periaqueductal gray. *Brain Res* 1156, 133–138.

Bertoglio, L.J., Zangrossi Jr., H. (2005) Involvement of dorsolateral periaqueductal gray cholecystokinin-2 receptors in the regulation of a panic-related behavior in rats. *Brain Res* 1059, 46–51.

Bielsky IF, Hu SB, Ren, X., Terwilliger, E.F., Young, L.J. (2005) The V1a vasopressin receptor is necessary and sufficient for normal social recognition: a gene replacement study. Neuron. 47:503–13. (2005) The V1a vasopressin receptor is necessary and sufficient for normal social recognition: a gene replacement study. *Neuron* 47, 503–513.

Bills LJ, Kreisler K (1993) Treatment of flashbacks with naltrexone. *Am J Psychiatry* 150, 1430.

Binder EB, Bradley RG, Liu W et al. (2008) Association of FKBP5 polymorphisms and childhood abuse with risk of posttraumatic stress disorder symptoms in adults. *JAMA* 299, 1291-305.

Bing O, Moller C, Engel, J.A., Soderpal, B., and Heilig, M. (1993) Anxiolytic-like action of centrally administered galanin. *Neurosci. Lett.* 164:17–20. (1993)

Bing, O., Moller, C., Engel, J.A., Soderpal, B., and Heilig, M. (1993) Anxiolytic-like action of centrally administered galanin. Neurosci. Lett. 164:17–20. *Neurosci Lett* 164, 17–20.

Blanchard EB, Kolb LC, Gerardi RJ et al. (1986) Cardiac response to relevant stimuli as an adjunctive tool for diagnosing post-traumatic stress disorder in Vietnam veterans. *Behav Ther* 17, 592–606.

Blanchard EB, Kolb LC, Pallmeyer TP et al. (1982) A psychophysiological study of post-traumatic stress disorder in Vietnam veterans. *Psychiatr Q* 54, 220–229.

Blanchard EB, Kolb LC, Prins A et al. (1991) Changes in plasma norepinephrine to combat-related stimuli among Vietnam veterans with posttraumatic stress disorder. *J Nerv Ment Dis* 179, 371–373.

Bonne O, Gill JM, Luckenbaugh DA et al. (2011) Corticotropin-releasing factor, interleukin-6, brain-derived neurotrophic factor, insulin-like growth factor-1, and substance P in the cerebrospinal fluid of civilians with posttraumatic stress disorder before and after treatment with paroxetine. *J Clin Psychiatry* 72, 1124–1128.

Borovikova LV, Ivanova S, Zhang M et al. (2000) Vagus nerve stimulation attenuates the systemic inflammatory response to endotoxin. *JNature* 405, 458–462.

Bouthillier A, De Montigny C (1988) Long-term benzodiazepine treatment reduces neuronal responsiveness to cholecystokinin: an electrophysiological study in the rat. *Eur J Pharmacol* 151, 135–138.

Brannon N, Labbate L, Huber M (2000) Gabapentin treatment for posttraumatic stress disorder. *Can J Psychiat* 45, 84.

Braun P, Greenberg D, Dasberg H et al. (1990) Core symptoms of posttraumatic stress disorder unimproved by alprazolam treatment. *J Clin Psychiatry* 51, 236–238.

Bremner JD (2003) Functional neuroanatomical correlates of traumatic stress revisited 7 years later, this time with data. *Psychopharmacol Bull* 37, 6–25.

Bremner JD (2005) The neurobiology of childhood sexual abuse in women with posttraumatic stress disorder. In: Kendall-Tackett KA (ed.) *Handbook of Women, Stress and Trauma*. Brunner-Routledge, New York, pp. 181–206.

Bremner JD (2007) Functional neuroimaging in posttraumatic stress disorder. *Expert Reviews in Neurotherapeutics* 7, 393–405.

Bremner JD (2011) Stress and human neuroimaging studies. In: Conrad CD (ed.) *The Handbook of Stress: Neuropsychological Effects on the Brain*. Wiley-Blackwell.

Bremner JD, Charney DS (2010) Neural circuits in fear and anxiety. In: Stein DJ, Hollander E, Rothbaum BO (eds) *Textbook of Anxiety Disorders*. 2 edn. American Psychiatric Publishing, Arlington, VA, pp. 55–71.

Bremner JD, Elzinga B, Schmahl C et al. (2008) Structural and functional plasticity of the human brain in posttraumatic stress disorder. *Prog Brain Res* 167, 171–186.

Bremner JD, Fani N, Ashraf A et al. (2005a) Functional brain imaging alterations in acne patients treated with isotretinoin. *Am J Psychiatry* 162, 983–991.

Bremner JD, Innis RB, Ng CK et al. (1997a) PET measurement of cerebral metabolic correlates of yohimbine administration in posttraumatic stress disorder. *Arch Gen Psychiatry* 54, 246–256.

Bremner JD, Innis RB, Southwick SM et al. (2000) Decreased benzodiazepine receptor binding in frontal cortex in combat-related posttraumatic stress disorder. *Am J Psychiatry* 157, 1120–1126.

Bremner JD, Krystal JH, Southwick SM et al. (1996a) Noradrenergic mechanisms in stress and anxiety: I. *Preclinical studies. Synapse* 23, 28–38.

Bremner JD, Krystal JH, Southwick SM et al. (1996b) Noradrenergic mechanisms in stress and anxiety: II. *Clinical studies. Synapse* 23, 39–51.

Bremner JD, Licinio J, Darnell A et al. (1997b) Elevated CSF corticotropin-releasing factor concentrations in posttraumatic stress disorder. *Am J Psychiatry* 154, 624–629.

Bremner JD, McCaffery P (2008) The neurobiology of retinoic acid in affective disorders. *Prog Neuropsychopharmacol Biol Psychiatry* 32, 315–331.

Bremner JD, Mletzko T, Welter S et al. (2005b) Effects of phenytoin on memory, cognition and brain structure in posttraumatic stress disorder: A pilot study. *J Psychopharmacol* 19, 159–165.

Bremner JD, Mletzko T, Welter S et al. (2004a) Treatment of posttraumatic stress disorder with phenytoin: An open label pilot study. *J Clin Psychiatry* 65, 1559–1564.

Bremner JD, Shearer KD, McCaffery PJ (2012) Retinoic acid and affective disorders: the evidence for an association. *J Clin Psychiatry* 73, 37–50.

Bremner JD, Southwick SM, Darnell A et al. (1996c) Chronic PTSD in Vietnam combat veterans: Course of illness and substance abuse. *Am J Psychiatry* 153, 369–375.

Bremner JD, Vermetten E, Kelley ME (2007) Cortisol, dehydroepiandrosterone, and estradiol measured over 24 hours in women with childhood sexual abuse-related posttraumatic stress disorder. *J Nerv Ment Dis* 195, 919–927.

Bremner JD, Vythilingam M, Vermetten E et al. (2003b) Cortisol response to a cognitive stress challenge in posttraumatic stress disorder (PTSD) related to childhood abuse. *Psychoneuroendocrinology* 28, 733–750.

Bremner JD, Vythilingam M, Vermetten E et al. (2004b) Effects of dexamethasone on declarative memory function in posttraumatic stress disorder (PTSD). *Psychiatry Res* 129, 1–10.

Bremner JD, Vythilingam M, Vermetten E et al. (2003a) MRI and PET study of deficits in hippocampal structure and function in women with childhood sexual abuse and posttraumatic stress disorder. *Am J Psychiatry* 160, 924–932.

Broekman BF, Olff M, Boer F (2007) The genetic background to PTSD. *Neurosci Biobehav Rev* 31, 348–362.

Brown GL, Linnoila ML (1990) CSF metabolite (5-HIAA) studies in depression, impulsivity, and violence. *J Clin Psychiatry* 51, 31–41.

Bruchfeld A, Goldstein RS, Chavan S et al. (2010) Whole blood cytokine attenuation by cholinergic agonists ex vivo and relationship to vagus nerve activity in rheumatoid arthritis. *Journal of internal medicine* 268, 94–101.

Brunson KL, Avishai-Eliner S, Hatalski CG et al. (2001a) Neurobiology of the stress response early in life: evolution of a concept and the role of corticotropin releasing hormone. *Mol Psychiatry* 6, 647–656.

Brunson KL, Eghbal-Ahmadi M, Bender R et al. (2001b) Long-term, progressive hippocampal cell loss and dysfunction induced by early-life administration of corticotrophin-releasing hormone reproduce the effects of early-life stress. *Proc Natl Acad Sci USA* 15, 8856–8861.

Bryant RA, Felmingham KL, Falconer EM et al. (2010) Preliminary evidence of the short allele of the serotonin transporter gene predicting poor response to cognitive behavior therapy in posttraumatic stress disorder. *Biol Psychiatry* 67, 1217–1219.

Bunevicius R, Prange AJ, Jr, (2006) Psychiatric manifestations of Graves' hyperthyroidism: pathophysiology and treatment options. *CNS Drugs* 20, 897–909.

Cabib S, Ventgura R, Puglisi-Allegra S (2002) Opposite imbalances between mesocortical and mesoaccumbens dopamine responses to stress by the same genotype depending on living conditions. *Behav Brain Res* 129, 179–185.

Carlson LE, Sherwin BB, Chertkow HM (2000) Relationships between mood and estradiol (E2) levels in Alzheimer's disease (AD) patients. *J Gerontol Psychol Sci Soc Sci* 55, 47–53.

Chambers RA, Bremner JD, Moghaddam B et al. (1999) Glutamate and posttraumatic stress disorder: Toward a psychobiology of dissociation. *Semin Clin Neuropsychiatry* 4, 274–281.

Chambon P (1996) A decade of molecular biology of retinoic acid receptors. *Faseb Journal* 10, 940–954.

Charney DS, Bremner JD (1999) The neurobiology of anxiety disorders. In: Charney DS, Nestler EJ, Bunney SS (eds) *Neurobiology of Mental Illness*. Oxford University Press, Oxford, UK, pp. 494–517.

Charney DS, Nagy LM, Bremner JD et al. (2000) Neurobiological mechanisms of human anxiety. In: Fogel BS, Schiffler RB, Rao SM (eds) *Synopsis of Neuropsychiatry*. Lippincott Williams & Wilkins, Baltimore, MD, pp. 273–288.

Chen X-N, Meng Q-Y, Bao A-M et al. (2009) The involvement of retinoic acid receptor-alpha in corticotropin-releasing hormone gene expression and affective disorders. *Biol Psychiatry* 66, 832–839.

Chiang MY, Misner D, Kempermann G et al. (1998) An essential role for retinoid receptors RAR beta and RXR gamma in long- term potentiation and depression. *Neuron* 21, 1353–1361.

Chuang JC, Perello M, Sakata I et al. (2011) Ghrelin mediates stress-induced food-reward behavior in mice. *J Clin Invest* 121, 2684–2692.

Cicchetti D, Rogosch FA (2001) The impact of child maltreatment and psychopathology on neuroendocrine functioning. *Dev Psychopathol* 13, 783–804.

Cocco S, Diaz G, Stancampiano R et al. (2002) Vitamin A deficiency produces spatial learning and memory impairment in rats. *Neuroscience* 115, 475–582.

Cohen H, Kaplan Z, Kotler M (1999) CCK-antagonists in a rat exposed to acute stress: implication for anxiety associated with post-traumatic stress disorder. *Depress Anxiety* 10, 8–17.

Colbert MC, Linney E, LaMantia AS (1993) Local sources of retinoic acid coincide with retinoid-mediated transgene activity during embryonic development. *Proc Natl Acad Sci USA* 90, 6572–6576.

Comings DE, Muhleman D, Gysin R (1996) Dopamine D2 receptor (DRD2) gene and susceptibility to posttraumatic stress disorder: a study and replication. *Biol Psychiatry* 40, 368–372.

Coplan JD, Andrews MW, Rosenblum LA et al. (1996) Persistent elevations of cerebrospinal fluid concentrations of corticotropin-releasing factor in adult nonhuman primates exposed to early-life stressors: Implications for the pathophysiology of mood and anxiety disorders. *Proc Natl Acad Sci USA* 93, 1619–1623.

Corcoran C, Connor T, O'keane V et al. (2004) The effects of vagus nerve stimulation on pro-and anti-inflammatory cytokines in humans: a preliminary report. *Neuroimmunomodulation* 12, 307–309.

Crandall J, Sakai Y, Zhang J et al. (2004) 13-cis-retinoic acid suppresses hippocampal cell division and hippocampal-dependent learning in mice. *Proc Natl Acad Sci USA* 101, 5111–5116.

Czeh B, Michaelis T, Watanabe T et al. (2001) Stress-induced changes in cerebral metabolites, hippocampal volume, and cell proliferation are prevented by antidepressant treatment with tianeptine. *Proc Natl Acad Sci USA* 98, 12796–12801.

D'Sa C, Duman RS (2002) Antidepressants and neuroplasticity. *Bipolar Disorder* 4, 183–194.

Das UN (2007) Vagus nerve stimulation, depression, and inflammation. *Neuropsychopharmacology* 32, 2053–2054.

Davidson J, Lipper S, Kilts CD et al. (1985) Platelet MAO activity in posttraumatic stress disorder. *Am J Psychiatry* 142, 1341–1343.

Davis LL, Suris A, Lambert MT et al. (1997) Posttraumatic stress disorder and serotonin: new directions for research and treatment. *J Psychiatry Neurosci* 22, 318–326.

Davis M (1992) The role of the amygdala in fear and anxiety. *Annu Rev Neurosci* 15, 353–375.

Davis M, Myers KM, Chhatwal JP et al. (2006) Pharmacological treatments that facilitate extinction of fear: relevance to psychotherapy. *NeuroRx: The Journal of the American Society for Experimental NeuroTherapeutics* 3, 82–96.

De Bellis MD, Baum AS, Keshavan MS et al. (1999) A.E. Bennett Research Award: Developmental traumatology: Part I: Biological stress systems. *Biol Psychiatry* 45, 1259–1270.

De Bellis MD, Chrousos GP, Dorn LD et al. (1994a) Hypothalamic pituitary adrenal dysregulation in sexually abused girls. *J Clin Endocrinol Metab* 78, 249–255.

De Bellis MD, Lefter L, Trickett PK et al. (1994b) Urinary catecholamine excretion in sexually abused girls. *J Am Acad Child Adolesc Psychiatry* 33, 320–327.

De Cuyper H (1987) (Auto)aggression and serotonin: a review of human data. *Acta Psychiatr Belg* 87, 325–331.

De Herdt V, Bogaert S, Bracke KR et al. (2009) Effects of vagus nerve stimulation on pro-and anti-inflammatory cytokine induction in patients with refractory epilepsy. *J Neuroimmunol* 214, 104–108.

de Kloet C, Vermetten E, Lentjes E et al. (2008a) Differences in the response to the combined DEX-CRH test between PTSD patients with and without co-morbid depressive disorder. *Psychoneuroendocrinology* 33, 313–320.

de Kloet CS, Vermetten E, Bikker A et al. (2007a) Leukocyte glucocorticoid receptor expression and immunoregulation in veterans with and without post-traumatic stress disorder. *Mol Psychiatry* 12, 443–453.

de Kloet CS, Vermetten E, Geuze E et al. (2008b) Elevated plasma corticotrophin-releasing hormone levels in veterans with posttraumatic stress disorder. *Prog Brain Res* 167, 287–291.

de Kloet CS, Vermetten E, Heijnen CJ et al. (2007b) Enhanced cortisol suppression in response to dexamethasone administration in traumatized veterans with and without posttraumatic stress disorder. *Psychoneuroendocrinology* 32, 215–226.

de Kloet ER, Oitzl MS, Joels M (1999) Stress and cognition: are corticosteroids good or bad guys? *Trends Neurosci* 22, 422–426.

Delahanty DL, Bogart LM, Figler JL (2004) Posttraumatic stress disorder symptoms, salivary cortisol, medication adherence, and CD4 levels in HIV-positive individuals. *AIDS Care* 16, 247–260.

Delahanty DL, Raimonde AJ, Spoonster E et al. (2003) Injury severity, prior trauma history, urinary cortisol levels, and acute PTSD in motor vehicle accident victims. *J Anxiety Disord* 17, 149–164.

Deutch AY, Bean AJ, Bissette G et al. (1987) Stress-induced alterations in neurotensin, somatostatin and corticotropin-releasing factor in mesotelencephalic dopamine system regions. *Brain Res* 417, 350–354.

Deutch AY, Roth RH (1990) The determinants of stress-induced activation of the prefrontal cortical dopamine system. *Prog Brain Res* 85, 367–402.

Deutch AY, Tam SY, Roth RH (1985) Footshock and conditioned stress increase 3,4-dihydroxyphenylacetic acid (DOPAC) in the ventral tegmental area but not substantia nigra. *Brain Res* 333, 143–146.

Dhabhar FS (2014) Effects of stress on immune function: the good, the bad, and the beautiful. *Immunol Res* 58, 193–210.

Diamond DM, Fleshner M, Ingersoll N et al. (1996) Psychological stress impairs spatial working memory: Relevance to electrophysiological studies of hippocampal function. *Behav Neurosci* 110, 661–672.

Dinan TG (1996) Serotonin and the regulation of hypothalamic pituitary-adrenal axis function. *Life Sci* 58, 1683–1694.

Dinan TG, Barry S, Yatham LN et al. (1990) A pilot study of a neuroendocrine test battery in posttraumatic stress disorder. *Biol Psychiatry* 28, 665–672.

Dobson H, Tebble JE, Phogat JB et al. (1999) Effect of transport on pulsatile and surge secretion of LH in ewes in the breeding season. *J Reprod Fertil* 116, 1–8.

Donnerer J, Amann R, Skofitsch G LFSP et al. (1991) Substance P afferents regulate ACTH-corticosterone release. *Ann NY Acad Sci* 632, 296–303.

Dorow R, Horowski R, Paschelke G et al. (1983) Severe anxiety induced by FG7142, a -carboline ligand for benzodiazepine receptors. *The Lancet*.

Drake RG, Davis LL, Cates ME et al. (2003) Baclofen treatment for chronic posttraumatic stress disorder. *Annals of Pharmacotherapy* 37, 1177–1181.

Drugan RC, Basile AC, Crawley JN et al. (1986) Inescapable shock reduces [3H]Ro 5–4864 binding to peripheral type benzodiazepine receptors in the rat. *Pharmacol Biochem Behav* 24, 1673–1677.

Drugan RC, Crawley JN, Paul SM et al. (1987) Buspirone attenuates learned helplessness behavior in rats. *Drug Develop Res* 10, 63–67.

Drugan RC, Morrow AL, Weizman R et al. (1989) Stress-induced behavioral depression in the rat is associated with a decrease in GABA receptor-mediated chloride ion flux and brain benzodiazepine receptor occupancy. *Brain Res* 487, 45–51.

Duman RS (2004) Depression: a case of neuronal life and death? *Biol Psychiatry* 56, 140–145.

Duman RS, Heninger GR, Nestler EJ (1997) A molecular and cellular theory of depression. *Arch Gen Psychiatry* 54, 597–606.

Duman RS, Malberg JE, Nakagawa S (2001) Regulation of adult neurogenesis by psychotropic drugs and stress. *J Pharmacol Exp Ther* 299, 401–407.

Egashira N, Tanoue A, Matsuda T et al. (2007) Impaired social interaction and reduced anxiety-related behavior in vasopressin V1a receptor knockout mice. *Behav Brain Res* 178, 123–127.

Elzinga BM, Bremner JD (2002) Are the neural substrates of memory the final common pathway in PTSD? *J Affect Disord* 70, 1–17.

Elzinga BM, Schmahl CS, Vermetten E et al. (2003) Higher cortisol levels following exposure to traumatic reminders in abuse-related PTSD. *Neuropsychopharmacology* 28, 1656–1665.

Eraly SA, Nievergelt CM, Maihofer AX et al. (2014) Assessment of plasma C-reactive protein as a biomarker of posttraumatic stress disorder risk. *JAMA Psychiatry* 71, 423–431.

Fanselow MS (1986) Conditioned fear-induced opiate analgesia: a competing motivational state theory of stress analgesia. *Ann NY Acad Sci* 467, 40–54.

Farooqui SM (1994) Induction of adenylate cyclase sensitive dopamine D2 receptors in retinoic acid induced differentiated human neuroblastoma SHSY-5Y cells. *Life Sci* 55, 1887–1893.

Fehder WP, Sachs J, UM, Douglas SD (1997) Substance P as an immune modulator of anxiety. *Neuroimmunomodulation* 4, 42–48.

Ferguson SA, Berry KJ (2007) Oral accutane (13-cis-retinoic acid) has no effects on spatial learning and memory in male and femal Sprague-Dawley rats. *Neurotoxicol Teratol* 29, 219–227.

Ferguson SA, Cisneros FJ, Goug BJ et al. (2005a) Four weeks of oral isotretinoin treatment causes few signs of general toxicity in male and female Sprague-Dawley rats. *Food Chem Toxicol* 43, 1289–1296.

Ferguson SA, Cisneros FJ, Gough B et al. (2005b) Chronic oral treatment with 13-cis-retinoic acid (isotretinoin) or all - trans - retinoic acid does not alter depression-like behaviors in rats. *Toxicol Sci* 87, 451–459.

Fichtner CG, Arora RC, O'Connor FL et al. (1994) Platelet paroxetine binding and fluoxetine pharmacotherapy in posttraumatic stress disorder: Preliminary observations on a possible predictor of clinical treatment response. *Life Sci* 54, 39–44.

Fichtner CG, O'Connor FL, Yeoh HC et al. (1995) Hypodensity of platelet serotonin uptake sites in posttraumatic stress disorder: Associated clinical features. *Life Sci* 57, 37–44.

Finlay JM, Zigmond MJ, Abercrombie ED (1995) Increased dopamine and norepinephrine release in medial prefrontal cortex induced by acute and chronic stress: effects of diazepam. *Neuroscience* 64, 619–628.

Foote SL, Bloom FE, Aston-Jones G (1983) Nucleus locus coeruleus: new evidence of anatomical and physiological specificity. *Physiol Behav* 63, 844–914.

Francis DD, Young LJ, Meaney MJ et al. (2002) Naturally occurring differences in maternal care are associated with the expression of oxytocin and vasopression (V1a) receptors: gender differences. *J Neuroendocrinol* 14, 349–353.

Fujita M, Southwick SM, Denucci CC et al. (2004) Central type benzodiazepine receptors in Gulf War veterans with posttraumatic stress disorder. *Biol Psychiatry* 56, 95–100.

Fuller GB, Hobson WC, Reyes FI et al. (1984) Influence of restraint and ketamine anesthesia on adrenal steroids, progesterone, and gonadotropins in rhesus monkeys. *Proc Soc Exp Biol Med* 175, 487–490.

Garakani A, Murrough J, Mathew SJ et al. (2011) The neurobiology of anxiety disorders. In: Charney DS, Nestler EJ (eds) *Neurobiology of Mental Illness*.

Garcia R (2002) Stress, metaplasticity, and antidepressants. *Current Mol Med* 2, 629–638.

Gavish M, Laor N, Bidder M et al. (1996) Altered platelet peripheraltype benzodiazepine receptor in posttraumatic stress disorder. *Neuropsychopharmacology* 14, 181–186.

Gelernter J, Southwick S, Goodson S et al. (1999) No association between D2 dopamine receptor (DRD2) "A" system alleles, or DRD2 haplotypes, and posttraumatic stress disorder. *Biol Psychiatry* 45, 620–625.

Gelpin E, Bonne O, Peri T et al. (1996) Treatment of recent trauma survivors with benzodiazepines: a prospective study. *J Clin Psychiatry* 57, 390–394.

Geracioti TD, Jr.,, Carpenter LL, Owens MJ et al. (2006) Elevated cerebrospinal fluid substance p concentrations in posttraumatic stress disorder and major depression. *Am J Psychiatry* 163, 637–643.

Geracioti TDJ, Baker DG, Ekhator NN et al. (2001) CSF norepinephrine concentrations in posttraumatic stress disorder. *Am J Psychiatry* 158, 1227–1230.

Geracioti TDJ, Jefferson-Wilson L, Strawn JR et al. (2013) Effect of traumatic imagery on cerebrospinal fluid dopamine and serotonin metabolites in posttraumatic stress disorder. *J Psychiatr Res* 47, 995–998.

Gibbs DM (1986) Stress-specific modulation of ACTH secretion by oxytocin. *Neuroendocrinology* 42, 456–458.

Gill JM, Saligan L, Woods S et al. (2009) PTSD is associated with an excess of inflammatory immune activities. *Perspect Psychiatr Care* 45, 262–277.

Glover H (1993) A preliminary trial of nalmefene for the treatment of emotional numbing in combat veterans with post-traumatic stress disorder. *Israel J Psychiatry Rel Sci* 30, 255–263.

Goenjian AK, Yehuda R, Pynoos RS et al. (1996) Basal cortisol, dexamethasone suppression of cortisol, and MHPG in adolescents after the 1988 earthquake in Armenia. *Am J Psychiatry* 153, 929–934.

Goldman PR, Vogel WH (1985) Plasma estradiol and prolactin levels and their response to stress in two strains of rat with different sensitivities to 7,12-dimethylbenz[a]anthracene -induced tumors. *Cancer Lett* 25, 277–282.

Goncharov NP, Taranov AG, Antonichev AV et al. (1979) Effect of stress on the profile of plasma steroids in baboons (Papio hamadryas). *Acta Endocrinol* 90, 372–384.

Goodman AB (1995) Chromosomal locations and modes of action of genes in the retinoid (vitamin A) system support their involvement in the etiology of schizophrenia. *Am J Med Genet* 60, 335–348.

Goodman AB (1998) Three independent lines of evidence suggest retinoids as causal to schizophrenia. *Proc Natl Acad Sci USA* 95, 7240–7244.

Gottsch ML, Zeng H, Hohmann JG et al. (2005) Phenotypic analysis of mice deficient in the type 2 galanin receptor (GALR2). *Mol Cell Biol* 25, 4804–4811.

Gould E, Tanapat P, McEwen BS et al. (1998) Proliferation of granule cell precursors in the dentate gyrus of adult monkeys is diminished by stress. *Proc Natl Acad Sci USA* 95, 3168–3171.

Grabe HJ, Spitzer C, Schwahn C et al. (2009) Serotonin transporter gene (SLC6A4) promoter polymorphisms and the susceptibility to posttraumatic stress disorder in the general population. *Am J Psychiatry* 166, 926–933.

Graeff FG (1993) Role of 5-HT in defensive behavior and anxiety. *Reviews in Neuroscience* 4, 181–211.

Grau JW, Hyson RL, Maier SF et al. (1981) Long-term stress-induced analgesia and activation of the opiate system. *Science* 213, 1409–1411.

Gudelsky GA, Berry SA, H.Y. M (1989) Neurotensin activates tuberoinfundibular dopamine neurons and increases serum corticosterone concentrations in the rat. *Neuroendocrinology* 49, 604–609.

Gunnar MR, Morison SJ, Chisolm K et al. (2001) Salivary cortisol levels in children adopted from Romanian orphanages. *Dev Psychopathol* 13, 611–628.

Gustafson EL, Smith KE, Durkin MM et al. (1996) Distribution of a rat galanin receptor mRNA in rat brain. *Neuroreport* 7, 953–957.

Hamner M, Gold P (1998) Plasma dopamine beta-hydroxylase activity in psychotic and non-psychotic post-traumatic stress disorder. *Psychiatry Res* 77, 175–181.

Hamner MB, Diamond BI (1993) Elevated plasma dopamine in posttraumatic stress disorder: a preliminary report. Biol. Psychiatry 33:304–306. *Biol Psychiatry* 33, 304–306.

Hamner MB, Hitri A (1992) Plasma beta-endorphin levels in posttraumatic stress disorder: a preliminary report on response to exercise-induced stress. *J Neuropsychiatry Clin Neurosci* 4, 59–63.

Hart J, Gunnar M, Cicchetti D (1996) Altered neuroendocrine activity in maltreated children related to symptoms of depression. *Dev Psychopathol* 8, 201–214.

Havoundjian H, Paul SM, Skolnick P (1986) Rapid, stress-induced modification of the benzodiazepine receptor-coupled chloride ionophore. *Brain Res* 375, 401–406.

Heilig M, McLeod S, Brot M et al. (1993) Anxiolytic-like action of neuropeptide Y: mediation by Y1 receptors in amygdala, and dissociation from food intake effects. *Neuropsychopharmacology* 8, 357–363.

Heim C, Newport DJ, Bonsall R et al. (2001) Altered pituitary-adrenal axis responses to provocative challenge tests in adult survivors of childhood abuse. *Am J Psychiatry* 158, 575–581.

Heim C, Newport DJ, Heit S et al. (2000) Pituitary-adrenal and autonomic responses to stress in women after sexual and physical abuse in childhood. *JAMA* 284, 592–597.

Heinsbroek RPW, Van Haaven F, Fecustra MGP et al. (1991) Controllable and uncontrollable footshock and monoaminergic activity in the frontal cortex of male and female rats. *Brain Res* 551, 247–255.

Henn FA, Vollmayr B (2004) Neurogenesis and depression: etiology or epiphenomenon? *Biol Psychiatry* 56, 146–150.

Heresco-Levy U, Kremer I, Javitt DC et al. (2002) Pilot-controlled trial of D-cycloserine for the treatment of post-traumatic stress disorder. *Int J Neuropsychopharmacol* 5, 301–307.

Hertting A, Theorell T (2002) Physiological changes associated with downsizing of personnel and reorganisation in the health care sector. *Psychother Psychosom* 71, 117–122.

Hodgson RA, Higgins GA, Guthrie DH et al. (2007) Comparison of the V1b antagonist, SSR149415, and the CRF1 antagonist, CP-154,526, in rodent models of anxiety and depression. *Pharmacol Biochem Behav* 86, 431–440.

Hoffman L, Watsgon PD, Wilson G et al. (1989) Low plasma endorphin in posttraumatic stress disorder. *Aus NZ J Psychiatry* 23, 268–273.

Holmes A, Kinney JW, Wrenn CC et al. (2003a) Galanin GAL-R1 receptor null mutant mice display increased anxiety-like behavior specific to the elevated plus-maze. *Neuropsychopharmacology* 28, 1031–1044.

Holmes A, Murphy DL, Crawley JN (2003b) Abnormal behavioral phenotypes of serotonin transporter knockout mice: Parallels with human anxiety and depression. *Biol Psychiatry* 54, 953–959.

Holmes A, Yang RJ, Murphy DL et al. (2002) Evaluation of antidepressant-related behavioral responses to mice lacking the serotonin transporter. *Neuropsychopharmacology* 27, 914–923.

Idres N, Marill J, Flexor MA et al. (2002) Activation of retinoic acid receptor-dependent transcription by all-trans-retinoic acid metabolites and isomers. *J Biol Chem* 277, 31491–31498.

Inoue T, Tsuchiya K, Koyama T (1994) Regional changes in dopamine and serotonin activation with various intensity of physical and psychological stress in the rat brain. *Pharmacol Biochem Behav* 49, 911–920.

Jedema HP, Finlay JM, Sved AF et al. (2001) Chronic cold exposure potentiates CRH-evoked increases in electrophysiologic activity of locus coeruleus neurons. *Biol Psychiatry* 49, 351–359.

Jessop DS, Renshaw D LP, Chowdrey HS et al. (2000) Substance P is involved in terminating the hypothalamopituitary-adrenal axis response to acute stress through centrally located neurokinin-1 receptors. *Stress* 3, 209–220.

Kaehler ST, Singewald N, Sinner C et al. (2000) Conditioned fear and inescapable shock modify the release of serotonin in the locus coeruleus. *Brain Res* 859, 249–254.

Kalivas PW, Abhold R (1987) Enkephalin release in to the ventral tegmental area in response to stress: modulation of mesocortical dopamine. *Biol Psychiatry* 339–348.

Kalivas PW, Duffy P (1989) Similar effects of daily cocaine and stress on mesocorticolimbic dopamine neurotransmission in the rat. *Biol Psychiatry* 25, 913–928.

Kalivas PW, Jennes L, Nemeroff CB et al. (1982) Neurotensin: topographical distribution of brain sites involved in hypothermia and antinociception. *J Comp Neurol* 210, 225–238.

Kam KY, Park Y, Cheon M et al. (2000) Effects of immobilization stress on estrogen-induced surges of luteinizing hormone and prolactin in ovariectomized rats. *Endocrine* 12, 279–287.

Kam KY, Park YB, Cheon MS et al. (2002) Influence of GnRH agonist and neural antagonists on stress-blockade of LH and prolactin surges induced by 17beta-estradiol in ovariectomized rats. *Yonsei Med J* 43, 482–490.

Kaminska M, Harris J, Gijsbers K et al. (2000) Dehydroepiandrosterone sulfate (DHEAS) counteracts decremental effects of corticosterone on dentate gyrus LTP: implications for depression. *Brain Res Bull* 52, 229–234.

Kanter ED, Wilkinson CW, Radant AD et al. (2001) Glucocorticoid feedback sensitivity and adrenocortical responsiveness in posttraumatic stress disorder. *Biol Psychiatry* 50, 238–245.

Karlsson RM, Holmes A (2006) Galanin as a modulator of anxiety and depression and a therapeutic target for affective disease. *Amino Acids* 31, 231–239.

Karlsson RM, Holmes A, Heilig M et al. (2005) Anxiolytic-like actions of centrally-administered neuropeptide Y, but not galanin, in C57BL/6J mice. *Pharmacol Biochem Behav* 80, 427–436.

Kasckow JW, Parkes DG, Owens MJ et al. (1994) The BE (2)-M17 neuroblastoma cell line synthesizes and secretes corticotropin-releasing factor. *Brain Res* 654, 159–162.

Katz RJ, Roth KA, Carroll BJ (1981) Acute and chronic stress effects on open field activity in the rat: Implications for a model of depression. *Neurosci Biobehav Rev* 5, 247–251.

Kellner M, Wiedemann K, Yassouridis A et al. (2000) Behavioral and endocrine response to cholecystokinin tetrapeptide in patients with posttraumatic stress disorder. *Biol Psychiatry* 47, 107–111.

Kenna GA, Roder-Hanna N, Leggio L et al. (2012) Association of the 5-HTT gene-linked promoter region (5-HTTLPR) polymorphism with psychiatric disorders: review of psychopathology and pharmacotherapy. *Pharmacogenomics Personalized Med* 5, 19–35.

Khoshbouei H, Cecchi M, Dove S et al. (2002a) Behavioral reactivity to stress: Amplification of stress-induced noradrenergic activation elicits a galanin-mediated anxiolytic effect in central amygdala. *Pharmacol Biochem Behav* 71, 407–417.

Khoshbouei H, Cecchi M, Morilak, D.A. (2002) Modulatory effects of galanin in the lateral bed nucleus of the stria terminalis on behavioral and neuroendocrine responses to acute stress. *Neuropsychopharmacology* 27, 25–34.

Kimonides VG, Khatibi NH, Svendsen CN et al. (1998) Dehydroepiandrosterone (DHEA) and DHEA-sulfate (DHEAS) protect hippocampal neurons against excitatory amino acid-induced neurotoxicity. *Proc Natl Acad Sci USA* 95, 1852–1857.

Kinney JW, Starosta G, Holmes A et al. (2002) Deficits in trace cued fear conditioning in galanin-treated rats and galanin-overexpressing transgenic mice. *Learn Mem* 9, 178–190.

Klemenhagen KC, Gordon JA, David DJ et al. (2006) Increased fear response to contextual cues in mice lacking the 5-HT1A receptor. *Neuropsychopharmacology* 31, 101–111.

Koenen KC, Amstadter AB, Nugent NR (2009) Gene-environment interaction in posttraumatic stress disorder: an update. *J Trauma Stress* 22, 416–426.

Kosten TR, Wahby V, Giller EJ et al. (1990) The dexamethasone suppression test and thyrotropin-releasing hormone stimulation test in posttraumatic stress disorder. *Biol Psychiatry* 28, 657–664.

Krahl SE, Clark KB, Smith DC et al. (1998) Locus coeruleus lesions suppress the seizure-attenuating effects of vagus nerve stimulation. *Epilepsia* 39, 709–714.

Krezel W, Ghyselinck N, Samad TA et al. (1998) Impaired locomotion and dopamine signaling in retinoid receptor mutant mice. *Science* 279, 863–867.

Krezel W, Kastner P, Chambon P (1999) Differential expression of retinoid receptors in the adult mouse central nervous system. *Neuroscience* 89, 1291–1300.

Krisch B (1981) Somatostatin-immunoreactive fiber projections into the brain stem and the spinal cord of the rat. *Cell Tissue Res* 217, 531–552.

Krystal JH, Karper LP, Seibyl JP et al. (1994) Subanesthetic effects of the non-competitive NMDA antagonist, ketamine, in humans: Psychotomimetic, perceptual, cognitive, and neuroendocrine responses. *Arch Gen Psychiatry* 51, 199–214.

Kuteeva E, Wardi T, Hokfelt T et al. (2007) Galanin enhances and a galanin antagonist attenuates depression-like behaviour in the rat. *Neuropsychopharmacology* 17, 64–69.

Kuzelova H, Ptacek R, Macek M (2010) The serotonin transporter gene (5-HTT) variant and psychiatric disorders: review of current literature. *Neuro Endocrinol Lett* 31, 4–10.

Lähdesmäki J, Sallinen J, MacDonald E et al. (2004) Alpha2A-adrenoceptors are important modulators of the effects of D-amphetamine on startle reactivity and brain monoamines. *Neuropsychopharmacology* 29, 1282–1293.

Lahdesmaki J, Sallinen J, MacDonald, E., Kobilka, B.K., Fagerholm, V., Scheinin, M. (2002) Behavioral and neurochemical characterization of alpha(2A)-adrenergic receptor knockout mice. *Neuroscience* 113, 289–299.

LaMantia AS (1999) Forebrain induction, retinoic acid, and vulnerability to schizophrenia: insights from molecular and genetic analysis in developing mice. *Biol Psychiatry* 46, 19–30.

Lane MA, Bailey SJ (2005) Role of retinoid signalling in the adult brain. *Prog Neurobiol* 75, 275–293.

Lee H, Kim JW, Yim SV et al. (2001) Fluoxetine enhances cell proliferation and prevents apoptosis in dentate gyrus of maternally separated rats. *Mol Psychiatry* 6, 725–728.

Lee HJ, Lee MS, Kang RH et al. (2005) Influence of the serotonin transporter promoter gene polymorphism on susceptibility to posttraumatic stress disorder. *Depress Anxiety* 21, 135–139.

Lemieux AM, Coe CL (1995) Abuse-related posttraumatic stress disorder: Evidence for chronic neuroendocrine activation in women. *Psychosom Med* 57, 105–115.

Lerer B BA, Bennett ER, Ebstein RP et al. (1990) Platelet adenylate cyclase and phospholipase C activity in posttraumatic stress disorder. *Biol Psychiatry* 27, 735–740.

Lerer B, Ebstein RP, Shestatsky M et al. (1987) Cyclic AMP transduction in posttraumatic stress disorder. *Am J Psychiatry* 144, 1324–1327.

Levine ES, Litto WJ, Jacobs BL (1990) Activity of cat locus coeruleus noradrenergic neurons during the defense reaction. *Brain Res* 531, 189–195.

Levine S, Weiner SG, Coe CL (1993) Temporal and social factors influencing behavioral and hormonal responses to separation in mother and infant squirrel monkeys. *Psychoneuroendocrinology* 4, 297–306.

Li W, Olshansky B (2011) Inflammatory cytokines and nitric oxide in heart failure and potential modulation by vagus nerve stimulation. *Heart Failure Rev* 16, 137–145.

Liberzon I, Taylor SF, Phan KL et al. (2007) Altered central micro-opioid receptor binding after psychological trauma. *Biol Psychiatry* 61, 1030–1038.

Lippa AS, Klepner CA, Yunger L et al. (1987) Relationship between benzodiazepine receptors and experimental anxiety in rats. *Pharmacol Biochem Behav* 9, 853–856.

Loh HH, Smith AP (1990) Molecular characterization of opioid receptors. *Annual Review of Pharmacol Toxicol* 30, 123–147.

Luby JL, Heffelfinger A, Mrakotsky C et al. (2003) Alterations in stress cortisol reactivity in depressed preschoolers relative to psychiatric and no-disorder comparison groups. *Arch Gen Psychiatry* 60, 1248–1255.

Lucassen PJ, Fuchs E, Czeh B (2004) Antidepressant treatment with tianeptine reduces apoptosis in the hippocampal dentate gyrus and temporal cortex. *Eur J Neurosci* 14, 161–166.

Luine V, Villages M, Martinex C et al. (1994) Repeated stress causes reversible impairments of spatial memory performance. *Brain Res* 639, 167–170.

Luo T, Wagner E, Grun F et al. (2004) Retinoic acid signaling in the brain marks formation of optic projections, maturation of the dorsal telencephalon, and function of limbic sites. *J Comp Neurol* 470, 297–316.

Maes M, Lin A, Bonaccorso S et al. (1998) Increased 24-hour urinary cortisol excretion in patients with post-traumatic stress disorder and patients with major depression, but not in patients with fibromyalgia. *Acta Psychiatr Scand* 98, 328–335.

Maes M, Lin AH, Verkerk R et al. (1999) Serotonergic and noradrenergic markers of post-traumatic stress disorder with and without major depression. *Neuropsychopharmacology* 20, 188–197.

Magarinos AM, McEwen BS, Flugge G et al. (1996) Chronic psychosocial stress causes apical dendritic atrophy of hippocampal CA3 pyramidal neurons in subordinate tree shrews. *J Neurosci* 16, 3534–3540.

Maier SF (1986) Stressor controllability and stress induced analgesia. *Ann NY Acad Sci* 467, 55–72.

Majoie H, Rijkers K, Berfelo M et al. (2011) Vagus nerve stimulation in refractory epilepsy: effects on pro-and anti-inflammatory cytokines in peripheral blood. *Neuroimmunomodulation* 18, 52–56.

Makino S, Baker RA, Smith MA et al. (2000) Differential regulation of neuropeptide Y mRNA expression in the accurate nucleus and locus coeruleus by stress and antidepressants. *J Neuroendocrinol* 12, 387–395.

Makino S, Schulkin J, Smith MA et al. (1995a) Regulation of corticotropin-releasing hormone receptor messenger-ribonucleic acid in the rat-brain and pituitary by glucocorticoids and stress. *Endocrinology* 136, 4517–4525.

Makino S, Smith MA, Gold PW (1995b) Increased expression of corticotropin-releasing hormone and vasopressin messenger-ribonucleic acid (messenger RNA) in the hypothalamic paraventricular nucleus during repeated stress-association with reduction in glucocorticoid messenger-RNA levels. *Endocrinology* 136, 3299–3309.

Malberg JE, Eisch AJ, Nestler EJ et al. (2000) Chronic antidepressant treatment increases neurogenesis in adult rat hippocampus. *J Neurosci* 20, 9104–9110.

Malloy PF, Fairbank JA, Keane TM (1983) Validation of a multimethod assessment of posttraumatic stress disorders in Vietnam veterans. *J Clin Consult Psychol* 51, 488–494.

Mann JJ, Arango V, Marzuk PM (1989) Evidence for the 5-HT hypothesis of suicide: A review of post-mortem studies. *Br J Psychiatry* 155, 7–14.

Mann JJ, Stanley M, McBride A et al. (1986) Increased serotonin-2 and beta-adrenergic receptor binding in the frontal cortices of suicide victims. *Arch Gen Psychiatry* 43, 954–959.

Martin P, Soubrie P, Puech AJ (1990) Reversal of helpless behavior by serotonin uptake blockers in rats. *Psychopharmacology* 101, 403–407.

Mason J, Southwick S, Yehuda R et al. (1994) Elevation of serum free triiodothyronine, total triiodothyronine, thyroxine-binding globulin, and total thyroxine levels in combat-related posttraumatic stress disorder. *Arch Gen Psychiatry* 51, 629–641.

Mason J, Wang S, Yehuda R et al. (2002) Marked lability of urinary free cortisol levels in sub-groups of combat veterans with posttraumatic stress disorder. *Psychosom Med* 64, 238–246.

Mason JW, Giller EL, Kosten TR (1988) Elevation of urinary norepinephrine/cortisol ratio in posttraumatic stress disorder. *J Nerv Ment Dis* 176, 498–502.

Mason JW, Giller EL, Kosten TR et al. (1986) Urinary free cortisol levels in post-traumatic stress disorder patients. *J Nerv Ment Dis* 174, 145–149.

Mason JW, Mougey EH BJ, Tolliver GA (1968) Thyroid, avoidance pb-eirt-h et al. (1968) Thyroid (plasma butanol-extractable iodine) responses to 72-hr avoidance sessions in the monkey. *Psychosom Med* 30, 682–695.

Mathew SJ, Vythilingam M, Murrough JW et al. (2011) A selective neurokinin-1 receptor antagonist in chronic PTSD: a randomized, double-blind, placebo-controlled, proof-of-concept trial. *Eur Neuropsychopharmacol* 21, 221–229.

McCaffery P, Drager UC (1994a) High levels of a retinoic acid-generating dehydrogenase in the meso-telencephalic dopamine system. *Proc Natl Acad Sci USA* 91, 7772–7776.

McCaffery P, Drager UC (1994b) Hot spots of retinoic acid synthesis in the developing spinal cord. *Proc Natl Acad Sci USA* 91, 7194–7197.

McCaffery P, Zhang J, Crandall JE (2006) Retinoic acid signaling and function in the adult hippocampus. *J Neurobiol* 66, 780–791.

McEwen BS, Angulo J, Cameron H et al. (1992) Paradoxical effects of adrenal steroids on the brain: Protection versus degeneration. *Biol Psychiatry* 31, 177–199.

McEwen BS, Chattarji S (2004) Molecular mechanisms of neuroplasticity and pharmacological implications: the example of tianeptine. *Eur Neuropsychopharmacol* 14 Suppl 5, S497–502.

McFall ME, Murburg MM, Ko GN et al. (1990) Autonomic responses to stress in Vietnam combat veterans with posttraumatic stress disorder. *Biol Psychiatry* 27, 1165–1175.

McFall ME, Veith RC, Murburg MM (1992) Basal sympathoadrenal function in posttraumatic stress disorder. *Biol Psychiatry* 31, 1050–1056.

McKittrick CR, Blanchard DC, Blanchard RJ et al. (1995) Serotonin receptor binding in a colony model of chronic social stress. *Biol Psychiatry* 37, 383–393.

McNally GP, Cole S (2006) Opioid receptors in the midbrain periaqueductal gray regulate prediction errors during Pavlovian fear conditioning. *Behav Neurosci* 120, 313–323.

Medina JH, Novas ML, De Robertis E (1983a) Changes in benzodiazepine receptors by acute stress: different effect of chronic diazepam or Ro15–1788 treatment. *Eur J Pharmacol* 96, 181–185.

Medina JH, Novas ML, Wolfman CNV et al. (1983b) Benzodiazepine receptors in rat cerebral cortex and hippocampus undergo rapid and reversible changes after acute stress. *Neuroscience* 9, 331–335.

Mellman TA, Alim T, Brown DD et al. (2009) Serotonin polymorphisms and posttraumatic stress disorder in a trauma exposed African American population. *Depress Anxiety* 26, 993–997.

Mellman TA, Kumar A, Kulick-Bell R et al. (1995) Nocturnal/daytime urine norepinephrine measures and sleep in combat-related PTSD. *Biol Psychiatry* 38, 174–179.

Mellman TA, Kumar AM (1994) Platelet serotonin measures in posttraumatic stress disorder. *Psychiatry Res* 53, 99–101.

Mendelsohn C, Lohnes D, Decimo D et al. (1994) Function of the retinoic acid receptors (RARs) during development (II). *Multiple abnormalities at various stages of organogenesis in RAR double mutants. Development* 120, 2749–2771.

Mendelson SD, McEwen BS (1991) Autoradiographic analyses of the effects of restraint-induced stress on 5-HT1A, 5-HT1C, and 5-HT2 receptors in the dorsal hippocampus of male and female rats. *Neuroendocrinology* 54, 454–461.

Mey J, McCaffery P (2004) Retinoic acid signaling in the nervous system of adult vertebrates. *Neuroscientist* 10, 409–421.

Meyer RM, Burgos-Robles A, Liu E et al. (2014) A ghrelin-growth hormone axis drives stress-induced vulnerability to enhanced fear. *Mol Psychiatry* 19, 1284–1294.

Miller LG, Thompson ML, Greenblatt DJ et al. (1987) Rapid increase in brain benzodiazepine receptor binding following defeat stress in mice. *Brain Res* 414, 395–400.

Miner LH, Jedema HP, Moore FW et al. (2006) Chronic stress increases the plasmalemmal distribution of the norepinephrine transporter and the coexpression of tyrosine hydroxylase in norepinephrine axons in the prefrontal cortex. *J Neurosci* 26, 1571–1578.

Misner DL, Jacobs S, Shimizu Y et al. (2001) Vitamin A deprivation results in reversible loss of hippocampal long-term synaptic plasticity. *Proc Natl Acad Sci USA* 98, 11714–11719.

Moghaddam B, Adams B, Verma A et al. (1997) Activation of glutamatergic neurotransmission by ketamine: a novel step in the pathway from NMDA receptor blockade to dopaminergic and cognitive disruptions associated with the prefrontal cortex. *J Neurosci* 17, 2912–2127.

Moller C, Sommer W, Thorsell A et al. (1999) Anxiogenic-like action of galanin after intra-amygdala administration in the rat. *Neuropsychopharmacology* 21, 507–512.

Mushtaq D, Ali A, Margoob MA et al. (2012) Association between serotonin transporter gene promoter-region polymorphism and 4- and 12-week treatment response to sertraline in post-traumatic stress disorder. *J Affect Disord* 136, 955–962.

Nemeroff CB, Hernandez DE, Orlando RC et al. (1982) Cytoprotective effect of centrally administered neurotensin on stress- induced gastric ulcers. *Am J Phys* 242, 342–346.

Neylan TC, Brunet A, Pole N et al. (2005) PTSD symptoms predict waking salivary cortisol levels in police officers. *Psychoneuroendocrinology* 30, 373–381.

Nibuya M, Morinobu S, Duman RS (1995) Regulation of BDNF and trkB mRNA in rat brain by chronic electroconvulsive seizure and antidepressant drug treatments. *J Neurosci* 15, 7539–7547.

Ninan PT, Insel TM, Cohen RM et al. (1982) Benzodiazepine receptor-mediated "anxiety" in primates. *Science* 218, 1332–1334.

Nisenbaum LK, Abercrombie ED (1993) Presynaptic alterations associated with enhancement of evoked release and synthesis of NE in hippocampus of chemically cold stressed rats. *Brain Res* 608, 280–287.

Nisenbaum LK, Zigmond MJ, Sved AF et al. (1991) Prior exposure to chronic stress results in enhanced synthesis and release of hippocampal norepinephrine in response to a novel stressor. *J Neurosci* 11, 1478–1484.

Nishith P, Griffin MG, Poth TL (2002) Stress-induced analgesia: prediction of posttraumatic stress symptoms in battered versus nonbattered women. *Biol Psychiatry* 51, 867–874.

Nutt DJ, Malizia AL (2001) New insights into the role of the GABA-A-benzodiazepine receptor in psychiatric disorder. *Br J Psychiatry* 179, 390–396.

O'Reilly KC, Shumaker J, Gonzalez-Lima F et al. (2006) Chronic administration of 13-cis-retinoic acid increases depression-related behavior in mice. *Neuropsychopharmacology* 31, 1919–1927.

O'Reilly KC, Trent S, Bailey SJ et al. (2007) 13-cis-retinoic acid alters intracellular serotonin, increases 5-HT1a receptor, and serotonin reuptake transporter levels in vitro. *Exp Biol Med* 232, 1195–1203.

Oquendo MA, Echavarria G, Galfalvy HC et al. (2003) Lower cortisol levels in depressed patients with comorbid post-traumatic stress disorder. *Neuropsychopharmacology* 28, 591–598.

Orr SP, Lasko NB, Metzger LJ et al. (1998) Psychophysiological assessment of women with posttraumatic stress disorder resulting from childhood sexual abuse. *J Consult Clin Psychol* 66, 906–913.

Orr SP, Lasko NB, Shalev AY et al. (1995) Physiological responses to loud tones in Vietnam veterans with posttraumatic stress disorder. *J Abnorm Psychology* 104, 75–82.

Orr SP, Pitman RK, Lasko NB et al. (1993) Psychophysiological assessment of posttraumatic stress disorder imagery in World War II and Korean combat veterans. *J Abnorm Psychology* 102, 152–159.

Orr SP, Roth WT (2000) Psychophysiological assessment: clinical applications for PTSD. *J Affect Disord* 61, 225–240.

Osadchuka LV, Braastad BO, Huhtaniemi I et al. (2000) Alterations of the pituitary-gonadal axis in the neonatal blue fox (Alopex lagopus) exposed to prenatal handling stress. *Reprod Fertil Dev* 12, 119–126.

Ottenweller JE, Natelson BH, Pitman DL et al. (1989) Adrenocortical and behavioral responses to repeated stressors: Toward an animal model of chronic stress and stress-related mental illness. *Biol Psychiatry* 26, 829–841.

Pande AC, Pollack MH, Crockatt J et al. (2000) Placebo-controlled study of gabapentin treatment of panic disorder. *J Clin Psychopharmacol* 20, 457–471.

Pavlov V, Tracey K (2006) Controlling inflammation: the cholinergic anti-inflammatory pathway. *Biochem Soc Trans* 34, 1037–1040.

Pei Q, Zetterstrom T, Fillenz M (1990) Tail pinch-induced changes in the turnover and release of dopamine and 5-hydroxytryptamine in different brain regions of the rat. *Neuroscience* 35, 133–138.

Penner SB, Smyth DD, Glavin GB (1993) Effects of neuropeptide Y on experimental gastric lesion formation and gastric secretion in the rat. *J Pharmacol Exp Ther* 266, 339–343.

Perry BD, Southwick SM, Giller EJ (1991) Adrenergic receptor regulation in posttraumatic stress disorder. In: Giller EJ (ed.) *Biological Assessment and Treatment of Posttraumatic Stress Disorder*. American Psychiatric Press, Washington, DC.

Pettibone DJ, Williams M (1984) Serotonin-releasing effects of substituted piperazine in vitro. *Biochem Pharmacol* 33, 1531–1535.

Petty F, Kramer G, Wilson L (1992) Prevention of learned helplessness: in vivo correlation with cortical serotonin. *Pharmacol Biochem Behav* 43, 361–367.

Petty F, Kramer G, Wilson L et al. (1993) Learned helplessness and in vivo hippocampal norepinephrine release. *Pharmacol Biochem Behav* 46, 231–235.

Petty F, Kramer GL, Wu J (1997) Serotonergic modulation of learned helplessness. *Ann NY Acad Sci* 821, 538–541.

Petty F, Sherman AD (1983) Learned helplessness induction decreases in vivo cortical serotonin release. *Pharmacol Biochem Beh* 18, 649–650.

Phelix CF, Liposits Z, Paull WK (1992) Serotonin-CRF interaction in the bed nucleus of the stria terminalis: a light microscopic double-label immunocytochemical analysis. *Brain Res Bull* 28, 943–948.

Pietrzak RH, Galea S, Southwick SM et al. (2012) Examining the relation between the serotonin transporter 5-HTTPLR genotype x trauma exposure interaction on a contemporary phenotypic model of posttraumatic stress symptomatology: A pilot study. *J Affect Disord* 148, 123–128.

Pitman RK, Orr SP (1990) Twenty-four hour urinary cortisol and catecholamine excretion in combat-related posttraumatic stress disorder. *Biol Psychiatry* 27, 245–247.

Pitman RK, Orr SP, Lasko NB (1993) Effects of intranasal vasopressin and oxytocin on physiologic responding during personal combat imagery in Vietnam veterans with posttraumatic stress disorder. *Psychiatry Res* 48, 107–117.

Pitman RK, van der Kolk BA, Orr SP et al. (1990) Naloxone-reversible analgesic response to combat-related stimuli in posttraumatic stress disorder. A pilot study. *Arch Gen Psychiatry* 47, 541–544.

Plotsky PM, Meaney MJ (1993) Early, postnatal experience alters hypothalamic corticotropin-releasing factor (CRF) mRNA, median eminence CRF content and stress-induced release in adult rats. *Mol Brain Res* 18, 195–200.

Pollack MH, Matthews J, Scott EL (1998) Gabapentin as a potential treatment for anxiety disorders [letter]. *Am J Psychiatry* 155, 992–993.

Prasad A, Imamura M, Prasad C (1997) Dehydroepiandrosterone decreases behavioral despair in high- but not low-anxiety rats. *Physiol Behav* 62, 1053–1057.

Przegalinski E, Moryl E, Papp M (1995) The effect of 5-HT1A receptor ligands in a chronic mild stress model of depression. *Neuropharmacology* 34, 1305–1310.

Rajarao SJ, Platt B, Sukoff SJ et al. (2007) Anxiolytic-like activity of the non-selective galanin receptor agonist, galnon. *Neuropeptides* 41, 307–329.

Randall PK, Bremner JD, Krystal JH et al. (1995) Effects of the benzodiazepine receptor antagonist flumazenil in PTSD. *Biol Psychiatry* 38, 319–324.

Rasmusson AM, Hauger RL, Morgan CA et al. (2000) Low baseline and yohimbine-stimulated plasma neuropeptide Y (NPY) response in combat-related posttraumatic stress disorder. *Biol Psychiatry* 47, 526–539.

Rasmusson AM, Pinna G, Paliwal P et al. (2006) Decreased cerebrospinal fluid allopregnanolone levels in women with posttraumatic stress disorder. *Biol Psychiatry* 60, 704–713.

Rasmusson AM, Vasek J, Lipschitz DS et al. (2004) An increased capacity for adrenal DHEA release is associated with decreased avoidance and negative mood symptoms in women with PTSD. *Neuropsychopharmacology* 29, 1546–1157.

Reddy DS, O'Malley BW, Rogawski MA (2005) Anxiolytic activity of progesterone in progesterone receptor knockout mice. *Neuropharmacology* 48, 14–24.

Redmond D, Huang Y (1979) New evidence for a locus coeruleus-norepinephrine connection with anxiety. *Life Sci* 25, 2149–2162.

Rivier C, Vale W (1987) Diminished responsiveness of the hypothalamic-pituitary-adrenal axis of the rat during exposure to prolonged stress: A pituitary-mediated mechanism. *Endocrinology* 121, 1320–1328.

Robertson HA, Martin IL, Candy JM (1978) Differences in benzodiazepine receptor binding in Maudsley-reative and nonreactive rats. *Eur J Pharmacol* 50, 455–457.

Ronan PJ, Steciuk M, Kramer GL et al. (2000) Increased septal 5-HIAA efflux in rats that do not develop learned helplessness after inescapable stress. *J Neurosci Res* 61, 101–106.

Roosevelt RW, Smith DC, Clough RW et al. (2006) Increased extracellular concentrations of norepinephrine in cortex and hippocampus following vagus nerve stimulation in the rat. *Brain* 1119, 124–132.

Roth RH, Tam SY, Ida Y et al. (1988) Stress and the mesocorticolimbic dopamine systems. *Ann NY Acad Sci* 537, 138–147.

Roy-Byrne PP (2005) The GABA-benzodiazepine receptor complex: Structure, function, and role in anxiety. *J Clin Psychiatry* 66, 14–20.

Rupprecht R (2003) Neuroactive steroids: mechanism of action and neuropharmacological properties. *Psychoneuroendocrinology* 28, 139–168.

Sakai Y, Crandall JE, Brodsky J et al. (2004) 13-cis Retinoic acid (accutane) suppresses hippocampal cell survival in mice. *Ann NY Acad Sci* 1021, 436–440.

Sanchez MM, Young LJ, Plotsky PM et al. (1999) Autoradiographic and in situ hybridization localization of corticotrophin-releasing factor 1 and 2 receptors in nonhuman primate brain. *J Comp Neurol* 408, 365–377.

Santarelli L, Saxe M, Gross C et al. (2003a) Requirement of hippocampal neurogenesis for the behavioral effects of antidepressants. *Science* 301, 805–809.

Santarelli L, Saxe M, Gross C et al. (2003b) Requirement of hippocampal neurogenesis for the behavioral effects of antidepressants. *Science* 301, 805–809.

Sapolsky RM (1996) Why stress is bad for your brain. *Science* 273, 749–750.

Sapolsky RM, Uno H, Rebert CS et al. (1990) Hippocampal damage associated with prolonged glucocorticoid exposure in primates. *J Neurosci* 10, 2897–2902.

Sautter FJ, Bissette G, Wiley J et al. (2003) Corticotropin-releasing factor in posttraumatic stress disorder (PTSD) with secondary psychotic symptoms, nonpsychotic PTSD, and healthy control subjects. *Biol Psychiatry* 54, 1382–1388.

Saxe G, Stoddard F, Courtney D et al. (2001) Relationship between acute morphine and the course of PTSD in children with burns. *J Am Acad Child Adolesc Psychiatry* 40, 915–921.

Saxe GN, Stoddard F, Hall E et al. (2005) Pathways to PTSD, part I: Children with burns. *Am J Psychiatry* 162, 1299–1304.

Schmahl C, Kleindienst N, Limberger M et al. (2012) Evaluation of naltrexone for dissociative symptoms in borderline personality disorder. *Int Clin Psychopharmacol* 27:61–68.

Schmahl C, Meinzer M, Zeuch A et al. (2010) Pain sensitivity is reduced in borderline personality disorder, but not in posttraumatic stress disorder and bulimia nervosa. *World J Biol Psychiatry* 11, 364–371.

Schmidt PJ, Nieman L, Danaceau MA et al. (2000) Estrogen replacement in perimenopause-related depression: a preliminary report. *Am J Obstet Gynecol* 183, 414–420.

Schmidt PJ, Roca CA, Bloch M et al. (1997) The perimenopause and affective disorders. *Semin Reprod Endocrinol* 15, 91–100.

Seedat S, Stein MB, Kennedy CM et al. (2003) Plasma cortisol and neuropeptide Y in female victims of intimate partner violence. *Psychoneuroendocrinology* 28, 796–808.

Segal M (1979) Serotonergic innervation of the locus coeruleus from the dorsal raphe and its action on responses to noxious stimuli. *J Physiol* 286, 401–415.

Sevcik J, Finta EP, Illes P (1993) Galanin receptors inhibit the spontaneous firing of locus coeruleus neurons and interact with mu-opioid receptors. *Eur J Pharmacol* 230, 223–230.

Shalev AY, Sahar T, Freedman S et al. (1998) A prospective study of heart rate responses following trauma and the subsequent development of posttraumatic stress disorder. *Arch Gen Psychiatry* 55, 553–559.

Shearer KD, Goodman TH, Ross AW et al. (2010) Photoperiodic regulation of retinoic acid signalling in the hypothalamus. *J Neurochem* 112, 246–257.

Sherman AD, Petty F (1980) Neurochemical basis of the action of antidepressants on learned helplessness. *Behav Neural Biol* 30, 119–134.

Sherman AD, Petty F (1982) Additivity of neurochemical changes in learned helplessness and imipramine. *Behav Neurol Biol* 35, 344–353.

Sherwin BB, Gelfand MM (1985) Sex steroids and affect in the surgical menopause: a double-blind, cross-over study. *Psychoneuroendocrinology* 10, 325–335.

Silverman MN, Pearce BD, Miller AH (2002) Cytokines and HPA Axis Regulation. In: Kronfol Z (ed.) *Cytokines and Mental Health*. Kluwer, Norwell.

Skerritt JH, Trisdikoon P, Johnston GAR (1981) Increased GABA binding in mouse brain following acute swim stress. *Brain Res*, 398–403.

Sloan RP, McCreath H, Tracey KJ et al. (2007) RR interval variability is inversely related to inflammatory markers: the CARDIA study. *Mol Med* 13, 178.

Smith MA, Davidson R, Ritchie JC et al. (1989) The corticotropin-releasing hormone test in patients with posttraumatic stress disorder. *Biol Psychiatry* 26, 349–355.

Smith MA, Kim SY, Van Oers HJJ et al. (1997) Maternal deprivation and stress induce immediate early genes in the infant rat brain. *Endocrinology* 138, 4622–4628.

Soares CN, Almeida OP, Joffe H et al. (2001) Efficacy of estradiol for the treatment of depressive disorders in perimenopausal women: a double-blind, randomized, placebo-controlled trial. *Arch Gen Psychiatry* 58, 529–534.

Southwick SM, Krystal JH, Bremner JD et al. (1997) Noradrenergic and serotonergic function in posttraumatic stress disorder. *Arch Gen Psychiatry* 54, 749–758.

Southwick SM, Krystal JH, Morgan CA et al. (1993) Abnormal noradrenergic function in posttraumatic stress disorder. *Arch Gen Psychiatry* 50, 295–305.

Southwick SM, Paige S, Morgan CA et al. (1999) Neurotransmitter alterations in PTSD: Catecholamines and serotonin. *Semin Clin Neuropsychiatry* 4, 242–248.

Spencer SJ, Xu L, Clarke MA et al. (2012) Ghrelin regulates the hypothalamic-pituitary-adrenal axis and restricts anxiety after acute stress. *Biol Psychiatry* 72, 457–465.

Spivak B, Maayan R, Kotler M et al. (2000) Elevated circulatory level of GABA-A antagonistic neurosteroids in patients with combat-related posttraumatic stress disorder. *Psychol Med* 30, 1227–1231.

Stanley M, Mann JJ (1983) Increased serotonin-2 binding sites in frontal cortex of suicide victims. *Lancet* 1, 214–216.

Stanly M, Stanley B (1990) Postmortem evidence for serotonin's role in suicide. *J Clin Psychiatry* 51, 22–28.

Stanton ME, Gutierrez YR, Levine S (1988) Maternal deprivation potentiates pituitary-adrenal stress responses in infant rats. *Behav Neurosci* 102, 692–700.

Steffen AM, Thompson LW, Gallagher-Thompson D et al. (1999) Physical and psychosocial correlates of hormone replacement therapy with chronically stressed postmenopausal women. *J Aging Health* 11, 3–26.

Stein MB, Koverola C, Hanna C et al. (1997a) Hippocampal volume in women victimized by childhood sexual abuse. *Psychol Med* 27, 951–959.

Stein MB, Yehuda R, Koverola C et al. (1997b) Enhanced dexamethasone suppression of plasma cortisol in adult women traumatized by childhood sexual abuse. *Biol Psychiatry* 42, 680–686.

Stengel A, Wang L, Tache Y (2011) Stress-related alterations of acyl and desacyl ghrelin circulating levels: mechanisms and functional implications. *Peptides* 32, 2208–2217.

Stern RA, Robinson B TA, Arruda JE et al. (1996) A survey study of neuropsychiatric complaints in patients with Graves' disease. *J Neuropsychiatry Clin Neurosci* 8, 181–185.

Stone TW, Stoy N, Darlington LG (2013) An expanding range of targets for kynurenine metabolites of tryptophan. *Trends Pharmacol Sci* 34, 136–143.

Strawn JR, Ekhator NN, Horn PS et al. (2004) Blood pressure and cerebrospinal fluid norepinephrine in combat-related posttraumatic stress disorder. *Psychosom Med* 66, 757–750.

Strömberg J, Haage D, Taube M et al. (2006) Neurosteroid modulation of allopregnanolone and GABA effect on the GABA-A receptor. *Neuroscience* 143, 73–81.

Stuckey J, Marra S, Minor T et al. (1989) Changes in m-opiate receptors following inescapable shock. *Brain Res* 476, 167–169.

Tanaka M, Yoshida M, Emoto H et al. (2000) Noradrenaline systems in the hypothalamus, amygdala and locus coeruleus are involved in the provocation of anxiety: basic studies. *Eur J Pharmacol* 405, 397–406.

Taylor FB (2003) Tiagabine for posttraumatic stress disorder: a case series of 7 women. *J Clin Psychiatry* 64, 1421–1425.

Terman GW, Shavit Y, Lewis JW et al. (1984) Intrinsic mechanisms of pain inhibition: activation by stress. *Science* 226, 1270–1277.

Thompson Haskell G, Maynard TM, Shatzmiller RA et al. (2002) Retinoic acid signaling at sites of plasticity in the mature central nervous system. *J Comp Neurol* 452, 228–241.

Thorsell A, Michalkiewicz M, Dumont Y et al. (2000) Behavioral insensitivity to restraint stress, absent fear suppression of behavior and impaired spatial learning in transgenic rats with hippocampal neuropeptide Y overexpression. *Proc Natl Acad Sci USA* 97, 12852–12857.

Tilbrook AJ, Canny BJ, Serapiglia MD et al. (1999) Suppression of the secretion of luteinizing hormone due to isolation/restraint stress in gonadectomized rams and ewes is influenced by sex steroids. *J Endocrinol* 160, 469–481.

Torda T, Kvetnansky R, Petrikova M (1984) Effect of repeated immobilization stress on rat central and peripheral adrenoceptors. In: Usdin E, Kvetnansky R, Axelrod J (eds) *Stress: The Role of Catecholamines and Other Neurotransmitters*. Gordon & Breach, New York, pp. 691–701.

Toresson H, Mata de Urquiza A, Fagerstrom C et al. (1999) Retinoids are produced by glia in the lateral ganglionic eminence and regulate striatal neuron differentiation. *Development* 126, 1317–1326.

Tuncel N, Erkasap N, Sahinturk V et al. (1998) Stress-induced inhibition of reproductive functions: role of endogenous corticotropin-releasing factor. *Science* 231, 607–609.

Vaccarino AL, Olson GA, Olson RD et al. (1999) Endogenous opiates: 1988. *Peptides* 20, 1527–1574.

van der Kolk BA, Greenberg MS, Orr SP et al. (1989) Endogenous opioids, stress induced analgesia, and posttraumatic stress disorder. *Psychopharmacol Bull* 25, 417–421.

Van Praag HM, Asnis GM, Kahn RS et al. (1990) Monoamines and abnormal behaviour: a multi-aminergic perspective. *Br J Psychiatry* 157, 723–734.

van Zuiden M, Geuze E, Willemen HL et al. (2011a) Pre-existing high glucocorticoid receptor number predicting development of posttraumatic stress symptoms after military deployment. *Am J Psychiatry* 168, 89–96.

van Zuiden M, Kavelaars A, Rademaker AR et al. (2011b) A prospective study on personality and the cortisol awakening response to predict posttraumatic stress symptoms in response to military deployment. *J Psychiatr Res* 45, 713–719.

Vanover KE, Rosenzweig-Lipson S, Hawkinson JE et al. (2000) Characterization of the anxiolytic properties of a novel neuroactive steroid, Co 2-6749 (GMA-839; WAY-141839; 3alpha, 21-dihydroxy-3beta-trifluoromethyl-19-nor-5beta-pregnan-20-one), a selective modulator of gamma-aminobutyric acid(A)receptors. *J Pharmacol Exp Ther* 295, 337–345.

Vecsei L, Kiraly C, Bollok I et al. (1984) Comparative studies with somatostatin and cysteamine in different behavioral tests on rats. *Pharmacol Biochem Behav* 21, 833–837.

Ventura R, Cabib S, Puglisi-Allegra S (2002) Genetic susceptibility of mesocortical dopamine to stress determines liability to inhibition of mesoaccumbens dopamine and to behavioral despair in a mouse model of depression. *Neuroscience* 115, 999–1007.

Vermetten E (2008) Epilogue: neuroendocrinology of PTSD. *Prog Brain Res* 167, 311–313.

Vermetten E, Bremner JD (2002a) Circuits and systems in stress. I. Preclinical studies. *Depress Anxiety* 15, 126–147.

Vermetten E, Bremner JD (2002b) Circuits and systems in stress. II. Applications to neurobiology and treatment of PTSD. *Depress Anxiety* 16, 14–38.

Vythilingam M, Anderson E, Owens MJ et al. (2000) Norepinephrine and opioid regulation of cerebrospinal fluid corticotropin releasing factor (CRF) in healthy humans. *J Clin Endocrinol Metab* 85, 4138–4145.

Waclaw RR, Wang B, Campbell KA (2004) The homeobox gene Gsh2 is required for retinoid production in the embryonic mouse telencephalon. *Development* 131, 4013–4020.

Wahlestedt C, Grundemar L, Hakanson R et al. (1990) Neuropeptide Y receptor subtypes, Y1 and Y2. *Ann NY Acad Sci* 611, 7–26.

Wang C, Marx CE, Morrow AL et al. (2007) Neurosteroid modulation of GABAergic neurotransmission in the central amygdala: a role for NMDA receptors. *Neurosci Lett* 415, 118–123.

Wang Z, Baker DG, Harrer J et al. (2011) The relationship between combat-related posttraumatic stress disorder and the 5-HTTLPR/rs25531 polymorphism. *Depress Anxiety* 28, 1067–1073.

Watanabe Y, Gould E, Daniels DC et al. (1992a) Tianeptine attenuates stress-induced morphological changes in the hippocampus. *Eur J Pharmacol* 222, 157–162.

Watanabe Y, Sakai RR, McEwen BS et al. (1993) Stress and antidepressant effects on hippocampal and cortical 5-HT1A and 5-HT2 receptors and transport sites for serotonin. *Brain Res* 615, 87–94.

Watanabe YE, Gould H, Cameron D et al. (1992b) Phenytoin prevents stress and corticosterone induced atrophy of CA3 pyramidal neurons. *Hippocampus* 2, 431–436.

Watkins LR, Maier SF, Goehler LE (1995) Cytokine-to-brain communication: a review and analysis of alternative mechanisms. *Life Sci* 57, 1011–1026.

Weiss JM, Bonsall RW, Demetrikopoulos MK et al. (1998) Galanin: A significant role in depression? *Ann NY Acad Sci* 863, 364–384.

Weiss JM, Goodman PA, Losito BG et al. (1981) Behavioral depression produced by an uncontrollable stressor: Relationship to norepinephrine, dopamine, and serotonin levels in various regions of rat brain. *Brain Res Rev* 3, 167–2015.

Weizman A, Weizman R, Kook KA et al. (1990) Adrenalectomy prevents the stress-induced decrease in in vivo [3H]Ro 15–1788 binding to GABAA benzodiazepine receptors in the mouse. *Brain Res* 519, 347–350.

Weizman R, Weizman A, Kook KA et al. (1989) Repeated swim stress alters brain benzodiazepine receptors measured in vivo. *J Pharmacol Exp Ther* 249, 701–707.

Weizmann R, Gur E, Laor N et al. (1994a) Platelet adenylate cyclase activity in Israeli victims of Iraqi Scud missile attacks with posttraumatic stress disorder. *Psychopharmacology* 114, 509–512.

Weizmann R, Laor N, Karp L et al. (1994b) Alteration of platelet benzodiazepine receptors by stress of war. *Am J Psychiatry* 151, 766–767.

Weizmann R, Tanne Z, Granek M et al. (1987) Peripheral benzodiazepine binding sites of platelet membranes are increased during diazepam treatment of anxious patients. *Eur J Pharmacol* 138, 289–292.

Wessa M, Rohleder N, Kirschbaum C et al. (2006) Altered cortisol awakening response in posttraumatic stress disorder. *Psychoneuroendocrinology* 31, 209–215.

Wolf M (1991) Plasma methionine enkephalin in PTSD. *Biol Psychiatry* 29, 295–308.

Wu J, Kramer GL, Kram M et al. (1999) Serotonin and learned helplessness: a regional study of 5-HT1A, 5-HT2A receptors and the serotonin transport site in rat brain. *J Psychiatr Res* 33, 17–22.

Xie P, Kranzler HR, Poling J et al. (2009) Interactive effect of stressful life events and the serotonin transporter 5-HTTLPR genotype on posttraumatic stress disorder diagnosis in 2 independent populations. *Arch Gen Psychiatry* 66, 1201–1209.

Yehuda R (2006) Advances in understanding neuroendocrine alterations in PTSD and their therapeutic implications. *Ann NY Acad Sci* 1071, 137–166.

Yehuda R, Boisoneau D, Lowy MT et al. (1995a) Dose response changes in plasma cortisol and lymphocyte glucocorticoid receptors following dexamethasone administration in combat veterans with and without posttraumatic stress disorder. *Arch Gen Psychiatry* 52, 583–593.

Yehuda R, Brand S, Yang RK (2006) Plasma neuropeptide Y concentrations in combat exposed veterans: relationship to trauma exposure, recovery from PTSD, and coping. *Biol Psychiatry* 59, 660–663.

Yehuda R, Golier J, Kaufman S (2005) Circadian rhythm of salivary cortisol in Holocaust survivors with and without PTSD. *Am J Psychiatry* 162, 998–1000.

Yehuda R, Kahana B, Binder-Brynes K et al. (1995b) Low urinary cortisol excretion in holocaust survivors with posttraumatic stress disorder. *Am J Psychiatry* 152, 982–986.

Yehuda R, Levengood RA, Schmeidler J et al. (1996a) Increased pituitary activation following metyrapone administration in posttraumatic stress disorder. *Psychoneuroendocrinology* 21, 1–16.

Yehuda R, Lowry MT, Southwick SM et al. (1991a) Lymphocyte glucocorticoid receptor number in posttraumatic stress disorder. *Am J Psychiatry* 149, 499–504.

Yehuda R, Siever LJ, Teicher MH (1998) Plasma norepinephrine and 3-methoxy-4-hydroxyphenylglycol concentrations and severity of depression in combat posttraumatic stress disorder and major depressive disorder. *Biol Psychiatry* 44, 56–63.

Yehuda R, Southwick SM, Krystal JH et al. (1993) Enhanced suppression of cortisol with low dose dexamethasone in posttraumatic stress disorder. *Am J Psychiatry* 150, 83–86.

Yehuda R, Southwick SM, Nussbaum EL et al. (1991b) Low urinary cortisol in PTSD. *J Nerv Ment Dis* 178, 366–369.

Yehuda R, Teicher MH, Levengood RA et al. (1994) Circadian regulation of basal cortisol levels in posttraumatic stress disorder. *Ann NY Acad Sci*, 378–380.

Yehuda R, Teicher MH, Trestman RL et al. (1996b) Cortisol regulation in posttraumatic stress disorder and major depression: a chronobiological analysis. *Biol Psychiatry* 40, 79–88.

Yildiz BO, Suchard MA, Wong ML et al. (2004) Alterations in the dynamics of circulating ghrelin, adiponectin, and leptin in human obesity. *Proc Natl Acad Sci USA* 101, 10 434–10 439.

Young BR, Lawford EP, Noble B et al. (2002) Harmful drinking in military veterans with post-traumatic stress disorder: association with the D2 dopamine receptor A1 allele, Alcohol and Alcoholism 37:451–456. *Alcohol Alcoholism* 37, 451–456.

Young EA, Akil H (1985) Corticotropin-releasing factor stimulation of adrenocorticotropin and beta-endorphin release: Effects of acute and chronic stress. *Endocrinology* 117, 23–30.

Young EA, Breslau N (2004a) Cortisol and catecholamines in posttraumatic stress disorder: An epidemiological community study. *Arch Gen Psychiatry* 61, 394–401.

Young EA, Breslau N (2004b) Salivary cortisol in posttraumatic stress disorder: A community epidemiologic study. *Biol Psychiatry* 56, 205–209.

Young EA, Toman T, Witkowski K et al. (2004) Salivary cortisol and posttraumatic stress disorder in a low-income community sample of women. *Biol Psychiatry* 55, 621–626.

Zetterstrom RH, Lindqvist E, Mata de Urquiza A et al. (1999) Role of retinoids in the CNS: differential expression of retinoid binding proteins and receptors and evidence for presence of retinoic acid. *Eur J Neurosci* 11, 407–416.

Zetterström RH, Tomac A, Eriksdotter-Nilsson M et al. (1994) Localization of retinoid-binding proteins and retinoid receptors suggests a function for retinoic acid in developing and adult dopamine-innervated brain areas. *Soc Neurosci Abstracts* 20, 1688.

Zhang J, Smith D, Yamamoto M et al. (2003) The meninges is a source of retinoic acid for the late-developing hindbrain. *J Neurosci* 23, 7610–7620.

Zuo Y, Smith DC, Jensen RA (2007) Vagus nerve stimulation potentiates hippocampal LTP in freely-moving rats. *Physiol Behav* 90, 583–589.

CHAPTER 10

Genomics of PTSD

Anthony S. Zannas, Elisabeth Binder & Divya Mehta

Department of Translational Research in Psychiatry, Max Planck Institute of Psychiatry, Munich, Germany

10.1 Introduction

The role of genetic influences in the pathogenesis of posttraumatic stress disorder (PTSD) has been recognized for over half a century (Cornelis et al., 2010), but the first molecular genetic study in PTSD wasn't reported until 1996 (Comings et al., 1996). Proof of the genetic contribution to PTSD came from compelling evidence from twin and family studies conducted largely in war veterans demonstrating that PTSD is influenced by genetic factors, and indicating a genetic vulnerability to PTSD independent of the effects of combat exposure and the genetic influences determining that exposure (Goldberg et al., 2002; True et al., 1993). These studies provided the impetus for the evaluation of pre-existing risk factors that might play an important role in the onset and trajectory of PTSD.

The last decade has seen a significant amount of research focused on the identification of genetic risk factors for PTSD. The condition is an enormous health burden not just for individuals, but also for their family and society, and hence an understanding of risk factors for PTSD is crucial for treatment, prevention, and the fostering of well-being. This chapter summarizes available literature on the genetics of PTSD and highlights scientific research in animal models and humans related to the identification of genetic risk factors for PTSD. These studies contribute to a better understanding of the disorder. Since trauma exposure is a prerequisite for diagnosis of PTSD, we will discuss how genetic predisposition can moderate the environmental impact on disease. This chapter presents an overview of candidate-based and genome-wide association studies as well as gene-environment interaction studies performed in humans to date. Additionally, we describe potential epigenetic mechanisms in tandem with gene expression results that provide new models for how the environment (e.g., stress) influences PTSD risk by modification of genetic contributions to PTSD.

Posttraumatic Stress Disorder: From Neurobiology to Treatment, First Edition.
Edited by J. Douglas Bremner.
© 2016 John Wiley & Sons, Inc. Published 2016 by John Wiley & Sons, Inc.

10.2 Genetic studies in PTSD

Complex disorders such as PTSD generally have a polygenic architecture whereby a large number of genes with small effects contribute in a variable and interactive way towards disease susceptibility. Assigning causality to specific genes is complicated as these disorders typically depend on a cumulative combination of multiple genetic and non-genetic factors. Genetic studies are usually carried out using either linkage- or association-based approaches. Linkage-based approaches in PTSD rely upon family pedigrees with multiple affected family members, requiring that they share exposure to an uncommon traumatic event or exposure. Obtaining large and, moreover, trauma-exposed samples of affected family members for a linkage-based study is difficult, and therefore the most widely used approach in PTSD has been the alternative association-based study design. As we discuss in this section, several lines of evidence support the role of genetic factors in the pathogenesis of PTSD.

10.2.1 Family and twin studies on the heritability of PTSD

A genetic contribution to PTSD risk is supported by studies examining heritability of the disorder. Risk for PTSD is increased in families where at least one member has the diagnosis of PTSD, but there is also increased risk with the presence of other psychopathology, including mood, anxiety, and substance-use disorders (Davidson et al., 1985, 1998; Koenen et al., 2002; Yehuda et al., 2008). However, this transmitted risk could be due to either genetic factors or exposure to trauma secondary to presence of psychopathology in the family, or both.

Twin studies allow a differentiation between the contribution of genetic and environmental risk factors in the etiopathogenesis of PTSD. Twin studies typically examine differences in PTSD risk between monozygotic and dizygotic twin pairs that have been exposed to similar traumatic experiences. Monozygotic twins have identical genetic backgrounds, whereas dizygotic twins only share half of their genes. Thus, difference in the degree of phenotypic similarity between monozygotic and dizygotic twin pairs in the presence of similar environments supports heritability of the phenotype. Alternately, twin studies allow comparisons of phenotypic differences between monozygotic co-twins who have identical genetic background but are exposed to different levels of trauma. By such comparisons, twin studies can provide an estimate of disorder heritability, i.e., the proportion of interindividual differences in PTSD risk that can be explained by genetic factors (Kendler, 2001).

Heritability estimates for PTSD vary widely across twin studies. Studies of male twin veterans estimate heritability to be between 26% and 35% (Koenen et al., 2008a; True et al., 1993; Xian et al., 2000), with some variation observed across different clusters of PTSD symptomatology (True et al., 1993). However, heritability has been found to be as high as 72% in studies confined to female–female twin pairs (Sartor et al., 2011). On the other hand, twin studies on both male and female twin pairs found PTSD heritability to range between 23% and 46% (Sartor et al., 2012; Stein et al., 2002; Tambs et al., 2009). Thus, there exists considerable variation in heritability estimates for PTSD, and these estimates cannot be easily generalized across populations, or even within the same population at different points in time (Kendler, 2001).

An additional complicating factor is the fact that genetics also influences the risk for exposure to trauma. Heritability for trauma exposure ranges between 30% and 60% (Ehlers et al., 2013; Lyons et al., 1993; Sartor et al., 2012; Stein et al., 2002). Considerable variation has been observed for various types of trauma. Sartor et al. (2012) differentiated high-risk from low-risk traumatic events based on the risk for PTSD associated with each event and noted heritability ratios of 60% for high-risk events and 47% for low-risk events. Similarly, Stein et al. (2002) found 53% heritability of assaultive traumatic events but no evidence for heritability of non-assaultive events. It has been suggested that genetic factors may confer risk for stressor exposure by contributing to the development of certain personality traits, such as antisocial personality trains, neuroticism, and sensation and novelty-seeking, which may predispose individuals to stressful experiences (Amstadter et al., 2012; Jang et al., 2003; Kendler, 2001; Stein et al., 2002). Thus, it is important to differentiate between genetic factors that confer risk for exposure to trauma exposure and those that increase susceptibility for development of the disorder after traumatic exposure.

Another question is whether and to what extent heritability for PTSD is specific for this disorder. In other words, do certain genes contribute risk specifically for the development of PTSD or, rather, is genetic risk shared among distinct psychiatric phenotypes? Studies examining the genetic overlap between major depressive disorder (MDD) and PTSD suggest that genetic risk factors are mostly shared between these disorders (Koenen et al., 2008a; Sartor et al., 2012). Similarly, studies comparing PTSD with other anxiety disorders noted that genetic risk is largely common for these disorders, with only a small proportion of genetic risk being specific for PTSD (Chantarujikapong et al., 2001; Tambs et al., 2009). Considerable overlap in genetic risk has also been found between PTSD and substance-use disorders (Sartor et al., 2011; Xian et al., 2000). Therefore, twin studies overall support a model of non-specific contribution by genetic factors to PTSD risk. These data are consistent with two possible explanations. First, it is possible that the same genetic factors lead to the development of distinct phenotypes in different individuals via entirely independent pathogenetic pathways. Second, genetic factors may contribute to the development of vulnerability endophenotypes that then lead to distinct psychiatric phenotypes. In both cases, the specific repertoire of expressed symptoms probably depends on the environmental context, genetic background, and epigenetic state of the individual.

Endophenotypes relevant for PTSD have been examined by a number of twin studies. PTSD endophenotypes that have been shown to be heritable include lower cognitive functioning (Gilbertson et al., 2006; Kremen et al., 2007), fear conditioning (Hettema et al., 2003; Lanius et al., 2010), hypothalamic–pituitary–adrenal (HPA) axis dysregulation (Binder et al., 2008; Ferguson et al., 2012; Yehuda et al., 2004), smaller hippocampal volumes (Gilbertson et al., 2002; Pitman et al., 2006), neurological soft signs (Gurvits et al., 2006; Pitman et al., 2006), abnormalities of the cavum septum pellucidum (May et al., 2004; Pitman et al., 2006), and hyper-responsive dorsal anterior cingulate (Shin et al., 2011). Refinement and clinical validation of such measures may have important implications for the early identification and targeting of intervention and possible treatment interventions for individuals at increased risk for developing PTSD.

In summary, studies on heritability of PTSD have important strengths but also considerable limitations. An additional consideration is their inherent inability to identify specific genetic loci that confer vulnerability for PTSD and thus to elucidate biological pathways involved in pathogenesis of the disorder. Furthermore, these studies differentiate between environmental and genetic risk factors, but with the advent of epigenetics it has become evident that these factors interact at multiple levels. Despite these limitations, family and twin studies support a central role for genetics in the etiopathogenesis of PTSD.

10.2.2 Candidate gene association studies in PTSD

Several biological alterations such as altered HPA axis activity, abnormal heart rate reactivity, enhanced adrenergic response and intrusive memory imprinting to stress, elevated response to startle tones, increased autonomic response to threat and memory impairments have been associated with PTSD (Cornelis et al., 2010). These findings have constituted a hypothesis-driven search for biologically plausible candidates involved in PTSD. An overview of published candidate gene studies assessing the main genetic effects in PTSD is provided in Table 10.1.

10.2.2.1 HPA axis-related genes

The HPA axis is one of the main systems that regulate the physiological stress response in mammals (Sapolsky et al., 2000) and alterations of the HPA axis are one of the most consistent neurobiological findings in PTSD (see Chapter 11 in this volume). Neuroendocrine abnormalities such as lowered cortisol levels and increased sensitivity to glucocorticoids suggested the possible involvement of glucocorticoid-related genes in predisposition to PTSD (Mehta & Binder, 2012; Yehuda et al., 2011). One polymorphism in intron 2 (*Bcl1*) of the glucocorticoid receptor (GR) gene was associated with increased glucocorticoid sensitivity and greater cortisol suppression following a low-dose dexamethasone suppression

Table 10.1 Gene–environment interaction studies in posttraumatic stress disorder (PTSD).

Genetic locus	Reference	N	Ethnicity (%)	Outcome (instrument)	Trauma (instrument)	Polymorphism	P-value	Primary finding
SLC6A4	Kilpatrick et al. (2007)	589	White (90), Black (4), Hispanic (4), other (2)	PTSD diagnosis (National Women's Study PTSD module)	Hurricane exposure (computer-assisted structured telephone interview)	5-HTTLPR	$P < 0.03$	S-allele carriers with low social support were at higher PTSD risk than LL homozygotes
	Koenen et al. (2009)	590	White (90), other (10)	PTSD diagnosis (National Women's Study PTSD module)	Hurricane exposure (computer-assisted structured telephone interview)	5-HTTLPR	$P = 0.03$ for interaction with crime; $P = 0.007$ for interaction with unemployment	S-allele increased PTSD risk in presence of high crime/ unemployment rates but decreased PTSD risk in presence of low crime/ unemployment
	Xie et al. (2009)	1,252	White (47), Black (53)	PTSD diagnosis (SSADDA)	Childhood and adult trauma (SSADDA)	5-HTTLPR	$P = 0.01$ for gene × adult trauma; $P = 0.046$ for gene × childhood trauma; $P < 0.001$ for gene × both adult and child trauma	S-allele carriers exposed to childhood or adult trauma had higher risk for lifetime PTSD as compared to the LL homozygotes
	Xie et al. (2012)	5,178	White (54), Black (46)	PTSD diagnosis (SSADDA)	Childhood trauma (SSADDA)	5-HTTLPR	$P = 0.019$ in Caucasians; $P = 0.62$ in AAs	Only in Caucasians, S-allele carriers exposed to child trauma had higher PTSD risk

(continued)

Table 10.1 (*Continued*)

Genetic locus	Reference	N	Ethnicity (%)	Outcome (instrument)	Trauma (instrument)	Polymorphism	P-value	Primary finding
	Mercer et al. (2012)	204	White (78), Black (14), Hispanic (2), Asian (3), Assyrian (1), Multiracial (3), unknown (1)	PTSD symptoms (DEQ)	Life trauma and shooting exposure (modified Virginia Tech shooting exposure measure, TLEQ, DEQ)	5-HTTLPR rs25531 STin2	P = 0.03	L_A carriers had lower PTSD symptom scores after the shooting when compared with the other genotype groups
	Grabe et al. (2009)	3,045	White	PTSD diagnosis (SCID)	Life trauma (SCID)	5-HTTLPR rs25531	P < 0.05	L_A carriers had higher risk for PTSD with increasing number of traumatic events
	Pietrzak et al. (2013)	149	White (71), Black (10), Hispanic (10), other (10)	PTSD symptoms (PCL)	Exposure to Hurricane Ike (interview)	5-HTTLPR	P < 001	S-allele carriers with increasing trauma had more symptoms in the arousal and re-experiencing clusters but not in other clusters
FKBP5	Binder et al. (2008)	762	White (2.2), Black (95.2), Hispanic (0.6), Asian (0.1), mixed (0.9), other (1.0)	PTSD diagnosis (CAPS) and severity (mPSS)	Childhood (CTQ) and adult (TEI) trauma	rs3800373 rs9296158 rs1360780 rs9470080	P < 0.002 P < 0.001 P < 0.002 P < 0.002	Four SNPs interact with childhood but not adulthood trauma to predict PSS scores
	Xie et al. (2010)	2427	Black (52.9), White (47.1)	PTSD diagnosis (SSADDA)	Childhood trauma (SSADDA)	rs9470080	P = 0.004	Only in AAs, the T-allele predicted increased PTSD risk following trauma but decreased risk in individuals not exposed to trauma

Gene	Study	N	Ethnicity	Outcome measure	Trauma measure	SNP	P value	Findings
	Boscarino et al. (2012)	410	White	Lifetime and early-onset PTSD (clinical interview)	Childhood trauma (ACES)	rs9470080	$P = 0.026$ (lifetime PTSD); $P = 0.016$ (early-onset PTSD)	The T-allele interacts, cumulatively with other genes, with early trauma to predict lifetime and early-onset PTSD
	White et al. (2012)	139	White	Amygdala reactivity (fMRI)	Childhood trauma (CTQ)	rs3800373 rs9296158 rs1360780 rs9470080 rs7748266 rs9394309	$P = 0.003$ $P = 0.002$ $P = 0.002$ $P = 0.011$ $P = 0.011$ $P = 0.097$	SNPs interacted with childhood emotional neglect to predict dorsal amygdala reactivity
COMT	Kolassa et al. (2010b)	424	Rwandese	PTSD diagnosis (structured interview based on PDS)	War- and non-war-related traumatic events (checklist)	Rs4680 (COMT Val^{158}Met)	$P = 0.04$	Met allele homozygotes were all at high PTSD risk, whereas Val allele carriers showed a dose–response relationship depending on the number of traumatic events
	Clark et al. (2013)	236	White	PTSD diagnosis and symptoms (CAPS, PTSD Checklist)	Life trauma (DRRI)	Rs4680 (COMT Val^{158}Met)	$P < 0.05$	Heterozygous Iraq War veterans were more resilient to trauma than either homozygous genotype
APOE	Lyons et al. (2013)	172	White (92), Black (4), other (4)	PTSD diagnosis and symptoms (DIS)	Combat exposure (Combat Experiences Scale)	Presence or absence of E4 allele	$P < 0.014$	E4 carriers have higher PTSD risk and symptom scores than non-carriers

(continued)

Table 10.1 (*Continued*)

Genetic locus	Reference	N	Ethnicity (%)	Outcome (instrument)	Trauma (instrument)	Polymorphism	P-value	Primary finding
ADCYAP1R1	Uddin et al. (2013)	495	White (12), Black (83) Other (5)	PTSD diagnosis and symptoms (CAPS)	Childhood maltreatment (CTQ, CTS, Wyatt's eight-item interview guide)	rs2267735	$P = 0.037$	Female C-allele carriers exposed to childhood trauma have higher PTSD risk and symptom severity
RGS2	Amstadter et al. (2009)	607	White (90), Black (4), Hispanic (4), other (2)	PTSD diagnosis (National Women's Study PTSD module)	Hurricane exposure (computer-assisted structured telephone interview)	rs4606	$P = 0.029$ for post-hurricane symptoms; $P < 0.001$ for lifetime PTSD symptoms	The C-allele interacted with trauma and low social support to predict higher post-hurricane and lifetime PTSD symptoms
	Dunn et al. (2014)	205	Black	PTSD (IES-R) PTG (PTG-I)	Exposure to hurricane Katrina (8-item scale)	rs4606	$P = 0.006$ for PTG	Individuals carrying the minor G-allele that were exposed to higher levels of hurricane showed higher PTG scores

ACES, Adverse Childhood Experiences Study Scale; CAPS, Clinician Administered PTSD Scale; CTQ, Child Trauma Questionnaire; CTS, Conflict Tactics Scale; DEQ, Distressing Events Questionnaire; DES, Dissociative Experiences Scale; DIS, Diagnostic Interview Scale; DRRI, Deployment Risk and Resilience Inventory; fMRI, functional magnetic resonance imaging; IES-R, Impactof EventsScale-Revised; PCL, PTSD Checklist-Specific Stressor Version; PDS, Posttraumatic Diagnostic Scale; PTGI, Post-Traumatic Growth Inventory; SCID, Structured Clinical Interview for DSM-IV; SSADDA, Semi-Structured Assessment for Drug Dependence and Alcoholism; TEI, Traumatic Events Inventory; TLEC, Traumatic Life Events Questionnaire.

N, number of subjects included in the gene–environment interaction analyses in each study.

test (Panarelli et al., 1998; van Rossum et al., 2004) and the same polymorphism was also associated with diminished cortisol response to stress (Wust et al., 2004) and an increased risk for PTSD after cardiac surgery (Hauer et al., 2011). Another study explored the association between these polymorphisms in the GR and PTSD in Vietnam veterans with PTSD and non-PTSD controls matched for combat exposure (Bachmann et al., 2005). The allelic and genotype frequencies of both polymorphisms were not significantly different between PTSD veterans and controls and no clear relationship was observed between the genotypes and glucocorticoid sensitivity by the low-dose dexamethasone test and the dermal vessel vasocontrictor assay. In contrast to previous findings, the authors did not observe significant differences in basal plasma cortisol levels between PTSD veterans and controls, and the low-dose dexamethasone suppression test resulted in similar levels of cortisol suppression in both groups. Only a subgroup of probands with the *BclI* GG genotype were responsive to dermal vessel vasoconstrictor assay and had higher PTSD symptom scores that were significantly and negatively correlated with basal levels of plasma cortisol.

Other studies have been conducted in the gene encoding FK506 binding protein 51 (FKBP5), a co-chaperone of the steroid receptor complex which, among other functions, regulates sensitivity of the GR (Grad & Picard, 2007; Pratt & Toft, 1997). Polymorphisms in *FKBP5* were associated with peri-traumatic dissociation, a known risk factor for PTSD, in medically injured children (Koenen et al., 2005) and with PTSD itself in other studies (Boscarino et al., 2011, 2012). In addition to the main genetic effects, these polymorphisms have also been assessed within the framework of gene–environment (G × E) interactions, which will be detailed in a later section. Boscarino et al. (2011) assessed the cumulative burden of polymorphisms within four candidate loci previously reported to be associated with PTSD, including *FKBP5*, *COMT*, *CHRNA5*, and *CRHR1*. The authors observed that while the individual single nucleotide polymorphism (SNP) markers within these four genes were associated with PTSD, combining these SNPs into a cumulative risk allele model significantly predicted both lifetime and early-onset PTSD. The multimarker cumulative risk model suggested up to nine-fold and 14-fold increased risk for lifetime PTSD and early-onset PTSD, respectively, among individuals harboring six or more risk alleles.

A recent study reported a significant association between SNPs within the corticotropin-releasing hormone receptor 1 gene (*CRHR1*) and post-disaster PTSD symptoms and diagnosis in adults exposed to 2004 Florida hurricanes (White et al., 2013). The pituitary adenylate cyclase-activating polypeptide (PACAP) gene, known to widely regulate the cellular stress response, has also been investigated for its role in PTSD (Ressler et al., 2011). A significant sex-specific association between a SNP in a putative estrogen response element within the PACAP receptor encoded by the *ADCYAP1R1* gene and PTSD diagnosis and symptoms was observed only in females. The same SNP was also associated with fear discrimination, *ADCYAP1R1* mRNA expression, and DNA methylation of the gene in DNA from peripheral blood. These findings suggest that perturbations in the PACAP/PAC1 pathway are involved in abnormal stress responses underlying PTSD and may exhibit sex-specific effects.

10.2.2.2 Non-HPA axis-related genes

The first candidate tested for association with PTSD was the dopamine D2 receptor (DRD2) gene. Comings et al. (1991, 1996) found higher frequency of the A1 allele of the restriction fragment length polymorphism site near the dopamine D2 receptor gene among veterans with alcohol and substance dependence and comorbid PTSD compared with veterans with alcohol and substance dependence without PTSD. These findings, however, were not replicated in a subsequent study with a larger sample size (Gelernter et al., 1999). Young et al. (2002) later reported significantly higher frequency of the A1 allele in Vietnam combat veterans of the Australian armed forces with PTSD compared with matched controls, although these findings were seen only in PTSD subjects with comorbid alcohol abuse. Subsequent studies implicated the A1 allele of the DRD2 gene in general psychopathological symptoms, including depression, anxiety, alcohol dependency, and social dysfunction, suggesting that this genetic variant is not specific to the diagnosis of PTSD (Heinz et al., 2004; Lawford et al., 2003; Noble et al., 1991).

The role of the serotonin transporter (5-HTT), a key protein in serotonin neurotransmission, has been extensively studied in PTSD. A functional polymorphism in the 5′ regulatory promoter (5-HTTLPR) of this gene was initially implicated in decreased 5-HTT transcriptional activity and reduced serotonin uptake (Lesch et al., 1996). This, combined with the fact that 5-HTT is the prime target for selective serotonin reuptake inhibitors, antidepressants commonly used for psychiatric disorders including PTSD, resulted in a plethora of studies subsequently testing for association of this gene with a range of psychiatric disorders. Despite this, the results of association studies of 5-HTTLPR with PTSD have been mixed. Several studies have found evidence for a significant association of the short form (s/s) of the 5-HTTLPR with PTSD risk (Kolassa et al., 2010a; Lee et al., 2005; Mercer et al., 2012; Wang et al., 2011), whereas other studies have reported a lack of association with PTSD (Mellman et al., 2009; Valente et al., 2011). These results should be interpreted with caution owing to the small sample sizes of the studies and the fact that the risk for PTSD might be driven by an interaction of this polymorphism with stressful life events, as is seen in the case of depression (Caspi et al., 2003; Kendler et al., 2005). In a recent study, a meta-analysis was performed across all 12 published association studies in PTSD that included trauma-exposed controls (Gressier et al., 2013).

Taking into account all these 12 studies, the authors found no association between 5-HTTLPR and PTSD, with evidence of heterogeneity between the studies partly due to gender differences. Still, interestingly, the 5-HTTLPR has been associated with differences in treatment response among PTSD patients with the short form/low-expression alleles predicting poor response (Bryant et al., 2010; Mushtaq et al., 2012). Nevertheless, the exact role of 5-HTTLPR in PTSD still remains to be elucidated.

The gene encoding the brain-derived neurotrophic factor (*BDNF*) plays an important role in the maintenance of neuronal plasticity (McAllister, 1999) and has been frequently studied in stress-related disorders. Zhang et al. (2006) screened a new SNP (G-712A) and two known SNPs (Val66Met and C270T) in patients with Alzheimer's, schizophrenia, substance-abuse disorders, affective disorders and PTSD. The authors observed no significant differences in allele, genotype, or haplotype frequencies of the SNPs between PTSD subjects and normal controls. These findings were confirmed by another study that also found no significant differences in allele and genotype frequencies between PTSD subjects and healthy controls in a Korean sample (Lee et al., 2005). In summary, no study to date has revealed clear evidence for a major role of *BDNF* in susceptibility to PTSD.

Several other well-studied candidates for psychiatric disorders have also been assessed with regard to their relationship with PTSD. For instance, one study tested the role of a polymorphism within the NPY gene (Leu7Pro) and found a significantly higher frequency of the Pro7 allele in alcohol-dependent patients but not PTSD patients as compared with controls (Lappalainen et al., 2002). This and other studies examining other candidate genes are reported in Table 10.1.

10.2.3 Genome-wide association studies in PTSD

In contrast to focusing on known candidates, a genome-wide approach is a hypothesis-free method that allows an unbiased comprehensive scan of genetic variants associated with the disorder. The advent of high-throughput technologies such as microarrays facilitated the investigation of genome-wide association studies (GWAS) that allowed for thousands of genes to be tested for simultaneously in a large number of samples at a reasonable cost. GWAS have been very successful in uncovering new loci for many complex traits, including psychiatric traits such as bipolar disorder, schizophrenia, and attention-deficit hyperactivity disorder (Hindorff et al., 2009). Nevertheless, until the beginning of this year, there was an absence of any GWAS of PTSD, but three studies have been published by the end of 2013. The first GWAS of PTSD was conducted in trauma-exposed, white non-Hispanic veterans and their intimate partners and was reported in 2013 (Logue et al., 2013). Logue and colleagues identified several SNPs that yielded evidence of association with PTSD, with one SNP located in the retinoid-related orphan receptor alpha gene (*RORA*), reaching genome-wide statistical significance. The authors went on to replicate their findings in an independent sample of African-Americans and found other SNPs within the *RORA* gene to be nominally significantly associated with PTSD. The *RORA* gene has been implicated in previous GWAS studies of psychiatric disorders and is known to play an important role in neuroprotection and other behavioral processes, and the retinoid system has been implicated in stress-related mental disorders (see Chapter 9). Albeit the samples in these studies were small, they represent an important initial step in identifying the genetic underpinnings of PTSD using a genome-wide approach.

Another recent genome-wide analysis was conducted in European-Americans to find novel common risk alleles for PTSD (Xie et al., 2013). The authors observed one SNP on chromosome 7p12, rs406001 that exceeded genome-wide significance. The SNP mapped to the first intron of the Tolloid-Like 1 gene (*TLL1*). Although no SNPs at this locus reached genome-wide significance, the authors successfully replicated the findings in an independent sample and one SNP, rs6812849 in the TLL1 gene, then reached genome-wide significance in the combined sample. The mammalian TLL1 (mTll1) protein is expressed at high levels in the cerebellum (Takahara et al., 1994) and hippocampus of mice (Tamura et al., 2005). Moreover, *in vitro* functional studies have suggested that glucocorticoids decrease *mTll1* expression (Tamura et al., 2005). This and involvement of TLL1 in cleaving the BDNF gene precursor into its mature form in reptiles (Keifer et al., 2009) suggest that *TLL1* might be a plausible candidate for PTSD.

Guffanti et al. (2013) performed a GWAS of PTSD in a primarily African-American cohort of women from the Detroit Neighborhood Health Study and tested the findings in a replication cohort of primarily European-American women from the Nurses Health Study II. One SNP mapping to a novel long non-coding RNA gene, lincRNA AC068718.1, of unknown function, was found to be associated with PTSD at the genome-wide significance level. Network-based analysis of the top associated results indicated an enrichment of transcripts implicated for pathways related to telomerase maintenance and immune function.

In summary, only three genome-wide, modest-sized association studies have been reported to date and there is a growing need for larger and well-powered GWAS to allow identification of novel genes in the etiology of PTSD. This will be achieved within the work group for PTSD of the Psychiatric Genomics Consortium. With regard to future genetic investigations of PTSD, several non-genetic factors such as environmental variables need to be taken into context when assessing the contributions of each of the reported genetic variants towards risk for PTSD. For example, in the above described case–control association studies, it is important to control for environmental factors by comparing trauma-exposed controls with PTSD cases. This allows for the dissection of genetic from environmental influences. However, obtaining controls adequately matched for trauma exposure is often very difficult. In this context, G × E interaction studies in PTSD that carefully assess details about types of traumas, and the intensity and duration of the trauma, and how these interact with the genetic variant(s) are likely to yield more useful information (Mehta & Binder, 2012). Therefore, the next section of this chapter will expand on genetic studies in PTSD by focusing on G × E interactions found to moderate risk of PTSD.

10.3 Gene–environment interaction studies in PTSD

As we discussed in previous sections, efforts to identify specific genes with consistent main effects on PTSD risk have met with little success. This may be attributed to the phenotypic heterogeneity and multifactorial etiology of PTSD that, like every complex phenotype, results from multiple genes and environmental exposures, each conferring modest risk for the development of the disorder. Furthermore, in contrast to other psychiatric phenotypes that are defined solely based on phenomenology, the diagnosis of PTSD requires exposure to a potentially traumatizing event. This requirement has evolved over the years and differs across diagnostic manuals, but in general includes a stressor of high intensity (American Psychiatric Association, 2013). However, beyond the mere presence of a traumatizing event, there are other important factors, including the type of event, its duration, and the number of cumulative exposures over the individual's lifetime. Such interindividual variability in environmental exposure could account for the observed phenotypic heterogeneity, and may decrease statistical power to identify risk genes. Thus, it is important to examine the interaction of specific environmental exposures with risk genes using a G × E interaction framework (Caspi et al., 2010; Koenen et al., 2008b). Despite these theoretical implications, it was not until recently that G × E interaction studies were conducted on a number of genetic loci in PTSD.

The first locus studied within the G × E interaction framework was the gene encoding the serotonin transporter (*SLC6A4*). A commonly examined polymorphism at this locus is the promoter polymorphic region (5-HTTLPR) that has two functional variants, the low-expression S (short) and the high-expression L (long) alleles (Heils et al., 1996). As noted earlier, the S-allele has been associated in a number of studies with heightened vulnerability for PTSD following exposure to hurricane disasters (Kilpatrick et al., 2007; Koenen et al., 2009; Pietrzak et al., 2013), childhood adversity (Xie et al., 2009, 2012), and adulthood trauma (Xie et al., 2009). Furthermore, expression of 5-HTTLPR can be modulated by a functional SNP (rs25531) at the *SLC6A4* locus (Hu et al., 2005). Specifically, 5-HTTLPR L-allele carriers with the A-allele of the rs25531 (L$_A$)

have high expression of the serotonin transporter, whereas L_G carriers have low expression levels similar to S-allele carriers. Mercer et al. (2012) examined the effects of a university campus shooting on PTSD and found that high-expression L_A carriers had lower PTSD symptom scores after the shooting when compared with the other genotype groups. On the other hand, Grabe et al. (2009) examined the effects of trauma in a general population sample and found the opposite direction for this interaction, with L_A carriers exhibiting a higher risk for PTSD following increasing numbers of traumatic events. The presence of moderating factors in different populations might attenuate or even reverse the observed G × E interactions. For example, Koenen et al. (2009) found that, among individuals exposed to Hurricane Katrina, the S-allele of the 5-HTTLPR polymorphism was associated with greater PTSD risk in the presence of high levels of crime and unemployment rates, but with decreased PTSD risk in the presence of low crime and unemployment. Similarly, Xie et al. (2012) found that the G × E interaction was present only in European-Americans and not in African-Americans. Thus, it is important to take into account such additional factors that might moderate the effects of G × E interaction.

Another genetic locus that has received increasing attention in G × E interaction studies in PTSD is *FKBP5*, the gene encoding FK506 binding protein 51 (*FKBP5*), a co-chaperone of the steroid receptor complex that, among other functions, regulates sensitivity of the GR (Grad & Picard, 2007; Pratt & Toft, 1997). Several *FKBP5* polymorphisms have been examined in relevant G × E interaction studies. Binder et al. (2008) studied eight *FKBP5* SNPs and showed that four SNPs (rs3800373, rs9296158, rs1360780, and rs9470080) moderated the effects of childhood adversity on severity of PTSD symptomatology in adulthood. These four SNPs were also found to moderate the effects of childhood emotional neglect on amygdala reactivity (White et al., 2012), a neuroimaging measure thought to represent an endophenotype of PTSD (Shin et al., 2005). On the other hand, Xie et al. (2010) showed that presence of the T-allele of rs9470080 is associated with increased PTSD risk in individuals exposed to childhood trauma but decreased risk in individuals not exposed to trauma. Similarly, Klengel et al. (2013) found that carriers of the T-allele of rs1360780 are at increased risk for lifetime PTSD if exposed to childhood sexual and physical abuse, but at lower risk for PTSD if not exposed to childhood abuse. These findings are in line with a "plasticity gene" hypothesis, which posits that some alleles traditionally viewed as risk variants in G × E interaction studies may also confer benefits in the presence of supportive environments (Belsky et al., 2009).

An important conclusion drawn from G × E interaction studies at the *FKBP5* locus is the presence of sensitive developmental periods during which G × E interaction s exert their effects. In particular, studies suggest that childhood but not adult trauma interacts with *FKBP5* risk variants to predict phenotypes during adulthood (Binder et al., 2008; Zannas & Binder, 2014). This is in accordance with animal studies showing that stressors occurring early in development have stronger and more enduring effects when compared with adult stressors (Hoffmann & Spengler, 2014; Russo et al., 2012). Our group explored the mechanism for this developmentally restricted G × E interaction by examining allele-specific effects of early trauma on DNA methylation of cytosine-phosphate-guanosine sites (CpGs) located in functional glucocorticoid response elements (GREs) of the *FKBP5* locus. These effects were examined on the rs1360780 SNP that is a functional variant associated with differential induction of *FKBP5* expression following activation of the GR (Binder et al., 2004). Specifically, the rarer T-allele of the rs1360780 has been associated with greater induction of *FKBP5* mRNA following GR activation and heightened glucocorticoid resistance (Klengel et al., 2013). We found that, in T-allele carriers, but not in non-carriers, childhood abuse was associated with demethylation of CpGs in intron 7 of the *FKBP5* gene (Klengel et al., 2013). This demethylation was observed only following exposure to childhood abuse, but not exposure to adult trauma (Klengel et al., 2013). Furthermore, using experiments of chromatin conformation capture in lymphoblastoid cell lines, we found that the T-allele is associated with enhanced physical contact of the intron 2 GRE with the transcription start site of the *FKBP5* gene. This allele-specific change in 3D conformation is probably promoted by the higher affinity of the T-allele sequence for the TATA-box binding protein (Klengel et al., 2013). Overall, these experiments showed that the developmentally restricted G × E interaction involving the *FKBP5* gene could be explained by allele-specific epigenetic modifications that are induced only by early trauma (Klengel & Binder, 2013).

A number of other genetic loci have been examined by G × E interaction studies. The gene encoding catechol-O-methyltransferase (*COMT*), an enzyme involved in the metabolism of catecholamines, has been shown to moderate the relationship between trauma exposure and PTSD risk. Kolassa et al. (2010b) found that survivors of the Rwandan genocide that were homozygous for the Met allele of the *COMT* Val[158]Met genotype were all at high risk for development of PTSD, whereas Val allele carriers showed a dose–response relationship that depended on the number of traumatic events. On the other hand, Clark et al. (2013) found that Iraq War veterans heterozygous for the polymorphism were more resilient to trauma exposure as compared with individuals with either homozygous genotype. Variation of the apolipoprotein E gene (*APOE*) was also found to moderate vulnerability for exposure to combat in Vietnam War veterans, with carriers of the E4 variant exhibiting greater risk for PTSD diagnosis and higher symptom scores than non-carrier veterans (Lyons et al., 2013). Similarly, a variant of the pituitary adenylate cyclase activating polypeptide 1 receptor type I gene (*ADCYAP1R1*) has been found to interact with childhood maltreatment and shape the risk for PTSD diagnosis and severity in women (Uddin et al.,

2013). Finally, a polymorphism (rs4606) of the gene encoding RGS2, a protein that regulates signaling through G-protein-coupled receptors (Manzur & Ganss, 2009), was shown to increase PTSD symptoms and lifetime PTSD risk via interactions with traumatic exposure and low social support (Amstadter et al., 2009). However, the same gene variant was also found to moderate the development of posttraumatic growth (PTG) in individuals exposed to the hurricane Katrina, with those carrying the minor G-allele and exposed to higher levels of hurricane showing higher PTG scores (Dunn et al., 2014). The exact mechanisms of these G × E interactions are currently not clear, but exploring such G × E interactions at the molecular level may offer particular insights into the pathogenesis of PTSD.

The G × E interaction studies in PTSD are summarized in Table 10.1. Besides their aforementioned strengths, these studies also have considerable limitations. For instance, although G × E interaction studies have the advantage of examining interactions between specific environmental exposures and biologically plausible genetic loci, they are reductionist in nature and usually do not account for the genetic background or the general environmental context in which these G × E interactions occur. This renders these studies prone to spurious findings, and concerns have been raised that most of the published G × E interaction studies have not controlled sufficiently for potential confounders (Keller, 2014). Furthermore, phenotypic specificity of the observed G × E interactions is essential for elucidating the molecular underpinnings of PTSD, but studies have shown contradictory findings. Some studies examining both PTSD and MDD as outcomes have noted these interactions to be specific for PTSD (Binder et al., 2008; Uddin et al., 2013) or even specific for some PTSD symptom clusters but not others (Mercer et al., 2012; Pietrzak et al., 2013). Nonetheless, G × E interactions involving the aforementioned *SLC6A4* and *FKBP5* variants have also been observed for MDD and other psychiatric phenotypes (Caspi et al., 2003; Kilpatrick et al., 2007; Zannas & Binder, 2014; Zimmermann et al., 2011). These findings suggest that factors beyond gene variation and environmental exposure may be contributing to the phenotypic heterogeneity observed with G × E interactions. As we discuss in the next section, epigenetics is one such contributing factor that has provided new insights into the molecular underpinnings of PTSD.

10.4 Epigenetic and gene expression studies in PTSD

One way for the environment to modify gene function in an enduring manner is via altered gene expression, which can be mediated by long-lasting changes in epigenetic marks. Over recent years, the understanding of psychiatric disorders has been improved with the advent of technologies that allow for the measurement of epigenetic changes. Epigenetic mechanisms consist of a wide range of biochemical processes, including DNA methylation and posttranslational histone modifications, which regulate gene transcription without changing the underlying genetic code. We refer the interested reader to a detailed description of these processes published elsewhere (Fazzari & Greally, 2010; Khan & Krishnamurthy, 2005). The relevance of epigenetic modifications for psychiatric disorders lies in their role in mediating the lasting effects of environmental exposure on gene expression (Feil & Fraga, 2011). In particular, a number of studies in animals have showed that epigenetic signatures can be embedded by adverse life experiences (Hoffmann & Spengler, 2014; McGowan et al., 2008; Weaver et al., 2004). Given the causal link of PTSD with traumatic experiences, epigenetic mechanisms may be particularly relevant for this disorder. Furthermore, variation in genetic sequences can affect the extent of epigenetic modifications (Feil & Fraga, 2011) and, as we discussed in the previous section, allele-specific epigenetic modifications may mediate G × E interactions (Klengel & Binder, 2013; Klengel et al., 2013). Thus, epigenetic mechanisms may act in concert with genetic and environmental factors to shape risk or resilience for PTSD.

The epigenetic modification most studied in this context is change in the methylation status of cytosine residues of genomic DNA. The pattern of DNA methylation may be modified by a number of environmental and neuroendocrine factors (Feil & Fraga, 2011; Hoffmann & Spengler, 2014; Li et al., 2003; McGowan et al., 2008; Telese et al., 2013). In particular, studies in rodents and humans showed that the methylation status of genes involved in the stress response can be altered by stressor exposure and may shape subsequent vulnerability or resilience to stressors (Hoffmann & Spengler, 2014; McGowan et al., 2008, 2009; Murgatroyd et al., 2009; Weaver et al., 2004). Although previously considered a non-reversible modification, DNA methylation has been shown to be a dynamic process induced by DNA methyltransferases and reversed by enzymatic demethylation (Telese et al., 2013). Despite this dynamic regulation, some stressor-induced changes in methylation have also been suggested to be stable and potentially heritable (Dias & Ressler, 2014; Franklin et al., 2010; Hoffmann & Spengler, 2014; Rodgers et al., 2013). Identifying and characterizing such methylation markers may offer particular insights into the pathogenesis of PTSD.

10.4.1 DNA methylation studies in PTSD

A number of studies have associated PTSD with changes in DNA methylation of genes important for neurotransmission and regulation of stress responses. DNA methylation in two genetic loci that regulate neurotransmission, the genes encoding the dopamine transporter (*SLC6A3*) and the serotonin transporter (*SLC6A4*), were found to moderate risk for PTSD in humans (Chang et al., 2012;

Koenen et al., 2011). Higher methylation levels of the *SLC6A3* promoter were shown to interact with the 9R allele of *SLC6A3* to predict increased lifetime risk for PTSD (Chang et al., 2012). Methylation levels of the *SLC6A4* promoter were similarly found to interact with traumatic events and predict PTSD diagnosis. In the presence of low *SLC6A4* methylation levels, greater numbers of traumatic events predicted increased risk for PTSD, whereas at high methylation levels greater traumatic exposure predicted lower PTSD risk (Koenen et al., 2011).

Changes in DNA methylation in relation to PTSD have also been observed in genes involved in glucocorticoid signaling. As previously discussed, we found allele-specific demethylation of the intron 7 of the *FKBP5* gene in response to childhood but not adulthood trauma (Klengel et al., 2013). *FKBP5* demethylation has been associated with GR resistance (Klengel et al., 2013), which leads to aberrant feedback regulation of the HPA axis and prolonged stressor-induced increases in HPA activity (Zannas & Binder, 2014). Similarly, converging evidence from rodent and human studies has linked early life adversity with increased methylation both in peripheral blood and in brain tissue of the promoter region of the gene encoding GR (*Nr3c1*), a molecular marker that has been shown to predict heightened HPA responsiveness and worse behavioral outcomes in adulthood (Hoffmann & Spengler, 2014; McGowan et al., 2008, 2009; Oberlander et al., 2008; Perroud et al., 2011; Weaver et al., 2004). DNA methylation levels in these genetic loci have been suggested as promising biomarkers for PTSD. A recent pilot study found that higher pre-treatment methylation levels of the *Nr3c1* promoter predicted favorable response to prolonged exposure psychotherapy, whereas successful response to treatment correlated with longitudinal decrease in methylation of the *FKBP5* promoter (Yehuda et al., 2013). While these findings await validation by larger studies, refinement of such measures offer promise as biomarkers for predicting outcomes and monitoring treatment response in PTSD.

Several other DNA methylation markers have been linked with PTSD. As compared with comparison subjects, patients with PTSD were found to have differences in the methylation status of several genes with immune function, along with differences in plasma cytokine levels and cytomegalovirus antibody titers (Rusiecki et al., 2013; Smith et al., 2011; Uddin et al., 2010). Greater peripheral blood methylation levels at a CpG site (cg04008455) of the gene encoding mannosidase alpha class 2C member 1 (*MAN2C1*), an enzyme involved in the clearance of oligosaccharides (Suzuki et al., 2006), interacted with traumatic events to predict greater risk for lifetime PTSD (Uddin et al., 2011). Further studies are warranted in order to clarify the exact role of these molecular markers and to elucidate possible common biological pathways involved in the pathogenesis of the disorder.

In summary, an exponentially increasing number of studies support a role for epigenetic modifications in PTSD. Despite the excitement associated with these studies, most of the findings so far come from animal studies or peripheral blood. Given the tissue specificity of epigenetic modifications, it is currently unclear whether these modifications will also be observed in the tissue of interest, i.e., the human brain. An additional consideration is to what extent these modifications can be said to apply for all patients with PTSD. Like other psychiatric phenotypes, PTSD is defined phenomenologically, and clinical heterogeneity raises challenges in linking molecular findings with specific phenotypes. The wide range of social environmental exposures contributes to this phenotypic variation and identification of such ecophenotypic variation within diagnostic entities is important for elucidating the molecular underpinnings of this psychiatric disorder (Teicher & Samson, 2013). For example, our group found that patterns of DNA methylation and gene expression vary markedly among subjects with similar PTSD symptoms, depending on the presence or absence of exposure to childhood abuse (Mehta et al., 2013). These findings suggest the presence of a number of PTSD subtypes with distinct molecular phenotypes and pathophysiologies. Identification of these subtypes will be an important step towards the development of personalized therapeutic interventions for patients suffering from PTSD.

10.4.2 Gene expression studies in PTSD

Several studies have further examined gene expression profiles in PTSD, using mostly peripheral blood cells as the target tissue. These studies are summarized in Table 10.2 and described in the following sections.

10.4.3 Prospective vs. cross-sectional studies

Prospective studies are studies that attempt to predict the outcome of the disease by assessing gene expression profiles before the disease has manifested, while cross-sectional studies examine gene expression profiles that track with the disease and give a snapshot of the disease at the time of the study.

Segman et al. (2005) performed the first genome-wide prospective gene expression study in PTSD where they correlated transcriptional response of peripheral blood mononuclear cells with PTSD occurring among trauma survivors. They observed a substantial number of differentially expressed transcripts that encoded for proteins involved in stress response, transcriptional activation, immune pathways, cell cycle and proliferation, signal transduction and apoptosis. Interestingly, the majority of the differentially expressed transcripts are expressed in brain areas and neuroendocrine systems involved in the stress response, including the amygdala, hippocampus, and HPA axis. This study demonstrated the value of using blood biomarkers for identification of PTSD-related gene expression signatures and paved the way for other gene expression studies in PTSD. In another study, van Zuiden et al. (2012) examined

Table 10.2 Gene expression studies in posttraumatic stress disorder (PTSD).

Reference	Study type	Tissue	Subjects	Outcome
Segman et al. (2005)	Genome-wide	Peripheral blood mononuclear cells	24	Several differentiating genes having a role in stress response
Zieker et al. (2007)	Stress/immune genes	Peripheral blood	16	The majority of genes belonged to ROS-related metabolism
Yehuda et al. (2009)	Genome-wide	Peripheral blood	40	Several genes involved in GR regulation, signal transduction, brain and immune function associated with PTSD
O'Donovan et al. (2011)	Genome-wide	Monocytes	67	Gender-specific differences in genes within inflamamtory pathways
Neylan et al. (2011)	Genome-wide	Monocytes	67	Male PTSD subjects had an overall pattern of under-expression of genes
Mehta et al. (2011)	Genome-wide	Peripheral blood	211	FKBP5 polymophisms revealed distinct gene expression patterns in PTSD
van Zuiden et al. (2012)	Candidate-gene tests	Peripheral blood mononuclear cells	448	Significantly low FKBP5 and high GILZ expression associated with PTSD
Glatt et al. (2013)	Genome-wide	Peripheral blood	50	Significantly enrichment of immune genes, 70% prediction accuracy based on the expression of 23 transcripts and 80% accuracy based on the expression of one exon from each of five genes
Mehta et al. (2013)	Genome-wide	Peripheral blood	169	Gene expression in PTSD with or without child abuse is distinct
Hollifield et al. (2013)	qPCR	Peripheral blood	17	Genes within inflammatory and the adrenergic system differentially expressed in PTSD

ROS, reactive oxygen species; GR, glucocorticoid receptor; qPCR, quantitative polymerase chain reaction.

soldiers before military deployment and assessed whether GR pathway components in leukocytes characterized pre-existing vulnerability factors for the development of PTSD symptoms following military deployment. The authors assessed male soldiers before and 6 months after deployment to a combat zone for differences in gene expression of GR candidate genes, including *FKBP5*, *GILZ* and *SGK1*, SNPs within the *Nr3c1* and *FKBP5* genes, as well as plasma cortisol and level of childhood trauma. They identified low *FKBP5* expression, high *GILZ* expression and high number of GRs from peripheral blood mononuclear cells as independent prospective predictors of PTSD symptoms. A recent study investigated US Marines before and after deployment overseas to war zones in Iraq or Afghanistan and reported a panel of biomarkers dysregulated in peripheral blood cells that was significantly enriched for immune genes (Glatt et al., 2013). In an independent sample, using gene expression levels of five genes within this panel of biomarkers, the authors could predict with up to 80% accuracy which individuals would go on to develop PTSD. While the results should be interpreted with caution, owing to the small samples, these findings parallel previous findings of the role of immune-related genes in PTSD. These findings have implications for early intervention and prevention in individuals at high risk for PTSD.

The remaining gene expression studies in PTSD have been cross-sectional by nature. Yehuda and colleagues also identified lower gene expression levels of *FKBP5* among other genes in the 9/11 World Trade Center attack survivors who subsequently developed PTSD, as compared with those who did not (Sarapas et al., 2011; Yehuda et al., 2009).

A series of studies have been conducted examining the role of immune-related genes in PTSD. Zieker et al. (2007) assessed peripheral gene expression signatures in subjects with PTSD following the Ramstein air show catastrophe using customized "stress immune arrays." A large number of differentially regulated genes were involved in immune function or reactive oxygen species and the fact that these changes were observed even 16 years after the catastrophe highlighted the enduring nature of gene expression changes in immune-related genes after experiencing a traumatic event. Another study identified altered transcriptional control of immune cell gene expression in PTSD by examining the prevalence of specific transcription factor binding motifs in promoter regions of differentially expressed genes in monocytes from PTSD subjects and matched controls (O'Donovan et al., 2011). The results indicated possible gender differences in PTSD, with increased inflammatory and adrenergic signaling in conjunction with decreased glucocorticoid signaling in men and increased inflammatory and decreased adrenergic signaling in women. These findings allow a better understanding of the role of components of the immune system in regulation of brain function at the cellular and systems levels and how these may underlie the pathology of PTSD and possibly other stress-related psychiatric disorders.

10.4.3.1 Studies accounting for risk factors

Gene expression levels can vary depending on genetic and/or environmental risk factors and it is only recently that the influence of these risk factors in altering gene expression has been investigated. For instance, taking *FKBP5* as an example, we have demonstrated that, depending on *FKBP5* genotype, distinct gene expression differences are observed in PTSD cases vs. controls. While we did identify a number of genes regulated by PTSD symptom severity itself, these data suggested that a distinct network of genes was differentially regulated depending on *FKBP5* genotype and related differences in GR sensitivity. These results suggest that depending on the genotype, individuals may represent biologically distinct subgroups within PTSD (Mehta et al., 2011). This study underlines the importance of considering genotype information when assessing gene expression. In our recent work, we performed a genome-wide gene expression analysis to identify differences in transcriptional patterns between PTSD cases and controls (Mehta et al., 2013). Taking the history of child abuse into account, we questioned whether the underlying biology between PTSD with or without child abuse was similar or distinct. While we identified a large number of transcripts differentially expressed between PTSD cases and controls, there was almost no overlap between gene expression differences in PTSD cases with and without child abuse as compared with trauma-matched controls. One of the genes differentially expressed between PTSD cases with child abuse and controls was the *MAN2C1* gene, previously reported to show differential gene expression (Yehuda et al., 2009) and different DNA methylation patterns (Uddin et al., 2011) in PTSD. Among the differentially expressed transcripts in both PTSD with and without child abuse, several non-overlapping pathways were also enriched, suggesting differences in the underlying biology between the two PTSD groups. Remarkably, even among the differentially expressed genes, only for the PTSD cases with child abuse, DNA methylation changes seemed to underlie and even modulate the observed gene expression differences up to 12-fold higher than for PTSD cases with no history of child abuse. This study underscores the importance of taking the environment into account even when assessing gene expression signatures in PTSD.

10.4.3.2 Focus on one candidate

In addition to evidence from genetic association studies, several candidate-based gene expression studies have also pointed towards the role of the FKBP5 gene, a co-chaperone of the mature GR complex, in PTSD. The initial gene expression study by Segman et al. (2005) in a small study sample of emergency room-admitted individuals demonstrated that FKBP5 gene expression within a few hours after emergency room admission correlated significantly with the amount of acute PTSD symptoms. Yehuda and colleagues also identified lower gene expression levels of the FKBP5 gene among other genes in the 9/11 World

Trade Center attack survivors who subsequently developed PTSD compared with those who did not (Sarapas et al., 2011; Yehuda et al., 2009). These findings were replicated by van Zuiden et al. (2012), who also observed that both low FKBP5 and high GILZ gene expression prior to deployment were risk factors for developing PTSD in an independent sample. We, too, observed lower FKBP5 gene expression in PTSD subjects; however, the gene expression levels were consistently and significantly lower, especially for PTSD probands who carried the risk allele of a functional polymorphism within the FKBP5 gene (Mehta et al., 2011). In summary, these studies point towards the role of the FKBP5 gene in the etiology of PTSD.

All these gene expression studies in PTSD have been performed using peripheral blood or peripheral blood cell subtypes. Owing to the tissue-specific nature of gene expression patterns, assessing the most informative tissue for gene expression profiling is crucial. Nevertheless, as it is very difficult to obtain brain samples for experimental purposes, peripheral blood acts as a good surrogate for assessment of gene expression levels. A large number of gene expression studies in psychiatric diseases have been performed using peripheral blood cells, indicating the reliability of using peripheral blood for gene expression studies in psychiatry (Mehta et al., 2010). The ultimate goal would be to have a large repository of gene expression profiles from a range of cells and tissue from both healthy and disease samples to allow a comprehensive scan of gene expression profiles relevant to disease. Until this is achieved, studies assessing gene expression profiles in psychiatric disorders such as PTSD will continue to benefit from the ease and accessibility of peripheral blood in the hope that what we observe in peripheral blood is a reflection, even in part, of gene expression changes in the brain.

10.5 Conclusions

In this chapter we have highlighted evidence supporting a central role of genomics in the pathogenesis of PTSD. We have underlined studies that have examined the role of genetic variants alone or in combination with environmental factors, gene expression profiles and epigenetic marks in the susceptibility to the development of PTSD. The genetic contributors identified in the etiology of PTSD to date are largely involved in the regulation of neurotransmission, HPA axis activity, emotion and cognition. As heuristically depicted in Figure 10.1, a complex interplay among these genetic loci, potentially traumatizing events and epigenetic regulation may alter gene expression and ultimately shape distinct phenotypes. Given the complexity of PTSD, identifying and refining endophenotypes linked with the disorder, but also with resilient phenotypes such as PTG, will be essential in future endeavors. The complexity and heterogeneity of these phenotypes further dictate that multiple genes, rather than single loci, in combination with multiple environmental risk factors are involved in their

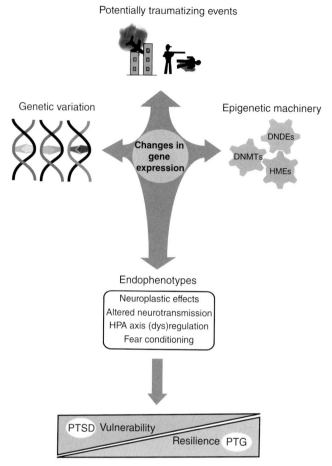

Figure 10.1 Simplified heuristic representation of the mechanisms leading to the development of posttraumatic stress disorder (PTSD) and posttraumatic growth (PTG). A complex interplay among potentially traumatizing events, multiple gene variants, and epigenetic mechanisms results in changes in the expression of genes that are involved in the regulation of neurotransmission, hypothalamic–pituitary–adrenal (HPA) axis activity, emotion and cognition. This shapes endophenotypes and, ultimately, vulnerability or resilience phenotypes. DNDEs, DNA demthylating enzymes; DNMTs, DNA methyltransferases; HMEs, histone-modifying enzymes. (*See color plate section for the color representation of this figure.*)

genesis. The genetic basis of PTSD is highly complex and there remain many unanswered questions. Future studies will offer a systems-level understanding of how multiple genes and biological pathways interact with traumatic events to determine distinct outcomes among individuals. Such integrative studies will hopefully pave the way for a better understanding of genomics and subsequently treatment of PTSD.

References

American Psychiatric Association (2013) *Diagnostic and Statistical Manual of Mental Disorders*, 5th edn, Washington DC.

Amstadter AB, Aggen SH, Knudsen GP et al. (2012) A population-based study of familial and individual-specific environmental contributions to traumatic event exposure and posttraumatic stress disorder symptoms in a Norwegian twin sample. *Twin Res Hum Genet* 15, 656–662.

Amstadter AB, Koenen KC, Ruggiero KJ et al. (2009) Variant in RGS2 moderates posttraumatic stress symptoms following potentially traumatic event exposure. *J Anxiety Disord* 23, 369–373.

Bachmann AW, Sedgley TL, Jackson RV et al. (2005) Glucocorticoid receptor polymorphisms and post-traumatic stress disorder. *Psychoneuroendocrinology* 30, 297–306.

Belsky J, Jonassaint C, Pluess M et al. (2009) Vulnerability genes or plasticity genes? *Mol Psychiatry* 14, 746–754.

Binder EB, Bradley RG, Liu W et al. (2008) Association of FKBP5 polymorphisms and childhood abuse with risk of posttraumatic stress disorder symptoms in adults. *JAMA* 299, 1291–1305.

Binder EB, Salyakina D, Lichtner P et al. (2004) Polymorphisms in FKBP5 are associated with increased recurrence of depressive episodes and rapid response to antidepressant treatment. *Nat Genet* 36, 1319–1325.

Boscarino JA, Erlich PM, Hoffman SN et al. (2011) Association of FKBP5, COMT and CHRNA5 polymorphisms with PTSD among outpatients at risk for PTSD. *Psychiatry Res* 188, 173–174.

Boscarino JA, Erlich PM, Hoffman SN et al. (2012) Higher FKBP5, COMT, CHRNA5, and CRHR1 allele burdens are associated with PTSD and interact with trauma exposure: implications for neuropsychiatric research and treatment. *Neuropsychiatr Dis Treat* 8, 131–139.

Bryant RA, Felmingham KL, Falconer EM et al. (2010) Preliminary evidence of the short allele of the serotonin transporter gene predicting poor response to cognitive behavior therapy in posttraumatic stress disorder. *Biol Psychiatry* 67, 1217–1219.

Caspi A, Hariri AR, Holmes A et al. (2010) Genetic sensitivity to the environment: the case of the serotonin transporter gene and its implications for studying complex diseases and traits. *Am J Psychiatry* 167, 509–527.

Caspi A, Sugden K, Moffitt TE et al. (2003) Influence of life stress on depression: moderation by a polymorphism in the 5-HTT gene. *Science* 301, 386–389.

Chang SC, Koenen KC, Galea S et al. (2012) Molecular variation at the SLC6A3 locus predicts lifetime risk of PTSD in the Detroit Neighborhood Health Study. *PloS one* 7, e39184.

Chantarujikapong SI, Scherrer JF, Xian H et al. (2001) A twin study of generalized anxiety disorder symptoms, panic disorder symptoms and post-traumatic stress disorder in men. *Psychiatry Res* 103, 133–145.

Clark R, Deyoung CG, Sponheim SR et al. (2013) Predicting post-traumatic stress disorder in veterans: Interaction of traumatic load with COMT gene variation. *J Psychiatr Res* 47, 1849–1856.

Comings DE, Comings BG, Muhleman D et al. (1991) The dopamine D2 receptor locus as a modifying gene in neuropsychiatric disorders. *JAMA* 266, 1793–1800.

Comings DE, Muhleman D, Gysin R (1996) Dopamine D2 receptor (DRD2) gene and susceptibility to posttraumatic stress disorder: a study and replication. *Biol Psychiatry* 40, 368–372.

Cornelis MC, Nugent NR, Amstadter AB et al. (2010) Genetics of post-traumatic stress disorder: review and recommendations for genome-wide association studies. *Current psychiatry reports* 12, 313–326.

Davidson J, Swartz M, Storck M et al. (1985) A diagnostic and family study of posttraumatic stress disorder. *Am J Psychiatry* 142, 90–93.

Davidson JR, Tupler LA, Wilson WH et al. (1998) A family study of chronic post-traumatic stress disorder following rape trauma. *J Psychiatr Res* 32, 301–309.

Dias BG, Ressler KJ (2014) Parental olfactory experience influences behavior and neural structure in subsequent generations. *Nature Neurosci* 17, 89–96.

Dunn EC, Solovieff N, Lowe SR et al. (2014) Interaction between genetic variants and exposure to Hurricane Katrina on post-traumatic stress and post-traumatic growth: A prospective analysis of low income adults. *J Affect Disord* 152–154, 243–249.

Ehlers CL, Gizer IR, Gilder DA et al. (2013) Lifetime history of traumatic events in an American Indian community sample: heritability and relation to substance dependence, affective disorder, conduct disorder and PTSD. *J Psychiatr Res* 47, 155–161.

Fazzari MJ, Greally JM (2010) Introduction to epigenomics and epigenome-wide analysis. *Methods Mol Biol* 620, 243–265.

Feil R, Fraga MF (2011) Epigenetics and the environment: emerging patterns and implications. *Nat Rev Genet* 13, 97–109.

Ferguson B, Hunter JE, Luty J et al. (2012) Genetic load is associated with hypothalamic-pituitary-adrenal axis dysregulation in macaques. *Genes Brain Behav* 11, 949–945.

Franklin TB, Russig H, Weiss IC et al. (2010) Epigenetic transmission of the impact of early stress across generations. *Biol Psychiatry* 68, 408–415.

Gelernter J, Southwick S, Goodson S et al. (1999) No association between D2 dopamine receptor (DRD2) "A" system alleles, or DRD2 haplotypes, and posttraumatic stress disorder. *Biol Psychiatry* 45, 620–625.

Gilbertson MW, Paulus LA, Williston SK et al. (2006) Neurocognitive function in monozygotic twins discordant for combat exposure: relationship to posttraumatic stress disorder. *J Abnorm Psychol* 115, 484–495.

Gilbertson MW, Shenton ME, Ciszewski A et al. (2002) Smaller hippocampal volume predicts pathologic vulnerability to psychological trauma. *Nat Neurosci* 5, 1242–1247.

Glatt SJ, Tylee DS, Chandler SD et al. (2013) Blood-based gene-expression predictors of PTSD risk and resilience among deployed marines: a pilot study. *Am J Med Genet Part B* 162B, 313–326.

Goldberg J, True WR, Eisen SA et al. (1990) A twin study of the effects of the Vietnam War on posttraumatic stress disorder. *JAMA* 263, 1227–1232.

Grabe HJ, Spitzer C, Schwahn C et al. (2009) Serotonin transporter gene (SLC6A4) promoter polymorphisms and the susceptibility to posttraumatic stress disorder in the general population. *Am J Psychiatry* 166, 926–933.

Grad I, Picard D (2007) The glucocorticoid responses are shaped by molecular chaperones. *Mol Cell Endocrinol* 275, 2–12.

Gressier F, Calati R, Balestri M et al. (2013) The 5-HTTLPR Polymorphism and Posttraumatic Stress Disorder: A Meta-Analysis. *J Trauma Stress* 26, 645–653.

Guffanti G, Galea S, Yan L et al. (2013) Genome-wide association study implicates a novel RNA gene, the lincRNA AC068718.1, as a risk factor for post-traumatic stress disorder in women. *Psychoneuroendocrinology* 38, 3029–3038.

Gurvits TV, Metzger LJ, Lasko NB et al. (2006) Subtle neurologic compromise as a vulnerability factor for combat-related posttraumatic stress disorder: results of a twin study. *Arch Gen Psychiatry* 63, 571–576.

Hauer D, Weis F, Papassotiropoulos A et al. (2011) Relationship of a common polymorphism of the glucocorticoid receptor gene to traumatic memories and posttraumatic stress disorder in patients after intensive care therapy. *Critical Care Med* 39, 643–650.

Heils A, Teufel A, Petri S et al. (1996) Allelic variation of human serotonin transporter gene expression. *J Neurochem* 66, 2621–2624.

Heinz A, Siessmeier T, Wrase J et al. (2004) Correlation between dopamine D(2) receptors in the ventral striatum and central processing of alcohol cues and craving. *Am J Psychiatry* 161, 1783–1789.

Hettema JM, Annas P, Neale MC et al. (2003) A twin study of the genetics of fear conditioning. *Arch Gen Psychiatry* 60, 702–708.

Hindorff LA, Sethupathy P, Junkins HA et al. (2009) Potential etiologic and functional implications of genome-wide association loci for human diseases and traits. *Proc Natl Acad Sci USA* 106, 9362–9367.

Hoffmann A, Spengler D (2014) DNA memories of early social life. *Neuroscience* 264, 64–75.

Hu X, Oroszi G, Chun J et al. (2005) An expanded evaluation of the relationship of four alleles to the level of response to alcohol and the alcoholism risk. *Alcohol Clin Exp Res* 29, 8–16.

Jang KL, Stein MB, Taylor S et al. (2003) Exposure to traumatic events and experiences: aetiological relationships with personality function. *Psychiatry Res* 120, 61–69.

Keifer J, Sabirzhanov BE, Zheng Z et al. (2009) Cleavage of proBDNF to BDNF by a tolloid-like metalloproteinase is required for acquisition of in vitro eyeblink classical conditioning. *J Neurosci* 29, 14956–14964.

Keller MC (2014) Gene × Environment Interaction Studies Have Not Properly Controlled for Potential Confounders: The Problem and the (Simple) Solution. *Biol Psychiatry* 75, 18–24.

Kendler KS (2001) Twin studies of psychiatric illness: an update. *Arch Gen Psychiatry* 58, 1005–1014.

Kendler KS, Kuhn JW, Vittum J et al. (2005) The interaction of stressful life events and a serotonin transporter polymorphism in the prediction of episodes of major depression: a replication. *Archiv Gen Psychiatry* 62, 529–535.

Khan AU, Krishnamurthy S (2005) Histone modifications as key regulators of transcription. *Front Biosci* 10, 866–872.

Kilpatrick DG, Koenen KC, Ruggiero KJ et al. (2007) The serotonin transporter genotype and social support and moderation of posttraumatic stress disorder and depression in hurricane-exposed adults. *Am J Psychiatry* 164, 1693–1699.

Klengel T, Binder EB (2013) Allele-specific epigenetic modification: a molecular mechanism for gene-environment interactions in stress-related psychiatric disorders? *Epigenomics* 5, 109–112.

Klengel T, Mehta D, Anacker C et al. (2013) Allele-specific FKBP5 DNA demethylation mediates gene-childhood trauma interactions. *Nat Neurosci* 16, 33–41.

Koenen KC, Aiello AE, Bakshis E et al. (2009) Modification of the association between serotonin transporter genotype and risk of posttraumatic stress disorder in adults by county-level social environment. *Am J Epidemiol* 169, 704–711.

Koenen KC, Fu QJ, Ertel K et al. (2008a) Common genetic liability to major depression and posttraumatic stress disorder in men. *J Affect Disord* 105, 109–115.

Koenen KC, Harley R, Lyons MJ et al. (2002) A twin registry study of familial and individual risk factors for trauma exposure and posttraumatic stress disorder. *J Nerv Ment Dis* 190, 209–218.

Koenen KC, Nugent NR, Amstadter AB (2008b) Gene-environment interaction in posttraumatic stress disorder: review, strategy and new directions for future research. *Eur Arch Psychiatry Clin Neurosci* 258, 82–96.

Koenen KC, Saxe G, Purcell S et al. (2005) Polymorphisms in FKBP5 are associated with peritraumatic dissociation in medically injured children. *Mol Psychiatry* 10, 1058–1059.

Koenen KC, Uddin M, Chang SC et al. (2011) SLC6A4 methylation modifies the effect of the number of traumatic events on risk for posttraumatic stress disorder. *Depress Anxiety* 28, 639–647.

Kolassa IT, Ertl V, Eckart C et al. (2010a) Association study of trauma load and SLC6A4 promoter polymorphism in posttraumatic stress disorder: evidence from survivors of the Rwandan genocide. *J Clin Psychiatry* 71, 543–547.

Kolassa IT, Kolassa S, Ertl V et al. (2010b) The risk of posttraumatic stress disorder after trauma depends on traumatic load and the catechol-o-methyltransferase Val(158)Met polymorphism. *Biol Psychiatry* 67, 304–308.

Kremen WS, Koenen KC, Boake C et al. (2007) Pretrauma cognitive ability and risk for posttraumatic stress disorder: a twin study. *Arch Gen Psychiatry* 64, 361–368.

Lanius RA, Frewen PA, Vermetten E et al. (2010) Fear conditioning and early life vulnerabilities: two distinct pathways of emotional dysregulation and brain dysfunction in PTSD. *Eur J Psychotraumatol* 1.

Lappalainen J, Kranzler HR, Malison R et al. (2002) A functional neuropeptide Y Leu7Pro polymorphism associated with alcohol dependence in a large population sample from the United States. *Archiv Gen Psychiatry* 59, 825–831.

Lawford BR, Mc DYR, Noble EP et al. (2003) D2 dopamine receptor gene polymorphism: paroxetine and social functioning in posttraumatic stress disorder. *Eur Neuropsychopharmacol* 13, 313–320.

Lee HJ, Lee MS, Kang RH et al. (2005) Influence of the serotonin transporter promoter gene polymorphism on susceptibility to posttraumatic stress disorder. *Depression Anxiety* 21, 135–139.

Lesch KP, Heils A, Riederer P (1996) The role of neurotransporters in excitotoxicity, neuronal cell death, and other neurodegenerative processes. *J Mol Med (Berl)* 74, 365–378.

Li S, Hursting SD, Davis BJ et al. (2003) Environmental exposure, DNA methylation, and gene regulation: lessons from diethylstilbesterol-induced cancers. *Ann N Y Acad Sci* 983, 161–169.

Logue MW, Baldwin C, Guffanti G et al. (2013) A genome-wide association study of post-traumatic stress disorder identifies the retinoid-related orphan receptor alpha (RORA) gene as a significant risk locus. *Mol Psychiatry* 18, 937–942.

Lyons MJ, Genderson M, Grant MD et al. (2013) Gene-environment interaction of ApoE genotype and combat exposure on PTSD. *Am J Med Genet B Neuropsychiatr Genet* 162b, 762–769.

Lyons MJ, Goldberg J, Eisen SA et al. (1993) Do genes influence exposure to trauma? A twin study of combat. *Am J Med Genet* 48, 22–27.

Manzur M, Ganss R (2009) Regulator of G protein signaling 5: a new player in vascular remodeling. *Trends Cardiovasc Med* 19, 26–30.

May FS, Chen QC, Gilbertson MW et al. (2004) Cavum septum pellucidum in monozygotic twins discordant for combat exposure: relationship to posttraumatic stress disorder. *Biol Psychiatry* 55, 656–658.

McAllister AK (1999) Subplate neurons: a missing link among neurotrophins, activity, and ocular dominance plasticity? *Proc Natl Acad Sci USA* 96, 13600–13602.

McGowan PO, Meaney MJ, Szyf M (2008) Diet and the epigenetic (re)programming of phenotypic differences in behavior. *Brain Res* 1237, 12–24.

McGowan PO, Sasaki A, D'Alessio AC et al. (2009) Epigenetic regulation of the glucocorticoid receptor in human brain associates with childhood abuse. *Nat Neurosci* 12, 342–348.

Mehta D, Binder EB (2012) Gene × environment vulnerability factors for PTSD: the HPA-axis. *Neuropharmacology* 62, 654–662.

Mehta D, Gonik M, Klengel T et al. (2011) Using polymorphisms in FKBP5 to define biologically distinct subtypes of posttraumatic stress disorder: evidence from endocrine and gene expression studies. *Archiv Gen Psychiatry* 68, 901–910.

Mehta D, Klengel T, Conneely KN et al. (2013) Childhood maltreatment is associated with distinct genomic and epigenetic profiles in posttraumatic stress disorder. *Proc Natl Acad Sci USA* 110, 8302–8307.

Mehta D, Menke A, Binder EB (2010) Gene expression studies in major depression. *Curr Psychiatry Rep* 12, 135–144.

Mellman TA, Alim T, Brown DD et al. (2009) Serotonin polymorphisms and posttraumatic stress disorder in a trauma exposed African American population. *Depression Anxiety* 26, 993–997.

Mercer KB, Orcutt HK, Quinn JF et al. (2012) Acute and posttraumatic stress symptoms in a prospective gene x environment study of a university campus shooting. *Archiv Gen Psychiatry* 69, 89–97.

Murgatroyd C, Patchev AV, Wu Y et al. (2009) Dynamic DNA methylation programs persistent adverse effects of early-life stress. *Nat Neurosci* 12, 1559–1566.

Mushtaq D, Ali A, Margoob MA et al. (2012) Association between serotonin transporter gene promoter-region polymorphism and 4- and 12-week treatment response to sertraline in post-traumatic stress disorder. *J Affect Disord* 136, 955–962.

Neylan TC, Sun B, Rempel H et al. (2011) Suppressed monocyte gene expression profile in men versus women with PTSD. *Brain Behav Immun* 25, 524–531.

Noble EP, Blum K, Ritchie T et al. (1991) Allelic association of the D2 dopamine receptor gene with receptor-binding characteristics in alcoholism. *Archiv Gen Psychiatry* 48, 648–654.

O'Donovan A, Sun B, Cole S et al. (2011) Transcriptional control of monocyte gene expression in post-traumatic stress disorder. *Dis Markers* 30, 123–132.

Oberlander TF, Weinberg J, Papsdorf M et al. (2008) Prenatal exposure to maternal depression, neonatal methylation of human glucocorticoid receptor gene (NR3C1) and infant cortisol stress responses. *Epigenetics* 3, 97–106.

Panarelli M, Holloway CD, Fraser R et al. (1998) Glucocorticoid receptor polymorphism, skin vasoconstriction, and other metabolic intermediate phenotypes in normal human subjects. *J Clin Endocrinol Metab* 83, 1846–1852.

Perroud N, Paoloni-Giacobino A, Prada P et al. (2011) Increased methylation of glucocorticoid receptor gene (NR3C1) in adults with a history of childhood maltreatment: a link with the severity and type of trauma. *Transl Psychiatry* 1, e59.

Pietrzak RH, Galea S, Southwick SM et al. (2013) Examining the relation between the serotonin transporter 5-HTTPLR genotype x trauma exposure interaction on a contemporary phenotypic model of posttraumatic stress symptomatology: a pilot study. *J Affect Disord* 148, 123–128.

Pitman RK, Gilbertson MW, Gurvits TV et al. (2006) Clarifying the origin of biological abnormalities in PTSD through the study of identical twins discordant for combat exposure. *Ann NY Acad Sci* 1071, 242–254.

Pratt WB, Toft DO (1997) Steroid receptor interactions with heat shock protein and immunophilin chaperones. *Endocr Rev* 18, 306–360.

Ressler KJ, Mercer KB, Bradley B et al. (2011) Post-traumatic stress disorder is associated with PACAP and the PAC1 receptor. *Nature* 470, 492–497.

Rodgers AB, Morgan CP, Bronson SL et al. (2013) Paternal stress exposure alters sperm microRNA content and reprograms offspring HPA stress axis regulation. *J Neurosci* 33, 9003–9012.

Rusiecki JA, Byrne C, Galdzicki Z et al. (2013) PTSD and DNA Methylation in Select Immune Function Gene Promoter Regions: A Repeated Measures Case-Control Study of U.S. Military Service Members. *Front Psychiatry* 4, 56.

Russo SJ, Murrough JW, Han MH et al. (2012) Neurobiology of resilience. *Nat Neurosci* 15, 1475–1484.

Sapolsky RM, Romero LM, Munck AU (2000) How do glucocorticoids influence stress responses? Integrating permissive, suppressive, stimulatory, and preparative actions. *Endocrin Rev* 21, 55–89.

Sarapas C, Cai G, Bierer LM et al. (2011) Genetic markers for PTSD risk and resilience among survivors of the World Trade Center attacks. *Dis Markers* 30, 101–110.

Sartor CE, Grant JD, Lynskey MT et al. (2012) Common heritable contributions to low-risk trauma, high-risk trauma, posttraumatic stress disorder, and major depression. *Arch Gen Psychiatry* 69, 293–299.

Sartor CE, McCutcheon VV, Pommer NE et al. (2011) Common genetic and environmental contributions to post-traumatic stress disorder and alcohol dependence in young women. *Psychol Med* 41, 1497–1505.

Segman RH, Shefi N, Goltser-Dubner T et al. (2005) Peripheral blood mononuclear cell gene expression profiles identify emergent post-traumatic stress disorder among trauma survivors. *Mol Psychiatry* 10, 500–513, 425.

Shin LM, Bush G, Milad MR et al. (2011) Exaggerated activation of dorsal anterior cingulate cortex during cognitive interference: a monozygotic twin study of posttraumatic stress disorder. *Am J Psychiatry* 168, 979–985.

Shin LM, Wright CI, Cannistraro PA et al. (2005) A functional magnetic resonance imaging study of amygdala and medial prefrontal cortex responses to overtly presented fearful faces in posttraumatic stress disorder. *Arch Gen Psychiatry* 62, 273–281.

Smith AK, Conneely KN, Kilaru V et al. (2011) Differential immune system DNA methylation and cytokine regulation in post-traumatic stress disorder. *Am J Med Genet B Neuropsychiatr Genet* 156b, 700–708.

Stein MB, Jang KL, Taylor S et al. (2002) Genetic and environmental influences on trauma exposure and posttraumatic stress disorder symptoms: a twin study. *Am J Psychiatry* 159, 1675–1681.

Suzuki T, Hara I, Nakano M et al. (2006) Man2C1, an alpha-mannosidase, is involved in the trimming of free oligosaccharides in the cytosol. *Biochem J* 400, 33–41.

Takahara K, Lyons GE, Greenspan DS (1994) Bone morphogenetic protein-1 and a mammalian tolloid homologue (mTld) are encoded by alternatively spliced transcripts which are differentially expressed in some tissues. *The J biol Chem* 269, 32572–32578.

Tambs K, Czajkowsky N, Roysamb E et al. (2009) Structure of genetic and environmental risk factors for dimensional representations of DSM-IV anxiety disorders. *Br J Psychiatry* 195, 301–307.

Tamura G, Olson D, Miron J et al. (2005) Tolloid-like 1 is negatively regulated by stress and glucocorticoids. *Brain Res Mol Brain res* 142, 81–90.

Teicher MH, Samson JA (2013) Childhood maltreatment and psychopathology: A case for ecophenotypic variants as clinically and neurobiologically distinct subtypes. *Am J Psychiatry* 170, 1114–1133.

Telese F, Gamliel A, Skowronska-Krawczyk D et al. (2013) "Seq-ing" insights into the epigenetics of neuronal gene regulation. *Neuron* 77, 606–623.

True WR, Rice J, Eisen SA et al. (1993) A twin study of genetic and environmental contributions to liability for posttraumatic stress symptoms. *Archiv Gen Psychiatry* 50, 257–264.

Uddin M, Aiello AE, Wildman DE et al. (2010) Epigenetic and immune function profiles associated with posttraumatic stress disorder. *Proc Natl Acad Sci USA* 107, 9470–9475.

Uddin M, Chang SC, Zhang C et al. (2013) Adcyap1r1 genotype, posttraumatic stress disorder, and depression among women exposed to childhood maltreatment. *Depress Anxiety* 30, 251–258.

Uddin M, Galea S, Chang SC et al. (2011) Gene expression and methylation signatures of MAN2C1 are associated with PTSD. *Dis Markers* 30, 111–121.

Valente NL, Vallada H, Cordeiro Q et al. (2011) Candidate-gene approach in posttraumatic stress disorder after urban violence: association analysis of the genes encoding serotonin transporter, dopamine transporter, and BDNF. *J Mol Neurosci : MN* 44, 59–67.

van Rossum EF, Roks PH, de Jong FH et al. (2004) Characterization of a promoter polymorphism in the glucocorticoid receptor gene and its relationship to three other polymorphisms. *Clinical Endocrin* 61, 573–581.

van Zuiden M, Geuze E, Willemen HL et al. (2012) Glucocorticoid receptor pathway components predict posttraumatic stress disorder symptom development: a prospective study. *Biol Psychiatry* 71, 309–316.

Wang Z, Baker DG, Harrer J et al. (2011) The relationship between combat-related posttraumatic stress disorder and the 5-HTTLPR/rs25531 polymorphism. *Depression Anxiety* 28, 1067–1073.

Weaver IC, Cervoni N, Champagne FA et al. (2004) Epigenetic programming by maternal behavior. *Nat Neurosci* 7, 847–854.

White MG, Bogdan R, Fisher PM et al. (2012) FKBP5 and emotional neglect interact to predict individual differences in amygdala reactivity. *Genes Brain Behav* 11, 869–878.

White S, Acierno R, Ruggiero KJ et al. (2013) Association of CRHR1 variants and posttraumatic stress symptoms in hurricane exposed adults. *J Anxiety Disord* 27, 678–683.

Wust S, Van Rossum EF, Federenko IS et al. (2004) Common polymorphisms in the glucocorticoid receptor gene are associated with adrenocortical responses to psychosocial stress. *J Clin Endocrinol Metab* 89, 565–573.

Xian H, Chantarujikapong SI, Scherrer JF et al. (2000) Genetic and environmental influences on posttraumatic stress disorder, alcohol and drug dependence in twin pairs. *Drug Alcohol Depend* 61, 95–102.

Xie P, Kranzler HR, Farrer L et al. (2012) Serotonin transporter 5-HTTLPR genotype moderates the effects of childhood adversity on posttraumatic stress disorder risk: a replication study. *Am J Med Genet B Neuropsychiatr Genet* 159b, 644–652.

Xie P, Kranzler HR, Poling J et al. (2009) Interactive effect of stressful life events and the serotonin transporter 5-HTTLPR genotype on posttraumatic stress disorder diagnosis in 2 independent populations. *Arch Gen Psychiatry* 66, 1201–1209.

Xie P, Kranzler HR, Poling J et al. (2010) Interaction of FKBP5 with childhood adversity on risk for post-traumatic stress disorder. *Neuropsychopharmacology* 35, 1684–1692.

Xie P, Kranzler HR, Yang C et al. (2013) Genome-wide association study identifies new susceptibility loci for posttraumatic stress disorder. *Biol Psychiatry* 74, 656–663.

Yehuda R, Bell A, Bierer LM et al. (2008) Maternal, not paternal, PTSD is related to increased risk for PTSD in offspring of Holocaust survivors. *J Psychiatr Res* 42, 1104–1111.

Yehuda R, Cai G, Golier JA et al. (2009) Gene expression patterns associated with posttraumatic stress disorder following exposure to the World Trade Center attacks. *Biol Psychiatry* 66, 708–711.

Yehuda R, Daskalakis NP, Desarnaud F et al. (2013) Epigenetic Biomarkers as Predictors and Correlates of Symptom Improvement Following Psychotherapy in Combat Veterans with PTSD. *Front Psychiatry* 4, 118.

Yehuda R, Golier JA, Yang RK et al. (2004) Enhanced sensitivity to glucocorticoids in peripheral mononuclear leukocytes in posttraumatic stress disorder. *Biol Psychiatry* 55, 1110–1116.

Yehuda R, Koenen KC, Galea S et al. (2011) The role of genes in defining a molecular biology of PTSD. *Dis Markers* 30, 67–76.

Young RM, Lawford BR, Noble EP et al. (2002) Harmful drinking in military veterans with post-traumatic stress disorder: association with the D2 dopamine receptor A1 allele. *Alcohol Alcohol* 37, 451–456.

Zannas AS, Binder EB (2014) Gene-environment interactions at the FKBP5 locus: sensitive periods, mechanisms and pleiotropism. *Genes Brain Behav* 13, 25–3.

Zhang H, Ozbay F, Lappalainen J et al. (2006) Brain derived neurotrophic factor (BDNF) gene variants and Alzheimer's disease, affective disorders, posttraumatic stress disorder, schizophrenia, and substance dependence. *Am J Med Genet Part B* 141B, 387–393.

Zieker J, Zieker D, Jatzko A et al. (2007) Differential gene expression in peripheral blood of patients suffering from post-traumatic stress disorder. *Mol Psychiatry* 12, 116–118.

Zimmermann P, Bruckl T, Nocon A et al. (2011) Interaction of FKBP5 gene variants and adverse life events in predicting depression onset: results from a 10-year prospective community study. *Am J Psychiatry* 168, 1107–1116.

CHAPTER 11

Cortisol and the Hypothalamic–Pituitary–Adrenal Axis in PTSD

Amy Lehrner, Nicolaos Daskalakis & Rachel Yehuda
Department of Psychiatry, Icahn School of Medicine at Mount Sinai, New York, NY, USA

11.1 Introduction

Initial conceptualizations of posttraumatic stress disorder (PTSD) framed the condition as a normative response to extremely traumatic events that evoked horror, helplessness, or fear, and that included posttraumatic reactions such as nightmares, intrusive memories, difficulty sleeping, and irritability. Accordingly, initial research focused on a link between PTSD and biological mechanisms associated with stress. The physiological response to acute stress involves the activation of the sympathetic nervous system (SNS) and the release of epinephrine, preparing the organism for "fight, flight or freeze" in response to a perceived threat. The acute stress response also includes activation of the hypothalamic–pituitary–adrenal (HPA) axis, which leads to the release of cortisol, a glucocorticoid. Through negative feedback inhibition at the pituitary, cortisol ultimately acts to contain the stress response and return the body to homeostasis once safety is established. However, early neuroendocrine studies of PTSD found that while catecholamines and corticotropin-releasing factor (CRF) appeared to be elevated in PTSD, cortisol levels were unexpectedly found to be lower than in controls (Bremner et al., 1997; Mason, 1986; Yehuda, 2009).

Hypocortisolism and HPA axis alterations have now been widely associated with PTSD, although there are mixed findings regarding whether these alterations reflect PTSD, trauma exposure, or adverse experiences earlier in development (Morris et al., 2012; Yehuda et al. 2010). The unanticipated direction of cortisol alterations paralleled unexpected epidemiological data showing that only a minority (generally < 10%) of those exposed to trauma develop PTSD (Breslau, 2009; Hidalgo & Davidson, 2000; de Vries & Olff, 2009). Indeed, early

Posttraumatic Stress Disorder: From Neurobiology to Treatment, First Edition.
Edited by J. Douglas Bremner.
© 2016 John Wiley & Sons, Inc. Published 2016 by John Wiley & Sons, Inc.

posttraumatic reactions, such as re-experiencing, avoidance and hyperarousal symptoms, are poor at predicting who will ultimately develop PTSD (McFarlane, 1997; Shalev et al., 1997). These findings spurred a reconceptualization of PTSD as a disorder of failed recovery – that is, as a failure of the normative recovery process following trauma exposure (e.g., Yehuda, 1996, 2002).

Biological investigations of PTSD have primarily made use of cross-sectional designs to identify correlates of PTSD and trauma exposure. More recently there has been an increased emphasis on implementing longitudinal designs that can identify pre-existing biological factors that may confer vulnerability, or resilience, to PTSD following trauma. Longitudinal designs are needed to investigate the potential interactions of posttraumatic stress symptoms and HPA axis responsiveness over time. For example, dynamic patterns of decreasing basal cortisol and increasing glucocorticoid sensitivity over time following trauma exposure have been identified in PTSD, highlighting the limitations of static, cross-sectional data (Yehuda et al., 2004; Morris et al., 2012). These patterns suggest that a traumatic experience may trigger initial increases in cortisol that eventually rebound, progressively sensitizing negative feedback inhibition and ultimately leading to hyposecretion of cortisol (Morris et al., 2012; Yehuda, 2002).

11.2 HPA axis and the stress response

The natural biological response to threat or fear involves complex interactions of the SNS and the HPA axis, allowing the organism to both prepare for threat and return to baseline once the threat is removed. The stress reaction is an instinctive, adaptive response to promote survival, and is not an inherently deleterious process. Indeed, the stress response is crucial to the organism's ability to react and adapt to changes in the environment. The HPA axis directs the body's neuroendocrine response to physical and emotional stressors through influences and feedback between the hypothalamus, the anterior pituitary and the cortex of the adrenal glands (Figure 11.1).

In response to a perceived threat, emotional, cognitive, and biological networks are activated, including the limbic system, which then initiates HPA axis activity through the hypothalamus. Parvocellular neurons in the paraventricular nucleus in the hypothalamus synthesize corticotropin-releasing hormone (CRH) and arginine vasopressin (AVP). These in turn stimulate the anterior pituitary gland to release to adrenocorticotropic hormone (ACTH). ACTH is released into the bloodstream and, upon reaching the adrenal cortex, binds to the type 2 melanocortin receptor (MC2R). The binding leads to a fast production and secretion of cortisol, the main glucocorticoid hormone, by the adrenal cortex. The resulting glucocorticoid signaling cascade ultimately acts on the hypothalamus and pituitary in a negative feedback loop, dampening further release of

Figure 11.1 Normal functioning of the hypothalamic–pituitary–adrenal axis. The normal reaction to acute or brief stress or threat involves increases in cortisol and corticotropin-releasing hormone (CRH) and arginine vasopressin (AVP). CRH stimulates the release of adrenocorticotropic hormone (ACTH) from the pituitary, which in turn stimulates the production of cortisol in the adrenal cortex. Cortisol provides negative feedback and inhibits the further release of CRH, AVP and ACTH, leading to the containment of the stress response and return to homeostasis. (*See color plate section for the color representation of this figure.*)

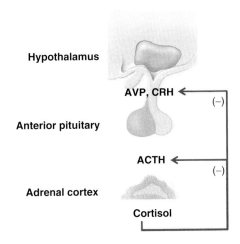

CRH, AVP and ACTH and subsequent release of glucocorticoids (de Kloet et al., 2005).

Glucocorticoid (which includes cortisol in humans and corticosterone in rodents) signaling is mediated by two kinds of receptors: the high-affinity mineralocorticoid receptor (MR) expressed predominantly in the limbic structures and the widely distributed low-affinity glucocortiocoid receptor (GR). MR in the limbic structures, particularly the hippocampus, is in charge of the maintenance of a basal state of stress system activity and is involved in initial phase of the stress response. The GR facilitates the termination of the stress response by negative feedback, and thus is central to the regulation of glucocorticoids levels.

In addition to helping coordinate the stress response system, cortisol is involved in the regulation of metabolic and immune systems. Although the stress response may be adaptive in the short term, if chronically engaged, the resulting allostatic overload may also lead to negative physical and mental health outcomes (McEwen & Wingfield, 2003; McEwen, 2012). HPA axis dysregulation has been associated with behavioral and cognitive deficits and brain changes across a large range of disorders (Chrousos, 2009).

11.3 HPA axis alterations in PTSD

Hypothalamic–pituitary–adrenal axis alterations are one of the most consistent neurobiological findings in PTSD (Mehta & Binder, 2012). Thirty years of biological research has led to evidence of alterations in the HPA axis in PTSD, with findings of lower cortisol and increased glucocorticoid sensitivity that efficiently suppress the HPA axis, leading some afferent pathways to have less exposure to cortisol and thus increased sympathetic activation (de Kloet et al. 2006; Raison &

Miller, 2003; Yehuda, 2002). This results in long-term increases in catecholamine levels that are associated with chronic symptoms of hyperarousal and distress. Such findings explain why patients with chronic PTSD have higher circulating levels of norepinephrine and greater reactivity of adrenergic receptors, as well as lower cortisol (Pervanidou, 2008; Yehuda et al., 1998; Southwick et al., 1999). They also explain why, although cortisol levels at baseline may be lower, enhanced responsiveness of glucocorticoid receptors (GRs) may render the person more responsive, or even hyper-responsive, to some types of provocations. For example, an exaggerated cortisol response to experimentally induced psychological stress has been observed in PTSD (Bremner et al., 2003; Elzinga et al., 2003; de Kloet et al., 2006).

Reduced cortisol in the face of trauma may reflect an adaptation to a hostile environment in which continued threat is anticipated. In this circumstance, low cortisol may facilitate an enhanced and possibly prolonged threat response, without dampening by cortisol induced negative feedback. For example, the chronicity, rather than severity, of intimate partner violence victimization was associated with low cortisol awakening response in sheltered battered women (Johnson et al., 2008). However, the failure to contain sympathetic activation impairs the ability to re-establish homeostasis after the traumatic experience and may interfere with the recovery process, increasing risk for PTSD and comorbid medical conditions related to inflammatory and immunosuppressive processes linked to allostatic load and glucocorticoid function, such as diabetes, fibromyalgia, cardiovascular and gastrointestinal diseases, rheumatoid arthritis, psoriasis, and thyroid disease (Boscarino, 2004; Qureshi et al., 2009).

Importantly, this biological signature differs from that found in response to acute or chronic stress, and in depression, where CRH and cortisol levels are higher, there is less cortisol suppression on the dexamethasone suppression test (DST), and GR responsiveness is reduced (Nemeroff, 1996; Pariante & Miller, 2001). HPA axis alterations in PTSD, including low cortisol, increased glucocorticoid sensitivity, and higher numbers of GRs, in association with higher levels of norepinephrine, CRH, and pro-inflammatory cytokines, are indicative of vulnerabilities in the glucocorticoid signaling pathway (Daskalakis et al., 2013; van Zuiden et al., 2013).

It has been hypothesized that enhanced sympathetic system activation might contribute to an over-consolidation of the trauma memory, as catecholamines and glucocorticoids are known to modulate memory formation (Elzinga et al., 2005; Finsterwald & Alberini, 2013; Roozendaal et al., 2006; van Stegeren, 2008). Prolonged arousal may also increase the likelihood of overgeneralized conditioning to fear-based stimuli. Furthermore, an attenuated cortisol response may contribute to the intensification and entrenchment of PTSD symptoms through the failure to effectively contain subsequent SNS activation in response to memories or traumatic stimuli. This failure could exacerbate intrusive and arousal symptoms, and indirectly contribute to greater avoidance strategies as the individual works harder to minimize the distress caused by trauma reminders (Yehuda, 2009).

11.3.1 Basal cortisol

Mason (1986) was the first to identify lower cortisol levels in PTSD, and numerous PTSD studies have replicated this finding (Yehuda, 2009). For example, low cortisol levels in PTSD have been found in samples of combat veterans (Kanter et al., 2001; de Kloet et al., 2006; Wahbeh & Oken, 2013), war refugees (Rohleder et al., 2004), Holocaust survivors (Yehuda et al., 1995), mothers of child cancer survivors (Glover & Poland, 2002), and adults with a history of childhood emotional (Yehuda et al., 2001) and sexual (Bremner et al., 2007) abuse. Cortisol levels have also been associated with dissociative symptoms in trauma exposed women (Basu et al., 2013), and with posttraumatic symptom severity (Aardal-Eriksson et al., 2001).

While HPA axis alterations have been robustly associated with PTSD, some have failed to observe lower activity (Morris et al., 2012; Zoladz & Diamond, 2013). A number of explanations have been suggested for this, including inconsistencies in defining comparison groups (i.e., allowing trauma exposure histories among control subjects), influences of frequently comorbid conditions such as major depressive disorder (MDD) and substance abuse, sensitivity of cortisol to circadian oscillations, and transient elevations in circulating cortisol in response to stressful experiences and other factors such as food intake, exercise, sex, and memory consolidation (Morris et al., 2012; Yehuda, 2002; van Zuiden et al., 2012). Basal cortisol levels are also affected by age and gender (Morris et al., 2012). Furthermore, cortisol can be measured in saliva, blood, urine, or cerebrospinal fluid, and levels will vary depending on the method of analysis, time of day, and context of the assessment. Cortisol is also synthesized in skin and hair through what has been called a "peripheral HPA axis" (Slominski et al., 2007), and hair cortisol may provide a method for retrospectively investigating chronic cortisol alterations in response to trauma or stress exposure (e.g., Meyer et al., 2012; Stalder & Kirschbaum, 2012; Steudte et al. 2013). However, more data regarding the influences of gender, age, diurnal rhythm, localization, transitory stressors, whether concentrations vary along the hair shaft, and whether they are dynamic or static over time are needed (Sharpley et al., 2011). The failure to observe uniform observations of low cortisol in PTSD is probably a result of the many influences on HPA axis functioning, including the presence of comorbid disorders, a history of previous trauma exposure, and circadian rhythm, as well as the result of methodological differences in the type and timing of assessment (both time of day and time since trauma) and the type of control group used.

A meta-analysis investigating HPA axis indicators related to trauma exposure, PTSD, and MDD pooled data from over 6,000 individuals who participated in

47 independent cross-sectional studies, taking into account the time and type of assessment (Morris et al., 2012). Lower daily cortisol output was uniquely associated with PTSD compared with both non-traumatized and trauma-exposed controls (i.e., trauma-exposed with no PTSD). It could not be concluded from cross-sectional data whether low cortisol represents a prior vulnerability factor, or emerges following trauma exposure and accelerates over time (Morris et al., 2012). Interestingly, trauma-exposed controls showed enhanced negative feedback comparable to those with PTSD. However, trauma-exposed persons had morning cortisol levels and daily cortisol output that were not different from non-traumatized controls. In cross-sectional studies there is the possibility of remitted PTSD that may explain this finding. The meta-analysis also showed lower afternoon cortisol levels for both PTSD and trauma-exposed control groups, but higher levels in the PTSD with MDD group, compared with non-trauma-exposed controls (Morris et al., 2012). Trauma exposure, PTSD, and MDD may therefore associate with different cortisol activity profiles, as was previously demonstrated by a comprehensive chronobiological analysis (Yehuda et al., 1996; see also Pinna et al., 2014).

Different cortisol profiles may also be associated with specific symptoms of PTSD (i.e., numbing vs. hyperarousal). This was shown in a recent longitudinal study of firefighters and police officers, populations at high risk for trauma exposure (Pineles et al., 2012). Low awakening cortisol at baseline was associated with peri-traumatic distress and mood and anxiety symptoms at follow-up, whereas high cortisol at awakening was associated with higher reactivity to a trauma-script at follow-up. These profiles also associated with different emotional and physiological reactivity profiles at baseline.

Importantly, lower levels of cortisol in PTSD do not appear to reflect an underactive HPA axis or functional impairment in the adrenal glands that produce cortisol. Cortisol oscillations due to circadian rhythm patterns, and hormonal responses to stressful provocations in PTSD have both demonstrated that adrenal production of cortisol is not impaired, and may even be exaggerated in some cases (Bremner et al. 2007; Yehuda et al. 1996, 2005a). For example, PTSD patients showed a more rapid decrease of plasma cortisol than healthy controls without PTSD following administration of the anxiogenic cholecystokinin tetrapeptide, indicative of increased glucocorticoid sensitivity (Kellner et al., 2000).

Longitudinal research is needed to capture the biological correlates of what are increasingly recognized as dynamic symptom trajectories in PTSD, with courses that improve or worsen over time, and with delayed onset of symptoms (Bonanno et al., 2012; Pietrzak et al., 2013). Furthermore, treatment-associated symptom change has been shown to affect HPA axis functioning. Olff et al. (2007) observed that, when controlling for depressive symptoms, levels of cortisol increased in responders to brief eclectic psychotherapy for PTSD, while levels decreased for non-responders. Non-responders to treatment for PTSD resulting from the 9/11 World Trade Center terrorist attacks had significant declines in post-treatment cortisol levels that distinguished them from responders (Yehuda et al., 2009). Among combat veterans treated with psychotherapy for PTSD, symptom change over time associated with changes in glucocorticoid sensitivity (Yehuda et al., 2014). Another study showed that treatment with paroxetine resulted in decreased cortisol response to a mental stress task in PTSD patients (Vermetten et al., 2006). Such findings provide some evidence that HPA axis function may change as a result of effective psychotherapy.

Basal cortisol levels may vary as a function of length of time since trauma exposure or onset of disorder (Bremner, 2001). Interestingly, among individuals with PTSD, time since the focal trauma has a moderating effect on cortisol secretion, such that increased HPA activity is observed closer to the trauma, whereas more distal trauma exposure is associated with decreased HPA activity (Morris et al., 2012). This pattern was observed for PTSD, but not for trauma-exposed individuals without PTSD, and thus may specifically reflect a pathogenic process. Similarly, analyses of hair cortisol levels have shown that PTSD is associated with an initial increase in cortisol, followed by a decrease to below baseline levels (Staufenbiel et al., 2013). The influence of time and developmental stage of exposure (i.e., trauma in childhood) point to the importance of longitudinal studies in PTSD, as different factors may be relevant for risk, onset, maintenance, and recovery from PTSD.

11.4 HPA feedback functioning and GR sensitivity

A contributor to reduced cortisol levels or signaling in PTSD is an enhanced negative feedback inhibition at the level of the pituitary, hypothalamus, hippocampus and amygdala. The most widely used measure of HPA feedback activity is the DST, in which cortisol levels are measured before and after oral ingestion of dexamethasone, a synthetic corticosteroid. Greater cortisol suppression on the DST, reflecting an enhanced negative feedback inhibition, has been widely observed in PTSD, although not universally (for reviews, see de Kloet et al., 2006; Yehuda, 2002). Mathematical modeling of urinary cortisol data supports the hypothesis that dysregulation of the negative feedback loop is responsible for low cortisol levels in PTSD (Sriram et al., 2012). This modeling further predicts that the transitions from conditions of health to PTSD and vice-versa are due to a disrupted negative feedback loop. However, meta-analytic analyses have found enhanced negative feedback inhibition in trauma-exposed individuals with and without PTSD, suggesting that enhanced HPA feedback may be a marker of trauma exposure rather than a specific risk factor for the development of the disorder (Klaassens et al., 2012; Morris et al., 2012).

An overly strong negative feedback inhibition in PTSD may result from excessive sensitivity of GRs (Yehuda, 2009). GR changes have been observed following the DST and other HPA axis challenges (e.g., Newport et al. 2004; Yehuda et al. 2002). Increased sensitivity might result in a heightened response to cortisol or, alternatively, in reduced cortisol signaling. In support of the former hypothesis, investigations of glucocorticoid challenge strategies have demonstrated that the administration of exogenous glucocorticoids results in an exaggerated suppression effect in PTSD (Vythilingam et al., 2006; Yehuda et al. 2006). PTSD has also been associated with enhanced glucocorticoid sensitivity assessed by *in vitro* assays of peripheral mononuclear blood cells (PBMCs; Matić et al., 2013; Rohleder et al., 2004; Yehuda et al., 2004), although T cells in veterans with PTSD show decreased glucocorticoid sensitivity compared with combat veterans without PTSD and healthy controls (de Kloet et al., 2007). Such reduced sensitivity in a measure of adaptive immune response was also observed in trauma-exposed veterans compared with non-exposed veterans. Patients with PTSD have also been found to have more GRs than patients with MDD, bipolar mania, PTSD, panic disorder, and schizophrenia (Yehuda et al., 1993). However, other studies have found lower or similar GR numbers in PTSD compared with controls (e.g., de Kloet et al., 2007; Yehuda et al., 2004).

11.5 Gender, PTSD, and HPA axis activity

Despite the fact that men experience more traumatic events than do women, lifetime rates of PTSD are twice as high in women as in men (Breslau, 2002; Breslau et al., 1998; Breslau & Anthony, 2007). Epidemiological research suggests that women have a higher risk of PTSD following violent assault than men, and that prior violent victimization increases risk for PTSD following subsequent, non-violent trauma for women only (Breslau & Anthony, 2007). Psychological theories for these increased rates have been proposed (e.g., the interpersonal nature of many forms of violence against women, gender differences in emotion regulation and cognitive style), but biological investigations of women's heightened vulnerability to PTSD have been limited (Pratchett et al., 2010). Interestingly, basal cortisol levels are lower in healthy women than in men (Van Cauter et al., 1996), and women demonstrate slower glucocorticoid negative feedback than men, a pattern also observed in female rodents (Bangasser, 2013). Under baseline conditions, women show greater expression of CRF, the stress hormone that activates the HPA axis in response to stress, than do men. Animal studies also indicate sex differences in CRF receptor binding, signaling, and trafficking (Bangasser, 2013).

Some gender differences have been observed in biological studies of PTSD. In a small pilot study, women with PTSD have shown lower salivary cortisol levels, which decreased through the afternoon and evening, whereas men with PTSD showed higher levels that increased over time (Freidenberg et al., 2010). This contrasts with a finding in children with PTSD, in which girls demonstrated higher cortisol than boys (Carrion et al., 2002). Higher salivary cortisol levels in response to trauma recollections have recently been associated with post-traumatic re-experiencing symptoms in male, but not female, survivors of the terrorist attacks on the World Trade Center (Dekel et al., 2013). Differences in catecholamines have also been observed. Men, but not women, demonstrated higher levels of catecholamines in relation to PTSD and posttraumatic symptoms (Hawk et al., 2000). Meta-analytic results regarding gender effects have been mixed. In one study, lower plasma cortisol levels were observed in women with PTSD compared with healthy female controls, whereas no differences were found in men (Meewisse et al., 2007). However, alterations in basal and post-DST cortisol associated with trauma exposure, PTSD, and MDD were found in both men and women in a more recent meta-analysis (Morris et al., 2012).

Estrogen may partly account for sex differences in basal cortisol and glucocorticoid negative feedback. Estrogen has been shown to slow negative feedback and GR expression in rodents. Interestingly, animal models show that stress during adolescence (when there is a surge of gonadal hormones) impacts HPA axis reactivity and is associated with different behavioral phenotypes in male and females (Viveros et al., 2012). Sex differences in CRF receptor binding emerge after puberty, implicating gonadal hormones (i.e., estrogen, progesterone, and androgen). Adolescent stress has been associated with higher reactivity in females compared with males in both animal and human research. In addition to its association with HPA axis functioning, estrogen and menstrual cycle position have been linked with intrusive memories (Cheung et al., 2013), fear inhibition, and extinction (Glover et al., 2012, 2013), and the development of posttraumatic stress symptoms following sexual assault (Ferree et al., 2012).

11.6 HPA alterations as a risk factor for PTSD

11.6.1 Basal cortisol

A critical question in PTSD research concerns why only a minority of trauma-exposed persons develop PTSD. Prospective studies increasingly suggest that HPA axis alterations associated with PTSD may represent pre-existing characteristics that increase vulnerability to the disorder following trauma exposure (Yehuda, 2009; van Zuiden et al., 2013). Furthermore, such risk factors may be longstanding, or they may emerge in the acute experience of the trauma (i.e., peri-traumatic reactions). For example, studies of individuals admitted to emergency rooms following trauma exposure find that low cortisol in the acute aftermath of trauma predicts the development of PTSD. For example, lower morning salivary (Aardal-Erikson et al., 2001; Ehring et al., 2008; McFarlane et al., 2011) and urinary (Delahanty et al., 2000) cortisol levels following motor vehicle accidents predicted the subsequent development of PTSD. Enhanced cortisol suppression 1 month following the accident was also observed in survivors who developed PTSD compared with those who did not (McFarlane et al., 2011). In contrast with adult findings but consistent with cross-sectional findings of increased HPA axis closer to trauma exposure (Morris et al., 2012), higher urinary cortisol excretion levels in children, particularly boys, admitted to a level 1 trauma center predicted acute PTSD symptoms 6 weeks later (Delahanty et al., 2005). High afternoon and evening salivary cortisol up to 5 days following trauma exposure have also been associated with the development of PTSD (Aardal-Eriksson et al., 2001; Ehring et al., 2008; McFarlane et al., 2011; Pervanidou et al., 2007).

Low serum cortisol or hair cortisol alone post-trauma has not been predictive of PTSD (Bonne et al., 2003; Luo et al., 2012; McFarlane et al., 1997; Shalev et al., 2008), but a history of previous trauma may be associated with low cortisol, which together increase risk for PTSD after a subsequent traumatic experience. For example, the first prospective biological investigation of PTSD obtained plasma cortisol from women in the emergency room immediately after being raped (Resnick et al., 1995). Women with a history of sexual assault had lower cortisol levels and were three times more likely to develop PTSD by the 4-month follow-up than women with no sexual assault history. A recent replication study found that a history of prior assault was associated with reduced serum cortisol in the emergency room following sexual assault, and that assault history and cortisol levels interacted to predict higher initial posttraumatic symptoms with a slower decrease over 6 months (Walsh et al., 2013).

Research on the intergenerational transmission of the effects of trauma provides additional support for the role of low cortisol in increasing risk. Studies of traumatized parents and their offspring have found that parental PTSD is associated with lower offspring cortisol, and increased risk for PTSD among offspring. For example, adult children of Holocaust survivors with PTSD show reduced daily cortisol secretion (Yehuda et al., 2007) and increased glucocorticoid sensitivity (Lehrner et al., 2013) as well as higher rates of PTSD than comparable comparison subjects (Yehuda et al., 2007). Research with women who were pregnant and exposed to the 9/11 terrorist attacks on the World Trade Center also found lower salivary cortisol among the infants whose mothers subsequently developed PTSD compared with those who did not (Yehuda et al., 2005b).

The rapid introduction of cortisol (hydrocortisone in humans or corticosterone in animals) immediately following trauma exposure has been found to reduce the incidence of PTSD and PTSD-like behaviors, providing additional evidence that reduced cortisol in the acute aftermath of trauma increases risk for PTSD (e.g., Delahanty et al., 2013; Schelling et al., 2004a, 2001). Similarly, rats previously treated with a high-dose corticosterone compared with a saline control have demonstrated a reduction in PTSD-like behaviors following a stressor (Cohen et al., 2008).

11.6.2 Glucocorticoid sensitivity

Heightened glucocorticoid sensitivity has been associated with trauma exposure (Morris et al., 2012), concurrent PTSD symptoms (Shalev et al., 2008), and with prospective risk for development of PTSD (van Zuiden et al., 2013). In an emergency room sample, negative feedback inhibition as assessed by the DST in the acute aftermath of trauma was not predictive of PTSD at follow-up, but DST results at 1 month were associated with concurrent PTSD symptoms, suggestive that negative feedback inhibition reflects clinical state rather than conferring vulnerability (Shalev et al., 2008). Furthermore, GR number in PBMCs in the acute aftermath of trauma exposure did not predict PTSD at follow-up. In contrast, recent prospective studies of male military personnel before and after combat zone deployment found that high glucocorticoid sensitivity and higher GR number in PBMCs before deployment predicted high levels of PTSD symptoms 6 months post-deployment (van Zuiden et al., 2011, 2012). This association was observed in a diagnostically heterogeneous sample that included high levels of fatigue and depression, and remained significant when covarying for pre-deployment PTSD, depression, and basal plasma cortisol (van Zuiden et al., 2012). These are the first published findings including pre-trauma baseline data supporting the hypothesis of increased glucocorticoid sensitivity as a pre-existing risk factor for the development of PTSD.

Interestingly, glucocorticoid sensitivity has been differentially associated with specific psychiatric profiles following deployment and trauma exposure. High pre-deployment glucocorticoid responsiveness in T cells predicted increased risk for high PTSD symptoms post-deployment only in the absence of comorbid depressive symptoms, whereas low responsiveness predicted high levels of depression with or without comorbid PTSD (van Zuiden, Heijnen et al., 2012). The predictive value of T-cell glucocorticoid sensitivity was independent of GR number. These results echo the cross-sectional findings reported earlier of differential basal cortisol profiles in association with PTSD and comorbid MDD.

11.7 Genetic and epigenetic influences on GR sensitivity

Findings of HPA axis dysregulation in PTSD have spurred recent research on more "upstream" molecular and genetic factors and pathways that may influence HPA axis functioning and thus the development and maintenance of the disorder (Yehuda et al., 2011). HPA axis regulation is influenced by genetic polymorphisms, epigenetic modifications affecting gene expression, and other transient changes in associated biological processes. Several genes associated with HPA axis function, including the GR (*NR3C1*), the CRH type 1 receptor (*CRHR1*), and FK506 binding protein 5 (*FKBP5*) genes, have been associated with PTSD. FKBP5 is implicated in glucocorticoid sensitivity and has been identified as differentially expressed in PTSD. As a co-chaperone of the GR cellular complex, FKBP5 inhibits the nuclear translocation of bound GR, thereby directly affecting GR sensitivity (Binder 2009). FKBP5 expression is up-regulated by glucocorticoids through glucocorticoid response elements and by glucocorticoid-induced demethylation of the gene (Binder 2009).

Single nucleotide polymorphisms (SNPs) in *CRHR1* have been associated with PTSD symptoms and diagnosis, providing evidence for the relevance of this gene in the development of PTSD. For example, a study of adult hurricane survivors identified an association of two SNPs in *CRHR1*, rs12938031 and rs4792887, with PTSD symptoms, and a third, rs12938031, with PTSD diagnosis (White et al., 2013). A prospective study of 103 children in the acute aftermath of a severe injury found an association of CRHR1 SNP rs12944712 with acute PTSD symptoms and with symptom trajectory over time (Amstadter et al., 2011). Genetic polymorphisms and gene expression of FKBP5, a modulator of GR sensitivity, have also been associated with PTSD in survivors of the 9/11 terrorist attack (Sarapas et al., 2011). Among those who developed PTSD, FKBP5 showed reduced expression, consistent with enhanced GR responsivenesss (Yehuda et al., 2009). PTSD has been associated with an interaction of childhood trauma and polymorphisms of FKBP5 (Binder et al., 2008). No association was found between two GR polymorphisms, N363S and BclI, with PTSD, although individuals with PTSD who were homozygous for BclI GG genotype demonstrated higher glucocorticoid sensitivity and more severe symptoms (Bachmann et al., 2005). However, van Zuiden et al. (2012) found an interaction of childhood trauma with the GR haplotype BclI, resulting in an increase in GR number.

Initial optimism regarding the identification of genetic risk factors for psychiatric disorders spurred by technological advances in genome-wide sequencing has shifted in response to limited findings and a recognition of the multifactorial nature of mental disorders. There is an increasing interest in epigenetic mechanisms, which represent flexible adaptations to environmental stimuli, as a potential source of vulnerability or resilience. Epigenetic changes are modifications to the genome but not to the DNA sequence, such as DNA methylation and histone acetylation, which influence the expression and function of genes, (Kim et al., 2009). Such mechanisms may define pathways through which environmental influences (such as childhood abuse or trauma exposure, or conversely, the presence of social support) alter the expression of a gene, providing a molecular basis for individual differences in a gene-related function, and potentially, vulnerability to disorder (Szyf et al., 2008; Toyokawa et al., 2012; Yehuda, 2009). Animal models have demonstrated that early life events, such as differences in maternal care, influence the expression of genes that regulate HPA activity through DNA methylation (Meaney, 2001). These findings are consistent with findings that adverse early life events, such as child abuse, are associated with both later PTSD and HPA alterations that characterize PTSD (Yehuda et al., 2010a).

Recent attention has focused on epigenetic programming of two genes central to glucocorticoid functioning, the NR3C1 (GR) gene and FKBP5. The GR gene has been shown to be differentially methylated in the rat hippocampus based on variations in maternal care, and in human hippocampal post-mortem tissue in association with child abuse. Childhood adversity is associated with increased methylation of the GR gene in adult lymphocytes (Perroud et al., 2011; Tyrka et al., 2012). Lower methylation of the NR3C1 1F promoter has been observed in combat veterans with PTSD compared with similarly exposed veterans who never developed PTSD (Yehuda et al., 2015a). Binder et al. (2008) have reported an association of FKBP5 intron 7 methylation and child abuse, and have specifically identified allele-specific DNA methylation of FKBP5 as increasing risk for stress-related psychiatric disorders in individuals exposed to childhood abuse (Klengel et al., 2013; for recent reviews of the relationship of early life adversity, PTSD, & epigenetics, see Skelton et al., 2012; Yehuda et al., 2010b; Zovkic et al., 2013).

In a genome-wide gene expression study in World Trade Center survivors, FKBP5 was differentially expressed in current PTSD compared with trauma-exposed/no PTSD and past PTSD groups, suggesting that FKBP5 gene expression may be a state marker of current PTSD status. The FKBP5 gene was also detected as differentially expressed in a genome-wide analysis of acute PTSD (Yehuda et al., 2009; Sarapas et al., 2011). Methylation of glucocorticoid-related genes may be differentially associated with risk or symptom severity. Higher levels of methylation of the GR gene (NR3C1) exon 1F promoter in veterans with PTSD at pre-treatment distinguished those who responded to trauma-focused psychotherapy from those who did not, whereas methylation of the FKBP5 gene (FKBP51) exon 1 promoter region decreased in association with recovery from PTSD (Yehuda et al., 2013) (Figure 11.2). In a separate study of veterans with PTSD, changes in symptom severity following treatment were associated with changes in glucocorticoid sensitivity (Yehuda et al., 2014).

11.8 Modifying glucocorticoid responsiveness: implications for prevention and treatment

If the HPA axis alterations observed in PTSD are mutable, they may represent potential treatment targets. These may be "downstream" targets such as cortisol, or more "upstream" targets such as DNA methylation. Primary prevention

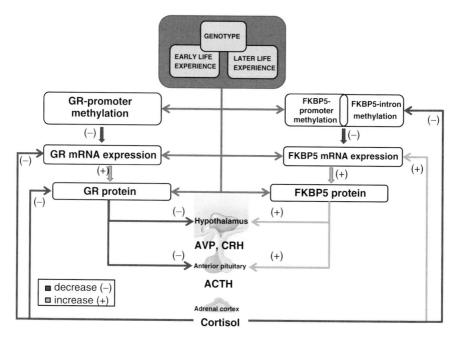

Figure 11.2 Conceptual model of hypothalamic–pituitary–adrenal axis regulation by glucocorticoid receptor (GR) and FK506 binding protein 5 (FKBP5). Early life experience (e.g., adversity) and later life stressors (e.g., trauma) may influence GR and FKBP5 methylation; these influences may interact with genotype to increase risk. Higher GR responsiveness and lower cortisol in PTSD may result from lower GR methylation and expression. Low cortisol levels probably contribute to higher *FKBP5* methylation and lower *FKBP5* gene expression, corresponding to lower *FKBP5* protein expression, and ultimately more GR responsiveness (glucocorticoid negative feedback) at the hypothalamus and pituitary. Green arrows indicate a positive influence (+) and red arrows a negative influence (−). Blue arrows depict a relationship. GR encoded by the *NR3C1* gene, *FKBP5* FK506 binding protein 5 encoded by the *FKBP5* gene. CRH, corticotropin-releasing hormone; AVP, arginine vasopressin; ACTH, adrenocorticotropic hormone. (*See color plate section for the color representation of this figure.*)

(i.e., to prevent the occurrence of the disorder) could include interventions either prior to or in the acute aftermath of trauma exposure in order to strengthen or boost the stress response system, thereby enhancing resilience. Interventions to increase circulating cortisol through treatment with glucocorticoids have been investigated as a potential preventative intervention (Yehuda, 2009). For example, preclinical studies have demonstrated that the administration of corticosterone prior to stress exposure reduces anxiety-like behavior in rats (Cohen et al., 2006; Rao et al., 2012). Because glucocorticoids have been shown to impair memory retrieval in animals and humans and have been implicated in fear extinction in animal models (de Bitencourt et al., 2013), it has been suggested that increasing cortisol may attenuate or prevent PTSD symptoms by disrupting memory consolidation or enhancing extinction of fear memories (de Bitencourt et al., 2013; Steckler & Risbrough, 2012).

Given findings in PTSD of high glucocorticoid sensitivity, an alternative approach is the use of GR antagonists to increase circulating cortisol levels. Animal studies have demonstrated that blocking molecular mechanisms implicated in HPA activity, thereby preventing an enhanced stress response, prevents the development of enhanced fear response and PTSD-like effects following stress exposure (Adamec et al., 1997, 2010; Kohda et al., 2007). However, findings of low cortisol in PTSD suggest that interventions to suppress HPA activity might in fact increase risk for PTSD by prolonging the SNS response. An important consideration regarding any pre-exposure prophylaxis is the potential impact of the intervention on the adaptive responses of individuals under extreme stress and threat (Fletcher et al., 2010).

Early intervention in the acute aftermath of trauma has been more widely investigated. In animals, a single, high dose of corticosterone in the immediate aftermath of predator scent stress leads to a reduction of PTSD-like behaviors in rats 30 days later (Cohen et al., 2008). Similar results have been demonstrated in humans. A fortuitous observation of reduced rates of PTSD in patients who received high doses of hydrocortisone in the context of a critical illness requiring hospitalization in an intensive care unit spurred further investigations of the potential effectiveness of hydrocortisone as a preventative intervention (Schelling et al., 1999, 2004b). A few clinical trials have provided preliminary support for such early intervention with hydrocortisone. In a randomized, double-blind study of septic shock patients, those treated with hydrocortisone had a significantly lower rate of PTSD approximately 2.5 years later than those given placebo (Schelling et al., 2001). High doses of hydrocortisone, compared with placebo, administered during cardiac surgery led to fewer posttraumatic stress symptoms and improved physical and mental health quality of life scores at 6 months follow-up (Weis et al., 2006). A qualification in the interpretation of these findings is that the effectiveness of hydrocortisone may have been partly due to its impact on the severe medical conditions of these patients, which could have attenuated the stressfulness of their experience.

However, initial studies with accident victims demonstrate similar results. For example, the administration of a single, high-dose bolus of hydrocortisone to victims within 6 hours of a trauma reduced the risk for the development of subsequent PTSD (Zohar et al., 2011). Similarly, a clinical trial of low-dose hydrocortisone treatment initiated within 12 hours of a traumatic injury led to fewer posttraumatic stress symptoms and lower rates of PTSD (Delahanty et al., 2013). These studies support the hypothesis that there is a "window of opportunity" for PTSD prophylaxis following a traumatic experience. Such findings support the theory that an increase in glucocorticoids, either preceding or immediately following a traumatic stressor, confers protection against the development of PTSD symptoms.

Glucocorticoids, including metyrapone, corticosterone, dexamethasone, spironolactone, and mifepristone, are also being investigated as possible treatments for PTSD. Such interventions are being tested alone and in conjunction with trauma-focused psychotherapy, based on evidence that glucocorticoids may enhance extinction learning in exposure therapies (Bentz et al., 2010; de Kleine et al, 2013). For example, a small pilot study of treatment with mifepristone for 1 week in combat veterans with PTSD found significant reductions in symptom severity at 1 month follow-up (Golier et al., 2012). A case report of glucocorticoid augmentation of prolonged exposure (PE) therapy described an accelerated improvement and greater decline in PTSD symptoms in the patient treated with hydrocortisone (Yehuda et al., 2010a). A randomized trial of hydrocortisone augmentation of PE therapy with combat veterans found that hydrocortisone administered 30 minutes prior to imaginal exposure may improve treatment retention (Yehuda et al., 2015b). Furthermore, augmentation was most effective among veterans with the highest levels of pre-treatment glucocorticoid sensitivity, suggesting that individuals with elevated pre-treatment sensitivity were most likely to respond to augmented trauma-focused therapy targeting glucocorticoid sensitivity. Glucocorticoids have also been found to enhance response to exposure therapy in phobic patients treated with cortisol prior to each session (de Quervain et al., 2011).

Glucocorticoid-driven memory impairment may also function to interrupt the reconsolidation of trauma memories that may happen as a result of re-experiencing symptoms such as intrusive memories and flashbacks. For example, a double-blind study of combat veterans demonstrated a temporary (<1 month) reduction of avoidance symptoms in those treated with hydrocortisone following imagery-triggered memory reactivation (Surís et al., 2010). A small case–control study found that a low dose of cortisol may reduce the severity of trauma memories (Aerni et al., 2004). Glucocorticoid treatment may thus function to prevent PTSD as well as to treat memory-dependent symptoms (e.g., re-experiencing symptoms) in patients with established PTSD. Randomized, double-blind studies of medication-enhanced psychotherapy using mifepristone and hydrocortisone are currently ongoing, as are prevention studies of hydrocortisone administered subsequent to trauma exposure (Dunlop et al., 2012).

Finally, treatment with oxytocin, a neuropeptide associated with glucocorticoid signaling as well as other processes associated with PTSD, has been investigated as a preventative and early intervention strategy (Olff, 2012). Administration of oxytocin has been associated with reduced PTSD-like behaviors, decreased GR translocation in the hippocampus, an increase in corticosterone following a stressor, and a faster return to baseline in a preclinical study (Cohen et al., 2010), but has also been associated with delayed fear extinction in rats (Eskandarian et al., 2013; Toth et al., 2012). Treatment with oxytocin in humans has been associated with attenuated physiological arousal to trauma cues and acute PTSD symptoms, and the facilitation of fear extinction in healthy controls (Acheson et al., 2013; Pitman et al., 1993).

Blood-based biomarkers of PTSD may ultimately be important in the development of individualized approaches to treatment (Lehrner & Yehuda, 2014; Schmidt et al., 2013) and correlate with brain signaling (Daskalakis et al., 2014). For example, some markers may predict who will benefit from different forms of treatment. The BCLI polymorphism of the GR gene, higher bedtime salivary cortisol and higher 24 h urinary cortisol excretion all predicted treatment gains in veterans with PTSD (Yehuda et al., 2014). As noted earlier, in veterans treated with PE, pre-treatment methylation of the GR gene (NR3C1) exon 1F promoter predicted treatment outcome (Yehuda et al., 2013). Findings suggestive of epigenetic regulation of glucocorticoid functioning in PTSD may also hold promise for the development of novel treatment targets or to help match patients to treatments. The pharmacological manipulation of DNA by histone demethyltransferases, histone deacetylases and other enzymes that affect the epigenome is an emerging field ("pharmaco-epigenetics"). For example, Weaver et al. (2005) have demonstrated a reversal of maternal programming of stress responses in adult rat offspring through methyl supplementation. Selective DNA methyltransferases or other nuclear enzymes can augment methylation or otherwise affect the epigenome to produce an increase in cytosine methylation (Bestor, 2000) and a decrease in GR gene transcription. This might be one mechanism of directly diminishing GR sensitivity and elevating basal circulating cortisol. Recently, Smith et al. (2011) demonstrated differential immune system DNA methylation and cytokine regulation in PTSD which might be related to HPA axis alterations. Currently available antidepressants such as escitalopram, fluoxetine, amitriptyline and imipramine have been shown to diminish methylation or increase histone acetylation (but not necessarily of the GR) (Tsankova et al., 2006, 2007; Robison et al., 2014). Furthermore, imipramine and resilience to social defeat stress, a putative animal model for PTSD/depression, exhibit a similar "epigenetic signature" on chromatin regulation (Wilkinson et al., 2009). New technical and analytic methods are rapidly advancing our understanding of epigenetic processes in conferring vulnerability and maintaining PTSD, but the translation of these findings to therapeutic interventions remains a goal for the future (McGowan, 2013).

11.9 Conclusion

Hypothalamic–pituitary–adrenal axis alterations, including low cortisol, enhanced negative feedback inhibition, and increased glucocorticoid sensitivity have been identified in PTSD. Cross-sectional and prospective studies are suggestive of a hypoactive HPA axis, leading to an elevated and prolonged SNS arousal to a threat and impairment in returning to baseline. These alterations may exist prior to trauma exposure and confer risk for development of PTSD, and they may also reflect the pathophysiology of ongoing PTSD symptoms. While there are individual differences in basal cortisol levels and HPA axis sensitivity, experiences throughout development may alter the "set point" in this dynamic system. Prior or chronic traumatic experiences, in childhood or adulthood, may sensitize the HPA axis and increase vulnerability to subsequent traumas. An elevated or prolonged response to trauma may lead to adaptations in the system that result in an attenuated cortisol response and sluggish HPA axis in response to later trauma (Morris et al., 2012). As PTSD is increasingly recognized to be a dynamic disorder, with varied symptom trajectories, biological correlates are also understood to be less static, and more dynamic, than initially conceived.

Technical and analytic advances in methods for investigation of genetic and epigenetic mechanisms hold promise for more complex, and more integrated, models of PTSD that incorporate neuroendocrine mechanisms with other biological pathways and networks. Glucocorticoids are implicated in inflammatory and immunosuppressive processes, and systems biology approaches that include metabolomics, proteomics, and genomics (i.e., "omics" approaches) represent the cutting edge of PTSD research (Neylan et al., 2014). Future research that incorporates a wide range of cellular and molecular indicators may identify more stable, "upstream" mechanisms that drive more variable functional neuroendocrine markers.

Translation of research findings on HPA axis functioning in PTSD to prevention and treatment is in the early stages. Glucocorticoids have been used as therapeutic agents prior to and in the immediate aftermath of trauma exposure, and they are currently being tested as stand-alone treatments or as supplements to trauma-focused psychotherapy. Successful psychotherapy has also been shown to impact biological markers of PTSD, an encouraging indication that physiological correlates of the disorder are malleable. The further elaboration of HPA axis dysfunction in PTSD, ideally through longitudinal research with heterogeneous populations, has the potential to ultimately inform treatment planning and the development of new pharmacological and psychological interventions.

References

Aardal–Eriksson E, Eriksson TE, Thorell LH (2001) Salivary cortisol, posttraumatic stress symptoms, and general health in the acute phase and during 9-month follow-up. *Biol Psychiatry* Dec 15;50, 986–93.

Acheson D, Feifel D, de Wilde S et al. (2013) The effect of intranasal oxytocin treatment on conditioned fear extinction and recall in a healthy human sample. *Psychopharmacology* 229, 199–208.

Aerni A, Traber R, Hock C et al. (2004) Low-dose cortisol for symptoms of posttraumatic stress disorder. *Am J Psychiatry* 161, 1488–90.

Amstadter AB, Nugent NR, Yang BZ et al. (2011) Corticotrophin-releasing hormone type 1 receptor gene (CRHR1) variants predict posttraumatic stress disorder onset and course in pediatric injury patients. *Dis Markers* 30(2–3), 89–99.

Bangasser DA. Sex differences in stress-related receptors: "micro" differences with "macro" implications for mood and anxiety disorders. *Biol Sex Differ* 4, 2.

Basu A, Levendosky AA, Lonstein JS (2013) Trauma sequelae and cortisol levels in women exposed to intimate partner violence. *Psychodyn Psychiatry* 41, 247–75.

Bentz D, Michael T, de Quervain DJ et al. (2010) Enhancing exposure therapy for anxiety disorders with glucocorticoids: from basic mechanisms of emotional learning to clinical applications. *J Anxiety Disord* 24, 223–30.

Bestor TH (2000) The DNA methyltransferases of mammals. *Hum Mol Genet* 9, 2395–2402.

Binder EB, Bradley RG, Liu W et al. (2008) Association of FKBP5 polymorphisms and childhood abuse with risk of posttraumatic stress disorder symptoms in adults. *JAMA* 299, 1291–305.

Binder EB (2009) The role of fkbp5, a co-chaperone of the glucocorticoid receptor in the pathogenesis and therapy of affective and anxiety disorders. *Psychoneuroendocrinology* 34 Suppl 1, S186–195.

Bonanno GA, Mancini AD, Horton JL et al. (2012) Trajectories of trauma symptoms and resilience in deployed U.S. military service members: prospective cohort study. *Br J Psychiatry* 200, 317–23.

Bonne O, Brandes D, Segman R et al. (2003) Prospective evaluation of plasma cortisol in recent trauma survivors with posttraumatic stress disorder. *Psychiatry Res* 119(1–2), 171–5.

Boscarino JA (2004) Posttraumatic stress disorder and physical illness: results from clinical and epidemiologic studies. *Ann NY Acad Sci* 1032, 141–53.

Bremner JD, Licinio J, Darnell A et al. (1997) Elevated CSF corticotropin-releasing factor concentrations in posttraumatic stress disorder. *Am J Psychiatry* 154, 624–9.

Bremner JD, Vermetten E, Kelley ME (2007) Cortisol, dehydroepiandrosterone, and estradiol measured over 24 hours in women with childhood sexual abuse-related posttraumatic stress disorder. *J Nerv Ment Dis* 195, 919–927.

Bremner JD, Vythilingam M, Vermetten E et al. (2003b) Cortisol response to a cognitive stress challenge in posttraumatic stress disorder (PTSD) related to childhood abuse. *Psychoneuroendocrinology* 28, 733–50.

Bremner JD (2001) Hypotheses and controversies related to effects of stress on the hippocampus: an argument for stress-induced damage to the hippocampus in patients with posttraumatic stress disorder. *Hippocampus* 11, 75–81.

Breslau N, Anthony JC (2007) Gender differences in the sensitivity to posttraumatic stress disorder: An epidemiological study of urban young adults. *J Abnorm Psychol* 116, 607–11.

Breslau N, Davis GC, Andreski P et al. Traumatic events and posttraumatic stress disorder in an urban population of young adults. *Arch Gen Psychiatry* 48, 216–222.

Breslau N, Kessler RC, Chilcoat HD et al. Trauma and posttraumatic stress disorder in the community: the 1996 Detroit Area Survey of Trauma. *Arch Gen Psychiatry* 55, 626–32.

Breslau N (2002) Gender differences in trauma and posttraumatic stress disorder. *J Gend Specif Med* 5, 34–40.

Breslau N (2009) The epidemiology of trauma, PTSD, and other posttrauma disorders. *Trauma Violence Abuse* 10, 198–210.

Carrion VG, Weems CF, Ray RD et al. (2002) Diurnal salivary cortisol in pediatric posttraumatic stress disorder. *Biol Psychiatry* 51, 575–82.

Cheung J, Chervonsky L, Felmingham KL et al. (2013) The role of estrogen in intrusive memories. *Neurobiol Learn Mem* 106C, 87–94.

Chrousos GP (2009) Stress and disorders of the stress system. *Nat Rev Endocrinol* 5, 374–381.

Cohen H, Kaplan Z, Kozlovsky N et al. (2010) Hippocampal microinfusion of oxytocin attenuates the behavioural response to stress by means of dynamic interplay with the glucocorticoid-catecholamine responses. *J Neuroendocrinol* 22, 889–904.

Cohen H, Matar MA, Buskila D et al. (2008) Early post-stressor intervention with high-dose corticosterone attenuates posttraumatic stress response in an animal model of posttraumatic stress disorder. *Biol Psychiatry* 64, 708–17.

Cohen H, Zohar J, Gidron Y et al. (2006) Blunted HPA axis response to stress influences susceptibility to posttraumatic stress response in rats. *Biol Psychiatry* 59, 1208–18.

Daskalakis NP, Lehrner A, Yehuda R (2013) Endocrine aspects of post-traumatic stress disorder and implications for diagnosis and treatment. *Endocrinol Metab Clin North Am* 42, 503–13.

Daskalakis NP, Cohen H, Cai G et al. (2014). Expression profiling associates blood and brain glucocorticoid receptor signaling with trauma-related individual differences in both sexes. *Proc Natl Acad Sci USA* 111, 13529–13534.

de Bitencourt RM, Pamplona FA, Takahashi RN (2013) A current overview of cannabinoids and glucocorticoids in facilitating extinction of aversive memories:potential extinction enhancers. *Neuropharmacology* 64, 389–95.

de Kleine RA, Rothbaum BO, van Minnen A (2013) Pharmacological enhancement of exposure-based treatment in PTSD: a qualitative review. *Eur J Psychotraumatol* Oct 17, 4.

de Kloet CS, Vermetten E, Bikker A et al. (2007) Leukocyte glucocorticoid receptor expression and immunoregulation in veterans with and without post-traumatic stress disorder. *Mol Psychiatry* 12, 443–53.

de Kloet CS, Vermetten E, Geuze E et al. (2006) Assessment of HPA-axis function in posttraumatic stress disorder: pharmacological and non-pharmacological challenge tests, a review. *J Psychiatr Res* 40, 550–67.

de Kloet ER, Joëls M, Holsboer F (2005) Stress and the brain: from adaptation to disease. *Nat Rev Neurosci* 6, 463–75.

de Quervain DJ, Bentz D, Michael T et al. (2011) Glucocorticoids enhance extinction-based psychotherapy. *Proc Natl Acad Sci USA* 108, 6621–5.

de Vries GJ, Olff M (2009) The lifetime prevalence of traumatic events and posttraumatic stress disorder in the Netherlands. *J Trauma Stress* 22, 259–67.

Dekel S, Ein–Dor T, Gordon KM et al. (2013) Cortisol and PTSD Symptoms Among Male and Female High-Exposure 9/11 Survivors. *J Trauma Stress* 26, 621–625.

Delahanty DL, Gabert–Quillen C, Ostrowski SA et al. (2013) The efficacy of initial hydrocortisone administration at preventing posttraumatic distress in adult trauma patients: a randomized trial. *CNS Spectr* 18, 103–11.

Delahanty DL, Nugent NR, Christopher NC et al. (2005) Initial urinary epinephrine and cortisol levels predict acute PTSD symptoms in child trauma victims. *Psychoneuroendocrinology* 30, 121–8.

Delahanty DL, Raimonde AJ, Spoonster E (2000) Initial posttraumatic urinary cortisol levels predict subsequent PTSD symptoms in motor vehicle accident victims. *Biol Psychiatry* 48, 940–7.

Dunlop BW, Mansson E, Gerardi M (2012) Pharmacological innovations for posttraumatic stress disorder and medication- enhanced psychotherapy. *Curr Pharm Des* 18, 5645–58.

Ehring T, Ehlers A, Cleare AJ et al. (2008) Do acute psychological and psychobiological responses to trauma predict subsequent symptom severities of PTSD and depression? *Psychiatry Res* 161, 67–75.

Elzinga BM, Bakker A, Bremner JD (2005) Stress-induced cortisol elevations are associated with impaired delayed, but not immediate recall. *Psychiatry Res* 134, 211–223.

Elzinga BM, Schmahl CS, Vermetten E et al. (2003) Higher cortisol levels following exposure to traumatic reminders in abuse-related PTSD. *Neuropsychopharmacology* 28, 1656–1665.

Eskandarian S, Vafaei AA, Vaezi GH et al. (2013) Effects of systemic administration of oxytocin on contextual fear extinction in a rat model of post-traumatic stress disorder. *Basic Clin Neurosci* 4, 315–22.

Ferree NK, Wheeler M, Cahill L (2012) The influence of emergency contraception on post-traumatic stress symptoms following sexual assault. *J Forensic Nurs* 8, 122–30.

Finsterwald C, Alberini CM (2013) Stress and glucocorticoid receptor-dependent mechanisms in long-term memory: From adaptive responses to psychopathologies. *Neurobiol Learn Mem* 112, 17–29.

Fletcher S, Creamer M, Forbes D (2010) Preventing post traumatic stress disorder: are drugs the answer? *Aust NZ J Psychiatry* 44, 1064–71.

Freidenberg BM, Gusmano R, Hickling EJ et al. (2010) Women with PTSD have lower basal salivary cortisol levels later in the day than do men with PTSD: a preliminary study. *Physiol Behav* 99, 234–6.

Glover DA, Poland RE (2002) Urinary cortisol and catecholamines in mothers of child cancer survivors with and without PTSD. *Psychoneuroendocrinology* 27, 805–19.

Glover EM, Jovanovic T, Mercer KB et al. (2012) Estrogen levels are associated with extinction deficits in women with posttraumatic stress disorder. *Biol Psychiatry* 72, 19–24.

Glover EM, Mercer KB, Norrholm SD et al. (2013) Inhibition of fear is differentially associated with cycling estrogen levels in women. *J Psychiatry Neurosci* 38, 341–8.

Golier JA, Caramanica K, Demaria R et al. (2012) A pilot study of mifepristone in combat-related PTSD. *Depress Res Treat*, 393251.

Hawk LW, Dougall AL, Ursano RJ et al. (2000) Urinary catecholamines and cortisol inrecent-onset posttraumatic stress disorder after motor vehicle accidents. *Psychosom Med* 62, 423–34.

Hidalgo RB, Davidson JR (2000) Posttraumatic stress disorder: epidemiology and health-related considerations. *J Clin Psychiatry* 61 Suppl 7, 5–13.

*Hongrong Luo, Xun Hu, Xiang Liu et al. (2012) Hair cortisol level as a biomarker for altered hypothalamic-pituitary-adrenal activity in female adolescents with posttraumatic stress disorder after the 2008 Wenchuan Earthquake. *Biol Psychiatry* 72, 65–69.

Johnson DM, Delahanty DL, Pinna K (2008) The cortisol awakening response as a function of PTSD severity and abuse chronicity in sheltered battered women. *J Anxiety Disord* 22, 793–800.

Kanter ED, Wilkinson CW, Radant AD et al. (2001) Glucocorticoid feedback sensitivity and adrenocortical responsiveness in posttraumatic stress disorder. *Biol Psychiatry* 50, 238–45.

Kellner M, Wiedemann K, Yassouridis A et al. (2000) Behavioral and endocrine response to cholecystokinin tetrapeptide in patients with posttraumatic stress disorder. *Biol Psychiatry* 47, 107–11.

Kendall-Tackett KA (2000) Physiological correlates of childhood abuse: chronic hyperarousal in PTSD, depression, and irritable bowel syndrome. *Child Abuse Negl* 24, 799–810.

Kim JK, Samaranayake M, Pradhan S. (2009) Epigenetic mechanisms in mammals. *Cell Mol Life Sci* 66, 596–612.

Klaassens ER, Giltay EJ, Cuijpers P et al. (2012) Adulthood trauma and HPA-axis functioning in healthy subjects and PTSD patients: a meta-analysis. *Psychoneuroendocrinology* 37, 317–31.

Klengel T, Mehta D, Anacker C, et al. (2013) Allele-specific *FKBP5* DNA demethylation mediates gene–childhood trauma interactions. *Nat Neurosci* 16, 33–41.

Lehrner A, Bierer LM, Passarelli V et al. (2014) Maternal PTSD associates with greater glucocorticoid sensitivity in offspring of Holocaust survivors. *Psychoneuroendocrinology* 40, 213–20.

Lehrner A, Yehuda R (2014) Biomarkers of PTSD: military applications and considerations. *Eur J Psychotraumatol* 5.

Luo H, Hu X, Liu X et al. (2012) Hair cortisol level as a biomarker for altered hypothalamic-pituitary-adrenal activity in female adolescents with posttraumatic stress disorder after the 2008 Wenchuan earthquake. *Biol Psychiatry* 72, 65–9.

Mason JW, Giller EL, Kosten TR et al. (1986) Urinary free-cortisol levels in posttraumatic stress disorder patients. *J Nerv Ment Dis* 174, 145–9.

Matić G, Milutinović DV, Nestorov J et al. (2013) Lymphocyteglucocorticoid receptor expression level and hormone-binding properties differ between war trauma-exposed men with and without PTSD. *Prog Neuropsychopharmacol Biol Psychiatry Jun* 3;43, 238–45.

McEwen BS, Wingfield JC (2003) The concept of allostasis in biology and biomedicine. *Horm Behav* 43, 2–15. Review.

McEwen BS (2012) Brain on stress: how the social environment gets under the skin. *Proc Natl Acad Sci USA* 109 Suppl 2, 17180–17185. Erratum in: *Proc Natl Acad Sci USA* 110, 1561.

McFarlane AC, Atchison M, Yehuda R (1997) The acute stress response following motor vehicle accidents and its relation to PTSD. *Ann NY Acad Sci* 821, 437–41.

McFarlane AC, Barton CA, Yehuda R et al. (2011) Cortisol response to acute trauma and risk of posttraumatic stress disorder. *Psychoneuroendocrinology* 36, 720–7.

McGowan PO (2013) Epigenomic mechanisms of early adversity and HPA dysfunction: considerations for PTSD research. *Front Psychiatry Sep* 4, 110.

Meaney MJ (2001) Maternal care, gene expression, and the transmission of individual differences in stress reactivity across generations. *Annu Rev Neurosci* 24, 1161–92.

Meewisse ML, Reitsma JB, de Vries GJ et al. (2007) Cortisol and post-traumatic stress disorder in adults: systematic review and meta-analysis. *BrJ Psychiatry* 191, 387–92. Review.

Mehta D, Binder EB (2012) Gene × environment vulnerability factors for PTSD: The HPA-axis. *Neuropharmacology* 62, 654–662.

Meyer JS, Novak MA (2012) Minireview: Hair cortisol: a novel biomarker of hypothalamic-pituitary-adrenocortical activity. *Endocrinology* 153, 4120–7.

Morris MC, Compas BE, Garber J (2012) Relations among posttraumatic stress disorder, comorbid major depression, and HPA function: a systematic review and meta-analysis. *Clin Psychol Rev* 32, 301–15.

Nemeroff CB (1996) The corticotropin-releasing factor (CRF) hypothesis of depression: new findings and new directions. *Mol Psychiatry* 1, 336–42. Review.

Newport DJ, Heim C, Bonsall R et al. (2004) Pituitary-adrenal responses to standard and low-dose dexamethasone suppression tests in adult survivors of child abuse. *Biol Psychiatry* 55, 10–20.

Neylan TC, Schadt EE, Yehuda R (2014) Biomarkers for combat-related PTSD: focus on molecular networks from high-dimensional data. *Eur J Psychotraumatol* Aug 14, 5.

Olff M, de Vries GJ, Güzelcan Y et al. (2007) Changes in cortisol and DHEA plasma levels after psychotherapy for PTSD. *Psychoneuroendocrinology* 32, 619–26.

Olff M (2012) Bonding after trauma: on the role of social support and the oxytocin system in traumatic stress. *Eur J Psychotraumatol* 3.

Pariante CM, Miller AH (2001) Glucocorticoid receptors in major depression: relevance to pathophysiology and treatment. *Biol Psychiatry* 49, 391–404.

Perroud N, Paoloni–Giacobino A, Prada P et al. (2011) Increased methylation of glucocorticoid receptor gene (NR3C1) in adults with a history of childhood maltreatment: a link with the severity and type of trauma. *Transl Psychiatry Dec* 1, e59.

Pervanidou P (2008) Biology of post-traumatic stress disorder in childhood and adolescence. *J Neuroendocrinol* 20, 632–8.

Pietrzak RH, Feder A, Schechter CB et al. (2013) Dimensional structure and course of post-traumatic stress symptomatology in World Trade Center responders. *Psychol Med Dec* 2, 1–14. [Epub 2013 Dec 2]

Pineles SL, Rasmusson AM, Yehuda R et al. (2013) Predicting emotional responses to potentially traumatic events from pre-exposure waking cortisol levels: a longitudinal study of police and firefighters. *Anxiety Stress Coping* 26, 241–53.

Pinna KL, Johnson DM, Delahanty DL. (2014) PTSD, comorbid depression, and the cortisol waking response in victims of intimate partner violence: preliminary evidence. *Anxiety Stress Coping* 27, 253–69.

Pitman RK, Orr SP, Lasko NB (1993) Effects of intranasal vasopressin and oxytocin on physiologic responding during personal combat imagery in Vietnam veterans with posttraumatic stress disorder. *Psychiatry Res* 48, 107–17.

Pratchett LC, Pelcovitz MR, Yehuda R. (2010) Trauma and violence: are women the weaker sex? *Psychiatr Clin North Am* 33, 465–74.

Qureshi SU, Pyne JM, Magruder KM et al. (2009) The link between post-traumatic stress disorder and physical comorbidities: a systematic review. *Psychiatr Q* 80, 87–97.

Raison CL, Miller AH. (2003) When not enough is too much: the role of insufficient glucocorticoid signaling in the pathophysiology of stress-related disorders. *Am J Psychiatry* 160, 1554–65. Review.

Resnick HS, Yehuda R, Pitman RK et al. (1995) Effect of previous trauma on acute plasma cortisol level following rape. *Am J Psychiatry* 152, 1675–7.

Robison AJ, Vialou V, Sun HS et al. (2014). Fluoxetine epigenetically alters the CaMKIIα promoter in nucleus accumbens to regulate ΔFosB binding and antidepressant effects.*Neuropsychopharmacology* 39, 1178–1186.

Rohleder N, Joksimovic L, Wolf JM et al. (2004) Hypocortisolism and increasedglucocorticoid sensitivity of pro-Inflammatory cytokine production in Bosnian war refugees with posttraumatic stress disorder. *Biol Psychiatry* 55, 745–51.

Roozendaal B, Okuda S, de Quervain DJ et al. (2006) Glucocorticoids interact with emotion-induced noradrenergic activation in influencing different memory functions. *Neuroscience* 138, 901–10.

Sarapas C, Cai G, Bierer LM et al. (2011) Genetic markers for PTSD risk and resilience among survivors of the World Trade Center attacks. *Dis Markers* 30(2–3), 101–10.

Schelling G, Briegel J, Roozendaal B et al. (2001) The effect of stress doses of hydrocortisone during septic shock on posttraumatic stress disorder in survivors. *Biol Psychiatry* 50, 978–85.

Schelling G, Kilger E, Roozendaal B et al. (2004b) Stress doses of hydrocortisone, traumatic memories, and symptoms of posttraumatic stress disorder in patients after cardiac surgery: a randomized study. *Biol Psychiatry* 55, 627–33.

Schelling G, Roozendaal B, De Quervain DJ (2004a) Can posttraumatic stress disorder be prevented with glucocorticoids? *Ann NY Acad Sci* 1032, 158–66.

Schelling G, Stoll C, Kapfhammer HP et al. (1999) The effect of stress doses of hydrocortisone during septic shock on posttraumatic stress disorder and health-related quality of life in survivors. *Crit Care Med* 27, 2678–83.

Schmidt U, Kaltwasser SF, Wotjak CT (2013). Biomarkers in posttraumatic stress disorder: overview and implications for future research. *Dis Markers* 35, 43–54.

Shalev AY, Freedman S, Peri T et al.(1997) Predicting PTSD in trauma survivors: prospective evaluation of self-report and clinician-administered instruments. *Br J Psychiatry* 170, 558–64.

Shalev AY, Videlock EJ, Peleg T et al. (2008) Stress hormones and post-traumatic stress disorder in civilian trauma victims: a longitudinal study. Part I: HPA axis responses. *Int J Neuropsychopharmacol* 11, 365–72.

Sharpley CF, McFarlane JR, Slominski A (2011) Stress-linked cortisol concentrations in hair: what we know and what we need to know. *Rev Neurosci Dec* 23, 111–21.

Skelton K, Ressler KJ, Norrholm SD et al.PTSD and gene variants: new pathways and new thinking. *Neuropharmacology* (2012) 62, 628–37.

Slominski A, Wortsman J, Tuckey RC et al. (2007) Differential expression of HPA axis homolog in the skin. *Mol Cell Endocrinol* 265–266, 143–149.

Smith AK, Conneely KN, Kilaru V et al. (2011) Differential immune system DNA methylation and cytokine regulation in post-traumatic stress disorder. *Am J Med Genet* 156, 700–708.

Southwick SM, Bremner JD, Rasmusson A et al. (1999) Role of norepinephrine in the pathophysiology and treatment of posttraumatic stress disorder. *Biol Psychiatry* 46, 1192–204.

Sriram K, Rodriguez–Fernandez M, Doyle FJ 3rd (2012) Modeling cortisol dynamics in the neuro-endocrine axis distinguishes normal, depression, and post-traumatic stress disorder (PTSD) in humans. *PLoS Comput Biol* 8, e1002379.

Stalder T, Kirschbaum C (2012) Analysis of cortisol in hair – state of the art and future directions. *Brain Behav Immun* 26, 1019–29.

Staufenbiel SM, Penninx BW, Spijker AT et al. (2013) Hair cortisol, stress exposure, and mental health in humans: a systematic review. *Psychoneuroendocrinology* 38, 1220–35.

Steckler T, Risbrough V (2012) Pharmacological treatment of PTSD – established and new approaches. *Neuropharmacology* 62, 617–27.

Steudte S, Kirschbaum C, Gao W et al. (2013) Hair cortisol as a biomarker of traumatization in healthy individuals and posttraumatic stress disorder patients. *Biol Psychiatry* 74, 639–46.

Surís A, North C, Adinoff B et al. (2010) Effects of exogenous glucocorticoid on combat-related PTSD symptoms. *Ann Clin Psychiatry* 22, 274–9.

Szyf M, McGowan P, Meaney MJ (2008) The social environment and the epigenome. *Environ Mol Mutagen* 49, 46–60.

Toth I, Neumann ID, Slattery DA (2012) Central administration of oxytocin receptor ligands affects cued fear extinction in rats and mice in a timepoint-dependent manner. *Psychopharmacology (Berl)* 223, 149–58.

Toyokawa S, Uddin M, Koenen KC et al. (2012) How does the social environment 'get into the mind'? Epigenetics at the intersection of social and psychiatric epidemiology. *Soc Sci Med* 74, 67–74.

Tsankova NM, Berton O, Renthal W et al. (2006) Sustained hippocampal chromatin regulation in a mouse model of depression and antidepressant action. *Nature Neurosci* 9, 519–525.

Tsankova, N., Renthal, W., Kumar, A., & Nestler, E. J. (2007). Epigenetic regulation in psychiatric disorders. *Nature Reviews Neuroscience*, 8(5), 355-367.

Tyrka AR, Price LH, Marsit C et al. (2012) Childhood adversity and epigenetic modulation of the leukocyte glucocorticoid receptor: preliminary findings in healthy adults. *PLoS One* 7, e30148.

Van Cauter E, Leproult R, Kupfer DJ (1996) Effects of gender and age on the levels and circadian rhythmicity of plasma cortisol. *J Clin Endocrinol Metab* 81, 2468–73.

van Stegeren AH (2008) The role of the noradrenergic system in emotional memory. *Acta Psychol (Amst)* 127, 532–41.

van Zuiden M, Geuze E, Willemen HL et al. (2011) Pre-existing high glucocorticoid receptor number predicting development of posttraumatic stress symptoms after military deployment. *Am J Psychiatry* 168, 89–96.

van Zuiden M, Geuze E, Willemen HL et al. (2012) Glucocorticoid receptor pathway components predict posttraumatic stress disorder symptom development: a prospective study. *Biol Psychiatry* 71, 309–16.

van Zuiden M, Heijnen CJ, Maas M et al. (2012) Glucocorticoid sensitivity of leukocytes predicts PTSD, depressive and fatigue symptoms after military deployment: A prospective study. *Psychoneuroendocrinology* 37, 1822–36.

van Zuiden M, Kavelaars A, Geuze E et al. (2013) Predicting PTSD: pre-existing vulnerabilities in glucocorticoid-signaling and implications for preventive interventions. *Brain Behav Immun* 30, 12–21.

Vermetten E, Vythilingam M, Schmahl C et al. (2006) Alterations in stress reactivity after long-term treatment with paroxetine in women with posttraumatic stress disorder. *Ann NY Acad Sci* 1071, 80–86.

Viveros MP, Mendrek A, Paus T et al. (2012) A comparative, developmental, and clinical perspectiveof neurobehavioral sexual dimorphisms. *Front Neurosci* 6, 84.

Vythilingam M, Lawley M, Collin C et al. (2006) Hydrocortisone impairs hippocampal-dependent trace eyeblink conditioning in post-traumatic stress disorder. *Neuropsychopharmacology* 31, 182–8.

Wahbeh H, Oken BS (2013) Salivary cortisol lower in posttraumatic stress disorder. *J Trauma Stress* 26, 241–8.

Walsh K, Nugent NR, Kotte A et al. (2013) Cortisol at the emergency room rape visit as a predictor of PTSD and depression symptoms over time. *Psychoneuroendocrinology* 38, 2520–8.

Weaver IC, Champagne FA, Brown SE et al. (2005) Reversal of maternal programming of stress responses in adult offspring through methyl supplementation: altering epigenetic marking later in life. *J Neurosci* 25, 11045–11054.

Weis F, Kilger E, Roozendaal B et al. (2006) Stress doses of hydrocortisone reduce chronic stress symptoms and improve health-related quality of life in high-risk patients after cardiac surgery: a randomized study. *J Thorac Cardiovasc Surg* 131, 277–82.

White S, Acierno R, Ruggiero KJ, Koenen KC, et al. (2013) Association of CRHR1 variants and posttraumatic stress symptoms in hurricane exposed adults. *J Anxiety Disord* 27, 678–83.

Wilkinson MB, Xiao G, Kumar A et al. (2009) Imipramine treatment and resiliency exhibit similar chromatin regulation in the mouse nucleus accumbens in depression models. *J Neurosci* 29, 7820–7832.

Yehuda R, Bierer LM, Pratchett L et al. (2010a) Glucocorticoid augmentation of prolonged exposure therapy: rationale and case report. *Eur J Psychotraumatol* 1.

Yehuda R, Bierer LM, Pratchett LC et al. (2015b) Cortisol augmentation of a psychological treatment for warfighters with posttraumatic stress disorder: Randomized trial showing improved treatment retention and outcome. *Psychoneuroendocrinology* 51, 589–97.

Yehuda R, Boisoneau D, Mason JW et al. (1993) Glucocorticoid receptor number and cortisol excretion in mood, anxiety, and psychotic disorders. *Biol Psychiatry* 34(1–2), 18–25.

Yehuda R, Cai G, Golier JA et al. (2009) Gene expression patterns associated with posttraumatic stress disorder following exposure to the World Trade Center attacks. *Biol Psychiatry* 66, 708–11.

Yehuda R, Daskalakis NP, Desarnaud F et al. (2013) Epigenetic biomarkers as predictors and correlates of symptom improvement following psychotherapy in combat veterans with PTSD. *Front Psychiatry* 4, 118.

Yehuda R, Engel SM, Brand SR et al. (2005) Transgenerational effects of posttraumatic stress disorder in babies of mothers exposed to the World Trade Center attacks during pregnancy. *J Clin Endocrinol Metab* 90, 4115–8.

Yehuda R, Flory JD, Bierer LM et al. (2015a) Lower methylation of glucocorticoid receptor gene promoter 1F in peripheral blood of veterans with posttraumatic stress disorder. *Biol Psychiatry* 77, 356–64.

Yehuda R, Flory JD, Pratchett LC et al. (2010b) *Psychopharmacology (Berl)* 212, 405–17.

Yehuda R, Golier JA, Kaufman S (2005a) Circadian rhythm of salivary cortisol in Holocaust survivors with and without PTSD. *Am J Psychiatry* 162, 998–1000.

Yehuda R, Halligan SL, Grossman R et al. (2002) The cortisol and glucocorticoid receptor response to low dose dexamethasone administration in aging combat veterans and holocaust survivors with and without posttraumatic stress disorder. *Biol Psychiatry Sep* 1;52, 393–403.

Yehuda R, Halligan SL, Grossman R (2001) Childhood trauma and risk for PTSD: relationship to intergenerational effects of trauma, parental PTSD, and cortisol excretion. *Dev Psychopathol* 13, 733–53.

Yehuda R, Kahana B, Binder-Brynes K et al. (1995) Low urinary cortisol excretion in Holocaust survivors with posttraumatic stress disorder. *Am J Psychiatry* 152, 982–6.

Yehuda R, Koenen KC, Galea S et al. (2011) The role of genes in defining a molecular biology of PTSD. *Dis Markers* 30(2–3), 67–76.

Yehuda R, McFarlane AC, Shalev AY (1998) Predicting the development of posttraumatic stress disorder from the acute response to a traumatic event. *Biol Psychiatry* 44, 1305–13.

Yehuda R, Pratchett LC, Elmes MW et al. (2014) Glucocorticoid-related predictors and correlates of post-traumatic stress disorder treatment response in combat veterans. *Interface Focus* 4, 20140048.

Yehuda R, Teicher MH, Trestman RL et al. (1996) Cortisol regulation in posttraumatic stress disorder and major depression: a chronobiological analysis. *Biol Psychiatry* 40, 79–88.

Yehuda R, Yang RK, Buchsbaum MS et al. (2006) Alterations in cortisol negative feedback inhibition as examined using the ACTH response to cortisol administration in PTSD. *Psychoneuroendocrinology* 31, 447–51.

Yehuda R (2002) Current status of cortisol findings in post-traumatic stress disorder. *Psychiatr Clin North Am* 25, 341–68.

Yehuda R (1997) Sensitization of the hypothalamic-pituitary-adrenal axis in posttraumatic stress disorder. *Ann NY Acad Sci* 821, 57–75.

Yehuda R (2009) Status of glucocorticoid alterations in post-traumatic stress disorder. *Ann N Y Acad Sci* 1179, 56–69.

Yehuda, R., Halligan, S. L., Golier, J. A., Grossman, R., & Bierer, L. M. (2004). Effects of trauma exposure on the cortisol response to dexamethasone administration in PTSD and major depressive disorder. *Psychoneuroendocrinology* 29, 389–404.

Zohar J, Yahalom H, Kozlovsky N et al. (2011) High dose hydrocortisone immediately after trauma may alter the trajectory of PTSD: interplay between clinical and animal studies. *Eur Neuropsychopharmacol* 21, 796–809.

Zoladz PR, Diamond DM. Current status on behavioral and biological markers of PTSD: a search for clarity in a conflicting literature. *Neurosci Biobehav Rev* 37, 860–95.

Zoladz PR, Diamond DM (2013) Current status on behavioral and biological markers of PTSD: a search for clarity in a conflicting literature. *Neurosci Biobehav Rev* 37, 860–95.

Zovkic IB, Meadows JP, Kaas GA et al. (2013) Interindividual variability in stress susceptibility: a role for epigenetic mechanisms in PTSD. *Front Psychiatry* 4, 60.

CHAPTER 12

Neuroimaging of PTSD

Carolina Campanella[1] & J. Douglas Bremner[2]

[1] *Department of Psychiatry & Behavioral Sciences, Emory University, Atlanta, GA, USA*
[2] *Departments of Psychiatry & Behavioral Sciences and Radiology, Emory University School of Medicine, and the Atlanta VA Medical Center, Atlanta, GA, USA*

12.1 History and background

The psychological consequences of exposure to trauma have been well recognized throughout the history of medicine. After World Wars I and II, terms such as "shell shock," "combat fatigue," and "war neurosis" were commonly used to describe the mental disturbances resulting from wartime trauma experienced amongst combatants and concentration camp survivors. After World War II, this psychological distress was more formally defined as *gross stress reaction* in the American Psychiatric Association's (APA) inaugural diagnostic manual for psychiatric disorders, the *Diagnostic and Statistical Manual I* (DSM-1) (Crocq & Crocq, 2000; Saigh & Bremner, 1999). Gross stress reaction was considered a relatively short-lived disorder resulting from acute and severe stress. If symptoms persisted, the assumption was that it was a result of pathology that preceded the war. Later, in the 1970s, it was observed that other traumatic life-stressors, such as rape, could produce similar mental disturbances in its victims, although in cases of rape the resulting disturbance was termed *rape trauma syndrome* (Burgess & Holmstrom, 1974).

Due to confusion resulting from the wide range of competing terms to describe and diagnose traumatic stress, the APA decided to formulate a more central list of diagnostic criteria, eventually leading to inclusion of posttraumatic stress disorder (PTSD) as a psychiatric disorder in the DSM-III in 1980. Moreover, the new diagnosis for traumatic stress recognized that psychological trauma could cause long-lasting disturbances, even in the absence of an accompanying physical injury (Saigh & Bremner, 1999). Subsequent research has since shown that PTSD is associated with lasting changes in the brain, cognition, and physiological responding. The formal diagnosis of PTSD in 1980, therefore, represented a departure from the previous view of psychological distress as a result of trauma being a transitory disorder.

Posttraumatic Stress Disorder: From Neurobiology to Treatment, First Edition.
Edited by J. Douglas Bremner.
© 2016 John Wiley & Sons, Inc. Published 2016 by John Wiley & Sons, Inc.

Although the diagnosis of PTSD was formally recognized in 1980 and there was a subsequent call for research into PTSD – to deal with ongoing mental health issues of Vietnam veterans – the diagnosis was rarely made until 1988 (Bremner et al., 1996c). The lack of PTSD diagnoses may have been a result of a delay in the education of clinicians or changes in diagnostic practice. However, since the late 1980s there has been an acceleration of research in PTSD, which has led to increased acceptance of the idea that psychological trauma can have lasting consequences on an individual.

Since the incorporation of PTSD in the diagnostic classification system, epidemiological studies document relatively high prevalence rates, with 7–8% of the general population in the United States being affected (Kessler et al., 1995, 2005). The prevalence rate of PTSD for women (10.4%) is almost double that of men (5.0%) (Kessler et al., 1995). In addition, for many trauma victims, PTSD can be a lifelong problem (Saigh & Bremner, 1999). Risk factors for the development of PTSD include lower education, young age, history of prior trauma, reaction at the time of the trauma, and the absence of social support (Brewin, 2001).

The current diagnosis of PTSD requires exposure to actual or threatened death, serious injury, or sexual violation, in which the individual directly experiences the traumatic event; witnesses the traumatic event in person; learns that the traumatic event occurred to a close family member or friend; or experiences first-hand repeated or extreme exposure to aversive details of the traumatic event (American Psychiatric Association, 2013). In addition, the diagnosis requires the presence of symptoms in four clusters, including *intrusions, avoidance, negative alterations in cognitions and mood* and *alterations in arousal and reactivity*. The diagnosis requires at least one symptom in the intrusion category, one in the avoidance category, two in the negative alterations in cognition and mood, and two in the alterations in arousal and reactivity category. Moreover, the persistence of symptoms must occur for more than 1 month. Intrusive symptoms include recurrent intrusive memories, traumatic nightmares, flashbacks, and prolonged and intense distress with reminders of the event, in addition to having increase physiological reactivity to stimuli related to the traumatic event. Avoidant symptoms include avoidance of external reminders of the event, and avoidance of thoughts and feelings related to the event. Negative alterations in cognition and mood symptoms include trouble remembering an important aspect of the trauma, persistent – and often distorted – negative beliefs and expectations about themselves and the world (i.e., "I am a terrible person" and "The world is a dangerous place"), persistent distorted blame for themselves or others for causing the traumatic event or resulting consequences, persistent negative emotions related to trauma (e.g., fear, horror, shame, anger, or guilt), decreased interest in things, feeling detached or cut off from others, emotional numbing, and a persistent inability to experience positive emotions. Alterations in arousal and reactivity symptoms include irritability or outbursts of anger, self-destructive or reckless behavior, hyper-vigilance, difficulty falling or staying asleep, difficulty concentrating, and exaggerated startle response.

12.2 Neural circuits of PTSD

Symptoms of PTSD are thought to be the behavioral manifestation of stress-induced changes in brain structure and function (Bremner et al., 2007). More specifically, stress results in acute and chronic changes in neuro-chemical systems and specific brain regions, which result in long-term changes in neural circuits involved in the stress response (Bremner, 2002a; Pitman et al., 2001; Vermetten & Bremner, 2002a,b). Brain regions implicated in the development of PTSD include the hippocampus, amygdala, and medial prefrontal cortex (including the anterior cingulate) (see Figure 12.1). The hypothalamic–pituitary–adrenal (HPA) axis, which produces cortisol, and noradrenergic systems are two neurochemical systems that are critical in the stress response (Bremner, 2005, 2007b; Bremner et al., 2007; see also Chapters 9 and 11).

12.2.1 Overview of brain regions implicated in PTSD

The hippocampus, which plays a critical role in declarative (or explicit) memory (Squire, 2004), is very sensitive to stress. Pre-clinical and clinical studies have shown that PTSD patients have alterations in memory function (Elzinga & Bremner, 2002). Animals studies corroborate such findings, demostrating that

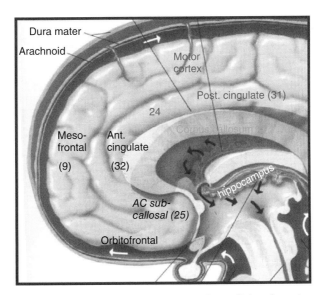

Figure 12.1 Brain regions involved stress and emotion. The medial prefrontal cortex includes parts of the prefrontal cortex, including mesofrontal cortex (Brodmann's area (BA 9), anterior cingulate (AC, BA 32), subcallosal gyrus (BA 25), and orbitofrontal cortex. Other areas shown include the motor cortex, posterior cingulate (BA 31), and hippocampus. (*See color plate section for the color representation of this figure.*)

exposure to repeated stress results in deficits to memory function (Luine et al., 1994) and damage to the hippocampus (Sapolsky et al., 1990; Uno et al., 1989). In addition, stress has been shown to interfere with hippocampal-based mechanisms of memory function, including long-term potentiation (LTP; Diamond et al., 1996; Luine et al., 1994) (see Chapter 6). Damage to hippocampal neurons may be a result of elevated levels of glucocorticoids (Lawrence & Sapolsky, 1994; Sapolsky, 1996), inhibition of brain-derived neurotrophic factor (BDNF; Nibuya et al., 1995; Smith et al., 1995), changes in serotonergic function (McEwen et al., 1992), or inhibition of neurogenesis (growth of new neurons) (Fowler et al., 2002; Gould et al., 1997) in the hippocampus.

However, animals studies have also demonstrated that several agents may reverse or block hippocampal damage due to stress. For example, antidepressant treatments have been shown to block the effects of stress and/or promote neurogenesis in the brain (Czéh et al., 2001; D'Sa & Duman, 2002; Duman et al., 1997, 2001; Garcia, 2002; Lucassen et al., 2004; Malberg et al., 2000; McEwen & Chattarji, 2004; Nibuya et al., 1995; Santarelli et al., 2003; Watanabe et al., 1992).

Other brain structures often implicated in the neural circuitry of stress, and stress-related disorders such as PTSD, include the amygdala and prefrontal cortex (McLaughlin et al., 2009). The amygdala is involved in processing of emotional stimuli, emotional memory, and plays a critical role in the acquisition of fear responses (Davis, 1992; Davis & Whalen, 2001; Phelps, 2006). The amygdala's role in fear conditioning is one possible explanation for the perseverance of biological and psychological fear responses in PTSD well after the end of the trauma (Hayes et al., 2012). One theory suggests that PTSD might reflect strong associative memory, similar to Pavlovian fear conditioning, where individuals initially react to a traumatic event with arousal and fear and then continue to show arousal when confronted with trauma-related cues, long after the initial trauma (Charney & Deutch, 1996; Pitman, 1989). Animal (LeDoux, 2003) and human studies (Phelps, 2006) both demonstrate that the amygdala plays a key role fear conditioning. Furthermore, studies of PTSD patients typically show increased activity in the amygdala in response to threat stimuli compared with individuals who did not experience trauma and individuals who experienced trauma but did not develop PTSD (Bremner, 2007a; Protopopescu et al., 2005; Rauch et al., 2006).

The final brain region implicated in the neural circuitry of PTSD is the medial prefrontal cortex, which includes the anterior cingulate gyrus (Brodmann's area 32), subcallosal gyrus (Brodmann's area 25), anterior prefrontal cortext (Brodmann's area 9), and the orbitofrontal cortex (Devinsky et al., 1995; Vogt et al., 1992). The medial prefrontal cortex is implicated in the appraisal and regulation of emotions (Etkin et al., 2011; Quirk & Beer, 2006). Animal studies have shown that the medial prefrontal cortex modulates emotional responsiveness by inhibiting fear responses mediated by the amygdala (Milad & Quirk, 2002; Milad et al., 2006; Morgan et al., 1993). Moreover, early stress exposure is associated with a decrease in branching of neurons in the medial prefrontal cortex (Brown et al., 2005; Cook & Wellman, 2004; Radley et al., 2004).

12.3 Changes in brain structure and cognitive functioning in PTSD

Declarative memory dysfuction exhibited by patients with PTSD is thought to be mediated in part by alterations in the hippocampus (Bremner et al., 1993, 1995a,b) (see Figure 12.2). Neuroimaging studies using magnetic resonance imaging (MRI) to measure hippocampal volume demonstrated that Vietnam veterans with PTSD have smaller right hippocampal volume, compared with controls, and that the decreases in hippocampal volume in the PTSD patients were associated with deficits in short-term memory (Bremner et al., 1995a). Reductions in left hippocampal volume have also been observed in patients with childhood abuse-related PTSD, when compared with case-matched controls (Bremner et al., 1997a). Smaller hippocampal volume and/or a reduction of N-acetyl aspartate (NAA) in the hippocampus (considered a marker of neuronal

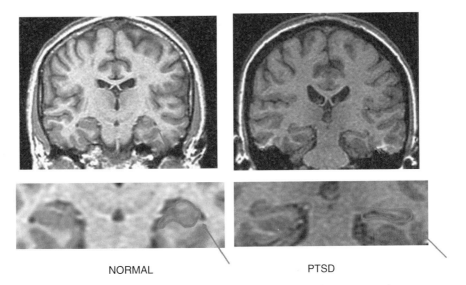

NORMAL   PTSD

Figure 12.2 Hippocampal volume on magnetic resonance imaging in posttraumatic stress disorder (PTSD). There is smaller hippocampal volume in this patient with PTSD compared with a control (from Bremner, 2005). (*See color plate section for the color representation of this figure.*)

integrity within the brain) in adults with chronic PTSD have also been observed in multiple studies (Bonne et al., 2008; Bossini et al., 2008; Bremner et al., 2003a; Emdad et al., 2006; Felmingham et al., 2007; Freeman et al., 1998; Gilbertson et al., 2002; Gurvits et al., 1996; Hedges et al., 2003; Irle et al., 2005; Kimbrell et al., 2005; Kitayama et al., 2005; Li et al., 2006; Lindauer et al., 2004b, 2005, 2006; Mahmutyazıcıouglu et al., 2005; Mohanakrishnan Menon et al., 2003; Pavić et al., 2007; Schuff et al., 1997, 2001, 2008; Shin et al., 2004b; Stein et al., 1997; Thomaes et al., 2010; Villarreal et al., 2002; Wang et al., 2010b, 2013; Woon et al., 2010). Furthermore, smaller hippocampal volume has been shown to be specific to PTSD and is not seen in panic disorder (Narayan et al., 1999).

However, not all adult studies observe the typical pattern of reduced hippocampal volume (Hedges et al., 2008; Jatzko et al., 2006; Landré et al., 2010; Pederson et al., 2004), suggesting a more complicated relationship between the two variables. Patients with new-onset PTSD (Bonne et al., 2001; Fennema-Notestine et al., 2002) and holocaust survivors with PTSD (Golier et al., 2005) did not show smaller hippocampal volume. When hippocampal volume of monozygotic twins – who differed in trauma exposure – were compared, a correlation emerged between PTSD symptoms and hippocampal volume, suggesting that hippocampal volume may, at least in part, be genetically determined and render the brain more vunerable to the development of PTSD (Gilbertson et al., 2002). Studies with cancer survivors, a population lacking neurological and psychiatric pathology, revealed a correlation between smaller hippocampal volume and intrusive memories (Hara et al., 2008; Nakano et al., 2002) and deficits in autobiographical retrieval (Bergouignan et al., 2011). Studies in children with PTSD have consistently not shown smaller hippocampal volume (Carrion et al., 2001; De Bellis et al., 1999, 2001), whereas women who were abused in childhood at specific periods of development were found to have smaller hippocampal volume in adulthood (Andersen et al., 2008).

Behaviorally, PTSD patients exhibit changes in learning and memory, which are likely to be mediated by the hippocampus (Brewin, 2001; Buckley et al., 2000; Elzinga & Bremner, 2002; Golier & Yehuda, 1998). Deficits in verbal declarative memory performance have been observed in Vietnam veterans with PTSD, with relative sparing of visual memory and IQ (Barrett et al., 1996; Bremner et al., 1993; Gilbertson et al., 2001; Golier et al., 1997; Roca & Freeman, 2001; Sachinvala et al., 2000; Uddo et al., 1993; Vasterling et al., 1998, 2002; Yehuda et al., 1995). Victims of rape (Jenkins et al., 1998), adults with early childhood abuse (Bremner et al., 1995b), and traumatized children (Moradi et al., 1999) show similar deficits in memory functioning. Moreover, evidence suggests that cognitive deficits are specifically associated with PTSD and are not due to the non-specific effects of trauma exposure (Bremner et al., 2004a; Jenkins et al., 1998). Some studies, however, have not observed specific deficits in verbal memory function (Stein et al., 1999; Zalewski et al., 1994), suggesting that memory deficits in PTSD may be somewhat limited. Furthermore, individuals with PTSD have even shown improvement in memory performance when cuing and recognition testing were used, as opposed to recall testing (Jenkins et al., 1998).

In addition to measuring changes in hippocampal volume, MRI has been used to measure brain volume changes in other structures implicated in PTSD. Thinner cortical volumes in frontal and temporal cortex have been observed in individuals with PTSD (Geuze et al., 2008d). Changes have also been observed in the anterior cingulate of individuals with PTSD. Specifically, smaller anterior cingulate volume (Kasai et al., 2008; Kitayama et al., 2005; Rauch et al., 2003; Rogers et al., 2009; Thomaes et al., 2010; Woodward et al., 2006; Yamasue et al., 2003) and reduced anterior cingulate NAA (De Bellis et al., 2000; Mahmutyazıcıouglu et al., 2005). However, select studies have not documented changes in anterior cingulate volume or NAA ratios for PTSD patients (Seedat et al., 2005). Other changes observed in individuals with PTSD include decreases in gray matter density (Corbo et al., 2005), smaller volume of the corpus callosum in neglected children (De Bellis et al., 2002; Teicher et al., 2004) and adults (Kitayama et al., 2007; Villarreal et al., 2004), reduced gray matter density in left posterior cingulate and left posterior parahippocampal gyrus (Nardo et al., 2009), and smaller volume of the insula (Chen et al., 2006), cavum septum pellucidum (May et al., 2004), and orbitofrontal cortex (Hakamata et al., 2007; Thomaes et al., 2010). Descreases in NAA have also been observed in the basal ganglia (Lim et al., 2003), whereas increased volume in the right caudate has also been reported (Looi et al., 2009). No difference in the volume of cerebellar vermis has been observed between monozygotic twins who are discordant for PTSD (Levitt et al., 2006).

With regard to the amygdala, there appears to be little consensus on whether there are structural differences in the amygdala. Although some studies observe smaller amygdala volume in individuals with PTSD (Rogers et al., 2009; Thomaes et al., 2010) and in cancer patients with intrusive memory recollections (Matsuoka et al., 2003), recent meta-analyses report no size reductions in amygdalar volume (Woon & Hedges, 2008, 2009). More recently, smaller amygdala volumes have been observed in PTSD patients in a study using a large case-controlled population (Morey et al., 2012). However, reductions in amygdalar volume did not correlate with trauma load and illness chronicity, suggesting that there may not be a dose–response relationship with amygdala (i.e., the more trauma there is, the smaller the amygdala), or that a smaller amygdala may only represent a vulnerability to developing PTSD. Damage to the amygdala and/or medial prefrontal cortex is shown to be associated with a decreased risk of developing PTSD, suggesting that the amygdala, along with the medial prefrontal cortex, plays a role in the development of the disorder after traumatic stress (Koenigs et al., 2007).

Along with measuring changes in brain volume, studies also utilize measures of fractional anisotropy (FA) to assess white matter integrity, with decreases in

FA corresponding to decreased white matter integrity in PTSD. Decreases in FA have been observed in the medial and posterior portions of the corpus callosum in children with PTSD (Jackowski et al., 2008). Adults with PTSD show decreases in FA in the hippocampus and cingulum bundle (Wang et al., 2010a), left side of rostral subgenual and dorsal cingulum bundle (Kim et al., 2007), and the left anterior cingulate (Kim et al., 2005, 2007). Voxel-based morphometry (VBM), an analysis that measures brain morphometry, shows that children with PTSD have increased gray matter volume in the right and left inferior and superior quandrants of the prefrontal cortex and smaller gray matter volume in the pons and posterior vermis areas (Carrion et al., 2009).

12.4 Neurohormonal responses to PTSD

In addition to investigating changes in brain structure in patients with PTSD, numerous studies have examined changes in the neurohormonal systems that play a role in PTSD and stress responses, including the noradrenergic system and the HPA/cortisol system. The noradrenergic system plays a critical role in stress and (Bremner et al., 1996a,b) and may facillitate emotional memory (for review, see Ferry et al., 1999). Norepinephrine, which is released through the noradrenergic system, sharpens the senses, focuses attention, raises the level of fear, quickens the heart rate and blood pressure, and helps organisms for "fight or flight" during a stressful or threatening situation. The noradrenergic system accomplishes this by focusing the senses by acitvating the neuronal systems that process sensory information in order to assess dangers in the environment rapidly and efficiently, although at the expense of more detailed processing of such information. At the same time, norepinephrine increases heart rate and blood pressure, allowing an "emergency" mobilization of oxygen and nutrients, essential for survival, to all cells in the body. Essentially, norepinephrine both activates the brain and stimulates the heart, and other bodily organs regulated by the autonomic nervous system, in order to faciliate behavioral responses important to survival in situations of threat or danger (Bremner et al., 1996a,b).

In the case of PTSD, studies have found long-term dysregulation of the noradrenergic system (Bremner et al., 1996b). Psychophysiology studies have observed an increase in sympathetic responses, measured by heart rate, blood pressure, and galvanic skin response, to traumatic reminders (i.e., traumatic slides and sounds, or traumatic scripts), in PTSD (Pitman et al., 1987). In addition, exposure to combat films, which served as a traumatic reminder, resulted in increased concentrations of plasma epinephrine, along with increases in autonomic activity, in combat veterans with PTSD (McFall et al., 1990). Administering yohimbineyohimbine, an α_2 antagonist, which results in an increase of norepinephrine in the brain, to PTSD patients resulted in an increase in symptoms specific to PTSD, as well as a greater release of norepinephrine metabolites in plasma (Southwick et al., 1993). In addition, positron emission tomography (PET) revealed changes in central metabolic responses to yohimbine in PTSD patients (Bremner et al., 1997b).

12.5 Functional neuroimaging studies in PTSD

Functional neuroimaging studies, performed to measure brain function in PTSD, are consistent with dysfunction in a network of related brain regions including the hippocampus, amygdala, and medial prefrontal cortex (Bremner, 1998, 2002b; Cannistraro & Rauch, 2003; Liberzon et al., 2003; Liberzon & Martis, 2006; Liberzon & Phan, 2003; Pitman et al., 2001; Rauch et al., 2006). This network mediates memory and the stress response, and may mediate symptoms of PTSD (Bremner, 2002b, 2003; Pitman et al., 2001). Studies of resting blood flow or metabolism with PET and single-photon emission computed tomography (SPECT) showed alterations at rest in medial prefrontal, temporal, and dorsolateral prefrontal cortex, cerebellum, amygdala (Bonne et al., 2003; Bremner et al., 1997b; Chung et al., 2006), thalamus (Kim et al., 2007), and mid-cingulate (Shin et al., 2009). A recent study comparing brain metabolism during wakefulness and rapid eye movement (REM) sleep showed that that the brain stem (which regulates both arousal and REM sleep), core limbic areas (including amygdala and hippocampus), and cortical areas (including anterior, posterior, and medial cingulate, and ventromedial and ventrolateral frontal cortex) are active both during wake and REM sleep, suggesting that alterations in brain function during either wakefulness and REM sleep may influence one another, which may have important implications related to treatment and/or persistence of PTSD symptomology (Germain et al., 2013). Patients with PTSD showed reduced coupling within the default mode network (DMN; brain regions active when an individual is not focused on external world and is at wakeful rest), greater coupling within the salience network (SN; network of brain regions tasked with priortizing processing of information based on importance, urgency, and task relevancy), and increased coupling between the DMN and the SN, suggesting a relative dominance of threat-sensitive circuitry in PTSD (Sripada et al., 2012). The disequilibrium between the salience and defult mode brain networks, favoring detection of salient stimuli over internally focused thought may account for PTSD pathophysiology.

The amygdala, as mentioned earlier, plays a central role in conditioned fear responses (Davis, 1992; LeDoux, 2003). The medial prefrontal cortex, which consists of several related areas including the orbitofrontal cortex, anterior cingulate and subcallosal gyrus, and anterior prefrontal cortex (Devinsky et al., 1995; Vogt et al., 1992), has inhibitory inputs to the amygdala that mediate the extinction of fear responding (Morgan & LeDoux, 1995; Quirk, 2002). Lesions in the medial prefrontal cortex result in a failure to build up the peripheral cortisol and sympathetic response to stress (Devinsky et al., 1995; Vogt et al., 1992). A meta-analysis of functional MRI (fMRI) and PET studies compared patients with PTSD to individuals with social anxiety disorder, specific phobias, and fear conditioning (but otherwise healthy) and found that only PTSD patients showed hypoactivation in regions of the prefrontal cortex (Etkin & Wager, 2007). More specifically, hypoactivations were observed in the dorsal and rostral anterior cingulate cortices and the ventromedial prefrontal cortex, which are structures linked to the experiencing and regulation of emotion. Early stress also affects the medial prefrontal cortex, resulting in a reduction in dendritic branching in that area (Radley et al., 2004). These findings suggest that medial prefrontal cortex dysfunction plays a role in mediating symptoms of PTSD.

Stimulating the noradrenergic system with yohimbine results in decreased activation in cortical regions, including dorsolateral, prefrontal, temporal, parietal, and orbitofrontal cortex, along with decreased activity in the hippocampus (Bremner et al., 1997b). PET, SPECT, or fMRI studies, where patients were exposed to traumatic reminders in the form of traumatic slides and/or sounds or traumatic scripts resulted in an increase in PTSD symptoms, decreased blood flow and/or decreased activation in the medial prefrontal cortex/anterior cingulate, including Brodmann's area 25, or subcallosal gyrus, area 32 and 24 (Bremner et al., 1999a,b; Britton et al., 2005; Fonzo et al., 2010; Hopper et al., 2007; Hou et al., 2007; Lanius et al., 2001, 2003; Liberzon et al., 1999; Lindauer et al., 2004a; Phan et al., 2006; Semple et al., 2000; Shin et al., 1997, 1999, 2001, 2004a, 2005; Yang et al., 2004) (see Figure 12.3). Traumatic reminder exposure

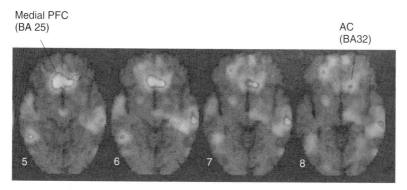

Figure 12.3 Medial prefrontal cortex (PFC) dysfunction in PTSD. There was a failure of medial prefrontal activation in a group of combat veterans with PTSD compared with combat veterans without PTSD during exposure to traumatic combat-related slides and sounds. The light areas represent decreased function in the medial PFC, which includes both Brodmann's rea (BA) 25 and anterior cingulate (AC) BA 32. Each image represents an adjacent slice of the brain, with the light areas representing a composite of areas of relative decrease in blood flow in PTSD patients compared with controls (from Bremner, 2005). (*See color plate section for the color representation of this figure.*)

has also been shown to decrease function in the hippocampus (Bremner et al., 1999a), thalamus (Lanius et al., 2001, 2003), visual association cortex (Bremner et al., 1999a; Lanius et al., 2001, 2003; Shin et al., 1997, 2004b), parietal cortex (Bremner et al., 1999a; Rauch et al., 1996; Sakamoto et al., 2005; Shin et al., 1997, 1999), and inferior frontal gyrus (Bremner et al., 1999a; Lanius et al., 2003; Rauch et al., 1996; Sakamoto et al., 2005; Shin et al., 1997, 1999, 2001). An increase in function is observed in the amygdala (Liberzon et al., 1999; Rauch et al., 1996; Shin et al., 2004a), insula (Fonzo et al., 2010; Hopper et al., 2007; Simmons et al., 2008), posterior cingulate cortex (Bremner et al., 1999a,b; Lanius et al., 2001; Shin et al., 1997), ventromedial prefrontal cortex (Morey et al., 2008), and parahippocampal gyrus (Bremner et al., 1999a; Liberzon et al., 1999).

Delving in more detail into the interplay between core limbic regions and prefrontal cortex, Shin et al. (2004a) found increased amygdala activation and decreased medial prefrontal function in Vietnam veterans who were exposed to traumatic reminders, suggesting that a failure by the medial prefrontal cortex to inhibit the amygdala could account for increased PTSD symptoms with exposure to traumatic reminders. Admon et al. (2009) showed that increased amygdala reactivity predicted increased stress symptom response to combat, whereas increased hippocampal activity paralleled the increase in stress symptoms. This indicates that there is a difference in the temporal trajectory in amygdala and hippocampal responses to stress. Other neuroimaging studies showed increased amygdala and parahippocampal function while performing an attention task (Felmingham et al., 2009; Semple et al., 2000), and increased amygdala activity at rest (Chung et al., 2006), during a working memory task (Bryant et al., 2005) and whilst recalling traumatic words (Protopopescu et al., 2005). Increased amygdala function is also observed with exposure to masked fearful faces (Armony et al., 2005; Bryant et al., 2008; Felmingham et al., 2010; Kemp et al., 2007, 2009; Rauch et al., 2000), overt fearful faces (Fonzo et al., 2010; Shin et al., 2005), negative pictures (Brohawn et al., 2010), neutral pictures (Brunetti et al., 2010), traumatic sounds (Liberzon et al., 1999; Pissiota et al., 2002), traumatic scripts (Rauch et al., 1996), extinction learning (Milad et al., 2009), and classical fear conditioning (Bremner et al., 2005a).

Children with posttraumatic stress symptoms show increased medial prefrontal cortex activation and decreased middle frontal gyrus activation with a response inhibition task (Carrion et al., 2008). In addition, children with posttraumatic stress symptoms, as a result of interpersonal trauma, also show reduced hippocampal activity during a verbal declarative memory task, which may serve as a neurofunctional marker of posttraumatic stress symptoms (Carrión et al., 2010).

In addition to looking at neural correlates of chronic PTSD (PTSD with symptoms persisting longer than 3 months), studies have also examined the neural correlates of PTSD during its acute phase, where symptoms have only presented for less than 3 months. Patients with acute PTSD from severe accident trauma showed increased activation in the hippocampus, anterior cingulate and amygdala when exposed to memories of the trauma (Piefke et al., 2007). Conversely, a PET study with acute motor vehicle accident survivors showed decreased amygdala blood flow during exposure to traumatic scripts (Osuch et al., 2008). Osuch et al. (2008) also observed negative correlation between symptom improvement at 3 months and hippocampal blood flow during exposure to traumatic scripts.

In addition to looking at the neural responses to traumatic reminders, several studies have examined the neural correlates of cognitive tasks in PTSD. Decreased activation in the hippocampus (Astur et al., 2006; Bremner et al., 2003a; Shin et al., 2004b) and insula (Chen et al., 2009; Whalley et al., 2009) was observed while PTSD patients performed specific declarative memory tasks. PTSD patients showed decreased inferior frontal cortex (Clark et al., 2003), parietal (Bryant et al., 2005; Clark et al., 2003), hippocampal and anterior cingulate function (Moores et al., 2008) during working memory tasks. PTSD patients peforming an executive processing task with emotional combat-related scenes interleaved in the task showed increased activation in the amygdala, ventrolateral prefrontal cortex, and fusiform gyrus, and decreased activation in the dorsolateral prefrontal cortex (Morey et al., 2008). When performing a same–different emotional conflict task, PTSD patients showed reduced anterior cingulate activation (Kim et al., 2008). Peri-amygdala areas, ventrolateral prefrontal cortex, and orbitofrontal cortex showed increased activation in patients with high symptomatology during an emotional oddball task (Hayes et al., 2009). While performing working memory tasks, PTSD patients showed a relative lack (compared with controls) of connectivity in the right inferior frontal gyrus and right inferior parietal lobule. PTSD patients, however, showed stronger connectivity between posterior cingulate cortex and right superior frontal gyrus, and between medial prefrontal cortex and the left parahippocampal gyrus during the working memory tasks (Daniels et al., 2010). Finally, during an emotional stroop task (e.g., naming the color of a word such as "rape"), PTSD patients showed decreased function in medial prefrontal cortex/anterior cingulate (Bremner et al., 2004b; Shin et al., 2001), visual association cortex and parietal cortex (Bremner et al., 2004b), and dorsolateral prefrontal cortex (Bremner et al., 2004b; Shin et al., 2001). Increased function, meanwhile, was observed in posterior cingulate and parahippocampal gyrus (Shin et al., 2001).

Memory studies, where women with PTSD from early abuse retrieved emotionally valenced words (e.g., "rape-mutilate") (Bremner et al., 2001), resulted in decreases in blood flow in areas including the orbitofrontal cortex, anterior cingulate, and medial prefrontal cortex (Brodmann's areas 25, 32, 9), left hippocampus, and fusiform gyrus/inferior temporal gyrus (Bremner et al., 2003a), thus lending further support to the theory of a dysfunctional network of brain regions, including areas implicated in memory, in PTSD. PTSD patients showed decreased frontal, temporal (Geuze et al., 2008c), and pre-cuneus activation (Geuze et al., 2008b) during neutral word encoding. Neutral word retrieval, on the other hand, was associated with decreased activation of hippocampus, middle temporal gyrus, frontal cortex (Geuze et al., 2008c) and parahippocampal gyrus (Hou et al., 2007). During an associative learning task, where participants had to pair faces with professions, PTSD patients showed increased hippocampal activation and decreased prefrontal activation. During retrieval of the face–profession pairs, patients showed decreased activation in left parahippocampal gyrus and other memory-related brain regions, despite showing no differences in memory accuracy, suggesting that PTSD might effect memory-related brain function without necessarily impairing memory performance (Werner et al., 2009).

With regard to emotional memory, results are mixed, although this could be explained by the stimuli used. Brohawn et al. (2010) showed enhanced hip-pocampal activity in patients with PTSD during encoding of emotional items rela-tive to controls. Increased activity in both the amygdala and hippcampus has also been observed in PTSD patients when contrasting remembered with forgotten stimuli (Dickie et al., 2008). A recent study, however, reported reduced amygdala and hippocampal activity during successful encoding of trauma-specific material, as opposed to general negative stimuli used in the previous studies, in patients with PTSD (Hayes et al., 2011). Moreoever, PTSD patients produced greater false alarms for the trauma-specific negative information, suggesting that the reduced activity in the hippocampus and amygdala may underlie distortions in memory observed in PTSD patients. Decreased function in the hippocampus and medial prefrontal cortex was also seen in women with childhood abuse-related PTSD during recall of trauma-related emotional word pairs (Bremner et al., 2003a).

Abnormalities in the neural circuitry involved in motivation and reward systems has also been observed in various functional imaging studies in PTSD patients. During a decision-making task, where neural response to gain and loss feedback was evaluated, PTSD patients showed lower activation in the nucleus accumbens and mesial PFC when processing gains feedback, suggesting that positive outcome information loses its salience in patients with PTSD, thereby reducing task-related motivation (Sailer et al., 2008). PTSD patients were also less successful at down-regulating emotional responses and showed a decrease in activity in the prefrontal cortex during down-regulating attempts, indicating that the ability to down-regulate emotion may be impaired after trauma (New et al., 2009). Other evidence demonstrating an impairment in motivation and reward neural pathways in PTSD patients include decreased insula activation during an affective set shifting task (Simmons et al., 2009), decreased right dorsolateral frontal activation and increased striatal activity during a go–no go task (Falconer et al., 2009), and a negative correlation between levels of emotional awareness and anterior cingulate activation (Frewen et al., 2008).

In addition to showing deficits in cognitive functioning, PTSD patients have exhibited decreased sensitivity to pain. Administration of painful heat stimulation corresponded to increased bilateral insula activation in PTSD patients (Geuze et al., 2007; Strigo et al., 2010) and dorsolateral prefrontal cortex activation (Strigo et al., 2010). Processing of pain stimuli also resulted in increased hippocampal and amygdala activation and decreased ventrolateral prefrontal activation (Geuze et al., 2007).

More recently, studies have looked at connectivity between different brain regions implicated in PTSD and have typically observed increased connectivity with the amygdala and other limbic regions. Increased connectivity between the amygdala and anterior cingulate was associated with current PTSD symptom severity and risk of chronicity of future PTSD symptoms in acutely traumatized patients (Lanius et al., 2010). Increased connectivity among the amygdala, anterior cingulate, visual cortex, and subcallosal gyrus has also been observed in PTSD (Gilboa et al., 2004). Other studies, on the other hand, show a decrease in resting state posterior cingulate/precuneus connectivity in PTSD patients (Bluhm et al., 2009).

Finally, various neuroimaging studies have looked at the neural correlates of pharmalogical treatment response in PTSD (see Chapter 17 for a review of the effects of psychotherapy on the brain in PTSD). PTSD patients treated with paroxetine (i.e., Paxil), a selective serotonin reuptake inhibitors (SSRI) antidepressant drug, for up to a year showed significant improvements in verbal declarative memory and a 4.6% increase in mean hippocampal volume (Vermetten et al., 2003). Increases in hippocampal volume were also observed following treament with setraline (i.e., Zoloft), another SSRI antidepressant (Bossini et al., 2007). PTSD patients treated with phenytoin (i.e., Dilantin), an antiepileptic drug that may be efficacious in treating PTSD through antiglutamatergic effects, has been shown to increase right hippocampal and cerebral cortical brain volume (Bremner et al., 2005b). In patients with PTSD randomized in a double-blind fashion to paroxetine or placebo, treatment with paroxetine, but not placebo, resulted in an increase in frontal cortical function in response to exposure to traumatic scripts of the individual's traumatic experience (Fani et al., 2011). In sum, mounting evidence suggests that successful treatment of PTSD is associated with changes in brain areas that have been implicated with PTSD, including the hippocampus and prefrontal cortex. In addition, circuitry involved in inhibitory control may be key to determining treatment outcome.

12.6 Neuroreceptor Studies in PTSD

A relatively small number of studies have begun to use PET and SPECT to measure neuroreceptors in PTSD. Some studies with combat veterans report reduced binding of benzodiazepine receptors – which may play an important role in regulating stress – in frontal cortex (Bremner et al., 2000; Geuze et al., 2008a), whereas others do not (Fujita et al., 2004). Binding of 5-hydroxytryptamine 1A (5-HT$_{1A}$) serotonin receptors – thought to play an important role in regulating mood and anxiety – was unchanged in PTSD patients, indicating that 5-HT$_{1AR}$ expression may not be altered in PTSD (Bonne et al., 2005), although serotonin transporter binding was reduced in the amygdala of PTSD patients (Murrough et al., 2011). Norepinephrine transporter availability was decreased in the locus coeruleus in patients with PTSD (Pietrzak et al., 2013). Other PET studies with PTSD patients found a reduction in anterior cingulate opiate receptor (which modulates anxiety) binding (Liberzon et al., 2007), increases in hippocampal beta2-nicotinic acetylcholine receptor binding (Czermak et al., 2008), and a general elevation of brain cannabinoid-1 receptor binding (Neumeister et al., 2013).

12.7 Conclusions

Since its formal classification, PTSD has been recognized as a common psychiatric disorder associated with long-term changes in the brain and stress response systems. Although some of the findings appear to be mixed, functional neuroimaging research implicates brain areas, including the amygdala, hippocampus, and frontal cortex. More specifically, the amygdala, which mediates emotional and fear responses, is hyper-responsive, whereas the frontal cortex, which is implicated in appraisal and regulation, is hypo-responsive. Functional and structural abnormalities in the hippocampus have been reported in PTSD patients, although the direction of the functional abnormalities vary across studies, depending on circumstances such as task and recency of the trauma. The observed changes in the highlighted brain regions may lead to deficits in memory and maintenance of abnormal fear responses, as well as other symptoms of PTSD. Recent evidence suggests that specific treatments may affect the hippocampus and prefrontal cortex, possibly by facilitating an extinction of fear responses and intrusive memories, thereby facilitating recovery. Future studies should consist of meta-analyses, which will help to identify patterns of brain function across data sets and help to resolve some of the mixed findings between studies. In addition, future studies need to delve further into the neurochemical substrates of PTSD and response to treatment.

References

Admon R, Lubin G, Stern O et al. (2009) Human vulnerability to stress depends on amygdala's predisposition and hippocampal plasticity. *Proc Natl Acad Sci USA* 106, 14120–14125.
American Psychiatric Association (2013) Diagnostic and statistical manual of mental disorders, 5th edn. American Psychiatric Publishing, Arlington, VA.

Andersen S, Tomada A, Vincow E et al. (2008) Preliminary evidence for sensitive periods in the effect of childhood sexual abuse on regional brain development. *J Neuropsychiatry Clin Neurosci* 20, 292–301.

Armony JL, Corbo V, Clément M-H et al. (2005) Amygdala response in patients with acute PTSD to masked and unmasked emotional facial expressions. *Am J Psychiatry* 162, 1961–1963.

Astur RS, St. Germain SA, Tolin D et al. (2006) Hippocampus function predicts severity of post-traumatic stress disorder. *Cyberpsychol Behav* 9, 234–240.

Barrett DH, Green ML, Morris R et al. (1996) Cognitive functioning and posttraumatic stress disorder. *Am J Psychiatry* 153, 1492–1494.

Bergouignan L, Lefranc JP, Chupin M et al. (2011) Breast cancer affects both the hippocampus volume and the episodic autobiographical memory retrieval. *PloS One* 6, e25349.

Bluhm RL, Williamson PC, Osuch EA et al. (2009) Alterations in default network connectivity in posttraumatic stress disorder related to early-life trauma. *J Psychiatry Neurosci JPN* 34, 187.

Bonne O, Bain E, Neumeister A et al. (2005) No change in serotonin type 1A receptor binding in patients with posttraumatic stress disorder. *Am J Psychiatry* 162, 383–385.

Bonne O, Brandes D, Gilboa A et al. (2001) Longitudinal MRI study of hippocampal volume in trauma survivors with PTSD. *Am J Psychiatry* 158, 1248.

Bonne O, Gilboa A, Louzoun Y et al. (2003) Resting regional cerebral perfusion in recent post-traumatic stress disorder. *Biol Psychiatry* 54, 1077–1086.

Bonne O, Vythilingam M, Inagaki M et al. (2008) Reduced posterior hippocampal volume in posttraumatic stress disorder. *J Clin Psychiatry* 69, 1087–1091.

Bossini L, Tavanti M, Calossi S et al. (2008) Magnetic resonance imaging volumes of the hippocampus in drug-naïve patients with post-traumatic stress disorder without comorbidity conditions. *J Psychiatr Res* 42, 752–762.

Bossini L, Tavanti M, Lombardelli A et al. (2007) Changes in hippocampal volume in patients with post-traumatic stress disorder after sertraline treatment. *J Clin Psychopharmacol* 27, 233–235.

Bremner JD (1998) Neuroimaging of posttraumatic stress disorder. *Psychiatr Ann* 28, 445-450.

Bremner JD (2002a) Neuroimaging of childhood trauma. *Sem Clin Neuropsychiatry* 7, 104.

Bremner JD (2002b) Does stress damage the brain?: Understanding trauma-related disorders from a mind-body perspective. WW Norton & Company.

Bremner JD (2003) Functional neuroanatomical correlates of traumatic stress revisited 7 years later, this time with data. *Psychopharmacol Bull* 37, 6–25.

Bremner JD (2005) *Brain Imaging Handbook*. WW Norton & Co.

Bremner JD (2007a) Neuroimaging in posttraumatic stress disorder and other stress-related disorders. *Neuroimaging Clin N Am* 17, 523–538.

Bremner JD (2007b) Functional neuroimaging in post-traumatic stress disorder. *Expert Rev Neurother* 7, 393-405.

Bremner JD, Elzinga B, Schmahl C, Vermetten E (2007) Structural and functional plasticity of the human brain in posttraumatic stress disorder. *Prog Brain Res* 167, 171–186.

Bremner JD, Innis RB, Ng CK et al. (1997a) Positron emission tomography measurement of cerebral metabolic correlates of yohimbine administration in combat-related posttraumatic stress disorder. *Arch Gen Psychiatry* 54, 246.

Bremner JD, Innis RB, Southwick SM et al. (2000) Decreased benzodiazepine receptor binding in prefrontal cortex in combat-related posttraumatic stress disorder. *Am J Psychiatry* 157, 1120–1126.

Bremner JD, Krystal JH, Southwick SM, Charney DS (1995a) Functional neuroanatomical correlates of the effects of stress on memory. *J Trauma Stress* 8, 527–553.

Bremner JD, Krystal JH, Southwick SM, Charney DS (1996a) Noradrenergic mechanisms in stress and anxiety: II. *Clinical studies. Synapse* 23, 39–51.

Bremner JD, Krystal JH, Southwick SM, Charney DS (1996b) Noradrenergic mechanisms in stress and anxiety: I. *Preclinical studies. Synapse* 23, 28–38.

Bremner JD, Mletzko T, Welter S et al. (2005a) Effects of phenytoin on memory, cognition and brain structure in post-traumatic stress disorder: a pilot study. *J Psychopharmacol (Oxf)* 19, 159–165.

Bremner JD, Narayan M, Staib LH et al. (1999a) Neural correlates of memories of childhood sexual abuse in women with and without posttraumatic stress disorder. *Am J Psychiatry* 156, 1787.

Bremner JD, Randall P, Scott TM et al. (1995b) Deficits in short-term memory in adult survivors of childhood abuse. *Psychiatry Res* 59, 97–107.

Bremner JD, Randall P, Scott TM et al. (1995c) MRI-based measurement of hippocampal volume in patients with combat-related posttraumatic stress disorder. *Am J Psychiatry* 152, 973.

Bremner JD, Randall P, Vermetten E et al. (1997b) Magnetic resonance imaging-based measurement of hippocampal volume in posttraumatic stress disorder related to childhood physical and sexual abuse – a preliminary report. *Biol Psychiatry* 41, 23–32.

Bremner JD, Scott TM, Delaney RC et al. (1993) Deficits in short-term memory in posttraumatic stress disorder. *Am J Psychiatry* 150, 1015–1015.

Bremner JD, Soufer R, McCarthy G et al. (2001) Gender differences in cognitive and neural correlates of remembrance of emotional words. *Psychopharmacol Bull* 35, 55–78.

Bremner JD, Southwick SM, Darnell A, Charney DS (1996c) Chronic PTSD in Vietnam combat veterans: course of illness and substance abuse. *Am J Psychiatry* 153, 369–375.

Bremner JD, Staib LH, Kaloupek D et al. (1999b) Neural correlates of exposure to traumatic pictures and sound in Vietnam combat veterans with and without posttraumatic stress disorder: a positron emission tomography study. *Biol Psychiatry* 45, 806–816.

Bremner JD, Vermetten E, Afzal N, Vythilingam M (2004a) Deficits in verbal declarative memory function in women with childhood sexual abuse-related posttraumatic stress disorder. *J Nerv Ment Dis* 192, 643–649.

Bremner JD, Vermetten E, Schmahl C et al. (2005b) Positron emission tomographic imaging of neural correlates of a fear acquisition and extinction paradigm in women with childhood sexual-abuse-related post-traumatic stress disorder. *Psychol Med* 35, 791–806.

Bremner JD, Vermetten E, Vythilingam M et al. (2004b) Neural correlates of the classic color and emotional stroop in women with abuse-related posttraumatic stress disorder. *Biol Psychiatry* 55, 612–620.

Bremner JD, Vythilingam M, Vermetten E et al. (2003a) Neural correlates of declarative memory for emotionally valenced words in women with posttraumatic stress disorder related to early childhood sexual abuse. *Biol Psychiatry* 53, 879–889.

Bremner JD, Vythilingam M, Vermetten E et al. (2003b) MRI and PET study of deficits in hippocampal structure and function in women with childhood sexual abuse and posttraumatic stress disorder. *Am J Psychiatry* 160, 924–932.

Bremner JD, Vythilingam M, Vermetten E et al. (2003c) Neural correlates of declarative memory for emotionally valenced words in women with posttraumatic stress disorder related to early childhood sexual abuse. *Biol Psychiatry* 53, 879–889.

Brewin CR (2001) A cognitive neuroscience account of posttraumatic stress disorder and its treatment. *Behav Res Ther* 39, 373–393.

Britton JC, Phan KL, Taylor SF et al. (2005) Corticolimbic blood flow in posttraumatic stress disorder during script-driven imagery. *Biol Psychiatry* 57, 832–840.

Brohawn KH, Offringa R, Pfaff DL et al. (2010) The Neural Correlates of Emotional Memory in Posttraumatic Stress Disorder. *Biol Psychiatry* 68, 1023–1030.

Brown SM, Henning S, Wellman CL (2005) Mild, short-term stress alters dendritic morphology in rat medial prefrontal cortex. *Cereb Cortex* 15, 1714–1722.

Brunetti M, Sepede G, Mingoia G et al. (2010) Elevated response of human amygdala to neutral stimuli in mild post traumatic stress disorder: neural correlates of generalized emotional response. *Neuroscience* 168, 670–679.

Bryant RA, Felmingham KL, Kemp AH et al. (2005) Neural networks of information processing in posttraumatic stress disorder: a functional magnetic resonance imaging study. *Biol Psychiatry* 58, 111–118.

Bryant RA, Kemp AH, Felmingham KL et al. (2008) Enhanced amygdala and medial prefrontal activation during nonconscious processing of fear in posttraumatic stress disorder: An fMRI study. *Hum Brain Mapp* 29, 517–523.

Bryant RA, Kemp AH, Felmingham KL et al. (2008). Enhanced amygdala and medial prefrontal activation during nonconscious processing of fear in posttraumatic stress disorder: An fMRI study. *Hum Brain Mapping* 29, 517–523.

Buckley TC, Blanchard EB, Neill WT (2000) Information processing and PTSD: A review of the empirical literature. *Clin Psychol Rev* 20, 1041–1065.

Burgess AW, Holmstrom LL (1974) Rape trauma syndrome. *Am J Psychiatry* 131, 981–986.

Cannistraro PA, Rauch SL (2003) Neural circuitry of anxiety: evidence from structural and functional neuroimaging studies. *Psychopharmacol Bull* 37, 8–25.

Carrion VG, Garrett A, Menon V et al. (2008) Posttraumatic stress symptoms and brain function during a response-inhibition task: an fMRI study in youth. *Depress Anxiety* 25, 514–526.

Carrión VG, Haas BW, Garrett A et al. (2010) Reduced hippocampal activity in youth with posttraumatic stress symptoms: an FMRI study. *J Pediatr Psychol* 35, 559–569.

Carrion VG, Weems CF, Eliez S et al. (2001) Attenuation of frontal asymmetry in pediatric posttraumatic stress disorder. *Biol Psychiatry* 50, 943–951.

Carrion VG, Weems CF, Watson C et al. (2009) Converging evidence for abnormalities of the prefrontal cortex and evaluation of midsagittal structures in pediatric posttraumatic stress disorder: An MRI study. *Psychiatry Res Neuroimaging* 172, 226–234.

Charney DS, Deutch A (1996) A functional neuroanatomy of anxiety and fear: implications for the pathophysiology and treatment of anxiety disorders. *Crit Rev Neurobiol* 10, 3–4.

Chen S, Li L, Xu B, Liu J (2009) Insular cortex involvement in declarative memory deficits in patients with post-traumatic stress disorder. *BMC Psychiatry* 9, 39.

Chen S, Xia W, Li L et al. (2006) Gray matter density reduction in the insula in fire survivors with posttraumatic stress disorder: a voxel-based morphometric study. *Psychiatry Res Neuroimaging* 146, 65–72.

Chung YA, Kim SH, Chung SK et al. (2006) Alterations in cerebral perfusion in posttraumatic stress disorder patients without re-exposure to accident-related stimuli. *Clin Neurophysiol* 117, 637–642.

Clark CR, McFarlane AC, Morris P et al. (2003) Cerebral function in posttraumatic stress disorder during verbal working memory updating: a positron emission tomography study. *Biol Psychiatry* 53, 474–481.

Cook SC, Wellman CL (2004) Chronic stress alters dendritic morphology in rat medial prefrontal cortex. *J Neurobiol* 60, 236–248.

Corbo V, Clément M-H, Armony JL et al. (2005) Size versus shape differences: contrasting voxel-based and volumetric analyses of the anterior cingulate cortex in individuals with acute posttraumatic stress disorder. *Biol Psychiatry* 58, 119–124.

Crocq M-A, Crocq L (2000) From shell shock and war neurosis to posttraumatic stress disorder: a history of Psychotraumatology. *Dialogues Clin Neurosci* 2, 47.

Czéh B, Michaelis T, Watanabe T et al. (2001) Stress-induced changes in cerebral metabolites, hippocampal volume, and cell proliferation are prevented by antidepressant treatment with tianeptine. *Proc Natl Acad Sci* 98, 12796–12801.

Czermak C, Staley JK, Kasserman S et al. (2008) Beta-2 nicotinic acetylcholine receptor availability in post-traumatic stress disorder. *Int J Neuropsychopharmacol* 11, 419-424.

D'Sa C, Duman RS (2002) Antidepressants and neuroplasticity. *Bipolar Disord* 4, 183–194.

Daniels JK, McFarlane AC, Bluhm RL et al. (2010) Switching between executive and default mode networks in posttraumatic stress disorder: alterations in functional connectivity. *J Psychiatry Neurosci JPN* 35, 258.

Davis M (1992) The role of the amygdala in fear and anxiety. *Annu Rev Neurosci* 15, 353–375.

Davis M, Whalen PJ (2001) The amygdala: vigilance and emotion. *Mol Psychiatry* 6, 13–34.

De Bellis MD, Hall J, Boring AM et al. (2001) A pilot longitudinal study of hippocampal volumes in pediatric maltreatment-related posttraumatic stress disorder. *Biol Psychiatry* 50, 305–309.

De Bellis MD, Keshavan MS, Clark DB et al. (1999) Developmental traumatology part II: Brain development. *Biol Psychiatry* 45, 1271–1284.

De Bellis MD, Keshavan MS, Shifflett H et al. (2002) Brain structures in pediatric maltreatment-related posttraumatic stress disorder: a sociodemographically matched study. *Biol Psychiatry* 52, 1066–1078.

De Bellis MD, Keshavan MS, Spencer S, Hall J (2000) N-Acetylaspartate concentration in the anterior cingulate of maltreated children and adolescents with PTSD. *Am J Psychiatry* 157, 1175–1177.

Devinsky O, Morrell MJ, Vogt BA (1995) Contributions of anterior cingulate cortex to behaviour. *Brain* 118, 279–306.

Diamond DM, Fleshner M, Ingersoll N, Rose G (1996) Psychological stress impairs spatial working memory: relevance to electrophysiological studies of hippocampal function. *Behav Neurosci* 110, 661.

Dickie EW, Brunet A, Akerib V, Armony JL (2008) An fMRI investigation of memory encoding in PTSD: Influence of symptom severity. *Neuropsychologia* 46, 1522–1531.

Duman RS, Heninger GR, Nestler EJ (1997) A molecular and cellular theory of depression. *Arch Gen Psychiatry* 54, 597.

Duman RS, Malberg J, Nakagawa S (2001) Regulation of adult neurogenesis by psychotropic drugs and stress. *J Pharmacol Exp Ther* 299, 401–407.

Elzinga BM, Bremner JD (2002) Are the neural substrates of memory the final common pathway in posttraumatic stress disorder (PTSD)? *J Affect Disord* 70, 1–17.

Emdad R, Bonekamp D, Söndergaard HP et al. (2006) Morphometric and psychometric comparisons between non-substance-abusing patients with posttraumatic stress disorder and normal controls. *Psychother Psychosom* 75, 122–132.

Etkin A, Egner T, Kalisch R (2011) Emotional processing in anterior cingulate and medial prefrontal cortex. *Trends Cogn Sci* 15, 85–93.

Etkin A, Wager TD (2007) Functional neuroimaging of anxiety: a meta-analysis of emotional processing in PTSD, social anxiety disorder, and specific phobia. *Am J Psychiatry* 164, 1476.

Falconer E, Bryant R, Felmingham KL et al. (2009) The neural networks of inhibitory control in posttraumatic stress disorder. *J Psychiatry Neurosci JPN* 33, 413.

Fani N, Ashraf A, Afzal N et al. (2011) Increased neural response to trauma scripts in posttraumatic stress disorder following paroxetine treatment: A pilot study. *Neuroscience Letters* 491, 196–201.

Felmingham K, Kemp A, Williams L et al. (2007) Changes in anterior cingulate and amygdala after cognitive behavior therapy of posttraumatic stress disorder. *Psychol Sci* 18, 127–129.

Felmingham K, Williams LM, Kemp AH et al. (2010) Neural responses to masked fear faces: Sex differences and trauma exposure in posttraumatic stress disorder. *J Abnorm Psychol* 119, 241–247.

Felmingham KL, Williams LM, Kemp AH et al. (2009) Anterior cingulate activity to salient stimuli is modulated by autonomic arousal in Posttraumatic Stress Disorder. *Psychiatry Res Neuroimaging* 173, 59–62.

Fennema-Notestine C, Stein MB, Kennedy CM et al. (2002) Brain morphometry in female victims of intimate partner violence with and without posttraumatic stress disorder. *Biol Psychiatry* 52, 1089–1101.

Ferry B, Roozendaal B, McGaugh JL (1999) Role of norepinephrine in mediating stress hormone regulation of long-term memory storage: a critical involvement of the amygdala. *Biol Psychiatry* 46, 1140–1152.

Fonzo GA, Simmons AN, Thorp SR et al. (2010) Exaggerated and disconnected insular-amygdalar blood oxygenation level-dependent response to threat-related emotional faces in women with intimate-partner violence posttraumatic stress disorder. *Biol Psychiatry* 68, 433–441.

Fowler CD, Liu Y, Ouimet C, Wang Z (2002) The effects of social environment on adult neurogenesis in the female prairie vole. *J Neurobiol* 51, 115–128.

Freeman TW, Cardwell D, Karson CN, Komoroski RA (1998) In vivo proton magnetic resonance spectroscopy of the medial temporal lobes of subjects with combat-related posttraumatic stress disorder. *Magn Reson Med* 40, 66–71.

Frewen P, Lane RD, Neufeld RWJ et al. (2008) Neural Correlates of Levels of Emotional Awareness During Trauma Script-Imagery in Posttraumatic Stress Disorder. *Psychosom Med* 70, 27–31.

Fujita M, Southwick SM, Denucci CC et al. (2004) Central type benzodiazepine receptors in Gulf War veterans with posttraumatic stress disorder. *Biol Psychiatry* 56, 95–100.

Garcia R (2002) Stress, metaplasticity, and antidepressants. *Curr Mol Med* 2, 629–638.

Germain A, James J, Insana S et al. (2013) A window into the invisible wound of war: functional neuroimaging of REM sleep in returning combat veterans with PTSD. *Psychiatry Res Neuroimaging* 211, 176–179.

Geuze E, Van Berckel BNM, Lammertsma AA et al. (2008d) Reduced GABAA benzodiazepine receptor binding in veterans with post-traumatic stress disorder. *Mol Psychiatry* 13, 74–83.

Geuze E, Vermetten E, de Kloet CS, Westenberg HGM (2008c) Precuneal activity during encoding in veterans with posttraumatic stress disorder. *Prog Brain Res* 167, 293–297.

Geuze E, Vermetten E, Ruf M et al. (2008b) Neural correlates of associative learning and memory in veterans with posttraumatic stress disorder. *J Psychiatr Res* 42, 659–669.

Geuze E, Westenberg HG, Jochims A et al. (2007) Altered pain processing in veterans with posttraumatic stress disorder. *Arch Gen Psychiatry* 64, 76–85.

Geuze E, Westenberg HGM, Heinecke A et al. (2008a) Thinner prefrontal cortex in veterans with posttraumatic stress disorder. *NeuroImage* 41, 675–681.

Gilbertson MW, Gurvits TV, Lasko NB et al. (2001) Multivariate assessment of explicit memory function in combat veterans with posttraumatic stress disorder. *J Trauma Stress* 14, 413–432.

Gilbertson MW, Shenton ME, Ciszewski A et al. (2002) Smaller hippocampal volume predicts pathologic vulnerability to psychological trauma. *Nat Neurosci* 5, 1242–1247.

Gilboa A, Shalev AY, Laor L et al. (2004) Functional connectivity of the prefrontal cortex and the amygdala in posttraumatic stress disorder. *Biol Psychiatry* 55, 263–272.

Golier J, Yehuda R (1998) Neuroendocrine activity and memory-related impairments in posttraumatic stress disorder. *Dev Psychopathol* 10, 857–869.

Golier J, Yehuda R, Cornblatt B et al. (1997) Sustained attention in combat-related posttraumatic stress disorder. *Integr Physiol Behav Sci* 32, 52–61.

Golier JA, Yehuda R, De Santi S et al. (2005) Absence of hippocampal volume differences in survivors of the Nazi Holocaust with and without posttraumatic stress disorder. *Psychiatry Res Neuroimaging* 139, 53–64.

Gould E, McEwen BS, Tanapat P et al. (1997) Neurogenesis in the dentate gyrus of the adult tree shrew is regulated by psychosocial stress and NMDA receptor activation. *J Neurosci* 17, 2492–2498.

Gurvits TV, Shenton ME, Hokama H et al. (1996) Magnetic resonance imaging study of hippocampal volume in chronic, combat-related posttraumatic stress disorder. *Biol Psychiatry* 40, 1091–1099.

Hakamata Y, Matsuoka Y, Inagaki M et al. (2007) Structure of orbitofrontal cortex and its longitudinal course in cancer-related post-traumatic stress disorder. *Neurosci Res* 59, 383–389.

Hara E, Matsuoka Y, Hakamata Y et al. (2008) Hippocampal and amygdalar volumes in breast cancer survivors with posttraumatic stress disorder. *J Neuropsychiatry Clin Neurosci* 20, 302–308.

Hayes JP, LaBar KS, McCarthy G et al. (2011) Reduced hippocampal and amygdala activity predicts memory distortions for trauma reminders in combat-related PTSD. *J Psychiatr Res* 45, 660–669.

Hayes JP, LaBar KS, Petty CM et al. (2009) Alterations in the neural circuitry for emotion and attention associated with posttraumatic stress symptomatology. *Psychiatry Res Neuroimaging* 172, 7–15.

Hayes JP, VanElzakker MB, Shin LM (2012) Emotion and cognition interactions in PTSD: a review of neurocognitive and neuroimaging studies. *Front Integr Neurosci* 6, 89.

Hedges DW, Allen S, Tate DF et al. (2003) Reduced hippocampal volume in alcohol and substance naive Vietnam combat veterans with posttraumatic stress disorder. *Cogn Behav Neurol* 16, 219–224.

Hedges DW, Thatcher GW, Bennett PJ et al. (2008) Brain Integrity and Cerebral Atrophy in Vietnam Combat Veterans with and without Posttraumatic Stress Disorder. *Neurocase* 13, 402–410.

Hopper JW, Frewen PA, van der Kolk BA, Lanius RA (2007) Neural correlates of reexperiencing, avoidance, and dissociation in PTSD: Symptom dimensions and emotion dysregulation in responses to script-driven trauma imagery. *J Trauma Stress* 20, 713–725.

Hou C, Liu J, Wang K et al. (2007) Brain responses to symptom provocation and trauma-related short-term memory recall in coal mining accident survivors with acute severe PTSD. *Brain Res* 1144, 165–174.

Irle E, Lange C, Sachsse U (2005) Reduced size and abnormal asymmetry of parietal cortex in women with borderline personality disorder. *Biol Psychiatry* 57, 173–182.

Jackowski AP, Douglas-Palumberi H, Jackowski M et al. (2008) Corpus callosum in maltreated children with posttraumatic stress disorder: A diffusion tensor imaging study. *Psychiatry Res Neuroimaging* 162, 256–261.

Jatzko A, Rothenhofer S, Schmitt A et al. (2006) Hippocampal volume in chronic posttraumatic stress disorder (PTSD): MRI study using two different evaluation methods. *J Affect Disord* 94, 121–126.

Jenkins MA, Langlais PJ, Delis D, Cohen R (1998) Learning and memory in rape victims with posttraumatic stress disorder. *Am J Psychiatry* 155, 278–279.

Kasai K, Yamasue H, Gilbertson MW et al. (2008) Evidence for Acquired Pregenual Anterior Cingulate Gray Matter Loss from a Twin Study of Combat-Related Posttraumatic Stress Disorder. *Biol Psychiatry* 63, 550–556.

Kemp AH, Felmingham K, Das P et al. (2007) Influence of comorbid depression on fear in posttraumatic stress disorder: An fMRI study. *Psychiatry Res Neuroimaging* 155, 265–269.

Kemp AH, Felmingham KL, Falconer E et al. (2009) Heterogeneity of non-conscious fear perception in posttraumatic stress disorder as a function of physiological arousal: an fMRI study. *Psychiatry Res Neuroimaging* 174, 158–161.

Kessler RC, Berglund P, Demler O et al. (2005) Lifetime prevalence and age-of-onset distributions of DSM-IV disorders in the National Comorbidity Survey Replication. *Arch Gen Psychiatry* 62, 593.

Kessler RC, Sonnega A, Bromet E et al. (1995) Posttraumatic stress disorder in the National Comorbidity Survey. *Arch Gen Psychiatry* 52, 1048.

Kim MJ, Chey J, Chung A et al. (2008) Diminished rostral anterior cingulate activity in response to threat-related events in posttraumatic stress disorder. *J Psychiatr Res* 42, 268–277.

Kim MJ, Lyoo IK, Kim SJ et al. (2005) Disrupted white matter tract integrity of anterior cingulate in trauma survivors. *Neuroreport* 16, 1049–1053.

Kim SJ, Jeong D-U, Sim ME et al. (2007) Asymmetrically altered integrity of cingulum bundle in posttraumatic stress disorder. *Neuropsychobiology* 54, 120–125.

Kimbrell T, Leulf C, Cardwell D et al. (2005) Relationship of in vivo medial temporal lobe magnetic resonance spectroscopy to documented combat exposure in veterans with chronic posttraumatic stress disorder. *Psychiatry Res Neuroimaging* 140, 91–94.

Kitayama N, Brummer M, Hertz L et al. (2007) Morphologic alterations in the corpus callosum in abuse-related posttraumatic stress disorder: a preliminary study. *J Nerv Ment Dis* 195, 1027.

Kitayama N, Vaccarino V, Kutner M et al. (2005) Magnetic resonance imaging (MRI) measurement of hippocampal volume in posttraumatic stress disorder: a meta-analysis. *J Affect Disord* 88, 79–86.

Koenigs M, Huey ED, Raymont V et al. (2007) Focal brain damage protects against post-traumatic stress disorder in combat veterans. *Nat Neurosci* 11, 232–237.

Landré L, Destrieux C, Baudry M et al. (2010) Preserved subcortical volumes and cortical thickness in women with sexual abuse-related PTSD. *Psychiatry Res Neuroimaging* 183, 181–186.

Lanius RA, Bluhm RL, Coupland NJ et al. (2010) Default mode network connectivity as a predictor of post-traumatic stress disorder symptom severity in acutely traumatized subjects. *Acta Psychiatr Scand* 121, 33–40.

Lanius RA, Williamson PC, Densmore M et al. (2001) Neural correlates of traumatic memories in posttraumatic stress disorder: a functional MRI investigation. *Am J Psychiatry* 158, 1920–1922.

Lanius RA, Williamson PC, Hopper J et al. (2003) Recall of emotional states in posttraumatic stress disorder: an fMRI investigation. *Biol Psychiatry* 53, 204–210.

Lawrence MS, Sapolsky RM (1994) Glucocorticoids accelerate ATP loss following metabolic insults in cultured hippocampal neurons. *Brain Res* 646, 303–306.

LeDoux J (2003) The emotional brain, fear, and the amygdala. *Cell Mol Neurobiol* 23, 727–738.

Levitt JJ, Chen QC, May FS et al. (2006) Volume of cerebellar vermis in monozygotic twins discordant for combat exposure: lack of relationship to post-traumatic stress disorder. *Psychiatry Res Neuroimaging* 148, 143–149.

Li L, Chen S, Liu J et al. (2006) Magnetic resonance imaging and magnetic resonance spectroscopy study of deficits in hippocampal structure in fire victims with recent-onset posttraumatic stress disorder. *Can J Psychiatry* 51, 431.

Liberzon I, Britton JC, Luan Phan K (2003) Neural correlates of traumatic recall in posttraumatic stress disorder. *Stress Int J Biol Stress* 6, 151–156.

Liberzon I, Martis B (2006) Neuroimaging studies of emotional responses in PTSD. *Ann NY Acad Sci* 1071, 87–109.

Liberzon I, Phan KL (2003) Brain-imaging studies of posttraumatic stress disorder. *CNS Spectr* 8, 641–650.

Liberzon I, Taylor SF, Amdur R et al. (1999) Brain activation in PTSD in response to trauma-related stimuli. *Biol Psychiatry* 45, 817–826.

Liberzon I, Taylor SF, Phan KL et al. (2007) Altered central micro-opioid receptor binding after psychological trauma. *Biol Psychiatry* 61, 1030–1038.

Lim MK, Suh CH, Kim HJ et al. (2003) Fire-related post-traumatic stress disorder: Brain 1H-MR spetroscopic findings. *Korean J Radiol* 4, 79–84.

Lindauer RJ, Booij J, Habraken J et al. (2004a) Cerebral blood flow changes during script-driven imagery in police officers with posttraumatic stress disorder. *Biol Psychiatry* 56, 853–861.

Lindauer RJ, Olff M, van Meijel EP et al. (2006) Cortisol, learning, memory, and attention in relation to smaller hippocampal volume in police officers with posttraumatic stress disorder. *Biol Psychiatry* 59, 171–177.

Lindauer RJ, Vlieger E-J, Jalink M et al. (2004b) Smaller hippocampal volume in Dutch police officers with posttraumatic stress disorder. *Biol Psychiatry* 56, 356–363.

Lindauer RJ, Vlieger E-J, Jalink M et al. (2005) Effects of psychotherapy on hippocampal volume in out-patients with post-traumatic stress disorder: a MRI investigation. *Psychol Med* 35, 1421–1432.

Looi JCL, Maller JJ, Pagani M et al. (2009) Caudate volumes in public transportation workers exposed to trauma in the Stockholm train system. *Psychiatry Res Neuroimaging* 171, 138–143.

Lucassen PJ, Fuchs E, Czéh B (2004) Antidepressant treatment with tianeptine reduces apoptosis in the hippocampal dentate gyrus and temporal cortex. *Biol Psychiatry* 55, 789–796.

Luine V, Villegas M, Martinez C, McEwen BS (1994) Repeated stress causes reversible impairments of spatial memory performance. *Brain Res* 639, 167–170.

Mahmutyazıcıo\uglu K, Konuk N, Özdemir H et al. (2005) Evaluation of the hippocampus and the anterior cingulate gyrus by proton MR spectroscopy in patients with post-traumatic stress disorder. *Evaluation* 11, 125–129.

Malberg JE, Eisch AJ, Nestler EJ, Duman RS (2000) Chronic antidepressant treatment increases neurogenesis in adult rat hippocampus. *J Neurosci* 20, 9104–9110.

Matsuoka Y, Yamawaki S, Inagaki M et al. (2003) A volumetric study of amygdala in cancer survivors with intrusive recollections. *Biol Psychiatry* 54, 736–743.

May FS, Chen QC, Gilbertson MW et al. (2004) Cavum septum pellucidum in monozygotic twins discordant for combat exposure: relationship to posttraumatic stress disorder. *Biol Psychiatry* 55, 656–658.

McEwen BS, Angulo J, Cameron H et al. (1992) Paradoxical effects of adrenal steroids on the brain: protection versus degeneration. *Biol Psychiatry* 31, 177–199.

McEwen BS, Chattarji S (2004) Molecular mechanisms of neuroplasticity and pharmacological implications: the example of tianeptine. *Eur Neuropsychopharmacol* 14, S497–S502.

McFall ME, Murburg MM, Ko GN, Veith RC (1990) Autonomic responses to stress in Vietnam combat veterans with posttraumatic stress disorder. *Biol Psychiatry* 27, 1165–1175.

McLaughlin KJ, Baran SE, Conrad CD (2009) Chronic stress-and sex-specific neuromorphological and functional changes in limbic structures. *Mol Neurobiol* 40, 166–182.

Milad MR, Pitman RK, Ellis CB et al. (2009) Neurobiological basis of failure to recall extinction memory in posttraumatic stress disorder. *Biol Psychiatry* 66, 1075–1082.

Milad MR, Quirk GJ (2002) Neurons in medial prefrontal cortex signal memory for fear extinction. *Nature* 420, 70–74.

Milad MR, Rauch SL, Pitman RK, Quirk GJ (2006) Fear extinction in rats: implications for human brain imaging and anxiety disorders. *Biol Psychol* 73, 61–71.

Mohanakrishnan Menon P, Nasrallah HA, Lyons JA et al. (2003) Single-voxel proton MR spectroscopy of right versus left hippocampi in PTSD. *Psychiatry Res Neuroimaging* 123, 101–108.

Moores KA, Clark CR, McFarlane AC et al. (2008) Abnormal recruitment of working memory updating networks during maintenance of trauma-neutral information in post-traumatic stress disorder. *Psychiatry Res Neuroimaging* 163, 156–170.

Moradi AR, Neshat Doost HT, Taghavi MR et al. (1999) Everyday memory deficits in children and adolescents with PTSD: Performance on the Rivermead Behavioural Memory Test. *J Child Psychol Psychiatry* 40, 357–361.

Morey RA, Gold AL, LaBar KS et al. (2012) Amygdala volume changes with posttraumatic stress disorder in a large case-controlled veteran group. *Arch Gen Psychiatry* 69, 1169–1178.

Morey RA, Petty CM, Cooper DA et al. (2008) Neural systems for executive and emotional processing are modulated by symptoms of posttraumatic stress disorder in Iraq War veterans. *Psychiatry Res Neuroimaging* 162, 59–72.

Morgan MA, LeDoux JE (1995) Differential contribution of dorsal and ventral medial prefrontal cortex to the acquisition and extinction of conditioned fear in rats. *Behav Neurosci* 109, 681.

Morgan MA, Romanski LM, LeDoux JE (1993) Extinction of emotional learning: contribution of medial prefrontal cortex. *Neurosci Lett* 163, 109–113.

Murrough JW, Huang Y, Hu J et al. (2011) Reduced amygdala serotonin transporter binding in posttraumatic stress disorder. *Biol Psychiatry* 70, 1033–1038.

Nakano T, Wenner M, Inagaki M et al. (2002) Relationship between distressing cancer-related recollections and hippocampal volume in cancer survivors. *Am J Psychiatry* 159, 2087–2093.

Narayan M, Bremner JD, Kumar A (1999) Neuroanatomic substrates of late-life mental disorders. *J Geriatr Psychiatry Neurol* 12, 95–106.

Nardo D, Högberg G, Looi JCL et al. (2009) Gray matter density in limbic and paralimbic cortices is associated with trauma load and EMDR outcome in PTSD patients. *J Psychiatr Res* 44, 477–485.

Neumeister A, Normandin MD, Pietrzak RH et al. (2013) Elevated brain cannabinoid CB1 receptor availability in post-traumatic stress disorder: a positron emission tomography study. *Mol Psychiatry* 18, 1034–1040.

New AS, Fan J, Murrough JW et al. (2009) A Functional Magnetic Resonance Imaging Study of Deliberate Emotion Regulation in Resilience and Posttraumatic Stress Disorder. *Biol Psychiatry* 66, 656–664.

Nibuya M, Morinobu S, Duman RS (1995) Regulation of BDNF and trkB mRNA in rat brain by chronic electroconvulsive seizure and antidepressant drug treatments. *J Neurosci* 15, 7539–7547.

Osuch EA, Willis MW, Bluhm R et al. (2008) Neurophysiological responses to traumatic reminders in the acute aftermath of serious motor vehicle collisions using [15O]-H2O positron emission tomography. *Biol Psychiatry* 64, 327–335.

Pavić L, Gregurek R, Radoš M et al. (2007) Smaller right hippocampus in war veterans with posttraumatic stress disorder. *Psychiatry Res Neuroimaging* 154, 191–198.

Pederson CL, Maurer SH, Kaminski PL et al. (2004) Hippocampal volume and memory performance in a community-based sample of women with posttraumatic stress disorder secondary to child abuse. *J Trauma Stress* 17, 37–40.

Phan KL, Britton JC, Taylor SF et al. (2006) Corticolimbic blood flow during nontraumatic emotional processing in posttraumatic stress disorder. *Arch Gen Psychiatry* 63, 184.

Phelps EA (2006) Emotion and cognition: insights from studies of the human amygdala. *Annu Rev Psychol* 57, 27–53.

Piefke M, Pestinger M, Arin T et al. (2007) The neurofunctional mechanisms of traumatic and non-traumatic memory in patients with acute PTSD following accident trauma. *Neurocase* 13, 342–357.

Pietrzak RH, Gallezot JD, Ding YS et al. (2013) Association of posttraumatic stress disorder with reduced in vivo norepinephrine transporter availability in the locus coeruleus. *JAMA Psychiatry* 70, 1199–1205.

Pissiota A, Frans Ö, Fernandez M et al. (2002) Neurofunctional correlates of posttraumatic stress disorder: a PET symptom provocation study. *Eur Arch Psychiatry Clin Neurosci* 252, 68–75.

Pitman RK (1989) Post-traumatic stress disorder, hormones, and memory. *Biol Psychiatry* 26, 221–223.

Pitman RK, Orr SP, Forgue DF et al. (1987) Psychophysiologic assessment of posttraumatic stress disorder imagery in Vietnam combat veterans. *Arch Gen Psychiatry* 44, 970.

Pitman RK, Shin LM, Rauch SL (2001) Investigating the pathogenesis of posttraumatic stress disorder with neuroimaging. *J Clin Psychiatry* 62 Suppl 17, 47–54.

Protopopescu X, Pan H, Tuescher O et al. (2005) Differential time courses and specificity of amygdala activity in posttraumatic stress disorder subjects and normal control subjects. *Biol Psychiatry* 57, 464–473.

Quirk GJ (2002) Memory for extinction of conditioned fear is long-lasting and persists following spontaneous recovery. *Learn Mem* 9, 402–407.

Quirk GJ, Beer JS (2006) Prefrontal involvement in the regulation of emotion: convergence of rat and human studies. *Curr Opin Neurobiol* 16, 723–727.

Radley JJ, Sisti HM, Hao J et al. (2004) Chronic behavioral stress induces apical dendritic reorganization in pyramidal neurons of the medial prefrontal cortex. *Neuroscience* 125, 1–6.

Rauch SL, Shin LM, Phelps EA (2006) Neurocircuitry models of posttraumatic stress disorder and extinction: human neuroimaging research—past, present, and future. *Biol Psychiatry* 60, 376–382.

Rauch SL, Shin LM, Segal E et al. (2003) Selectively reduced regional cortical volumes in post-traumatic stress disorder. *Neuroreport* 14, 913–916.

Rauch SL, van der Kolk BA, Fisler RE et al. (1996) A symptom provocation study of posttraumatic stress disorder using positron emission tomography and script-driven imagery. *Arch Gen Psychiatry* 53, 380.

Rauch SL, Whalen PJ, Shin LM et al. (2000) Exaggerated amygdala response to masked facial stimuli in posttraumatic stress disorder: a functional MRI study. *Biol Psychiatry* 47, 769–776.

Roca V, Freeman TW (2001) Complaints of impaired memory in veterans with PTSD. *Am J Psychiatry* 158, 1738–1739.

Rogers MA, Yamasue H, Abe O et al. (2009) Smaller amygdala volume and reduced anterior cingulate gray matter density associated with history of post-traumatic stress disorder. *Psychiatry Res Neuroimaging* 174, 210–216.

Sachinvala N, Von Scotti H, McGuire M et al. (2000) Memory, attention, function, and mood among patients with chronic posttraumatic stress disorder. *J Nerv Ment Dis* 188, 818–823.

Saigh PA, Bremner JD (1999) The history of posttraumatic stress disorder.

Sailer U, Robinson S, Fischmeister FPS et al. (2008) Altered reward processing in the nucleus accumbens and mesial prefrontal cortex of patients with posttraumatic stress disorder. *Neuropsychologia* 46, 2836–2844.

Sakamoto H, Fukuda R, Okuaki T et al. (2005) Parahippocampal activation evoked by masked traumatic images in posttraumatic stress disorder: a functional MRI study. *Neuroimage* 26, 813–821.

Santarelli L, Saxe M, Gross C et al. (2003) Requirement of hippocampal neurogenesis for the behavioral effects of antidepressants. *Science* 301, 805–809.

Sapolsky RM (1996) Why stress is bad for your brain. *Science* 273, 749–750.

Sapolsky RM, Uno H, Rebert CS, Finch CE (1990) Hippocampal damage associated with prolonged glucocorticoid exposure in primates. *J Neurosci* 10, 2897–2902.

Schuff N, Marmar CR, Weiss DS et al. (1997) Reduced hippocampal volume and N-acetyl aspartate in posttraumatic stress disorder. *Ann NY Acad Sci* 821, 516–520.

Schuff N, Neylan TC, Fox-Bosetti S et al. (2008) Abnormal N-acetylaspartate in hippocampus and anterior cingulate in posttraumatic stress disorder. *Psychiatry Res Neuroimaging* 162, 147–157.

Schuff N, Neylan TC, Lenoci MA et al. (2001) Decreased hippocampal *N*-acetylaspartate in the absence of atrophy in posttraumatic stress disorder. *Biol Psychiatry* 50, 952–959.

Seedat S, Videen JS, Kennedy CM, Stein MB (2005) Single voxel proton magnetic resonance spectroscopy in women with and without intimate partner violence-related posttraumatic stress disorder. *Psychiatry Res Neuroimaging* 139, 249–258.

Semple WE, Goyer PF, McCormick R et al. (2000) Higher brain blood flow at amygdala and lower frontal cortex blood flow in PTSD patients with comorbid cocaine and alcohol abuse compared with normals. *Psychiatry* 63, 65–74.

Shin LM, Kosslyn SM, McNally RJ et al. (1997) Visual imagery and perception in posttraumatic stress disorder: a positron emission tomographic investigation. *Arch Gen Psychiatry* 54, 233.

Shin LM, Lasko NB, Macklin ML et al. (2009) Resting metabolic activity in the cingulate cortex and vulnerability to posttraumatic stress disorder. *Arch Gen Psychiatry* 66, 1099–1107.

Shin LM, McNally RJ, Kosslyn SM et al. (1999) Regional cerebral blood flow during script-driven imagery in childhood sexual abuse-related PTSD: a PET investigation. *Am J Psychiatry* 156, 575–584.

Shin LM, Orr SP, Carson MA et al. (2004b) Regional cerebral blood flow in the amygdala and medial prefrontal cortex during traumatic imagery in male and female Vietnam veterans with PTSD. *Arch Gen Psychiatry* 61, 168–176.

Shin LM, Shin PS, Heckers S et al. (2004a) Hippocampal function in posttraumatic stress disorder. *Hippocampus* 14, 292–300.

Shin LM, Whalen PJ, Pitman RK et al. (2001) An fMRI study of anterior cingulate function in posttraumatic stress disorder. *Biol Psychiatry* 50, 932–942.

Shin LM, Wright CI, Cannistraro PA et al. (2005) A functional magnetic resonance imaging study of amygdala and medial prefrontal cortex responses to overtly presented fearful faces in posttraumatic stress disorder. *Arch Gen Psychiatry* 62, 273.

Simmons A, Strigo IA, Matthews SC et al. (2009) Initial Evidence of a Failure to Activate Right Anterior Insula During Affective Set Shifting in Posttraumatic Stress Disorder. *Psychosom Med* 71, 373–377.

Simmons AN, Paulus MP, Thorp SR et al. (2008) Functional activation and neural networks in women with posttraumatic stress disorder related to intimate partner violence. *Biol Psychiatry* 64, 681–690.

Smith MA, Makino S, Kvetnansky R, Post RM (1995) Stress and glucocorticoids affect the expression of brain-derived neurotrophic factor and neurotrophin-3 mRNAs in the hippocampus. *J Neurosci* 15, 1768–1777.

Southwick SM, Krystal JH, Morgan CA et al. (1993) Abnormal noradrenergic function in posttraumatic stress disorder. *Arch Gen Psychiatry* 50, 266.

Squire LR (2004) Memory systems of the brain: a brief history and current perspective. *Neurobiol Learn Mem* 82, 171–177.

Sripada RK, King AP, Welsh RC et al. (2012) Neural dysregulation in posttraumatic stress disorder: evidence for disrupted equilibrium between salience and default mode brain networks. *Psychosom Med* 74, 904–911.

Stein MB, Hanna C, Vaerum V, Koverola C (1999) Memory functioning in adult women traumatized by childhood sexual abuse. *J Trauma Stress* 12, 527–534.

Stein MB, Koverola C, Hanna C et al. (1997) Hippocampal volume in women victimized by childhood sexual abuse. *Psychol Med* 27, 951–959.

Strigo IA, Simmons AN, Matthews SC et al. (2010) Neural correlates of altered pain response in women with posttraumatic stress disorder from intimate partner violence. *Biol Psychiatry* 68, 442–450.

Teicher MH, Dumont NL, Ito Y et al. (2004) Childhood neglect is associated with reduced corpus callosum area. *Biol Psychiatry* 56, 80–85.

Thomaes K, Dorrepaal E, Draijer N et al. (2010) Reduced anterior cingulate and orbitofrontal volumes in child abuse-related complex PTSD. *J Clin Psychiatry* 71, 1636–1644.

Uddo M, Vasterling JJ, Brailey K, Sutker PB (1993) Memory and attention in combat-related post-traumatic stress disorder (PTSD). *J Psychopathol Behav Assess* 15, 43–52.

Uno H, Tarara R, Else JG et al. (1989) Hippocampal damage associated with prolonged and fatal stress in primates. *J Neurosci* 9, 1705–1711.

Vasterling JJ, Brailey K, Constans JI, Sutker PB (1998) Attention and memory dysfunction in posttraumatic stress disorder. *Neuropsychology* 12, 125.

Vasterling JJ, Duke LM, Brailey K et al. (2002) Attention, learning, and memory performances and intellectual resources in Vietnam veterans: PTSD and no disorder comparisons. *Neuropsychology* 16, 5.

Vermetten E, Bremner JD (2002a) Circuits and systems in stress. I. Preclinical studies. *Depress Anxiety* 15, 126–147.

Vermetten E, Bremner JD (2002b) Circuits and systems in stress. II. Applications to neurobiology and treatment in posttraumatic stress disorder. *Depress Anxiety* 16, 14–38.

Vermetten E, Vythilingam M, Southwick SM et al. (2003) Long-term treatment with paroxetine increases verbal declarative memory and hippocampal volume in posttraumatic stress disorder. *Biol Psychiatry* 54, 693–702.

Villarreal G, Hamilton DA, Graham DP et al. (2004) Reduced area of the corpus callosum in posttraumatic stress disorder. *Psychiatry Res Neuroimaging* 131, 227–235.

Villarreal G, Hamilton DA, Petropoulos H et al. (2002) Reduced hippocampal volume and total white matter volume in posttraumatic stress disorder. *Biol Psychiatry* 52, 119–125.

Vogt BA, Finch DM, Olson CR (1992) Functional heterogeneity in cingulate cortex: the anterior executive and posterior evaluative regions. *Cereb Cortex* 2, 435–443.

Wang H-H, Zhang Z-J, Tan Q-R et al. (2010b) Psychopathological, biological, and neuroimaging characterization of posttraumatic stress disorder in survivors of a severe coalmining disaster in China. *J Psychiatr Res* 44, 385–392.

Wang Z, Neylan TC, Mueller SG et al. (2010a) Magnetic resonance imaging of hippocampal subfields in posttraumatic stress disorder. *Arch Gen Psychiatry* 67, 296.

Wang Z, Zhou Y, Su S et al. (2013) 712–A longitudinal mri study of hippocampal subfields volume alteration in posttraumatic stress disorder following traffic accidents. *Eur Psychiatry* 28, 1.

Watanabe Y, Gould E, Cameron HA et al. (1992) Phenytoin prevents stress-and corticosterone-induced atrophy of CA3 pyramidal neurons. *Hippocampus* 2, 431–435.

Werner NS, Meindl T, Engel RR et al. (2009) Hippocampal function during associative learning in patients with posttraumatic stress disorder. *J Psychiatr Res* 43, 309–318.

Whalley MG, Rugg MD, Smith AP et al. (2009) Incidental retrieval of emotional contexts in post-traumatic stress disorder and depression: an fMRI study. *Brain Cogn* 69, 98–107.

Woodward SH, Kaloupek DG, Streeter CC et al. (2006) Decreased anterior cingulate volume in combat-related PTSD. *Biol Psychiatry* 59, 582–587.

Woon F, Hedges D (2009) Amygdala volume in adults with posttraumatic stress disorder: a meta-analysis. *J Neuropsychiatry Clin Neurosci* 21, 5–12.

Woon FL, Hedges DW (2008) Hippocampal and amygdala volumes in children and adults with childhood maltreatment-related posttraumatic stress disorder: A meta-analysis. *Hippocampus* 18, 729–736.

Woon FL, Sood S, Hedges DW (2010) Hippocampal volume deficits associated with exposure to psychological trauma and posttraumatic stress disorder in adults: a meta-analysis. *Prog Neuropsychopharmacol Biol Psychiatry* 34, 1181–1188.

Yamasue H, Kasai K, Iwanami A et al. (2003) Voxel-based analysis of MRI reveals anterior cingulate gray-matter volume reduction in posttraumatic stress disorder due to terrorism. *Proc Natl Acad Sci USA* 100, 9039–9043.

Yang P, Wu M-T, Hsu C-C, Ker J-H (2004) Evidence of early neurobiological alternations in adolescents with posttraumatic stress disorder: a functional MRI study. *Neurosci Lett* 370, 13–18.

Yehuda R, Keefe RS, Harvey PD, Levengood RA (1995) Learning and memory in combat veterans with posttraumatic stress disorder. *Am J Psychiatry* 152, 137–139.

Zalewski C, Thompson W, Gottesman I (1994) Comparison of neuropsychological test performance in PTSD, generalized anxiety disorder, and control Vietnam veterans. *Assessment* 1, 133–142.

PTSD and co-occuring conditions

CHAPTER 13

PTSD and mild traumatic brain injury

J. Douglas Bremner

Departments of Psychiatry & Behavioral Sciences and Radiology, Emory University School of Medicine, and the Atlanta VA Medical Center, Atlanta, GA, USA

13.1 Introduction

Posttraumatic stress disorder (PTSD) and mild traumatic brain injury (mTBI) overlap in a number of ways. PTSD and mTBI are often comorbid in combat veterans from Iraq and Afghanistan, and have been prioritized as two critically important priorities by the Veterans Administration (Brenner et al., 2010). Traumatic events, whether in the form of exposure to blasts in combat zones or motor vehicle accidents, can result in an impact to the head as well as being associated with psychological trauma. Several symptoms overlap between mTBI and PTSD, including problems with memory and concentration. In addition, headaches, sleep disturbances, and problems with chronic pain are frequently seen in both patient groups. Both diagnoses are currently based on clinical symptoms, and there are no objective diagnostic tests, including neuroimaging results, that can be used to corroborate the diagnosis in either disorder. However, research studies have found alterations in brain structure and function in both disorders, which in some areas have important overlaps (McAllister & Stein 2010; Stein & McAllister 2009). This chapter reviews the clinical overlap of PTSD and mTBI and differential diagnosis. It also reviews the use of neuroimaging in these disorders, which is primarily used now for research purposes and/or to exclude other diagnoses (Van Boven et al., 2009).

13.2 Mild TBI

Mild TBI is an important problem for soldiers deployed to Iraq and Afghanistan (Cifu et al., 2010; Jaffee et al., 2009; Kennedy et al., 2007). About 12% of soldiers

Posttraumatic Stress Disorder: From Neurobiology to Treatment, First Edition.
Edited by J. Douglas Bremner.
© 2016 John Wiley & Sons, Inc. Published 2016 by John Wiley & Sons, Inc.

returning from Iraq or Afghanistan have mTBI, and 11% have PTSD (Schneiderman et al., 2008). Mild TBI is defined as a loss of consciousness following a blow to the head or sudden acceleration/deceleration, loss of memory for events before or after the event, a change in mental state (feeling dazed, disoriented, or confused), or a focal neurological deficit that may or may not be transient (Mild Traumatic Brain Injury Committee of the Head Injury Interdisciplinary Special Interest Group of the American Congress of Rehabilitation Medicine, 1993). Mild TBI is ruled out if amnesia lasts longer than 24 hours, if the Glasgow Coma Scale Score after 30 minutes is less than 13, or if the loss of consciousness is more than 30 minutes. Mild TBI is not typically associated with structural brain changes on MRI or CT. Neurocognitive deficits (headache, confusion, problems with memory) can occur in the immediate aftermath of mTBI but most commonly resolve in the first 3 months (Levin et al., 1987). Brain injury from primary blast injury (in the absence of blunt trauma to the head) is actually quite rare and apparently fully reversible (Warden et al., 2009).

13.2.1 Brain Imaging in mTBI

Brain imaging has been used to study brain structure and function in patients with mTBI. Mollica et al. (2009) used magnetic resonance imaging (MRI) to study cortical thickness in 42 former political prisoners from Vietnam with a history of torture, with and without TBI. TBI was defined as loss of consciousness, post-event amnesia, and neurological symptoms. The TBI subjects showed cortical thinning in prefrontotemporal regions that were correlated with symptoms of depression after controlling for potential confounders. Koenigs et al. (2007) found that Vietnam veterans with brain damage involved ventral medial prefrontal cortex (PFC) and anterior temporal lobe (including amygdala) had reduced incidence of PTSD.

Studies have used magnetic resonance spectroscopy (MRS) measurement of N-acetyl aspartate (NAA, a marker of neuronal integrity) in the investigation of brain abnormalities in mTBI (Shutter et al., 2006). MRS studies showed decreased NAA/creatine in the splenium of the corpus callosum in mTBI patients compared with normal controls (Cecil et al., 1998). Other studies did not find significant reductions in NAA/creatine in frontal white matter of mTBI patients compared with controls, although reductions were seen in moderate and severe TBI (Garnett et al., 2000). Reductions in global NAA have been found to be predictive of outcome following severe head injury (Rutgers et al., 2008a). A study of patients with mTBI (GCS 13–15) and 30 seconds or more loss of consciousness found a significant reduction of 12% in whole-brain NAA. The authors reported no difference between subjects with and without MRI lesions (Cohen et al., 2007). There was also global and gray matter atrophy. Other studies of patients with mTBI (most of whom had abnormalities on CT or MRI) also showed decreased NAA in multiple brain regions (Govindaraju et al., 2004).

Studies have used MRI-based diffusion tensor imaging (DTI) to measure fractional anisotropy (FA), a measure of white matter integrity, in mTBI. FA measures movement of water, and a decrease in movement can be related to traumatic axonal injury of white matter fibers due to shearing effects. Several studies have shown reduced FA in white matter in mTBI (Rutgers et al., 2008b). Other DTI studies found initial increases in FA in acute mTBI in corpus callosum and several left hemisphere tracts (Mayer et al., 2011), while with the passage of time there is a decrease in white matter integrity in the corticospinal tract, sagittal stratum and superior longitudinal fasciculus but not the corpus callosum (Kraus et al., 2007). Changes were reversible for mTBI but not moderate or severe TBI (Kraus et al., 2007). Other studies have not shown differences in FA in mTBI although deficits in verbal memory as measured with the Selective Reminding Test were identified (Levin et al., 2010). Other studies found decreased FA in mTBI only in subjects with abnormalities on CT (Benson et al., 2007). A study of 46 mTBI and 26 controls showed no difference in whole-brain FA and a reduction in internal capsule and splenium of corpus callosum FA (Inglese et al., 2005). Patients with mTBI measured an average of 4 days after injury had decreased FA in centrum semiovale, corpus callosum, and internal capsule (Miles et al., 2008). Decreased FA was predictive of long-term cognitive function as measured by at least one outcome.

Lipton et al. (2008) compared FA measured with DTI in 17 patients with cognitive impairment related to mTBI and 10 controls. There was a decrease in subcortical white matter, corpus callosum, and internal capsule FA bilaterally (Lipton et al., 2008). A study of 34 adults with mTBI and persistent symptoms and 26 controls showed decreased FA in the anterior corona radiata, uncinate fasciculus, genu of the corpus callosum, inferior longitudinal fasiculus, and cingulum bundle; these changes correlated with cognitive function (Niogi et al., 2008). Another study showed reduced FA in the genu of the corpus callosum at less than 3 months after head injury but not after 3 months since the time of injury (Rutgers et al., 2008a). Iraq and Afghanistan veterans with mTBI had reduced FA in the corpus callosum, reduced macromolecular proton fraction in brain white matter tracts, and reduced glucose metabolism in parietal, somatosensory, and visual cortices (Petrie et al., 2014). In summary these studies are consistent with white matter abnormalities in mTBI that correlate with cognitive function and are reversible with time. Abnormal FA as measured with DTI, however, is highly nonspecific.

Mild TBI has also been associated with changes in brain function. Studies using magnetoencephalography found abnormal low-frequency activity in the brains of mTBI patients with post-concussive symptoms but not in those without symptoms (Lewine et al., 1999). Athletes tested within 1 week of a concussion showed increased blood flow during a finger-tapping task on functional MRI (fMRI) in parietal and lateral frontal and cerebellar regions (Jantzen et al., 2004). Studies performed during working memory tasks showed increased activation in mTBI patients during high-load working memory conditions in right parietal and right dorsolateral frontal regions (McAllister et al., 1999; McAllister et al., 2001).

Positron emission tomography (PET) and single photon emission computed tomography (SPECT) have been used to measure functional brain correlates of mTBI. SPECT has consistently been shown to be more sensitive in detection of abnormalities than computed tomography (CT) or MRI (Audenaert et al., 2003; Gray et al., 1992; Ichise et al., 2004; Nedd et al., 1993). About 60% of mTBI had cerebral cortical abnormalities on SPECT 6 months after the accident (Gray et al., 1992). SPECT imaging studies of brain blood flow showed decreased function in frontal (Abu-Judeh et al., 1998; Audenaert et al., 2003; Belanger et al., 2007; Bonne et al., 2003; Hofman et al., 2001; Ichise et al., 2004; Jacobs et al., 1994; Kant et al., 1997; Ruff et al., 1994; Umile et al., 2002; Varney & Bushnell, 1998), parietal (Hofman et al., 2001; Ichise et al., 2004), medial temporal (Belanger et al., 2007; Umile et al., 2002) and temporal regions (Audenaert et al., 2003; Bonne et al., 2003; Ichise et al., 2004; Jacobs et al., 1994; Kant et al., 1997) in patients with mTBI. Functional abnormalities were more commonly seen in mTBI patients with neuropsychological abnormalities (Ruff et al., 1994). An 18F-fluorodeoxyglucose (FDG) PET study showed a failure of activation in the right PFC during a working memory task in mTBI patients (Chen et al., 2003). Another FDG PET study of patients with mild or moderate TBI and normal CT scans scanned while performing a vigilance task showed significantly decreased function in medial temporal, posterior temporal, and posterior frontal cortices, as well as in the left caudate, and increased function in anterior temporal and anterior frontal cortices (Humayun et al., 1989). Normal SPECT brain scans after injury had a strong predictive value for favorable outcomes (Jacobs et al., 1994). In summary, a number of studies have shown abnormalities in multiple cortical regions in mTBI with functional imaging of the brain. In spite of this, PET and SPECT are not accepted for use in the diagnosis of mTBI.

13.3 Posttraumatic stress disorder

Posttraumatic stress disorder has debilitating effects on the individual, including potential changes in brain structure and function (see Chapter 17). As many as 30% of individuals will meet criteria for PTSD early after exposure to trauma; however, this goes on to chronic PTSD in about half (15%) of those patients (Kulka et al., 1990). Symptomatic responses to the trauma at the time it occurred, including dissociation (which can include symptoms like feeling you are out of your body or as if you are in a dream) (Bremner et al., 1992, 1998; Bremner & Marmar 1998; Cardena & Spiegel 1993; Koopman et al., 1994; Marmar et al., 1994; McFarlane 2000; Shalev et al., 1996), extreme feelings of panic (Bryant & Panasetis, 2005), or persistent elevations of heart rate (at 1 week but not 1 month), are associated with long-term psychopathology in trauma survivors (Bryant et al., 2004).

13.3.1 Brain structure and function in PTSD

There are a number of studies showing that psychological stress itself in the absence of physical injury can be associated with changes in memory and brain structures that mediate memory. As outlined in Chapter 6, the hippocampus plays a critical role in memory and is sensitive to stress. Animal studies showed that stress results in alterations to hippocampal morphology and deficits in hippocampal-based memory function (Diamond et al., 1996; Luine et al., 1994; Sapolsky et al., 1990; Uno et al., 1989) (see Chapter 6).

Neuropsychology studies demonstrated deficits in verbal declarative memory in PTSD (Elzinga & Bremner 2002). Memory deficits are seen in both combat veterans and civilians with PTSD(Barrett et al., 1996; Bremner et al., 1993, 1995; Brewin, 2001; Brewin et al., 2007; Buckley et al., 2000; Elzinga & Bremner 2002; Gil et al., 1990; Gilbertson et al., 2001; Golier & Yehuda 1998; Golier et al., 1997; Jenkins et al., 1998; Moradi et al., 1999; Roca & Freeman 2001; Sachinvala et al., 2000; Uddo et al., 1993; Vasterling et al., 1998, 2002; Yehuda et al., 1995) (although see Stein et al., 1999; Zalewski et al., 1994). Memory deficits were found in patients with PTSD but not in traumatized persons without PTSD (Bremner et al., 2004; Jenkins et al., 1998). This suggests that memory deficits are specific to PTSD, and not a non-specific response to trauma.

Neuroimaging studies showed alterations in the hippocampus in PTSD. Findings of smaller hippocampal volume measured with MRI in PTSD are described in detail in Chapter 17 (Bremner & Vermetten 2012). Studies in cancer survivors also found a correlation between intrusive memories and smaller hippocampal volume (Hara et al., 2008; Nakano et al., 2002). Meta-analyses that pooled data from all of the published studies found smaller hippocampal volume for both the left and right sides, equally in adult men and women with chronic PTSD, and no change in children (Kitayama et al., 2005; Smith 2005; Woon & Hedges 2008; Woon et al., 2010). Studies have also shown that PTSD patients have deficits in hippocampal activation while performing a verbal declarative memory task (Bremner et al., 2003; Shin et al., 2004) or a virtual water maze task (Astur et al., 2006). Hippocampal atrophy and hippocampal-based memory deficits reversed with treatment with the selective serotonin reuptake inhibitor, paroxetine, which has been shown to promote neurogenesis (the growth of neurons) in the hippocampus in preclinical studies (Vermetten et al., 2003).

Other brain imaging studies found volume reductions in the medial PFC. Studies in PTSD using MRI found thinner cortical volumes in the frontal and temporal cortex (Geuze et al., 2008b), smaller anterior cingulate volume (Kasai et al.,

2008; Kitayama et al., 2005; Rauch et al., 2003; Rogers et al., 2009; Thomaes et al., 2010; Woodward et al., 2006; Yamasue et al., 2003) and reduced NAA (De Bellis et al., 2000; Mahmutyazicioglu et al., 2005) (although see Seedat et al., 2005), decreased gray matter density (Corbo et al., 2005), smaller volume of the corpus callosum (De Bellis et al., 2002b; Kitayama et al., 2007; Teicher et al., 2004; Villarreal et al., 2004), reduced gray matter density in left posterior cingulate and the left posterior parahippocampal gyrus (Nardo et al., 2009), and smaller volume of the insula (Chen et al., 2006), cavum septum pellucidum (May et al., 2004), and orbitofrontal cortex in PTSD (Hakamata et al., 2007; Thomaes et al., 2010). Other studies showed no difference in volume of cerebellar vermis (Levitt et al., 2006) and increased volume of the right caudate (Looi et al., 2009); another study (Lim et al., 2003) showed decreased NAA in the basal ganglia in PTSD. Although some studies showed smaller amygdala volume in PTSD (Rogers et al., 2009; Thomaes et al., 2010) or in cancer patients with intrusive recollections (Matsuoka et al., 2003), a recent meta-analysis did not show smaller amygdala volumes in PTSD when results from multiple studies were combined (Woon & Hedges, 2008, 2009). Children with PTSD had increased gray matter volume in the right and left inferior and superior quadrants of the PFC and decreased pons and posterior vermis by volumetric MRI (Carrion et al., 2009). Other studies showed enlarged superior temporal gyrus volumes (De Bellis et al., 2002a) and reduced cerebral volume (De Bellis et al., 2002b) in children with PTSD.

Studies have used MRS measures of FA to assess white matter integrity, with a decrease in FA indicative of decreased white matter integrity in PTSD. Studies showed decreased FA in the medial and posterior portions of the corpus callosum in children with PTSD (Jackowski et al., 2008) and in the hippocampus, cingulum bundle (Wang et al., 2010), left side of rostral, subgenual and dorsal cingulum bundle (Kim et al., 2006) and left anterior cingulate (Kim et al., 2005, 2006) in adults with PTSD.

Imaging studies of brain function in PTSD are consistent with dysfunction of the medial PFC, amygdala, and hippocampus (Bremner, 1998, 2002, 2011; Cannistraro & Rauch, 2003; Liberzon & Martis, 2006; Liberzon & Phan, 2003; Liberzon et al., 2003; Pitman, 2001; Rauch et al., 2006). These studies, reviewed in Chapter 17, most consistently show failure of medial prefrontal activation during traumatic reminders, and increased amygdala activation with specific fear learning tasks. Studies show a failure of hippocampal activation with declarative memory and spatial memory tasks, and in some symptom provocation studies.

Studies have looked at neural correlates of acute traumatization. Patients with acute PTSD from surgical trauma had increased blood flow in the hippocampus, anterior cingulate and amygdala with exposure to traumatic memories (Piefke et al., 2007). One study of acute motor vehicle accident survivors showed decreased amygdala blood flow during exposure to traumatic scripts, and a negative correlation between symptom improvement at 3 months and hippocampal blood flow during exposure to traumatic scripts (Osuch et al., 2008).

Several studies have examined neural correlates of cognitive tasks in PTSD. Studies using specific declarative memory tasks found decreased activation of the hippocampus (Astur et al., 2006; Bremner et al., 2003; Shin et al., 2004) and insula (Chen et al., 2009; Whalley et al., 2009) in PTSD. During working memory tasks, PTSD patients showed decreased inferior frontal (Clark et al., 2003), parietal (Bryant et al., 2005; Clark et al., 2003), hippocampal and anterior cingulate function (Moores et al., 2008). In PTSD patients performing a working memory task, presentation of combat-related distractors was associated with increased activation in amygdala, ventrolateral PFC, and fusiform gyrus, and decreased activation in the dorsolateral PFC (Morey et al., 2008). An emotional oddball task was associated with activation in peri-amygdala areas, ventrolateral PFC, and orbitofrontal cortex (Pannu Hayes et al., 2009). PTSD patients showed reduced anterior cingulate activation during a same–different emotional conflict task (Kim et al., 2008). One study found a relative failure of connectivity during working memory tasks in PTSD in right inferior frontal gyrus and the right inferior parietal lobule, and stronger connectivity between the posterior cingulate cortex and the right superior frontal gyrus and between the medial PFC and the left parahippocampal gyrus during a working memory task (Daniels et al., 2010)

Functional imaging studies have also shown evidence of deficits in neural circuits involved in motivation and reward systems in PTSD. During the processing of gains in the late phase of learning, PTSD patients, as compared with controls, showed lower activation in the nucleus accumbens and the mesial PFC during a decision-making task (Sailer et al., 2008). PTSD patients showed a failure of PFC activation during attempts to diminish emotional responses to emotional pictures (New et al., 2009). Other studies showed decreased insula activation with an affective set shifting task (Simmons et al., 2009). One study showed a failure of right dorsolateral frontal and increased striatal activity in PTSD during a task involving inhibitory control (Falconer et al., 2009). Levels of emotional awareness were negatively correlated with activation of the anterior cingulate in PTSD patients (Frewen et al., 2008).

Studies have examined neural correlates of pain processing in PTSD. PTSD patients were shown to have decreased sensitivity to pain. During the processing of pain, PTSD subjects had increased insula (Geuze et al., 2007; Strigo et al., 2010) and dorsolateral PFC activation (Strigo et al., 2010), while other studies showed increased hippocampal and amygdala activation and decreased ventrolateral prefrontal function (Geuze et al., 2007).

More recently, studies have looked at connectivity between different brain areas in PTSD. Increased connectivity between amygdala and anterior cingulate in acutely traumatized patients was associated with current PTSD symptom severity as well as risk for chronicity of future PTSD symptoms (Lanius et al., 2010). PTSD patients showed increased connectivity between amygdala, anterior cingulate, visual cortex and subcallosal gyrus (Gilboa et al., 2004). Other studies showed a decrease in posterior cingulate/precuneus connectivity in a resting state in patients with PTSD (Bluhm et al., 2009).

Some positron emission tomography and SPECT receptor imaging studies showed reduced binding of benzodiazepine receptors in combat veterans in the frontal cortex (Bremner et al., 2000; Geuze et al., 2008a) but others did not (Fujita et al., 2004), while other studies found a reduction in anterior cingulate opiate receptor binding (Liberzon et al., 2007) and an increase in hippocampal beta2 nicotinic acetylcholine receptor binding in PTSD (Czermak et al., 2008) with no change in binding of the 5-hydroxytryptamine 1A serotonin receptor (Bonne et al., 2005).

13.4 Overlap between mTBI and PTSD

There is considerable overlap of symptoms between mTBI and PTSD, and the evaluation of these two disorders is considerably complex (see Table 13.1) (Bryant, 2011; Vasterling & Dikmen, 2012).

Estimates of the prevalence of PTSD in mTBI patients vary widely (0–56%) (Bryant, 2001; Bryant et al., 2003; McMillan, 1996). An early study of 24 patients

Table 13.1 Symptom overlap of posttraumatic stress disorder (PTSD) and mild traumatic brain injury (mTBI).

Symptom	PTSD	mTBI
Memory impairment	+	+
Poor concentration	+	+
Sleep disturbance	+	+
Headache	+	*
Dizziness	–	+
Flashbacks	+	–
Intrusive memories	+	–
Avoidance of reminders	+	–
Startle	+	–
Hypervigilance	+	–
Emotional numbing	+	–
Lack of interest in people/things	+	*

*Technically not a symptom, but frequently seen comorbidly.

with head injury showed that 33% had the diagnosis of PTSD. Eighty-two per cent of the patients had difficulty recalling some or all aspects of the trauma (Ohry et al., 1996). Gil et al. (2005) studied 120 subjects who presented with mTBI with hospitalization. They found that 14% developed PTSD at 6 months. Another study of TBI patients found that PTSD was more common in those who remembered the event, and affected only 3% of those with no memory of the accident (Glaesser et al., 2004). Bryant et al. (2000) studied 96 patients with severe TBI. PTSD was seen in 27%. Only 19% had intrusive memories of the trauma, but 96% had emotional reactivity. Patients with more PTSD symptoms had worse health and lower functioning (Bryant et al., 2001). Those with avoidant coping style had higher levels of PTSD (Bryant & Marosszeky, 2000). In another study by these authors, 1,084 traumatically injured persons who presented to emergency rooms were assessed. Patients with mTBI (defined as loss of consciousness without neurological deficits) showed a significant 1.9-fold increased risk of PTSD. Functional impairment, rather than mTBI, predicted the development of psychiatric illness (Bryant et al., 2010). PTSD rates were higher in patients with head injuries compared with other types of physical injuries following the Oklahoma City bombing (Walilko et al., 2009).

Creamer et al. (2005) looked at mTBI in 307 consecutive admissions to a level 1 trauma center. Over half of patients had at least partial recall of the event. Ten per cent of patients developed PTSD by 12 months post-injury, and there was no difference in PTSD symptoms between those with and without amnesia for the event. Hickling et al. (1998) studied 107 car accident victims with and without brain injury; in all, 38 (36%) of them developed PTSD. Patients who lost consciousness had greater impairment on neuropsychological testing of speed and verbal ability. PTSD was as common in TBI as non-TBI subjects. McMillan and colleagues studied 34 cases of TBI; 59% met criteria for PTSD by self-report measure, but only 3% had PTSD based on clinician-administered assessment with the Clinician Administered PTSD Scale (CAPS) (Sumpter & McMillan 2005). The authors concluded that the effects of head injury led to discrepancies in diagnosis. Williams et al. (2002) studied 66 patients with severe TBI. PTSD symptoms were not associated with severity of brain injury. Flesher et al. (2001) found that patients with amnesia had lower norepinephrine/cortisol ratios and fewer PTSD symptoms than non-amnesiacs.

Studies in children have not found increased PTSD rates in mTBI patients. A study of 43 children exposed to a motor vehicle accident with and without mTBI found no differences in PTSD rates in children with (86%) and without (69%) mTBI (Mather et al., 2003).

Both mTBI and PTSD are important problems for military personnel returning from Iraq and Afghanistan, and it is more common for the two disorders to present together than for either condition to present alone (Cifu et al., 2013; Lew et al., 2009, 2013). In a study of 1,680 active duty military personnel, 87%

of cases of deployment-related TBI were mTBI. Deployment-related mTBI raised the risk of deployment-related PTSD by 1.23, while moderate/severe TBI raised the PTSD risk by 1.71. TBI doubled the risk of PTSD in personnel with low pre-deployment PTSD symptoms, even when controlling for combat intensity and prior PTSD and TBI symptom history (Yurgil et al., 2014). Veterans with PTSD and comorbid mTBI had higher PTSD symptom levels and more functional impairment than veterans with PTSD alone (Ragsdale et al., 2013). Current suicidal ideation was associated with both TBI and increased PTSD symptoms following deployment to Iraq and Afghanistan (Wisco et al., 2014). The addition of a PTSD diagnosis to that of mTBI is associated with decreased health and cognitive function in comparison to mTBI patients without PTSD (Zatzick et al., 2010).

There is considerable overlap in returning Iraq and Afghanistan military personnel between mTBI and PTSD in post-concussion symptoms, PTSD symptoms, and chronic pain (Rosenfeld et al., 2013). Post-concussive symptoms, which include headache, dizziness, mood changes, sleep disturbance, and problems with memory and concentration, overlap with the clinical presentation of PTSD even in the absence of head injury. Comorbid PTSD and mTBI are associated with more post-concussive symptoms than either condition alone (Brenner et al., 2010; Wall, 2012). However, mTBI alone is not a good predictor of post-concussive syndrome (Meares et al., 2008). Veterans deployed to Iraq with PTSD showed more post-concussive syndrome symptoms than both non-deployed veterans and deployed veterans with mTBI (Soble et al., 2014).

Studies in soldiers returning from Iraq and Afghanistan show that post-concussive symptoms are linked more to PTSD than to mTBI (Schneiderman et al., 2008; Wilk et al., 2012). Hoge et al. (2008) surveyed 2,525 soldiers returning from Iraq; 44% of those with loss of consciousness had PTSD, compared with 27% with altered mental status, 16% with other injuries, and 9% with no injury. Physical health outcomes were primarily related to the presence of PTSD rather than mTBI. A study of 3,218 healthy male veterans injured in a motor vehicle accident, of whom 278 had mTBI, found mTBI to be associated with headaches, memory and sleep problems, even after controlling for PTSD. There was also an association between mTBI and diagnosis of PTSD. mTBI was not a moderator or mediator of the relationship between PTSD and symptoms (Vanderploeg et al., 2009). Hill et al. (2009) identified 94 combat veterans who screened positive for TBI using Veterans Affairs criteria. Eighty-five per cent were found to meet American Congress of Rehabilitation Medicine criteria for probable brain injury. The authors concluded that mTBI and PTSD could not be distinguished based on self-reported symptoms alone (Hill et al., 2009). Pietrzak et al. (2009) studied 277 OEF/OIF veterans and found higher rates of PTSD in those with mTBI. Furthermore, PTSD mediated the relationship between mTBI and psychosocial functioning. Kennedy et al. (2010) found that Operations Enduring Freedom and Iraqi Freedom veterans with blast-related mTBI

($N = 586$) had higher re-experiencing symptom levels than veterans with mTBI related to other causes ($N = 138$); overall there were no differences in total PTSD symptom scores between veterans with blast vs. non-blast TBI (Kennedy et al., 2010). In summary, the evidence does not support the ability of post-concussive symptoms to differentiate mTBI from PTSD.

There are a number of issues that complicate the diagnosis and treatment of PTSD in the face of possible mTBI in military personnel deployed to Iraq and Afghanistan. Hoge and colleagues have pointed out that merely having to be "dazed and confused" to merit diagnosis of mTBI meant that many who had merely experienced the "fog of war" would be classified as having a disorder that implies injury to the head as a cause of their symptoms, rather than another cause like PTSD (Bryant 2008; Hoge et al., 2008). Hoge et al. (2009, 2010) highlighted issues related to the use of vague screening questions without any requirement for a loss of function, persistence of symptoms, or functional impairment, for the diagnosis of mTBI. In summary, in military personnel deployed to Iraq and Afghanistan who experience a possible mTBI as defined by the current criteria, it is not possible to determine that functional impairments are primarily related to mTBI, and not PTSD.

A dilemma in the field of PTSD and mTBI has been the question of the diagnosis of PTSD in cases of mTBI where there has been a loss of memory regarding the accident (Bryant 2001, 2008). Up until the most recent version of the *Diagnostic and Statistical Manual* (DSM), in order for the diagnosis of PTSD to be made, it was necessary to experience the event with "intense fear, horror or helplessness." There is still the question of whether it is possible to encode a traumatic memory if there is no conscious memory for the event because of head injury.

Bryant (2001) argued that trace memories can exist for accidents that form the core of the memory that leads to PTSD, even if no explicit memory of the event exists. A number of cases have been reported of individuals who have no memory of the event, due to a blow to the head, where the victim nevertheless develops PTSD (Fani et al., 2006; McMillan, 1991). Currently there is a consensus that PTSD can occur in the aftermath of brain injury events (Bryant, 2001; Harvey et al., 2003; Jones et al., 2005; Mollica et al., 2002; Sumpter & McMillan, 2005), even with memory loss regarding the event. The prevalence of PTSD in which there is amnesia for the event, however, may be lower than that in those who remember the traumatic event (Flesher et al., 2001; Klein et al., 2003), primarily related to lower symptoms in the re-experiencing cluster (Gil et al., 2005).

Mild TBI is often associated with symptoms of memory disturbance or cognitive dysfunction. Studies showed that mTBI with comorbid PTSD was associated with greater errors on an executive function task than mTBI without PTSD (Amick et al., 2013). Other studies showed that PTSD patients from Iraq and Afghanistan with comorbid mTBI did not differ on measures testing a range of cognitive domains from veterans with PTSD alone (Soble et al., 2013).

Table 13.2 Changes in brain function in posttraumatic stress disorder (PTSD) and mild traumatic brain injury (mTBI).

Brain region	PTSD	mTBI
Amygdala	↑	↑
Hippocampus	↓	↓
Medial prefrontal cortex/anterior cingulate	↓	↓
Dorsolateral prefrontal cortex	–	↓

Memory symptoms in mTBI patients are often attributed to cognitive dysfunction as a result of brain injury, when there may or may not be evidence of head injury. It should also be considered that memory problems could potentially be related to early presentation of PTSD. As reviewed earlier, patients with PTSD exhibit a broad range of problems with memory, including gaps in memory, problems with declarative memory, attentional biases to trauma-related information, and intrusive memories (Elzinga & Bremner 2002).

Some brain imaging studies have been conducted in patients with PTSD and comorbid PTSD (Table 13.2). One study showed that FA was associated with PTSD symptom severity after controlling for diagnosis of mTBI (Bazarian et al., 2013). A meta-analysis of PTSD and mTBI fMRI functional activation studies showed increased activation in the amygdala and middle frontal gyrus compared with controls, and decreased activation in the anterior cingulate, in both PTSD and mTBI. mTBI patients were specific for a decreased activation in the middle frontal gyrus (Simmons & Matthews 2012).

13.5 Summary and conclusions

This chapter reviews the relationship between clinical and neuroimaging approaches to PTSD and mTBI. Cognitive problems can arise from either brain injury or PTSD, and a number of the symptoms of mTBI overlap. In addition, PTSD patients commonly suffer from symptoms like headache and minor neurological problems, which further complicate the differential diagnosis. Mild cognitive deficits are part of PTSD even without known brain injury; in patients with blows to the head where documented brain injury is not seen on MRI, it is difficult, if not impossible, to determine if the cognitive deficits are due to the PTSD or the head injury, or both. Studies to date, however, indicate that many of the functional problems seen in comorbid PTSD and mTBI, including symptoms of so-called "post-concussion syndrome," are primarily attributable to PTSD, at least in military personnel with these conditions who were deployed to Iraq and Afghanistan.

Studies have shown that many of the symptoms and functional impairments seen in mTBI patients may be more properly attributed to comorbid PTSD. In spite of this, mTBI patients, especially in military populations, often become categorized as primarily mTBI with symptoms attributed to that, and the contribution of comorbid PTSD is not emphasized. It might be more useful clinically to take a "more is worse" approach to comorbid mTBI and PTSD rather than trying to parcel out the relative contributions of the two separate conditions, which is often impractical, and in any case does not contribute to optimal clinical care of patients with these comorbid conditions.

Brain imaging studies show an overlap between PTSD and mTBI. Structural MRI, MRS, and functional MRI, SPECT and PET studies implicate a common network involving frontal cortex and hippocampus in both conditions. PTSD may be differentiated by more of an implication of increased amygdala function, while altered dorsolateral PFC function is more often seen in mTBI. DTI measurement of white matter integrity and corpus callosum appears to be a non-specific finding in both PTSD and mTBI. Future studies are needed to more fully evaluate brain structural and functional abnormalities in PTSD.

References

Abu-Judeh HH, Singh MAF, Masdeu JC et al. (1998) Discordance between FDG uptake and technetium-99m-HMPAO brain perfusion in acute traumatic brain injury. *J Nucl Med* 39, 1357–1359.

Amick MM, Clark A, Fortier CB et al. (2013) PTSD modifies performance on a task of affective executive control among deployed OEF/OIF veterans with mild traumatic brain injury. *J Int Neuropsychol Soc* 19, 792–801.

Astur RS, St Germain SA, Tolin D et al. (2006) Hippocampus function predicts severity of post-traumatic stress disorder. *Cyberpsychol Behav* 9, 234–240.

Audenaert K, Jansen HM, Otte A et al. (2003) Imaging of mild traumatic brain injury using 57Co and 99mTc HMPAO SPECT as compared to other diagnostic procedures. *Medical Science Monitor* 9, MT112–117.

Barrett DH, Green ML, Morris R et al. (1996) Cognitive functioning and posttraumatic stress disorder. *Am J Psychiatry* 153, 1492–1494.

Bazarian JJ, Donnelly K, Peterson DR et al. (2013) The relation between posttraumatic stress disorder and mild traumatic brain injury acquired during Operations Enduring Freedom and Iraqi Freedom. *J Head Trauma Rehabil* 28, 1–12.

Belanger HG, Vanderploeg R, Curtiss G et al. (2007) Recent neuroimaging techniques in mild traumatic brain injury. *J Neuropsychiatry Clin Neurosci* 19, 5–20.

Benson RR, Meda SA, Vasudevan S et al. (2007) Global white matter analysis of diffusion tensor images is predictive of injury severity in traumatic brain injury. *J Neurotrauma* 24, 446–459.

Bluhm RL, Williamson PC, Osuch EA et al. (2009) Alterations in default network connectivity in posttraumatic stress disorder related to early-life trauma. *J Psychiatry Neurosci* 34, 187–194.

Bonne O, Bain E, Neumeister A et al. (2005) No change in serotonin type 1A receptor binding in patients with posttraumatic stress disorder. *Am J Psychiatry* 162, 383–385.

Bonne O, Gilboa A, Louzoun Y et al. (2003) Cerebral blood flow in chronic symptomatic mild traumatic brain injury. *Psych Res: Neuroimaging* 124, 141–152.

Bremner JD (1998) Neuroimaging of posttraumatic stress disorder. *Psych Annal* 28, 445–450.

Bremner JD (2002) Neuroimaging of childhood trauma. *Semin Clin Neuropsychiatry* 7, 104–112.

Bremner JD (2011) Stress and human neuroimaging studies. In: Conrad CD (ed.) *The Handbook of Stress: Neuropsychological Effects on the Brain*. Wiley-Blackwell.

Bremner JD, Innis RB, White T et al. (2000) SPECT [I-123]iomazenil measurement of the benzodiazepine receptor in panic disorder. *Biol Psychiatry* 47, 96–106.

Bremner JD, Krystal JH, Putnam F et al. (1998) Measurement of dissociative states with the Clinician Administered Dissociative States Scale (CADSS). *J Trauma Stress* 11, 125–136.

Bremner JD, Marmar C (eds)(1998) *Trauma, Memory, and Dissociation*. American Psychiatric Press, Washington, DC.

Bremner JD, Randall PR, Capelli S et al. (1995) Deficits in short-term memory in adult survivors of childhood abuse. *Psychiatry Res* 59, 97–107.

Bremner JD, Scott TM, Delaney RC et al. (1993) Deficits in short-term memory in post-traumatic stress disorder. *Am J Psychiatry* 150, 1015–1019.

Bremner JD, Southwick SM, Brett E et al. (1992) Dissociation and posttraumatic stress disorder in Vietnam combat veterans. *Am J Psychiatry* 149, 328–332.

Bremner JD, Vermetten E (2012) The hippocampus and post-traumatic stress disorders. In: Bartsch T (ed.) The Clinical Neurobiology of the Hippocampus: An integrative view Oxford University Press, USA, New York, NY, pp. 262–272.

Bremner JD, Vermetten E, Nafzal N et al. (2004) Deficits in verbal declarative memory function in women with childhood sexual abuse-related posttraumatic stress disorder (PTSD). *J Nerv Ment Dis* 192, 643–649.

Bremner JD, Vythilingam M, Vermetten E et al. (2003) MRI and PET study of deficits in hippocampal structure and function in women with childhood sexual abuse and posttraumatic stress disorder (PTSD). *Am J Psychiatry* 160, 924–932.

Brenner LA, Ivins BJ, Schwab K et al. (2010) Traumatic brain injury, posttraumatics stress disorder, and postconcussive symptom reporting among troops returning from Iraq. *J Head Trauma Rehabil* 25, 307–312.

Brewin CR (2001) A cognitive neuroscience account of post-traumatic stress disorder and its treatment. *Behav Res Ther* 39, 373–393.

Brewin CR, Kleiner JS, Vasterling JJ et al. (2007) Memory for emotionally neutral information in posttraumatic stress disorder: A meta-analytic investigation. *J Abnorm Psychology* 116, 448–463.

Bryant RA (2001) Posttraumatic stress disorder and mild brain injury: controversies, causes and consequences. *J Clin Exper Neuropsychol* 23, 718–728.

Bryant RA (2008) Disentangling mild traumatic brain injury and stress reactions. *N Engl J Med* 385, 525–527.

Bryant RA (2011) Mental disorders and traumatic injury. *Depress Anxiety* 28, 99–102.

Bryant RA, Felmingham KL, Kemp AH et al. (2005) Neural networks of information processing in posttraumatic stress disorder: a functional magnetic resonance imaging study. *Biol Psychiatry* 58, 111–118.

Bryant RA, Marosszeky JE (2000) Coping style and post-traumatic stress disorder following severe traumatic brain injury. *Brain Injury* 14, 175–180.

Bryant RA, Marosszeky JE, Crooks J et al. (2001) Posttraumatic stress disorder and psychosocial functioning after severe traumatic brain injury. *J Nerv Ment Dis* 189, 109–113.

Bryant RA, Marosszeky JE, Crooks J et al. (2000) Posttraumatic stress disorder after severe traumatic brain injury. *Am J Psychiatry* 157, 629–631.

Bryant RA, Marosszeky JE, Crooks J et al. (2004) Elevated heart rate as a predictor of posttraumatic stress disorder after severe traumatic brain injury. *Psychosom Med* 66, 760–761.

Bryant RA, Moulds M, Guthrie R et al. (2003) Treating acute stress disorder following mild traumatic brain injury. *Am J Psychiatry* 160, 585–587.

Bryant RA, O'Donnell ML, Creamer M et al. (2010) The psychiatric sequelae of traumatic injury. *Am J Psychiatry* 167, 312–320.

Bryant RA, Panasetis P (2005) The role of panic in acute dissociative reactions following trauma. *Br J Clin Psychol* 44, 489–494.

Buckley TC, Blanchard EB, Neill WT (2000) Information processing and PTSD: A review of the empirical literature. *Clin Psychol Rev* 28, 1041–1065.

Cannistraro PA, Rauch SL (2003) Neural circuitry of anxiety: evidence from structural and functional neuroimaging studies. *Psychopharmacol Bull* 37, 8–25.

Cardena E, Spiegel D (1993) Dissociative reactions to the San Francisco Bay area earthquake of 1989. *Am J Psychiatry* 150, 474–478.

Carrion VG, Weems CF, Watson C et al. (2009) Converging evidence for abnormalities of the prefrontal cortex and evaluation of midsagittal structures in pediatric posttraumatic stress disorder: an MRI study. *Psychiatry Res* 172, 226–234.

Cecil KM, Hills EC, Sandel E et al. (1998) Proton magnetic resonance spectroscopy for detection of axonal injury in the splenium of the corpus callosum of brain-injured patients. *J Neurosurg* 88, 795–801.

Chen S, Li L, Xu B et al. (2009) Insular cortex involvement in declarative memory deficits in patients with post-traumatic stress disorder. *BMC Psychiatry* 9, 39.

Chen S, Xia W, Li L et al. (2006) Gray matter density reduction in the insula in fire survivors with posttraumatic stress disorder: a voxel-based morphometric study. *Psychiatry Res* 146, 65–72.

Chen SHA, Kareken DA, Fastenau PS et al. (2003) A study of persistent post-concussoin symptoms in mild head trauma using positron emission tomography. *J Neurol Neurosurg Psychiatr* 74, 326–332.

Cifu DX, Cohen SI, Lew HL et al. (2010) The history and evolution of traumatic brain injury rehabilitation in military service members and veterans. *Am J Phys Med Rehabil* 89, 688–694.

Cifu DX, Taylor BC, Carne WF et al. (2013) Traumatic brain injury, posttraumatic stress disorder, and pain diagnoses in OIF/OEF/OND Veterans. *J Rehabil Res Dev* 50, 1169–1176.

Clark CR, McFarlane AC, Morris P et al. (2003) Cerebral function in posttraumatic stress disorder during verbal working memory updating: A positron emission tomography study. *Biol Psychiatry* 53, 474–481.

Cohen BA, Inglese M, Rusinek H et al. (2007) Proton MR spectroscopy and MRI-volumetry in mild traumatic brain injury. *AJNR Am J Neuroradiol* 28, 907–913.

Corbo V, Clement MH, Armony JL et al. (2005) Size versus shape differences: contrasting voxel-based and volumetric analyses of the anterior cingulate cortex in individuals with acute posttraumatic stress disorder. *Biol Psychiatry* 58, 119–124.

Creamer M, O'Donnell ML, Pattison P (2005) Amnesia, traumatic brain injury, and posttraumatic stress disorder: a methodological inquiry. *Behav Res Ther* 43, 1383–1389.

Czermak C, Staley JK, Kasserman S et al. (2008) Beta-2 nicotinic acetylcholine receptor availability in post-traumatic stress disorder. *Int J Neuropsychopharmacol* 11, 419–424.

Daniels JK, McFarlane AC, Bluhm RL et al. (2010) Switching between executive and default mode networks in posttraumatic stress disorder: Alterations in functional connectivity. *J Psychiatry Neurosci* 35, 258–266.

De Bellis MD, Keshavan MS, Frustaci K et al. (2002a) Superior temporal gyrus volumes in maltreated children and adolescents with PTSD. *Biol Psychiatry* 51, 544–552.

De Bellis MD, Keshavan MS, Shifflett H et al. (2002b) Brain structures in pediatric maltreatment-related posttraumatic stress disorder: a sociodemographically matched study. *Biol Psychiatry* 52, 1066–1078.

De Bellis MD, Keshavan MS, Spencer S et al. (2000) N-acetylaspartate concentration in the anterior cingulate of maltreated children and adolescents with PTSD. *Am J Psychiatry* 157, 1175–1177.

Diamond DM, Fleshner M, Ingersoll N et al. (1996) Psychological stress impairs spatial working memory: Relevance to electrophysiological studies of hippocampal function. *Behav Neurosci* 110, 661–672.

Elzinga BM, Bremner JD (2002) Are the neural substrates of memory the final common pathway in PTSD? *J Affect Disord* 70, 1–17.

Falconer E, Bryant R, Felmingham KL et al. (2009) The neural networks of inhibitory control in posttraumatic stress disorder. *J Psychiatry Neurosci* 33, 413–422.

Fani N, Hampstead BM, Bremner JD (2006) PTSD in the emergency setting. *Psychiatr Issues Emerg Care Settings* 5, 17–22.

Flesher MR, Delahanty DL, Raimonde AJ et al. (2001) Amnesia, neuroendocrine levels and PTSD in motor vehicle accident victims. *Brain Injury* 15, 879–889.

Frewen P, Lane RD, Neufeld RW et al. (2008) Neural correlates of levels of emotional awareness during trauma script-imagery in posttraumatic stress disorder. *Psychosom Med* 70, 27–31.

Fujita M, Southwick SM, Denucci CC et al. (2004) Central type benzodiazepine receptors in Gulf War veterans with posttraumatic stress disorder. *Biol Psychiatry* 56, 95–100.

Garnett MR, Blamine AM, Rajagaopalan B et al. (2000) Evidence for cellular damage in noraml-appearing white matter correlates with injury severity in patients following traumatic brain injury: A magnetic resonance spectroscopy study. *Brain* 123, 1403–1409.

Geuze E, van Berckel BN, Lammertsma AA et al. (2008a) Reduced GABAA benzodiazepine receptor binding in veterans with post-traumatic stress disorder. *Mol Psychiatry* 13, 74–83, 73.

Geuze E, Westenberg HG, Heinecke A et al. (2008b) Thinner prefrontal cortex in veterans with posttraumatic stress disorder. *NeuroImage* 41, 675–681.

Geuze E, Westenberg HG, Jochims A et al. (2007) Altered pain processing in veterans with posttraumatic stress disorder. *Arch Gen Psychiatry* 64, 76–85.

Gil S, Caspi Y, Ben-Ari YZ et al. (2005) Does memory of a traumatic brain event increase the risk for posttraumatic stress disorder in patients with traumatic brain injury? A prospective study. *Am J Psychiatry* 162, 963–969.

Gil T, Calev A, Greenberg D et al. (1990) Cognitive functioning in posttraumatic stress disorder. *J Trauma Stress* 3, 29–45.

Gilbertson MW, Gurvits TV, Lasko NB et al. (2001) Multivariate assessment of explicit memory function in combat veterans with posttraumatic stress disorder. *J Trauma Stress* 14, 413–420.

Gilboa A, Shalev AY, Laor L et al. (2004) Functional connectivity of the prefrontal cortex and the amygdala in posttraumatic stress disorder. *Biol Psychiatry* 55, 263–272.

Glaesser J, Neuner F, Lutgehetmann R et al. (2004) Posttraumatic stress disorder in patients with traumatic brain injury. *BMC Psychiatry* 4.

Golier J, Yehuda R (1998) Neuroendocrine activity and memory-related impairments in post-traumatic stress disorder. *Dev Psychopathol* 10, 857–869.

Golier J, Yehuda R, Cornblatt B et al. (1997) Sustained attention in combat-related posttraumatic stress disorder. *Integr Physiol Behav Sci* 32, 52–61.

Govindaraju V, Gauger GE, Manley GT et al. (2004) Volumetric proton spectroscopic imaging of mild traumatic brain injury. *AJNR Am J Neuroradiol* 25, 730–737.

Gray BG, Ichise M, Chung D-G et al. (1992) Traumatic brain injury: A Comparison with X-ray computed tomography. *J Nucl Med* 33, 52–58.

Hakamata Y, Matsuoka Y, Inagaki M et al. (2007) Structure of orbitofrontal cortex and its longitudinal course in cancer-related post-traumatic stress disorder. *Neurosci Res* 59, 383–389.

Hara E, Matsuoka Y, Hakamata Y et al. (2008) Hippocampal and amygdalar volumes in breast cancer survivors with posttraumatic stress disorder. *J Neuropsychiatry Clin Neurosci* 20, 302–308.

Harvey AG, Brewin CR, Jones C et al. (2003) Coexistence of posttraumatic stress disorder and traumatic brain injury: towards a resolution of the paradox. *J Int Neuropsychol Soc* 9, 663–676.

Hickling EJ, Gillen R, Blanchard EB et al. (1998) Traumatic brain injury and posttraumatic stress disorder: a preliminary investigation of neuropsychological test results in PTSD secondary to motor vehicle accidents. *Brain Injury* 12, 265–274.

Hill JJ, Mobo BHP, Cullen MR (2009) Separating deployment-related traumatic brain injury and posttraumatic stress disorder in veterans. *Brain Injury* 88, 605–614.

Hofman PAM, Stapert SZ, van Kroonenburgh MJPG et al. (2001) MR imaging, single-photon emission CT, and neurocognitive performance after mild traumatic brain injury. *Am J Neuroradiol* 22, 441–449.

Hoge CW, Goldberg HM, Castro CA (2009) Care of war veterans with mild traumatic brain injury-- Flawed perspectives. *N Engl J Med* 360, 1588–1591.

Hoge CW, McGurk D, Thomas JL et al. (2008) Mild traumatic brain injury in U.S. Soldiers returning from Iraq. *N Engl J Med* 358, 453–463.

Hoge CW, Wilk JE, Herrell R (2010) Methodological issues in mild traumatic brain injury research. *Arch Phys Med Rehabil* 91, 963; author reply 963–964.

Humayun MS, Presty SK, LaFrance ND et al. (1989) Local cerebral glucose abnormalities in mild closed head injured patients with cognitive impairments. *Nucl Med Comm* 10, 335–344.

Ichise M, Chung D-G, Wortzman G et al. (2004) Technetium-99m-HMPAO SPECT, CT and MRI in the evaluatoin of patients with chronic traumatic brain injury: A correlations with neuropsychological performance. *J Nucl Med* 35, 217–226.

Inglese M, Makani S, Johnson G et al. (2005) Diffuse axonal injury in mild traumatic brain injury: a diffusion tensor imaging study. *J Neurosurg* 103, 298–303.

Jackowski AP, Douglas-Palumberi H, Jackowski M et al. (2008) Corpus callosum in maltreated children with posttraumatic stress disorder: a diffusion tensor imaging study. *Psychiatry Res* 162, 256–261.

Jacobs A, Put E, Ingels M et al. (1994) Prospective evaluation of technetium-99m-HMPAO SPECT in mild and moderate traumatic brain injury. *J Nucl Med* 35, 942–947.

Jaffee MS, Helmick KM, Girard PD et al. (2009) Acute clinical care and care coordination for traumatic brain injury within Department of Defense. *J Rehabil Dev* 46, 655–666.

Jantzen KJ, Anderson B, Steinberg FL et al. (2004) A prospective functional MR imaging study of mild traumatic brain injury in college football players. *American Journal of Neuroradiology* 25, 738–745.

Jenkins MA, Langlais PJ, Delis D et al. (1998) Learning and memory in rape victims with posttraumatic stress disorder. *Am J Psychiatry* 155, 278–279.

Jones C, Harvey AG, Brewin CR (2005) Traumatic brain injury, dissociation, and posttraumatic stress disorder in road traffic accident survivors. *J Trauma Stress* 18, 181–191.

Kant R, Smith-Seemiller L, Isaac G et al. (1997) Tc-HMPAO SPECT in persistent post-concussion syndrome after mild head injury: comparison with MRI/CT. *Brain Injury* 11, 115–124.

Kasai K, Yamasue H, Gilbertson MW et al. (2008) Evidence for acquired pregenual anterior cingulate gray matter loss from a twin study of combat-related posttraumatic stress disorder. *Biol Psychiatry* 63, 550–556.

Kennedy JE, Jaffee MS, Leskin GA et al. (2007) Posttraumatic stress disorder and posttraumatic stress disorder-like symptoms and mild traumatic brain injury. *J Rehabil Dev* 44, 895–920.

Kennedy JE, Leal FO, Lewis JD et al. (2010) Posttraumatic stress symptoms in OIF/OEF service members with blast-related and non-blast-related mild TBI. *Neurorehabilitation* 26, 223–231.

Kim MJ, Chey J, Chung A et al. (2008) Diminished rostral anterior cingulate activity in response to threat-related events in posttraumatic stress disorder. *J Psychiatr Res* 42, 268–277.

Kim MJ, Lyoo IK, Kim SJ et al. (2005) Disrupted white matter tract integrity of anterior cingulate in trauma survivors. *Neuroreport* 16, 1049–1053.

Kim SJ, Jeong DU, Sim ME et al. (2006) Asymmetrically altered integrity of cingulum bundle in posttraumatic stress disorder. *Neuropsychobiology* 54, 120–125.

Kitayama N, Brummer M, Hertz L et al. (2007) Morphologic alterations in the corpus callosum in abuse-related posttraumatic stress disorder: a preliminary study. *J Nerv Ment Dis* 195, 1027–1029.

Kitayama N, Vaccarino V, Kutner M et al. (2005) Magnetic resonance imaging (MRI) measurement of hippocampal volume in posttraumatic stress disorder: A meta-analysis. *J Affect Disord* 88, 79–86.

Klein E, Caspi Y, gil S (2003) The relation between memory of the traumatic event and PTSD: Evidence from studies of traumatic brain injury. *Can J Psychiat* 49, 28–33.

Koenigs M, huey ED, Raymont V et al. (2007) Focal brain damage protects against post-traumatic stress disorder in combat veterans. *Nat Neurosci* 11, 232–237.

Koopman C, Classen C, Spiegel D (1994) Predictors of posttraumatic stress symptoms among survivors of the Oakland/Berkeley, Calif., firestorm. *Am J Psychiatry* 151, 888–894.

Kraus MF, Susmaras T, Caughlin BP et al. (2007) White matter integrity and cognition in chronic traumatic brain injury: a diffusion tensor imaging study. *Brain* 130, 2508–2519.

Kulka RA, Schlenger WE, Fairbank JA et al. (1990) *Trauma and the Vietnam War Generation: Report of Findings from the National Vietnam Veterans Readjustment Study*. Brunner/Mazel, New York.

Lanius RA, Bluhm RL, Coupland NJ et al. (2010) Default mode network connectivity as a predictor of post-traumatic stress disorder. *Acta Psychiatr Scand* 121, 33–40.

Levin HS, Matis S, Ruff RM et al. (1987) Neurobehavioral outcome following minor head injury: a three-center study. *J Neurosurg* 66, 234–243.

Levin HS, Wilde E, Troyanskaya M et al. (2010) Diffusion tensor imaging of mild to moderate blast-related traumatic brain injury and its sequelae. *J Neurotrauma* 27, 583–594.

Levitt JJ, Chen QC, May FS et al. (2006) Volume of cerebellar vermis in monozygotic twins discordant for combat exposure: lack of relationship to post-traumatic stress disorder. *Psychiatry Res* 148, 143–149.

Lew HL, Cifu DX, Crowder T et al. (2013) National prevalence of traumatic brain injury, posttraumatic stress disorder, and pain diagnoses in OIF/OEF/OND Veterans from 2009 to 2011. *J Rehabil Res Dev* 50, xi–xiv.

Lew HL, Otis JD, Tun C et al. (2009) Prevalence of chronic pain, posttraumatic stress disorder, and persistent postconcussive symptoms in OIF/OEF veterans: Polytrauma clinical triad. *J Rehab Res Dev* 46, 697–702.

Lewine JD, Davis JT, Sloan JH et al. (1999) Neuromagnetic assessment of pathophysiologic brain activity induced by minor head trauma. *Am J Neuroradiol* 20, 857–866.

Liberzon I, Britton JC, Phan KL (2003) Neural correlates of traumatic recall in posttraumatic stress disorder. *Stress* 6, 151–156.

Liberzon I, Martis B (2006) Neuroimaging studies of emotional responses in PTSD. *Ann NY Acad Sci* 1071, 87–109.

Liberzon I, Phan KL (2003) Brain-imaging studies of posttraumatic stress disorder. *CNS Spectr* 8, 641–650.

Liberzon I, Taylor SF, Phan KL et al. (2007) Altered central micro-opioid receptor binding after psychological trauma. *Biol Psychiatry* 61, 1030–1038.

Lim MK, Suh CH, Kim HJ et al. (2003) Fire-related post-traumatic stress disorder: brain 1H-MR spectroscopic findings. *Korean J Radiol* 4, 79–84.

Lipton ML, Gellella E, Lo C et al. (2008) Multifocal white matter ultrastructural abnormalities in mild traumatic brain injury with cognitive disability: a voxel-wise analysis of diffusion tensor imaging. *J Neurotrauma* 25, 1335–1342.

Looi JCL, Maller JJ, Pagani M et al. (2009) Caudate volumes in public transportation workers exposed to trauma in the Stockholm train system. *Psych Res: Neuroimaging* 171, 138–143.

Luine V, Villages M, Martinex C et al. (1994) Repeated stress causes reversible impairments of spatial memory performance. *Brain Res* 639, 167–170.

Mahmutyazicioglu K, Konuk N, Ozdemir H et al. (2005) Evaluation of the hippocampus and the anterior cingulate gyrus by proton MR spectroscopy in patients with post-traumatic stress disorder. *Diagn Interv Radiol* 11, 125–129.

Marmar CR, Weiss DS, Schlenger DS et al. (1994) Peritraumatic dissociation and posttraumatic stress in male Vietnam theater veterans. *Am J Psychiatry* 151, 902–907.

Mather FJ, Tate RL, Hannan TJ (2003) Post-traumatic stress disorder in children following road traffic accidents: a comparison of those with and without mild traumatic brain injury. *Brain Injury* 17, 1077–1087.

Matsuoka Y, Yamawaki S, Inagaki M et al. (2003) A volumetric study of amygdala in cancer survivors with intrusive recollections. *Biol Psychiatry* 54, 736–743.

May FS, Chen QC, Gilbertson MW et al. (2004) Cavum septum pellucidum in monozygotic twins discordant for combat exposure: relationship to posttraumatic stress disorder. *Biol Psychiatry* 55, 656–658.

Mayer AR, Ling J, Mannell MV et al. (2011) A prospective diffusion tensor imaging study in mild traumatic brain injury. *Neurology* 74, 643–650.

McAllister TW, Saykin AJ, Flashman LA et al. (1999) Brain activation during working memory 1 month after mild traumatic brain injury: A functional MRI study. *Neurology* 53, 1300–1308.

McAllister TW, Sparling MB, Flashman LA et al. (2001) Differential working memory load effects after mild traumatic brain injury. *NeuroImage* 14, 1004–1012.

McAllister TW, Stein MB (2010) Effects of psychological and biomechanical trauma on brain and behavior. *Ann NY Acad Sci* 1208, 46–57.

McFarlane AC (2000) Posttraumatic stress disorder: A model of the longitudinal course and the role of risk factors. *J Clin Psychiatry* 61, 15–20.

McMillan T (1996) Post-traumatic stress disorder following minor and severe closed head injury: 10 single cases. *Brain Injury* 10, 749–758.

McMillan TM (1991) Post-traumatic stress disorder and severe head injury. *Br J Psychiatry* 159, 431–433.

Meares S, Shores EA, Taylor AJ et al. (2008) Mild traumatic brain injury does not predict acute postconcussion syndrome. *J Neurol Neurosurg Psychiatry* 79, 300–306.

Mild Traumatic Brain Injury Committee of the Head Injury Interdisciplinary Special Interest Group of the American Congress of Rehabilitation Medicine (1993) Definition of mild traumatic brain injury. *J Head Trauma Rehab* 8, 86–87.

Miles L, Grossman RI, Johnson G et al. (2008) Short-term DTI predictors of cognitive dysfunction in mild traumatic brain injury. *Brain Inj* 22, 115–122.

Mollica RF, Henderson DC, Tor S (2002) Psychiatric effects of traumatic brain injury events in Cambodian survivors of mass violence. *Br J Psychiatry* 181, 339–347.

Mollica RF, Lyoo IK, Chernoff MC et al. (2009) Brain structural abnormalities and mental health sequelae in South Vietnamese ex-political detainees who survived traumatic head injury and torture. *Arch Gen Psychiatry* 66, 1221–1232.

Moores KA, Clark CR, McFarlane AC et al. (2008) Abnormal recruitment of working memory updating networks during maintenance of trauma-neutral information in post-traumatic stress disorder. *Psychiatry Res* 163, 156–170.

Moradi AR, Doost HT, Taghavi MR et al. (1999) Everyday memory deficits in children and adolescents with PTSD: performance on the Rivermead Behavioural Memory Test. *J Child Psychol Psychiatr* 40, 357–361.

Morey RA, Petty CM, Cooper DA et al. (2008) Neural systems for executive and emotional processing are modulated by symptoms of posttraumatic stress disorder in Iraq War veterans. *Psychiatry Res* 162, 59–72.

Nakano T, Wenner M, Inagaki M et al. (2002) Relationship between distressing cancer-related recollections and hippocampal volume in cancer survivors. *Am J Psychiatry* 159, 2087–2093.

Nardo D, Högbert G, Looi JCL et al. (2009) Gray matter density in limbic and paralimbic cortices is associated with trauma load and EMDR outcome in PTSD patients. *J Psychiatr Res* 44, 477–485.

Nedd K, Sfakianakis G, Ganz W et al. (1993) Tc-99-m-HMPAO SPECT of the brain in mild to moderate traumatic brain injury patients: Comapres with CT- a prospective study. *Brain Injury* 7, 469–479.

New AS, Fan J, Murrough JW et al. (2009) A functional magnetic resonance imaging study of deliberate emotion regulation in resilience and posttraumatic stress disorder. *Biol Psychiatry* 66, 656–664.

Niogi SN, Mukherjee P, Ghajar J et al. (2008) Extent of microstructural white matter injury in postconcussive syndrome correlates with impaired cognitive reaction time: a 3T diffusion tensor imaging study of mild traumatic brain injury. *AJNR Am J Neuroradiol* 29, 967–973.

Ohry A, Rattock J, Solomon Z (1996) Post-traumatic stress disorder in brain injury patients. *Brain Injury* 10, 687–695.

Osuch EA, Willis MW, Bluhm R et al. (2008) Neurophysiological responses to traumatic reminders in the acute aftermath of serious motor vehicle collisions using [15O]-H2O positron emission tomography. *Biol Psychiatry* 64, 327–335.

Pannu Hayes J, Labar KS, Petty CM et al. (2009) Alterations in the neural circuitry for emotion and attention associated with posttraumatic stress symptomatology. *Psychiatry Res* 172, 7–15.

Petrie EC, Cross DJ, Yarnykh VL et al. (2014) Neuroimaging, behavioral, and psychological sequelae of repetitive combined blast/impact mild traumatic brain injury in Iraq and Afghanistan war veterans. *J Neurotrauma* 31, 425–436.

Piefke M, Pestinger M, Arin T et al. (2007) The neurofunctional mechanisms of traumatic and non-traumatic memory in patients with acute PTSD following accident trauma. *Neurocase* 13, 342–357.

Pietrzak RH, Johnson DC, Goldstein MB et al. (2009) Posttraumatic stress disorders mediates the relationship between mild traumatic brain injury and health and psychosocial functioning in veterans of Operations Enduring Freedom and Iraqi Freedom. *J Nervous Mental Dis* 197, 748–753.

Pitman RK (2001) Investigating the pathogenesis of posttraumatic stress disorder with neuroimaging. *J Clin Psychiatry* 62, 47–54.

Ragsdale KA, Neer SM, Beidel DC et al. (2013) Posttraumatic stress disorder in OEF/OIF veterans with and without traumatic brain injury. *J Anxiety Disord* 27, 420–426.

Rauch SL, Shin LM, Phelps EA (2006) Neurocircuitry models of posttraumatic stress disorder and extinction: human neuroimaging research – past, present, and future. *Biol Psychiatry* 60, 376–382.

Rauch SL, Shin LM, Segal E et al. (2003) Selectively reduced regional cortical volumes in post-traumatic stress disorder. *Neuroreport* 14, 913–916.

Roca V, Freeman TW (2001) Complaints of impaired memory in veterans with PTSD. *Am J Psychiatry* 158, 1738.

Rogers MA, Yamasue H, Abe O et al. (2009) Smaller amygdala volume and reduced anterior cingulate gray matter density associated with history of post-traumatic stress disorder. *Psychiatry Res* 174, 210–216.

Rosenfeld JV, McFarlane AC, Bragge P et al. (2013) Blast-related traumatic brain injury. *Lancet Neurol* 12, 882–893.

Ruff RM, Crouch JA, Tröster AI et al. (1994) Selected cases of poor outcome following a minor brain trauma: Comparing neuropsychological and positron emission tomography assessment. *Brain Injury* 8, 297–308.

Rutgers DR, Fillard P, Paradot G et al. (2008a) Diffusion tensor imaging characteristics of the corpus callosum in mild, moderate, and severe traumatic brain injury. *AJNR Am J Neuroradiol* 29, 1730–1735.

Rutgers DR, Toulgoat F, Cazejust J et al. (2008b) White matter abnormalities in mild traumatic brain injury: a diffusion tensor imaging study. *AJNR Am J Neuroradiol* 29, 514–519.

Sachinvala N, vonScotti H, McGuire M et al. (2000) Memory, attention, function, and mood among patients with chronic posttraumatic stress disorder. *J Nerv Ment Dis* 188, 818–823.

Sailer U, Robinson S, Fischmeister FP et al. (2008) Altered reward processing in the nucleus accumbens and mesial prefrontal cortex of patients with posttraumatic stress disorder. *Neuropsychologia* 46, 2836–2844.

Sapolsky RM, Uno H, Rebert CS et al. (1990) Hippocampal damage associated with prolonged glucocorticoid exposure in primates. *J Neurosci* 10, 2897–2902.

Schneiderman AI, Braver ER, Kang HK (2008) Understanding sequelae of injury mechanisms and mild traumatic brain injury incurred during the conflicts in Iraq and Afghanistan: Persistent postconcussive symptoms and posttraumatic stress disorder. *Am J Epidemiol* 167, 1446–1452.

Seedat S, Videen JS, Kennedy CM et al. (2005) Single voxel proton magnetic resonance spectroscopy in women with and without intimate partner violence-related posttraumatic stress disorder. *Psychiatry Res* 139, 249–258.

Shalev AY, Peri T, Canetti L et al. (1996) Predictors of PTSD in injured trauma survivors: A prospective study. *Am J Psychiatry* 153, 219–225.

Shin LM, Shin PS, Heckers S et al. (2004) Hippocampal function in posttraumatic stress disorder. *Hippocampus* 14, 292–300.

Shutter L, Tong KA, Lee A et al. (2006) Prognostic role of proton magnetic resonance spectroscopy in acute traumatic brain injury. *J Head Trauma Rehabil* 21, 334–349.

Simmons A, Strigo IA, Matthews SC et al. (2009) Initial evidence of a failure to activate right anterior insula during affective set shifting in posttraumatic stress disorder. *Psychosom Med* 71, 373–377.

Simmons AN, Matthews SC (2012) Neural circuitry of PTSD with or without mild traumatic brain injury: a meta-analysis. *Neuropharmacology* 62, 598–606.

Smith ME (2005) Bilateral hippocampal volume reduction in adults with post-traumatic stress disorder: a meta-analysis of structural MRI studies. *Hippocampus* 15, 798–807.

Soble JR, Silva MA, Vanderploeg RD et al. (2014) Normative Data for the Neurobehavioral Symptom Inventory (NSI) and post-concussion symptom profiles among TBI, PTSD, and nonclinical samples. *Clin Neuropsychol* 28, 614–632.

Soble JR, Spanierman LB, Fitzgerald Smith J (2013) Neuropsychological functioning of combat veterans with posttraumatic stress disorder and mild traumatic brain injury. *J Clin Exp Neuropsychol* 35, 551–561.

Stein MB, Hanna C, Vaerum V et al. (1999) Memory functioning in adult women traumatized by childhood sexual abuse. *J Trauma Stress* 12, 527–534.

Stein MB, McAllister TW (2009) Exploring the convergence of posttraumatic stress disorder and mild traumatic brain injury. *Am J Psychiatry* 166, 768–776.

Strigo IA, Simmons AN, Matthews SC et al. (2010) Neural correlates of altered pain response in women with posttraumatic stress disorder from intimate partner violence. *Biol Psychiatry* 68, 442–450.

Sumpter RE, McMillan TM (2005) Misdiagnosis of post-traumatic stress disorder following severe traumatic brain injury. *Br J Psychiatry* 186, 423–426.

Teicher MH, Dumont NL, Ito Y et al. (2004) Childhood neglect is associated with reduced corpus callosum area. *Biol Psychiatry* 56, 80–85.

Thomaes K, Dorrepaal E, Draijer N et al. (2010) Reduced anterior cingulate and orbitofrontal volumes in child abuse-related complex PTSD. *J Clin Psychiatry* 71, 1636–1644.

Uddo M, Vasterling JJ, Braily K et al. (1993) Memory and attention in posttraumatic stress disorder. *J Psychopathol Beh Assess* 15, 43–52.

Umile EM, Sandel ME, Alavai A et al. (2002) Dynamic imaging in mild traumatic brain injury: Support for the theory of medial temporal vulnerability. *Archiv Phys Med Rehabil* 83, 1506–1513.

Uno H, Tarara R, Else JG et al. (1989) Hippocampal damage associated with prolonged and fatal stress in primates. *J Neurosci* 9, 1705–1711.

Van Boven RW, Harrington GS, Hackney DB et al. (2009) Advances in neuroimaging of traumatic brain injury and posttraumatic stress disorder. *J Rehabil Res Dev* 46, 717–757.

Vanderploeg RD, Belanger HG, Curtiss G (2009) Mild traumatic brain injury and posttraumatic stress disorder and their associations with health symptoms. *Archiv Phys Med Rehabil* 90, 1084–1093.

Varney NR, Bushnell D (1998) NeuroSPECT findings in patients with posttraumatic anosmia: A quantitative analysis. *J Head Trauma Rehabil* 13, 63–72.

Vasterling JJ, Brailey K, Constans JI et al. (1998) Attention and memory dysfunction in post-traumatic stress disorder. *Neuropsychology* 12, 125–133.

Vasterling JJ, Dikmen S (2012) Mild traumatic brain injury and posttraumatic stress disorder: clinical and conceptual complexities. *J Int Neuropsychol Soc* 18, 390–393.

Vasterling JJ, Duke LM, Brailey K et al. (2002) Attention, learning, and memory performance and intellectual resources in Vietnam veterans: PTSD and no disorder comparisons. *Neuropsychology* 16, 5–14.

Vermetten E, Vythilingam M, Southwick SM et al. (2003) Long-term treatment with paroxetine increases verbal declarative memory and hippocampal volume in posttraumatic stress disorder. *Biol Psychiatry* 54, 693–702.

Villarreal G, Hamilton DA, Graham DP et al. (2004) Reduced area of the corpus callosum in posttraumatic stress disorder. *Psych Res: Neuroimaging* 131, 227–235.

Walilko T, North C, Young LA et al. (2009) Head injury as a PTSD predictor among Oklahoma City bombing survivors. *J Trauma* 67, 1311–1319.

Wall PL (2012) Posttraumatic stress disorder and traumatic brain injury in current military populations: a critical analysis. *J Am Psychiatr Nurse Assoc* 18, 278–298.

Wang H-H, Zhang Z-J, Tan Q-R et al. (2010) Psychopathological, biological, and neuroimaging characterization of posttraumatic stress disorder in survivors of a sever coalmining disaster in China. *J Psychiatr Res* 44, 385–392.

Warden DL, French LM, Shupenko L et al. (2009) Case report of a soldier with primary blast brain injury. *NeuroImage* 47, T152-T153.

Whalley MG, Rugg MD, Smith APR et al. (2009) Incidental retrieval of emotional contexts in post-traumatic stress disorder and depression: An fMRI study. *Brain and Cognition* 69, 98–107.

Wilk JE, Herrell RK, Wynn GH et al. (2012) Mild traumatic brain injury (concussion), post-traumatic stress disorder, and depression in U.S. soldiers involved in combat deployments: association with postdeployment symptoms. *Psychosom Med* 74, 249–257.

Williams WH, Evans JJ, Needham P et al. (2002) Neurological, cognitive and attributional predictors of posttraumatic stress symptoms after traumatic brain injury. *J Trauma Stress* 15, 397–400.

Wisco BE, Marx BP, Holowka DW et al. (2014) Traumatic brain injury, PTSD, and current suicidal ideation among Iraq and Afghanistan U.S. veterans. *J Trauma Stress* 27, 244–248.

Woodward SH, Kaloupek DG, Streeter CC et al. (2006) Decreased anterior cingulate volume in combat-related PTSD. *Biol Psychiatry* 59, 582–587.

Woon FL, Hedges DW (2008) Hippocampal and amygdala volumes in children and adults with childhood maltreatment-related posttraumatic stress disorder: a meta-analysis. *Hippocampus* 18, 729–736.

Woon FL, Hedges DW (2009) Amygdala volume in adults with posttraumatic stress disorder: a meta-analysis. *J Neuropsychiatry Clin Neurosci* 21, 5–12.

Woon FL, Sood S, Hedges DW (2010) Hippocampal volume deficits associated with exposure to psychological trauma and posttraumatic stress disorder in adults: a meta-analysis. *Prog Neuropsychopharmacol Biol Psychiatry* 34, 1181–1188.

Yamasue H, Kasai K, Iwanami A et al. (2003) Voxel-based analysis of MRI reveals anterior cingulate gray-matter volume reduction in posttraumatic stress disorder due to terrorism. *Proc Natl Acad Sci USA* 100, 9039–9043.

Yehuda R, Keefe RS, Harvey PD et al. (1995) Learning and memory in combat veterans with posttraumatic stress disorder. *Am J Psychiatry* 152, 137–139.

Yurgil KA, Barkauskas DA, Vasterling JJ et al. (2014) Association between traumatic brain injury and risk of posttraumatic stress disorder in active-duty Marines. *JAMA Psychiatry* 71, 149–157.

Zalewski C, Thompson W, Gottesman I (1994) Comparison of neuropsychological test performance in PTSD, generalized anxiety disorder, and control Vietnam veterans. *Assessment* 1, 133–142.

Zatzick DF, Rivara FP, Jurkovich GJ et al. (2010) Multisite investigation of traumatic brain injuries, posttraumatic stress disorder, and self-reported health and cognitive impairments. *Arch Gen Psychiatry* 67, 1291–1300.

CHAPTER 14

Stress-related psychopathology and pain

Sarah C. Reitz[1], Karl-Juergen Bär[2] & Christian Schmahl[1]

[1] Department of Psychosomatic Medicine and Psychotherapy, Central Institute of Mental Health Mannheim, Medical Faculty Mannheim, Heidelberg University, Mannheim, Germany

[2] Department of Psychiatry and Psychotherapy, University Hospital, Jena, Germany

14.1 Introduction

Pain is a multidimensional sensation comprising sensory information, affective processing and a cognitive-evaluative component. Furthermore, pain leads to changes in autonomic body functions (blood pressure, heart frequency, etc.). Pain perception can be substantially altered in different psychiatric disorders. Experimental studies have described different mechanisms for altered pain perception and processing in several psychiatric disorders.

This chapter reviews the relevant clinical and experimental knowledge with regard to pain processing in depression, schizophrenia, anorexia, borderline personality disorder, and posttraumatic stress disorder. The focus will be on changes in psychophysiology, neuroanatomy and neurochemistry.

Pain is understood to consist of a number of discrete components (Klossika et al., 2006; Price, 2000): a *sensory-discriminative* component (hereafter called "sensory"), representing the sensory information of the pain stimulus and giving information about its localization, quality, and intensity; *an affective motivational* component (hereinafter called "affective"), which is responsible for the emotional perception of the pain; and *a cognitive component*, which is associated with the anticipation, awareness and memory of the pain stimulus, comparing it with previous experiences (Melzack & Casey, 1968) and acting as a superordinated control for both of the other components. Specific disorders can be nicely differentiated and characterized in terms of dysfunctions of these individual components. Vegetative responses (e.g., the change of pupil diameter or blood pressure) to pain are caused by altered autonomic nervous system activity and are therefore referred to as autonomic components.

Posttraumatic Stress Disorder: From Neurobiology to Treatment, First Edition.
Edited by J. Douglas Bremner.
© 2016 John Wiley & Sons, Inc. Published 2016 by John Wiley & Sons, Inc.

The International Association for the Study of Pain (IASP) defines pain as "an unpleasant sensory and emotional experience associated with actual or potential tissue damage, or described in terms of such damage" (IASP, 1979). Nevertheless, not all people experience pain in the same way. Different cognitive mechanisms and central structures are involved in the processing and evaluation of pain and are sometimes disturbed due to psychopathological abnormalities. Changed perception or processing of pain can be symptoms of different psychiatric disorders and in some cases can constitute a substantial part of the actual disease itself. For example, patients suffering from borderline personality disorder (BPD) use non-suicidal self-injury to terminate states of aversive inner tension. In contrast, depressive patients often report an increase in pain complaints.

The ability to understand how pain perception and processing are affected in different disorders might help psychiatrists or psychologists dealing with their patients and could be essential in choosing an appropriate therapy. In this chapter, we describe five different psychiatric disorders, which to varying degrees are associated with exposure to stress, in terms of their pain components, and attempt to explain the diseases in terms of their neurobiology.

14.2 Depression

Around 45–75% of depressive in-patients suffer from pain symptoms, while 22% of those seeking primary care report chronic pain. Primary care patients suffering from pain are four times more likely to develop a comorbid anxiety disorder or depressive symptoms than patients without pain (Lepine & Briley, 2004). Furthermore, an increased prevalence of depressive disorders is known to exist in patients with chronic pain, which is why a notably higher rate of comorbidity has been found in specialized pain clinics. A British study found comorbid depression in 26 out of 36 (72%) patients with chronic pain (Poole et al., 2009).

14.2.1 Pain components

For many patients with depression, constant pain is an enormous strain. Pain complicates therapy and the severity of coincident pain influences the outcome of patient treatment (Bair et al., 2003). In healthy people, changes in mood are also associated with altered pain perception. For example, experimental induction of sad mood (Rainville et al., 2005) or loss of control as well as situations of helplessness are associated with an alteration in pain perception (Williams et al., 2004). Both loss of control and helplessness are important aspects perpetuating depression that also lead to increased pain sensitization.

Clinical experience and experimental results differ from one another: depressive patients show decreased pain sensitivity for heat pain stimuli (Bär et al.,

2003; Dickens et al., 2003) when exposed to simultaneously increased subjective pain experiences. On the other hand, increased sensitivity was found for deeper-lying pain. The latter was induced by inflating a blood pressure cuff above 200 mmHg and subjects were asked to perform continuous flexion of the right or left index finger using 50% of their maximum strength (Bär et al., 2005). Similar evidence for the difference between muscle and heat pain was found in patients with acute stress disorder (Bär et al., 2006b; Böttger & Bär, 2007).

During painful electrical or laser stimulation of a skeletal muscle, stronger activation of the anterior cingulate cortex could be shown. This region is associated with the affective pain component and a heightened awareness of painful stimuli (Mense, 2003).

But since, as described earlier, the induction of sadness leads to increased pain sensitivity in healthy participants as well as in depressive patients, it can be assumed that an increased pain threshold in depressive patients is due to a different mechanism of cortical processing compared with the short-term enhancement of pain sensitivity in induced sadness. No deficits or dysfunctions of the sensory component could be verified (Klauenberg et al., 2008). Furthermore, there was no indication that the autonomic component contributed to changed pain perception in depressive patients (Boettger et al., 2010).

14.2.2 Neuroanatomy

The dorsolateral prefrontal cortex (DLPFC) is assumed to be involved in the processing of pain and the generation of pain perception. In depressive patients, a reduced activity in the DLPFC is associated with a psychomotoric slowdown, an attention and memory deficit, and a positive correlation with the severity of the disorder (Mayberg, 2003).

The reduced activity and the assumption that the DLPFC is suppressing pain perception while simultaneously presenting cognitive or other tasks (Lorenz et al., 2003) suggests that reduced pain perception in depressive patients is due to changed cognitive processing of pain stimuli. This was shown in the DLPFC, pointing to a hyperactivation in patients compared with healthy controls (Bär et al., 2007).

The imagination of a pain stimulus led to increased amygdala activity in depressive patients (Strigo et al., 2008). In contrast, healthy persons showed a deactivation of the amygdala during the anticipation of pain (Petrovic et al., 2004).

14.2.3 Neurochemistry

As in other psychiatric disorders, the pathogenesis of depression is assumed to emanate from different neurochemical systems. Important targets of drug therapy (serotonin reuptake inhibitors, serotonin–norepinephrine reuptake inhibitors) are the neurotransmitters serotonin and norepinephrine, which are known to be involved in pain processing. In fact, these agents act in descending pain-regulating pathways, which are located in the brain stem (Bannister et al., 2009). A connection between pathogenesis of depression and altered pain perception might exist, but there are only a few studies on this topic. A relation between serotonergic dysfunction and altered pain perception in depressive patients has been shown (Kundermann et al., 2009): reduced serotonergic activation is correlated with reduced pain perception.

Serotonin–norepinephrine reuptake inhibitors are used to treat the physical symptoms of depressive patients (e.g., back pain, abdominal pain, musculoskeletal pain, etc.) (Brannan et al., 2005). Treatment with antidepressant drugs without noradrenergic components is not recommended.

In addition to changes in the serotonergic and noradrenergic systems, alterations in the opioid system have been shown (Frew & Drummond, 2009): An increased release of endogenous opioids has been postulated in depressive patients, potentially associated with reduced pain perception.

14.2.4 Summary

Clinically depressed patients are exposed to increased pain perception, and show increased physical symptoms such as back pain. Increased pain intensity was found experimentally, in particular in deep muscle pain, in contrast to superficial pain. Depression can primarily be related to dysfunctions of the affective and cognitive components, and less to the sensory component. An increased activation of the DLPFC is assumed to be involved in the reduced pain processing of external pain stimuli.

14.3 Schizophrenia

Although not as closely associated with stress exposure as the other mental disorders described in this chapter, there is some evidence for an association between stress and schizophrenia, and findings related to pain are presented to compare and contrast with these other disorders.

Patients with schizophrenia are known to have significantly reduced pain perception. They suffer much less from pain complaints than do healthy people (Kraepelin, 1919). Some patients injure themselves massively (e.g., eye enucleation, castration; Favazza, 1998) or they show reduced pain perception (e.g., after a bone fracture; Murthy et al., 2004).

In comparison to depressed patients, patients with schizophrenia rarely suffer from chronic pain. This apparently reduced pain sensitivity might lead to medical emergencies like acute abdomen conditions (e.g., peritonitis, ruptured appendix, etc.), during which these patients frequently mention little or even no pain (Geschwind, 1977; Rosenthal et al., 1990).

14.3.1 Pain components

Currently, research results on this topic are unclear: some authors found no differences in pain thresholds between patients and healthy controls (Collins & Stone, 1966; Guieu et al., 1994). Reduced pain sensitivity is associated with the main symptoms of the disorder (Singh et al., 2006), such as affective flattening (Dworkin, 1994), positive symptoms (Merskey et al., 1962), or disturbed cognition in acute disease conditions (Jochum et al., 2006). Patients in acute psychotic states are particularly limited in their cognition, which makes their ability to assess pain difficult. It can be assumed that the cognitive component of pain perception plays an important role in this disease.

Findings on reduced pain perception in patients with schizophrenia are often tied to therapeutic use of antipsychotic drugs (Jakubaschk & Boker, 1991). However, it could be shown that patients with schizophrenia who were not taking antipsychotics also show elevated pain thresholds compared with healthy controls and even tend to approach the thresholds of healthy controls when taking antipsychotic medication.

14.3.2 Summary

The cognitive component appears to be highly relevant for pain sensitivity of patients with schizophrenia. A precise statement about the affective and sensory pain components cannot currently be made. Furthermore, there remains no clear explanation of the neuroanatomical and neurochemical background of reduced pain perception in schizophrenia.

14.4 Anorexia nervosa

Patients with anorexia nervosa are known to have dysfunctions in several sensory systems, in addition to a dysfunction of the olfactory and gustatory system (Drewnowski et al., 1987). These patients also have a disturbance of body image, which is an important diagnostic criterion that might be related to impaired body-size perception (Berry et al., 1995; Skrzypek et al., 2001). Some patients suffer from anosognosia in their disease (Nunn et al., 2011).

An increased pain perception threshold has been found in the disease (Bär et al., 2006a, 2012; Lautenbacher & Krieg, 1994; Pauls et al., 1991; de Zwaan et al., 1996). Altered pain thresholds manifest in other eating disorders (e.g., bulimia nervosa) as well, but the mechanisms of disturbed pain processing appear to be different among different diseases (Lautenbacher et al., 1990).

14.4.1 Pain components

Until recently, subclinical neuropathy induced by malnutrition was suspected to underlie reduced pain perception in anorexia nervosa. However, this hypothesis could not be confirmed (Pauls et al., 1991) and a recent study by Goldzak-Kunik et al. (2012) has shown non-disturbed sensory perception.

It is assumed that reduced pain perception is caused by sympathetic dysregulation or altered receptor activity, for which there is currently no evidence (Lautenbacher et al., 1991). An activation of the parasympathetic system, determined by pupil diameter, is associated with an increased pain threshold (Bär et al., 2006a).

As already described in the section on depression, anorexic patients might suffer from physical pain symptoms as well (Coughlin et al., 2008). Association of the complaint's seriousness with depressive symptoms emphasizes the importance of the treatment of these symptoms in anorectic patients.

14.4.2 Neuroanatomy

Unfortunately, there are few data about neuroanatomical correlates of decreased pain threshold in anorexia nervosa. Several different characteristics of the disorder are assumed to be caused by an insular dysfunction. The insula contributes to dysfunctional processing and integration of autonomous, affective, and sensory stimuli (Nunn et al., 2008). A recent study showed a difference in central pain processing of patients with anorexia nervosa for the first time: by applying heat-pain stimuli on the right forearm by a thermode during functional magnetic resonance imaging (fMRI), increased activity of the left posterior insular cortex was found in healthy subjects compared with patients. According to Ianetti et al (2005), activation of this area of the cortex is correlated with perceived pain intensity. It can therefore be concluded that reduced activity of the left posterior insular cortex could be responsible for increased pain thresholds in anorectic patients.

A further dysfunction of the insula appears to influence pain perception in these patients: the right anterior insular cortex is believed to control effects of the sympathetic nervous system such as tachycardia or changes in blood pressure (Craig, 2005). Therefore, a stronger activation of the right anterior insular cortex, as well as a stronger activation of the pons (Bär et al., 2013), may be caused by stronger sympathetic modulation leading to increased adrenergic descending inhibition of pain. This may explain altered pain perception in patients with anorexia nervosa.

14.4.3 Neurochemistry

Anorexia nervosa is associated with variations in concentrations of several different hormonal systems. An increase in cortisol in anorexia nervosa (Misra et al.,

2004) is correlated with a decrease in pain perception (Bär et al., 2006a). Furthermore, there is an increase of corticotropin-releasing hormone (CRH), which induces the actual release of cortisol. CRH is produced by splitting from its precursor hormone, proopiomelanocortine, along with other opioid precursors. Central analgesia caused by opioids can be reversed by the opioidantagonist naloxone. A central reason for the decreased pain threshold in anorectic patients has been assumed to be a dysfunction of the opioid system due to an elevated opioid concentration in the CSF of anorectic patients. However, a normalization of pain thresholds under naloxone has not been confirmed (Lautenbacher et al., 1990).

Changes in thyroid hormone levels, induced by long-term fasting and malnutrition, cause symptoms of a hypothyroid metabolic condition: bradycardia, imbalance of themoregulation, and reduced metabolic rate. The observed correlation of free T3 with pain thresholds and an increase of pain thresholds in patients with hypothyroidism were confirmed by Bär et al. (2006).

14.4.4 Summary

In patients with anorexia nervosa, a pronounced decrease of pain perception can be found. This reduced sensitivity is specific for pain and there are no alterations in perception of coldness, warmth, touch, or vibration (Faris et al., 1992; Pauls et al., 1991). The lower the body mass index, the higher the pain thresholds found in these patients. However, these findings are reversible after treatment and achievement of a normal weight (Bär et al., 2006a). Besides a dysfunction of the sensory component, a dysfunction of the cognitive pain component can also be assumed. An involvement of the affective component may not be excluded, but should be clarified in future studies.

14.5 Borderline personality disorder

Non-suicidal self-injurious behavior is one of the criteria for the diagnosis of BPD and is frequently observed in combination with dissociative states and reduced pain perception. Further diagnostic criteria of BPD are affective instability, impulsivity, and a disturbance of self-image. Similarly to PTSD, traumatic events can frequently be found in the history of BPD patients, with approximately 60–62% reporting sexual abuse (Zanarini et al.. 2011).

14.5.1 Pain components

Several studies confirmed subjectively reduced pain sensitivity to cold-pressor tests (Bohus et al., 2000; Russ et al., 1992) and laser stimulation (Schmahl et al., 2004). Most probably, there is no dysfunction of the sensory pain component in BPD patients, as their spatial discrimination for painful stimuli is intact and laser-evoked potentials are not lower than in healthy controls (Schmahl et al., 2004). A positive correlation of pain thresholds and aversive tension in patients with BPD point, rather, to a disturbance of the affective pain component (Ludäscher et al., 2007).

A recent study shows that real tissue damage with a scalpel leads to a reduction of inner aversive tension and a decrease of heart rate after prior stress induction in BPD patients (Reitz et al., 2012). Further studies on this issue are necessary to obtain a better understanding of the relationship between pain and tissue damage.

14.5.2 Neuroanatomy

An fMRI investigation identified an apparent correlate of the antinociceptive mechanism in BPD: tonic heat pain stimulation with individually adapted temperatures led to a deactivation of the amygdala and the rostral anterior cingulate cortex, as well as to an increase of activation in the DLPFC in patients with BPD compared with healthy controls (Schmahl et al., 2006). Interestingly, in a follow-up study, this amygdala deactivation could only be found in patients with comorbid PTSD (Kraus et al., 2009a). This points to a connection between both trauma-associated disorders BPD and PTSD.

A recent finding, showing reduced experimentally induced activation of the amygdala by heat stimuli (Niedtfeld et al., 2012), suggests that hyperarousal in BPD patients can be reduced by strong painful stimuli such as self-injurious behavior. In the fMRI study mentioned above, emotionally negative pictures were used to induce stress. Painful and non-painful stimuli were then applied. After application of the heat stimuli, a deactivation of the insular cortex could be demonstrated, in addition to a decrease of activity in the amygdala. However, the reduction of activity was not specific to painful stimuli, as it was also found for neutral stimuli. In a recent follow-up study, an inhibitory connection between the amygdala and the prefrontal cortex could be demonstrated which was specifically related to painful (and not non-painful) stimuli (Niedtfeld et al., 2012).

In conclusion, these results point to an important impact of pain on disturbed emotion regulation in BPD. Dysfunctional behavior such as non-suicidal self-injury may have a substitute function of directing attention away from negative affective states and compensating for insufficient cognitive control mechanisms.

14.5.3 Neurochemistry

A dysfunction of the endogenous opioid system (EOS) has been assumed to be involved in reduced perception of pain in patients with BPD. In patients with both BPD and PTSD, treatment with naltrexone, an opioid antagonist, has a positive impact on symptoms such as derealization, depersonalization or analgesic states (Sharp & Harvey, 2001). Also, the therapeutic effect of naltrexone on self-injurious behavior (Sher & Stanley, 2009) and the clinical observation that patients with BPD often tend to overdose with opiates point to an involvement of the EOS. There are several explanations for this (cf. Bandelow et al., 2010; Tiefenbacher et al., 2005): On the one hand, we find the pain hypothesis, which suggests that an increased activity of the EOS combined with hypoalgesia can be terminated by patients only through strong painful stimuli such as during self-injury, and on the other we have the dependency hypothesis, which suggests that patients stimulate the EOS through self-injury and thereby induce a dependency. Altogether there is still a significant need for more studies in this area, particularly as findings regarding the EOS may help to shape further pharmacotherapy of non-suicidal, self-injurious behavior in BPD.

14.5.4 Summary

Reduced pain perception in BPD has been repeatedly demonstrated. The results of the individual studies point collectively to a dysregulation of the affective pain component. An involvement of the cognitive pain component may also be responsible for reduced pain perception. The disturbed processing of the affective and cognitive pain component is associated with alterations in limbic areas such as the amygdala, as well as in the DLPFC. In contrast, the sensory pain component seems to be intact.

Pain plays an important role in relation to disturbed emotion regulation in patients with BPD. Pain stimuli in experimental settings appear to significantly reduce aversive tension in BPD.

14.6 Post-traumatic stress disorder

Although chronic pain syndromes and PTSD are clearly differentiable disorders, there is a high comorbidity (Asmundson et al., 2004; Dobie et al., 2004; Norman et al., 2008). PTSD with comorbid chronic pain is associated with more depressive symptoms, reduced quality of life, and stronger psychosocial impairment (Bryant et al., 1999).

14.6.1 Pain components

Different approaches have been used to try to explain the relationship between PTSD and chronic pain. The "mutual maintenance theory" (Sharp & Harvey,

2001) explains the comorbidity between pain and PTSD in terms of mutual influence and perpetuation of symptoms. The interaction of different cognitive, affective, and behavioral mechanisms in processes such as rumination and catastrophizing, is found in patients with chronic pain as well as in patients with PTSD and plays an important role in the exacerbation and maintenance (Liedl et al., 2010) of the two disorders. It might be the case that the capacity to develop functional strategies to control pain is disturbed by dysfunctional cognition.

Different studies have shown increased thresholds for heat pain in male soldiers with PTSD (Kraus et al., 2009b; Pitman et al., 1990). A double influence of traumatization and PTSD was demonstrated in the latter study, in which thermal detection and pain thresholds were determined in 10 male combat-related PTSD patients, 10 combat control subjects (no PTSD), and 10 healthy controls without combat experience. Heat and cold pain thresholds in both combat groups (PTSD and combat controls) were significantly increased compared with healthy controls. However, these stimuli did not lead to a difference between these two groups due to ceiling effects (highest or lowest applicable temperature were reached). When using longer-lasting heat stimulation at different temperatures, a significantly lower frequency of pain reports was found in PTSD patients compared with both combat and healthy controls, as well as significantly lower pain ratings. In female PTSD patients with a history of sexual abuse, the reduction of pain sensitivity was found to be less pronounced than in patients with BPD (Schmahl et al., 2010).

14.6.2 Neuroanatomy

In a study using fMRI and the application of tonic heat pain and individually adapted stimuli, activation in the putamen and bilateral anterior insular cortex was found in PTSD patients, as well as a deactivation in the amygdala (Geuze et al., 2007). In contrast, in a study of female PTSD patients who suffered from domestic violence, no difference in the activation of the amygdala was found in comparison with healthy controls (Strigo et al., 2010). The amygdala plays an important role in pain processing (Neugebauer, 2007) as well as in PTSD (Etkin & Wager, 2007). More research is needed to identify altered amygdala activity in PTSD and its relation to specific symptoms of the disorder.

14.6.3 Neurochemistry

Trauma-relevant events, presented by video and combined with standardized heat pain stimuli, led to a decrease of pain intensity during placebo administration in Vietnam veterans with PTSD. During application of naloxone, pain tolerance did not differ from healthy controls (Pitman et al., 1990), who showed no change in pain perception after video exposure. This points to a stress-induced hypoalgesia in patients with PTSD, which is modulated by the EOS.

14.6.4 Summary

There is no dysfunction of the sensory pain component in PTSD, but, as with BPD, there is clearly reduced pain perception. This can be related to an involvement of the affective and cognitive pain components. Enhanced pain control has also been shown for these patients. The "mutual maintenance theory" clarifies to a certain extent the reciprocal perpetuation of pain symptoms and PTSD, but cannot explain the question of how comorbid disorders develop. The extent to which traumatic life events *per se* influence pain thresholds and central pain processing should be further examined.

14.7 Conclusion

Based on the studies outlined in this chapter, a tentative explanation can be offered in an attempt to delineate the different mechanisms and structures involved in alterations in pain processing in stress-related psychiatric disorders.

Common to the five described disorders is an experimental reduction of pain perception. With regard to this, contradictions between clinical description and experimental results appear: depressive patients often report chronic pain, although decreased pain sensitivity was found in experimental studies. In BPD patients, experimental studies verify that reduced sensitivity to pain, particularly in relation to self-injurious behavior, is frequent. Nonetheless, patients often suffer from reduced tolerance towards non-self-inflicted pain such as headaches. This is also reflected in increased use of pain medication (Saper & Lake, 2002). A distinction should be made for the individual localizations of pain, such as superficial and deeper-lying pain. Trauma-associated disorders such as BPD and PTSD show signs of a dysfunction of the affective pain component, while the sensory component seems to be intact. The severe cognitive restrictions created by the psychopathology of schizophrenia preclude obtaining reliable information regarding different pain components. However, a dysfunction of the cognitive pain component can be assumed. Disturbances in all three pain components can most likely be found in anorectic patients.

As altered pain perception is closely linked with all of these psychiatric conditions, as well as the level of psychopathology and patients' prognosis, further research in this field is urgently needed. A better understanding of the interconnection between pain and psychiatric disorders will be useful in the development of new treatments for both fields.

References

Asmundson GJ, Wright KD, Stein MB (2004) Pain and PTSD symptoms in female veterans. *Eur J Pain* 8, 345–350.

Bair MJ, Robinson RL, Katon W et al. (2003) Depression and pain comorbidity: a literature review. *Archives of internal medicine* 163, 2433–2445.

Bandelow B, Schmahl C, Falkai P et al. (2010) Borderline personality disorder: a dysregulation of the endogenous opioid system? *Psychol Rev* 117, 623–636.

Bannister K, Bee LA, Dickenson AH (2009) Preclinical and early clinical investigations related to monoaminergic pain modulation. *Neurotherapeutics* 6, 703–712.

Bär KJ, Berger S, Schwier C et al. (2013) Insular dysfunction and descending pain inhibition in anorexia nervosa. *Acta Psychiatr Scand* 127, 269–278.

Bär KJ, Böttger S, Wagner G et al. (2006a) Changes of pain perception, autonomic function, and endocrine parameters during treatment of anorectic adolescents. *J Am Acad Child Adolesc Psychiatry* 45, 1068–1076.

Bär KJ, Brehm S, Böttger MK et al. (2005) Pain perception in major depression depends on pain modality. *Pain* 117, 97–103.

Bär KJ, Brehm S, Böttger MK et al. (2006b) Decreased sensitivity to experimental pain in adjustment disorder. *Eur J Pain* 10, 467–471.

Bär KJ, Greiner W, Letsch A et al. (2003) Influence of gender and hemispheric lateralization on heat pain perception in major depression. *J Psychiatr Res* 37, 345–353.

Bär KJ, Wagner G, Koschke M et al. (2007) Increased prefrontal activation during pain perception in major depression. *Biol Psychiatry* 62, 1281–1287.

Berry EM, Fried S, Edelstein EL (1995) Abnormal oral sensory perception in patients with a history of anorexia nervosa and the relationship between physiological and psychological improvement in this disease. *Psychother Psychosom* 63, 32–37.

Boettger MK, Greiner W, Rachow T et al. (2010) Sympathetic skin response following painful electrical stimulation is increased in major depression. *Pain* 149, 130–134.

Bohus M, Limberger M, Ebner U et al. (2000) Pain perception during self-reported distress and calmness in patients with borderline personality disorder and self-mutilating behavior. *Psychiatry Res* 95, 251–260.

Böttger MK, Bär KJ (2007) Perception for ischemic pain shows similarities in adjustment disorder and major depression. *Eur J Pain* 11, 819–822.

Brannan SK, Mallinckrodt CH, Brown EB et al. (2005) Duloxetine 60 mg once-daily in the treatment of painful physical symptoms in patients with major depressive disorder. *Journal of psychiatric research* 39, 43–53.

Bryant RA, Marosszeky JE, Crooks J et al. (1999) Interaction of posttraumatic stress disorder and chronic pain following traumatic brain injury. *J Head Trauma Rehabil* 14, 588–594.

Collins GL, Stone LA (1966) Pain sensitivity, age and activity level in chronic schizophrenics and normals. *Br J Psychiatry* 112, 33–35.

Coughlin JW, Edwards R, Buenaver L et al. (2008) Pain, catastrophizing, and depressive symptomatology in eating disorders. *Clin J Pain* 24, 406–414.

Craig AD (2005) Forebrain emotional asymmetry: a neuroanatomical basis? *Trends Cogn Sci* 9, 566–571.

de Zwaan M, Biener D, Schneider C et al. (1996) Relationship between thresholds to thermally and to mechanically induced pain in patients with eating disorders and healthy subjects. *Pain* 67, 511–512.

Dickens C, McGowan L, Dale S (2003) Impact of depression on experimental pain perception: a systematic review of the literature with meta-analysis. *Psychosom Med* 65, 369–375.

Dobie DJ, Kivlahan DR, Maynard C et al. (2004) Posttraumatic stress disorder in female veterans: association with self-reported health problems and functional impairment. *Arch Intern Med* 164, 394–400.

Drewnowski A, Halmi KA, Pierce B et al. (1987) Taste and eating disorders. *Am J Clin Nutr* 46, 442–450.

Dworkin RH (1994) Pain insensitivity in schizophrenia: a neglected phenomenon and some implications. *Schizophr Bull* 20, 235–248.

Etkin A, Wager TD (2007) Functional neuroimaging of anxiety: a meta-analysis of emotional processing in PTSD, social anxiety disorder, and specific phobia. *Am J Psychiatry* 164, 1476–1488.

Faris PL, Raymond NC, De Zwaan M et al. (1992) Nociceptive, but not tactile, thresholds are elevated in bulimia nervosa. *Biol Psychiatry* 32, 462–466.

Favazza AR (1998) The coming of age of self-mutilation. *J Nerv Ment Dis* 186, 259–268.

Frew AK, Drummond PD (2009) Opposite effects of opioid blockade on the blood pressure-pain relationship in depressed and non-depressed participants. *Pain* 142, 68–74.

Geschwind N (1977) Insensitivity to pain in psychotic patients. *N Engl J Med* 296, 1480.

Geuze E, Westenberg HG, Jochims A et al. (2007) Altered pain processing in veterans with posttraumatic stress disorder. *Arch Gen Psychiatry* 64, 76–85.

Goldzak-Kunik G, Friedman R, Spitz M et al. (2012) Intact sensory function in anorexia nervosa. *Am J Clin Nutr* 95, 272–282.

Guieu R, Samuelian JC, Coulouvrat H (1994) Objective evaluation of pain perception in patients with schizophrenia. *The British Journal of Psychiatry* 164, 253–255.

Iannetti GD, Zambreanu L, Cruccu G et al. (2005) Operculoinsular cortex encodes pain intensity at the earliest stages of cortical processing as indicated by amplitude of laser-evoked potentials in humans. *Neuroscience* 131, 199–208.

IASP (1979) Pain terms: a list with definitions and notes on usage. Recommended by the IASP Subcommittee on Taxonomy. *Pain* 6, 249.

Jakubaschk J, Boker W (1991) [Disorders of pain perception in schizophrenia]. *Schweiz Arch Neurol Psychiatr* 142, 55–76.

Jochum T, Letzsch A, Greiner W et al. (2006) Influence of antipsychotic medication on pain perception in schizophrenia. *Psychiatry Res* 142, 151–156.

Klauenberg S, Maier C, Assion HJ et al. (2008) Depression and changed pain perception: hints for a central disinhibition mechanism. *Pain* 140, 332–343.

Klossika I, Flor H, Kamping S et al. (2006) Emotional modulation of pain: a clinical perspective. *Pain* 124, 264–268.

Kraepelin E (1919) *Dementia Praecox and Paraphrenia.* Chicago Medical Book Co., Chicago, IL.

Kraus A, Esposito F, Seifritz E et al. (2009a) Amygdala deactivation as a neural correlate of pain processing in patients with borderline personality disorder and co-occurrent posttraumatic stress disorder. *Biol Psychiatry* 65, 819–822.

Kraus A, Geuze E, Schmahl C et al. (2009b) Differentiation of pain ratings in combat-related posttraumatic stress disorder. *Pain* 143, 179–185.

Kundermann B, Hemmeter-Spernal J, Strate P et al. (2009) Pain sensitivity in major depression and its relationship to central serotoninergic function as reflected by the neuroendocrine response to clomipramine. *J Psychiatr Res* 43, 1253–1261.

Lautenbacher S, Krieg JC (1994) Pain perception in psychiatric disorders: a review of the literature. *J Psychiatr Res* 28, 109–122.

Lautenbacher S, Pauls AM, Strian F et al. (1990) Pain perception in patients with eating disorders. *Psychosom Med* 52, 673–682.

Lautenbacher S, Pauls AM, Strian F et al. (1991) Pain sensitivity in anorexia nervosa and bulimia nervosa. *Biol Psychiatry* 29, 1073–1078.

Lepine JP, Briley M (2004) The epidemiology of pain in depression. *Hum Psychopharmacol* 19 Suppl 1, S3–7.

Liedl A, O'Donnell M, Creamer M et al. (2010) Support for the mutual maintenance of pain and post-traumatic stress disorder symptoms. *Psychol Med* 40, 1215–1223.

Lorenz J, Minoshima S, Casey KL (2003) Keeping pain out of mind: the role of the dorsolateral prefrontal cortex in pain modulation. *Brain* 126, 1079–1091.

Ludäscher P, Bohus M, Lieb K et al. (2007) Elevated pain thresholds correlate with dissociation and aversive arousal in patients with borderline personality disorder. *Psychiatry Res* 149, 291–296.

Mayberg HS (2003) Positron emission tomography imaging in depression: a neural systems perspective. *Neuroimaging Clin N Am* 13, 805–815.

Melzack R, Casey KL (1968) Sensory, motivational, and central control determinants of pain. A new conceptual model. In: Kenshalo DR, Charles CT (eds) *The Skin Senses*. CC Thomas, Springfield, pp. 423–443.

Mense S (2003) [What is different about muscle pain?]. *Schmerz* 17, 459–463.

Merskey H, Gillis A, Marszalek KS (1962) A clinical investigation of reactions to pain. *J Ment Sci* 108, 347–355.

Misra M, Miller KK, Almazan C et al. (2004) Alterations in cortisol secretory dynamics in adolescent girls with anorexia nervosa and effects on bone metabolism. *J Clin Endocrinol Metab* 89, 4972–4980.

Murthy BV, Narayan B, Nayagam S (2004) Reduced perception of pain in schizophrenia: its relevance to the clinical diagnosis of compartment syndrome. *Injury* 35, 1192–1193.

Neugebauer V (2007) The amygdala: different pains, different mechanisms. *Pain* 127, 1–2.

Niedtfeld I, Kirsch P, Schulze L et al. (2012) Functional connectivity of pain-mediated affect regulation in Borderline Personality Disorder. *PLoS One* 7, e33293.

Norman SB, Stein MB, Dimsdale JE et al. (2008) Pain in the aftermath of trauma is a risk factor for post-traumatic stress disorder. *Psychol Med* 38, 533–542.

Nunn K, Frampton I, Fuglset TS et al. (2011) Anorexia nervosa and the insula. *Med Hypotheses* 76, 353–357.

Nunn K, Frampton I, Gordon I et al. (2008) The fault is not in her parents but in her insula--a neurobiological hypothesis of anorexia nervosa. *Eur Eat Disord Rev* 16, 355–360.

Pauls AM, Lautenbacher S, Strian F et al. (1991) Assessment of somatosensory indicators of polyneuropathy in patients with eating disorders. *Eur Arch Psychiatry Clin Neurosci* 241, 8–12.

Petrovic P, Carlsson K, Petersson KM et al. (2004) Context-dependent deactivation of the amygdala during pain. *J Cogn Neurosci* 16, 1289–1301.

Pitman RK, van der Kolk BA, Orr SP et al. (1990) Naloxone-reversible analgesic response to combat-related stimuli in posttraumatic stress disorder. A pilot study. *Arch Gen Psychiatry* 47, 541–544.

Poole H, White S, Blake C et al. (2009) Depression in chronic pain patients: prevalence and measurement. *Pain Pract* 9, 173–180.

Price DD (2000) Psychological and neural mechanisms of the affective dimension of pain. *Science* 288, 1769–1772.

Rainville P, Bao QV, Chretien P (2005) Pain-related emotions modulate experimental pain perception and autonomic responses. *Pain* 118, 306–318.

Reitz S, Krause-Utz A, Pogatzki-Zahn EM et al. (2012) *Stress Regulation and Incision in Borderline Personality Disorder – A Pilot Study Modeling Cutting Behavior*. *J Pers Disord*.

Rosenthal SH, Porter KA, Coffey B (1990) Pain insensitivity in schizophrenia. Case report and review of the literature. *Gen Hosp Psychiatry* 12, 319–322.

Russ MJ, Roth SD, Lerman A et al. (1992) Pain perception in self-injurious patients with borderline personality disorder. *Biol Psychiatry* 32, 501–511.

Saper JR, Lake AE, 3rd (2002) Borderline personality disorder and the chronic headache patient: review and management recommendations. *Headache* 42, 663–674.

Schmahl C, Bohus M, Esposito F et al. (2006) Neural correlates of antinociception in borderline personality disorder. *Arch Gen Psychiatry* 63, 659–667.

Schmahl C, Greffrath W, Baumgartner U et al. (2004) Differential nociceptive deficits in patients with borderline personality disorder and self-injurious behavior: laser-evoked potentials, spatial discrimination of noxious stimuli, and pain ratings. *Pain* 110, 470–479.

Schmahl C, Meinzer M, Zeuch A et al. (2010) Pain sensitivity is reduced in borderline personality disorder, but not in posttraumatic stress disorder and bulimia nervosa. *World J Biol Psychiatry* 11, 364–371.

Sharp TJ, Harvey AG (2001) Chronic pain and posttraumatic stress disorder: mutual maintenance? *Clin Psychol Rev* 21, 857–877.

Sher L, Stanley BH (2009) Biological models of non-suicidal self-injury. In: Nock MK (ed.) *Understanding Nonsuicidal Self-Injury: Origins, Assessment and Treatment.* American Psychological Association, Washington, DC, pp. 99–116.

Singh MK, Giles LL, Nasrallah HA (2006) Pain insensitivity in schizophrenia: trait or state marker? *J Psychiatr Pract* 12, 90–102.

Skrzypek S, Wehmeier PM, Remschmidt H (2001) Body image assessment using body size estimation in recent studies on anorexia nervosa. A brief review. *Eur Child Adolesc Psychiatry* 10, 215–221.

Strigo IA, Simmons AN, Matthews SC et al. (2008) Association of major depressive disorder with altered functional brain response during anticipation and processing of heat pain. *Arch Gen Psychiatry* 65, 1275–1284.

Strigo IA, Simmons AN, Matthews SC et al. (2010) Neural correlates of altered pain response in women with posttraumatic stress disorder from intimate partner violence. *Biol Psychiatry* 68, 442–450.

Tiefenbacher S, Novak MA, Lutz CK et al. (2005) The physiology and neurochemistry of self-injurious behavior: a nonhuman primate model. *Front Biosci* 10, 1–11.

Williams DC, Golding J, Phillips K et al. (2004) Perceived control, locus of control and preparatory information: effects on the perception of an acute pain stimulus. *Pers Individ Diff* 35, 1681–1691.

Zanarini MC, Laudate CS, Frankenburg FR et al. (2011) Predictors of self-mutilation in patients with borderline personality disorder: A 10-year follow-up study. *J Psychiatr Res* 45, 823–828.

CHAPTER 15

Stress and health

Viola Vaccarino[1], Emeran Mayer[2] & J. Douglas Bremner[3]

[1] *Department of Epidemiology, Emory University Rollins School of Public Health, and Department of Internal Medicine (Cardiology), Emory University School of Medicine, Atlanta, GA, USA*

[2] *UCLA School of Medicine, Los Angeles, CA, USA*

[3] *Departments of Psychiatry & Behavioral Sciences and Radiology, Emory University School of Medicine, and the Atlanta VA Medical Center, Atlanta, GA, USA*

15.1 Introduction

Stress not only leads to lasting changes in neurobiology as well as symptoms of posttraumatic stress disorder (PTSD), it also has lasting effects on physical health (Bremner, 2002; Proctor et al., 1998, 2001; Wagner et al., 2000; Zatzick et al., 1997). A number of studies reviewed in this chapter show that psychological stress results in an increased risk for a number of physical diseases, including cardiovascular disease (CVD), diabetes, asthma, infectious disease, cancer, functional gastrointestinal disorders and others. In addition, psychiatric disorders related to stress, such as PTSD and depression, are independently associated with a higher risk of CVD, ischemic heart disease in particular, and possibly other disorders as well. Studies have shown that this increased risk is not completely driven by adverse lifestyle factors such as smoking, obesity, and lack of exercise, although these risk factors are also associated with stress-related mental disorders.

Potential pathways linking stress-related psychiatric disorders and physical health conditions are numerous and complex. To use the example of CVD, PTSD and depression could cause CVD, or worsen pre-existing CVD; alternatively, they could be a consequence of CVD – they could, for example, be a psychological sequel of an acute myocardial infarction (heart attack). Moreover, there could be a common factor (e.g., genes) that leads to increased risk for both the physical disorder and the mental disorder, with or without exposure to stress (Mulle & Vaccarino, 2013; Steptoe & Kivimaki, 2012).

The exact mechanisms behind these relationships are also complex. Changes in behavior or attempted efforts to cope with altered neurobiology could clearly be implicated, e.g., alcohol use to decrease hyperarousal, or smoking to cope with negative mood states (Bremner et al., 1996c). However, direct effects are

Posttraumatic Stress Disorder: From Neurobiology to Treatment, First Edition.
Edited by J. Douglas Bremner.
© 2016 John Wiley & Sons, Inc. Published 2016 by John Wiley & Sons, Inc.

also possible. For example, childhood abuse is associated with increased obesity (Williamson et al., 2002), probably related to changes in metabolism in addition to behavioral changes. This in turn increases the risk for both CVD and diabetes. Therefore multiple factors converge and possibly interact to define trajectories of adverse physical health status in patients with stress-related psychiatric disorders.

This chapter reviews the complex relationship between exposure to stress, stress-related psychiatric disorders, and physical disease. Most research has been done in the area of CVD, which is the primary focus of this chapter, but we touch on other areas of physical health as well as on the functional disorders, i.e., physical disorders where a physical abnormality cannot be readily identified.

15.2 Stress and cardiovascular disease

Stress has long been associated in popular culture with CVD (Vaccarino & Bremner, 2011). This takes the form of common wisdom about a "broken heart," or popular stories where someone "drops dead" of fright (the assumption being that the person's heart stopped working). These anecdotes and the well-known link between sudden cardiac death and intense emotions, such as those experienced during earthquakes and sports events (Steptoe & Kivimaki, 2012), led to the field of "behavioral cardiology" (Rozanski et al., 2005). In this field, initially there was an emphasis on "type A personality," which was characterized as the high-achieving, time-pressured businessperson-type who was prone to outbursts of anger. As reviewed in the following, acute episodes of anger were themselves found to be associated with decreased blood flow to the heart, or myocardial ischemia. Studies using evoked anger led to the use of stress paradigms in the laboratory, and a growing realization that both stress and stress-related psychiatric disorders such as PTSD could play a role in promoting CVD or worsening its clinical course (Steptoe & Kivimaki, 2012; Vaccarino & Bremner, 2011). Although much of the epidemiological research in the last 20 years has moved away from the type A personality construct towards a focus on depression, more recently there is a growing appreciation for the independent role of childhood abuse in the etiology of CVD, as well as the diagnosis of PTSD.

Activation of the stress response results in a number of physiological events that are relevant to understanding the causes of CVD. The "fight or flight" response to threat is driven by the sympathoadrenal system and the hypothalamus–pituitary–adrenal (HPA) axis, with resulting release of cortisol and norepinephrine, as well as other neurohormonal mediators (Bremner et al., 1996a,b; Vermetten & Bremner, 2002a,b). This leads to increased heart rate and blood pressure, and an increase in the pumping demands of the heart, all responses that are adaptive in terms of rapidly increasing blood flow and hence energy to muscles and the brain that are required for quick and strong responses in order to survive (McEwen, 2012). In modern society, however, we are more likely to experience stress from being stuck in a traffic jam than from an attack by a tiger, so the stress response system is, in some ways, an obsolete one that may cause more harm than good (Bremner, 2006). Chronic activation of these stress-responsive systems can result in negative effects on hemodynamics, metabolism, inflammation, immune and heart function.

Studies in human subjects show an association between stress and acute heart events. A number of studies have shown that acute, intense stressful events are correlated with an increase in hospital admissions for acute coronary syndromes or an increased rate of sudden cardiac death around the time of the event (Steptoe & Brydon, 2009; Vaccarino & Bremner, 2011). These include, for example, natural and industrial disasters, terrorist attacks, sporting events, or sudden bereavement. For example, there was an increase in hospital admissions for myocardial infarction of 35% during the 1994 Northridge earthquake in Los Angeles, with an associated increase in cardiac deaths not related to physical exertion (Kloner, 2006). The start of the Gulf War was associated with an increase in myocardial infarctions in Tel Aviv, Israel (Vaccarino & Bremner, 2011). Sporting matches are similarly associated with an increase in cardiac events and death, primarily at the beginning of the match, and more frequently in men than in women (Kloner et al., 2009; Wilbert-Lampen et al., 2008). Acute stressors with an exaggerated sympathetic reaction have also been associated with acute stunning of the myocardium that causes a reversible left ventricular dysfunction in some individuals, usually women (Wittstein et al., 2005).

The perception of being stressed is also related to the risk of cardiac events. The INTERHEART study, an international case–control study including 15,152 patients with myocardial infarction and 14,820 controls from 52 countries worldwide, found an increased risk of heart attacks to be associated with financial stress and stress at work, as well as loss of control and symptoms of depression (Rosengren et al., 2004). Another study with 60,000 people from the general population in England found a relationship between measures of distress (anxiety, depression, self perceived stress and social dysfunction) and increased cardiac mortality (Russ et al., 2012).

Studies have also linked a number of emotional factors to CVD. For example, an association was found between intense episodes of anger and acute coronary events such as heart attacks (Lipovetzky et al., 2007; Mostofsky et al., 2013b; Steptoe & Brydon, 2009; Strike et al., 2006). Social isolation, loneliness, and lack of social support have also been related to cardiovascular risk (Barth et al., 2010; Steptoe & Kivimaki, 2012). These effects hold up even after adjusting for behavioral risk factors and cardiac disease severity.

Stress in the workplace has long been recognized to be a risk factor for CVD. Workers with a sudden increase in workload or a high pressure deadline had a six-fold increased risk of heart attack in the next 24 hours (Steptoe, 2006).

Factors associated with high work-related stress include elevated work demand, particularly in conjunction with low levels of control, poor social support at work, and low compensation for high work effort. All of these factors are associated with CVD risk (Backe et al., 2012; Kivimäki et al., 2006). Job insecurity also shows a modest relationship with CVD (Virtanen et al., 2013). Marital stress, especially in women, has also been linked to increased cardiac events (Orth-Gomér, 2007) and atherosclerosis progression (Wang et al., 2007). Other stressors associated with increased cardiac events include caregiving for an ill family member, especially in those who report psychological strain (Dimsdale, 2008; Haley et al., 2010), and low socioeconomic status, even after controlling for access to healthcare (Kumari et al., 2010; Shishehbor et al., 2006).

Recently there has been an increased appreciation for the role of childhood abuse and other childhood traumas in the development of CVD (Vaccarino & Bremner, 2011). Childhood trauma exposure is related to both adverse lifestyle, such as substance abuse, obesity, and smoking, and with CVD independent of these factors (Anda et al., 2006; Batten et al., 2004; Beckham, 1999; Butterfield et al., 2000; Dube et al., 2003; Rich-Edwards et al., 2012; Wegman & Stetler, 2009; Williamson et al., 2002). Obesity, in particular, which appears to be related to a primary effect of childhood abuse on metabolism (Williamson et al., 2002), leads to increased risk of both CVD and diabetes. Use of antipsychotic medications for the treatment of PTSD, which can be a consequence of childhood adversities, can further contribute to obesity and diabetes risk, which in turn increase the risk of CVD. In summary, chronic stress from a variety of sources, whether in the workplace or in marital relationships, or from traumatic events experienced in early life, is related to an increased risk of CVD. Acute emotions such as anger, or other forms of acute stress, are also related to the risk of cardiac events. The role of stress-related mental disorders, including PTSD and depression, in increasing the risk of heart disease, is discussed next.

15.3 Depression and cardiovascular disease

Depression, which often results from exposure to stress, is associated with an increased risk of CVD (Carney & Freedland, 2003; Evans et al., 2005; Meijer et al., 2011; Nicholson, 2006). Depression is three times more common among cardiac patients than in the general population, and 15–30% of cardiac patients have clinically significant depression (Vaccarino & Bremner, 2011). The increased risk of CVD is seen in both depressed patients with pre-existing CVD (Barefoot et al., 1996; Barth et al., 2004; Borowicz et al., 2002; Burg et al., 2003; Carney et al., 1988, 2003; Connerney et al., 2001; Frasure-Smith et al., 1993, 1999; Jenkins et al., 1994; Mallik et al., 2005; van Melle et al., 2004; Mendes de Leon et al., 1998; Perski et al., 1998; Rutledge et al., 2006) and those without pre-existing

CVD (Anda et al., 1993; Barefoot & Schroll, 1996; Carney & Freedland, 2003; de Jonge et al., 2006; Ford et al., 1998; Fredman et al., 1999; Hippisley-Cox et al., 1998; Pratt et al., 1996). Episodes of depressed mood or acute bereavement are associated with a triggering of myocardial ischemia (Gullette et al., 1997b) and acute myocardial infarction (Mostofsky et al., 2012b). Depression is also associated with an increased risk of mortality, which is primarily related to increased cardiovascular death (Anstey & Luszcz, 2002; Wulsin et al., 1999). Depression rates are higher in young women after a myocardial infarction than other age and gender groups (Mallik et al., 2006), and depression worsens outcomes in coronary artery disease patients, whether symptoms are present at the time of the heart attack or develop later (Parashar et al., 2006). Depression is also related to poor outcomes in congestive heart failure patients (Vaccarino et al., 2001).

Depression is a powerful predictor of CVD in young adults, and recent data suggest that this might be more so in women than in men. In the Third National Health and Nutrition Examination Survey (NHANES III), women with either major depression or a history of attempted suicide had a more than three times increased risk of cardiovascular death, after adjusting for conventional risk factors, and an almost 15-fold increased risk of ischemic heart disease death (Shah et al., 2011). Corresponding figures for men were 2.4 and 3.5. In the prospective Community Mental Health Epidemiology Study of Washington County, MD, depression increased cardiovascular risk in women younger than 40 years more than six-fold, while no association was found among men (Wyman et al., 2012).

15.4 PTSD and cardiovascular disease

Posttraumatic stress disorder has also been linked to CVD in prospective studies (Ahmadi et al., 2011; Boscarino, 2008; Kubzansky et al., 2007; Vaccarino et al., 2013). One pathway for the association is PTSD as a consequence of acute coronary syndromes, which occurs in about one in eight cases, particularly after out of hospital cardiac arrests, and is associated with a doubled risk for recurrent cardiac events and mortality (Edmondson et al., 2012). A recent study in twins showed an association between PTSD and ischemic heart disease that was not accounted for by traditional risk factors or depression, and was also independent of shared familial influences and genetic factors (Vaccarino et al., 2013).

15.5 Potential mechanisms linking stress to cardiovascular disease

Stress and other psychological factors can be both triggers of acute coronary events and promoters of the atherosclerotic process (Chi & Kloner, 2003; Kloner,

2006). The adverse effects of stress on the cardiovascular system have been modeled in animal models, particularly non-human primates (Kaplan et al., 2009; Shively et al., 2009). The possible mechanisms involved are numerous, and include stress-induced, repeated or sustained increases in blood pressure, heart rate, and myocardial ischemia, stress-induced metabolic abnormalities, enhancement of platelet activity, endothelial dysfunction, increased resistance in the peripheral circulation to blood flow, which increases the work of the heart (systemic vascular resistance), dysregulation of the inflammatory and immune response systems, autonomic dysfunction, and ventricular arrhythmias (Vaccarino & Bremner, 2011).

A number of studies have demonstrated a link between stress or acute emotions and myocardial ischemia (decreased blood flow to the heart) in coronary heart disease patients, among whom psychological stress or emotional factors can induce silent ischemia or trigger an heart attack. For example, depressive mood has been shown to trigger ischemia in patients with coronary disease (Gullette et al., 1997a), and acute bereavement or bursts of anger can precede an heart attack (Mostofsky et al., 2012a, 2013a). These effects, possibly mediated by the sympathetic nervous system, may be due to a sudden increase in oxygen demands on the heart or to stress-related constriction of coronary arteries, the vessels that supply blood to the heart.

Myocardial ischemia due to emotional factors can be studied experimentally through a standardized mental stress test (commonly referred to as "mental stress ischemia"; Arrighi et al., 2000, 2003; Blumenthal et al., 1995; Burg et al., 1993; Soufer, 2004; Soufer et al., 1998; Stone et al., 1999). In this method, subjects undergo a variety of stressors, such as mental arithmetic, public speaking, problem-solving, anger recall, or something similar, in conjunction with negative feedback. Mental stress-induced ischemia is a frequent phenomenon among cardiac patients, occurring in about half of them. Its stimulus is psychological, not physical (Becker et al., 1996; Deanfield et al., 1984; Jain et al., 1998; Krantz et al., 1991; LaVeau et al., 1989; Ramachandruni et al., 2006; Rozanski et al., 1988; Schang & Pepine, 1977; Schiffer et al., 1980). It is also not explained by emotion-induced increased heart rate and blood pressure, and typically occurs in the absence of pain. Mental stress-induced ischemia is related to abnormal constriction of coronary or peripheral arteries rather than coronary obstruction due to atherosclerotic disease (Dakak et al., 1995; Deanfield et al., 1984; Kop et al., 2001; Lacy et al., 1995; Ramadan et al., 2013; Sherwood et al., 1999; Wittstein et al., 2005; Yeung et al., 1991). Despite these unique features, mental stress-induced myocardial ischemia is associated with increased long-term risk for cardiac events, to a similar extent as exertion-related ischemia (Goldberg et al., 1996; Jain et al., 1995; Jiang et al., 1996; Krantz et al., 1999; Legault et al., 1995; Sheps et al., 2002). Psychological or emotional factors such as anger and depressed mood have also been linked to mental stress myocardial ischemia (Boltwood et al., 1993; Boyle et al., 2013; Burg et al., 1993; Gabbay et al., 1996; Mittleman et al., 1995; Strike & Steptoe, 2005; Strike et al., 2006).

In addition to the effects on ischemia, studies using the mental stress paradigm in the laboratory have found that increased hemodynamic activation (increase in blood pressure and heart rate; Chida & Steptoe, 2010) and cortisol (Hamer et al., 2012; Hamer & Steptoe, 2012) and catecholamine release (Flaa et al., 2008) in response to mental stress are associated with long-term increased risk of hypertension and future cardiovascular events. These effects reflect, in part, the key role of autonomic function, which is directly influenced by stress, in the regulation of body systems. Heart rate variability (HRV), the normal beat-to-beat fluctuation in heart rate that occurs with respiration and normal daily activities, is controlled by a balance of sympathetic and parasympathetic nervous system function, and thus serves as a useful marker of the overall health of the autonomic nervous system. Both mental stress in the laboratory and stress in daily life are associated with transient decreases in HRV (Steptoe & Brydon, 2009). In turn, decreased HRV associated with stress and emotion may affect myocardial electrical stability, potentially increasing the risk for cardiac arrhythmias (Kop et al., 2004; Lampert et al., 2002; Lane et al., 2005). Indeed, decreased HRV was associated with an increased risk for arrhythmia (Lampert et al., 1998), ischemic heart disease, and sudden cardiac death (Thayer & Lane, 2007). Therefore, stress-induced autonomic imbalance may heighten vulnerability to cardiac arrhythmias and sudden cardiac death.

The central nervous system plays a crucial role in the autonomic and vascular responses to stress and is implicated in the induction of mental stress-induced myocardial ischemia. Activation of specific brain regions with stress results in higher levels of peripheral catecholamines, which underlie, at least partially, the increased heart rate, blood pressure, and peripheral vascular resistance secondary to vasoconstriction seen with stress (Soufer, 2004; Soufer et al., 2009). Mental stress-induced coronary artery constriction is correlated with endothelial responses to acetylcholine infusion, and is blocked by intra-coronary infusion of the α-adrenergic blocker phentolamine, suggesting that endothelial dysfunction and increased activity of the sympathetic nervous system play a role in its genesis (Holmes et al., 2006; Soufer et al., 2009).

Stress may also increase the risk of CVD through inflammatory pathways. Activation of the noradrenergic/sympathetic system with stress leads to activation of the transcription factor nuclear factor kB (NF-kB) in circulating monocytes, which triggers the inflammation cascade, while the parasympathetic system has the opposite effect. Indeed, mental stress induced in the laboratory is associated with the release of inflammatory cytokines such as interleukin-6 and interleukin-1β (Steptoe et al., 2007). Several lines of evidence pinpoint inflammation as a key regulatory process that links multiple risk factors, including stress, with altered arterial biology, leading to atherosclerosis and its complications (Libby et al., 2009). Thus, stress-related repeated stimulation of the inflammatory system may lead to, or contribute to, increased risk of CVD.

One of the areas in which long-lasting mechanisms linking stress to somatic disease have been demonstrated most clearly is early life stress. Exposure to stress in early life, such as childhood abuse or neglect, may lead to a resetting of stress-responsive physiological systems that could increase the risk of CVD. Indeed, a number of studies have linked adverse childhood experiences to enduring changes in the nervous, endocrine, and immune systems (Danese & McEwen, 2012). A history of childhood maltreatment has been associated with smaller volumes of the prefrontal cortex and the hippocampus, greater activation of the HPA axis during stress, and elevated inflammation (Bremner, 2012). These changes may persist in adulthood. For example, in a prospective study (Danese et al., 2007), maltreated children showed higher inflammation 20 years later, which was not explained by other childhood exposures and health behaviors. These physiological alterations could increase the risk of CVD through multiple pathways and provide evidence for an enduring effect of early life stress on physical health.

15.6 Mechanisms through which depression and PTSD may increase CVD risk

As described earlier, a pathway by which stress may increase the risk of CVD is through the development of stress-related psychiatric disorders such as depression and PTSD. The association between depression and heart disease is not fully accounted for by the increase in CVD risk factors seen in these patients, including obesity, smoking, sedentary lifestyle, diabetes, and hypertension (Vaccarino & Bremner, 2011). Depressed patients, compared with those without depression, also exhibit poorer adherence to medications or preventive strategies, poorer health-seeking behavior, less adequate lifestyle risk factor modification, and poorer participation in cardiac rehabilitation (Whooley et al., 2008). These factors may all contribute to worse CVD outcomes.

Neurobiological responses in depressed patients may also contribute to CVD risk. Depression is characterized by overactivity of the HPA axis and the sympathoadrenal system, resembling the neuroendocrine response to stress, with increased, or prolonged, release of cortisol and norepinephrine and disruption of normal circadian patterns. These abnormalities may lead to repeated or sustained elevations in blood pressure, heart rate, and plasma glucose, resulting eventually in insulin resistance and dyslipidemia (Kent & PA., 2009). Depression is also associated with vagal withdrawal and decreased HRV (Carney & Freedland, 2009).

As for other CVD risk factors, depression is characterized by a pro-inflammatory state that may affect vascular function (Sherwood et al., 2005). A well replicated finding in depressed patients is an elevated level of acute-phase proteins, such as C-reactive protein, and of inflammatory cytokines, such as interleukin-6, in subjects with and without CVD, although it is unclear whether inflammation represents a mechanistic link between depression and cardiovascular outcomes (Vaccarino et al., 2007).

It is also possible that depression and heart disease are independently related to a common factor. Accumulating evidence suggests that depression and CVD may be different phenotypic expressions of the same genetic substrates (de Geus, 2006; Vaccarino et al., 2009).

The neurobiology of PTSD also suggests pathways by which the disorder could increase the risk for CVD. PTSD is associated with increased function of the nora-drenergic system, both at rest and with traumatic reminders, associated with increased heart rate, blood pressure, and peripheral and central catecholamine release (Bremner et al., 1996a,b; McFall et al., 1990; Orr et al., 1993; Pitman et al., 1987; Pitman & Orr, 1990; Shalev et al., 1992, 1993). PTSD is also associated with increased cortisol response with reminders of psychological trauma (Bremner et al., 2003; Elzinga et al., 2003), and chronic dysregulation of the HPA axis com-pared with controls, with a pattern of increased corticotropin-releasing factor concentrations (Baker et al., 1999; Bremner et al., 1997) and decreased periph-eral cortisol concentrations at rest (Bremner et al., 2007; Bremner & Charney, 2010; Yehuda et al., 1991, 1994). These alterations in stress response neuro-hormonal systems result in abnormal autonomic modulation in PTSD with a decrease in HRV (Shah et al., 2013), and may lead to disruption of immune func-tion, with associated increased inflammation (Plantinga et al., 2013), endothelial dysfunction, increased blood clotting, and cardiovascular hyperreactivity that increase CVD risk.

In summary, stress can increase the risk of CVD through its effects on neurohormonal systems, cardiac electrical instability, and metabolic, inflam-matory and coagulation pathways. Stress can also directly induce myocardial ischemia in susceptible individuals, mostly due to abnormal vasomotion of coronary or peripheral arteries. Finally, stress is a precedent of PTSD and depression, which are associated with enduring neurobiological and sys-temic changes that can affect cardiovascular risk through a multitude of mechanisms.

15.7 Stress, PTSD and functional pain disorders

Stress is associated with an increased risk for functional pain disorders and psy-chosomatic disorders (Bremner, 2009). Functional pain disorders are currently defined as physical disorders in which, after appropriate medical assessment, a specific medical or physiological etiology is not identifiable (Derbyshire et al., 2004; Drossman et al., 2000; Wessely et al., 1999). Functional pain disorders include irritable bowel syndrome (IBS), fibromyalgia, non-specific low back pain, chronic pelvic pain, temporomandibular pain, and chronic chest pain or sensitive heart (Mayer & Bushnell, 2009b). Even though functional pain disorders are responsible for the consumption of a great deal of medical resources, conventional medical treatments are unsatisfactory (Turk & Rudy, 1992; Turk, 2003; Wessely et al., 1999).

Alterations in stress response systems and interactions with disorders like PTSD are felt to contribute, at least in part, to the development of functional pain disorder (Mayer, 2000). There has been considerable attention, in particular, to the possible role of childhood abuse in the development of these disorders. However, the current medical consensus is that stress does not represent the entirety of the risk for functional pain disorders (Ballenger et al., 2001; Mayer & Collins, 2002; Mayer et al., 2001a,b). The development of functional pain disorders is probably related to a complex interplay among environmental events (including specific traumas in childhood and adulthood, as well as variables such as parenting style), genetics, central nervous system processing of sensory information, and autonomic nervous system modulation of the gut, heart, and other organs (McLean et al., 2005). There is a high comorbidity of the functional pain disorders with each other and with stress-related psychiatric disorders such as PTSD and depression, as well as chronic fatigue syndrome and headache (Schur et al., 2007). This may represent a common etiology (e.g., stress, a common genetic factor, or a common neural circuitry), or the fact that they are involved in each other's etiology (e.g., pain leads to depression, or depression is involved in maintenance of pain after minor injury).

Patients with PTSD are more likely to report chronic pain (Beckham et al., 1997), as well as increased somatization (Beckham et al., 1998) and poorer health (Schnurr & Spiro, 1999), and to show increased utilization of health resources (Zatzick et al., 1997). Although PTSD patients report more pain symptoms, they actually have a higher threshold for pain in laboratory settings, a finding that is associated with increased hippocampal and decreased amygdala and medial prefrontal brain activation (Geuze et al., 2006, 2007).

Another group of disorders related to stress, the dissociative disorders, are relevant to understanding the relationship between stress and somatic responses. Dissociative symptoms include feeling that one is in a dream or a sense of unreality (derealization), distortions of one's sense of one's own body (depersonalization), gaps in memory (amnesia), and other similar symptoms. Studies have examined the relationship between stress, dissociation, and somatization disorder, which is defined as having eight or more physical symptoms that cannot be explained by medical causes after a complete medical examination.

Compared with medical patients, somatization disorder patients were shown to have increased symptoms of dissociative amnesia (gaps in memory not due to ordinary forgetting), but not depersonalization (distortions in the sense of one's own body), derealization (experiences like you are in a dream) or identity confusion or alteration (Brown et al., 2005). Somatization patients were found more likely to have a history of emotional and physical abuse (but not sexual abuse), as well as more family conflict and less family cohesion.

15.7.1 Irritable bowel syndrome

Irritable bowel syndrome (IBS) is the most common functional pain disorder, with a prevalence of 10–15% worldwide, and a greater prevalence in women (Drossman et al., 2002). Like other functional pain disorders, IBS remains defined by symptom criteria (Longstreth et al., 2006). These diagnostic criteria require the chronic or recurrent presence of abdominal pain or discomfort related to altered bowel habits, in the absence of any established structural, biochemical or other "organic" findings (Longstreth et al., 2006). Despite these restrictive diagnostic criteria, the symptoms of IBS are not limited to the gastrointestinal tract. An extensive literature has demonstrated the high prevalence of so-called "comorbid" disorders, including other visceral or somatic complaints (such as other gastrointestinal symptoms, fibromyalgia, and interstitial cystitis/bladder pain syndrome) or alterations in mood and affect (Mayer & Bushnell, 2009a).

As in other functional syndromes and many psychiatric disorders, stress plays an important role in IBS, as 60% of IBS patients report an association of stressful life events with first onset or with the exacerbation of symptoms (Mayer, 2000). It has been suggested that in the genetically vulnerable individual, different types of stressors can play a role in enhancing stress sensitivity, promoting IBS symptom exacerbation, and perpetuating IBS symptom chronicity (Mayer et al., 2001b). Early life stress and trauma, in the form of abuse, neglect, or loss of the primary caregiver, play a major role in the vulnerability of individuals to develop functional gastrointestinal disorders later in life (Bradford et al., 2012). Acute, life-threatening stress episodes in adult life (e.g., rape, posttraumatic stress syndrome) are also important risk factors in the development of functional gastrointestinal disorders. For example, an association of trauma (sexual assault) with IBS onset was observed in female veterans (White et al., 2010). In another report, a three- to 46-fold increase in the odds of IBS or functional dyspepsia (an often comorbid condition) was observed in female veterans with PTSD, anxiety, or depression (Savas et al., 2009). In a civilian population, the prevalence of PTSD was found to be twice as high in IBS patients as in healthy individuals (Liebschutz et al., 2007), although another study did not find an increased PTSD prevalence in IBS (Cohen et al., 2006). "Physical" or interoceptive stressors of the digestive system (i.e., things affecting the gut wall), such as enteric infections, trauma, and surgery, may play a similar role in symptom exacerbation or first onset of symptoms in the predisposed individual. Interestingly, one of the strongest factors predicting the development of so-called post infectious IBS is a previous history of other pain disorder and preceding or concurring psychosocial stressors (Spiller & Garsed, 2009). Finally, in the affected patient, fear conditioning and interoceptive conditioning (the development of learned responses in the gut wall) are likely to play important roles in exacerbating symptoms in the context of stressful situations, and even in contexts that by themselves are not threatening or stressful (Mayer & Bushnell, 2009a). For a large number of IBS patients, the positive-feedback loop of conditioned fear responses to interoceptive stimuli (i.e., sensations coming from the gut) or conditioned responses to the context of situations where symptoms themselves become a stressor (e.g., the onset of IBS symptoms when there is not easy access to a restroom) may play a primary role in the development and maintenance of symptom chronicity. Functional brain imaging studies have revealed alterations in brain areas regulating emotion, arousal, and interpretation of external stimuli (Hong et al., 2013; Labus et al., 2013a,b), and recent results have demonstrated associated changes in brain structure (Ellingson et al., 2013; Jiang et al., 2013; Labus et al., 2014; Mayer et al., 2015).

15.7.2 Fibromyalgia

Fibromyalgia, which affects about 5% of women and 2% of men (White et al., 1999), is associated with chronic widespread pain, diffuse tenderness, fatigue and sleep disturbance; diagnostic criteria require at least 3 months of widespread pain and pain upon digital palpation at no fewer than 11 out of 18 characteristic tender points (Wolfe et al., 1990). Some studies have found an association with sexual assault in women or childhood abuse, although studies are not always consistent and the etiology is felt to be complex and multifactorial (Ciccone et al., 2005; Croft, 2000; Walker et al., 1997).

There is a strong connection between fibromyalgia and PTSD. About half of fibromyalgia patients have PTSD (Cohen et al., 2002; Sherman et al., 2000), and a fifth of PTSD patients have symptoms of fibromyalgia, which leads to an increase in psychological distress and decrease in quality of life (Amir et al., 1997; Culclasure et al., 1993). Fibromyalgia patients also have increased rates of anxiety, depression, and somatization (Goldenberg & Sandhu, 2002; Thieme et al., 2004). Soldiers deployed overseas in the Gulf War had an increase in self-reported fibromyalgia (19% vs. 10% non-deployed) (Iowa, 1997). Current models of fibromyalgia conceptualize it as a disorder that involves alterations in brain regions involved in pain, such as the anterior cingulate (Change et al., 2003; Derbyshire et al., 2004; Derbyshire & Bremner, 2009; Gracely et al., 2002, 2004). Fibromyalgia patients, especially those with a history of early trauma, also show a blunting of the cortisol diurnal rhythm similar to that seen in patients with PTSD (Griep et al., 1998; Weissbecker et al., 2006).

15.7.3 Other functional pain disorders

Non-specific low back pain is another disorder that is commonly associated with stress and PTSD. Back pain is the second leading symptomatic reason for physician visits in the United States (Lemrow et al., 1990). In many cases, there is no observable pathology to account for the symptoms (Derbyshire et al., 2002; Hadler, 1994; Jensen et al., 1994; Spitzer et al., 1987). About half of patients with low back pain have PTSD (DeCarvalho & Whealin, 2006). Back pain is a common problem in veterans of both the Vietnam and Iraq conflicts, with the latter complicated by the use of heavy flak jackets (Nice et al., 1996). Low back pain can exacerbate immobility and hence avoidance and isolation in PTSD patients.

Pelvic pain is another pain disorder that is more common in women with a history of childhood sexual abuse (Ehlert et al., 1999; Heim et al., 1997, 1998; Spinhoven et al., 2004). Another pain-related condition that has been linked to stress and PTSD is temporomandibular joint disorder (Buescher, 2007; Sherman et al., 2005).

Finally, there are several psychiatric disorders that are characterized by medically unexplained pain (APA, 2014) Somatoform disorders, for example, are disorders where physical symptoms are not attributable to a known organic etiology and are not secondary to anxiety or depression. Somatization disorder involves at least eight physical symptoms in four bodily systems. Other terms for this condition include psychogenic disease, chronic multisymptom illness, affective spectrum disorders, central sensitization syndrome, and functional pain disorder (Barsky & Borus, 1999; Clauw & Chrousos, 1997; Clauw et al., 1997; Hudson & Pope, 1989; Hudson et al., 1992; Wessely et al., 1999).

In summary, the role of stress in the development and maintenance of functional pain disorders is well established, although it is clear that the etiology is complex and involves other factors as well (Barsky & Borus, 1999; Wessely et al., 1999). The brain areas that mediate pain and other symptoms of these disorders have been shown to include the thalamus, insula cortex, prefrontal cortex, primary and secondary somatosensory cortex and the anterior cingulate (Change et al., 2003; Derbyshire et al., 2002, 2004; Geuze et al., 2007; Naliboff et al., 2001). These brain areas overlap with those implicated in the neural circuitry of stress and PTSD (Bremner, 2002; Bremner et al., 2008; Francati et al., 2007). However, the functional pain disorders have not been shown to share all the neurobiological alterations found in stress-related psychiatric conditions like depression and PTSD (see other chapters in this volume). For example, reduced hippocampal volume has not been reported in patients with long-standing chronic pain (Apkarian et al., 2004).

Although early abuse or trauma later in life is associated with functional pain disorders in some patients, in others the disorder itself becomes a source of continual stress, influenced by the patient's cognitions about pain as well as affective states (Turk & Rudy, 1992). One model is that stress and/or other factors initiate a process that leads to an increased general neuronal hypersensitization (Lane et al., 2009). This may manifest itself in different ways in different individuals (e.g., multiple sensitivity points in fibromyalgia, or increased sensitivity to one's own bowel contractions in IBS) (Turk & Rudy, 1992). Thus, the functional pain disorders are likely to result from a complex interplay among stress, genetics, other environmental factors, neuronal sensitization, and an interaction between central and peripheral nervous systems that are involved in the regulation of bodily organs, muscles, joints, and so on. The anterior cingulate and medial prefrontal cortex area, which have been implicated in both PTSD and depression, play an important role in pain processing and also in regulation of peripheral stress and physiological processes. Thus these brain areas represent a common connection between these different disorders that may account for their high comorbidity and the fact that they share many symptoms.

15.8 Conclusions

The increased risk of CVD and other physical disorders in patients with stress-related mental disorders like depression and PTSD, as well as the high degree of comorbidity of these psychiatric conditions with functional pain disorders suggest a pathophysiological connection between these diseases. The underlying mechanisms, however, are far from clear. It is likely that neuroendocrine, autonomic, and metabolic pathways involved in acute or chronic stress responses, as well as specific genetic factors, are implicated.

For some conditions, such as IBS, the role of fear and psychological stress is clear, given the known effects of the fear response on bowel motility. Similarly, the connection between acute stress and heart function is well established. For other disorders, such as fibromyalgia, the link with stress is not as obvious. The etiology of these disorders probably involves complex bidirectional effects linking the brain to peripheral organs, which in turn relay information back to the central nervous system, and interactions with environmental exposures such as stress and trauma. Common biological pathways could also underlie these conditions and explain their comorbidity. Brain areas (e.g., the anterior cingulate and the medial prefrontal cortex) and neuroendocrine systems (e.g., the noradrenergic system and the HPA axis) have been implicated in the etiology of stress-related psychiatric conditions, physical disorders like CVD, and functional pain disorders. Clearly, more studies are needed to better understand the interplay among stress,

stress-related psychiatric disorders, and physical health in order to improve the diagnosis, treatment, and prevention of these prevalent conditions.

References

Ahmadi N, Hajsadeghi F, Mirshkarlo HB et al. (2011) Post-traumatic stress disorder, coronary atherosclerosis, and mortality. *Am J Cardiol* 108, 29–33.

Amir M, Kaplan Z, Neumann L et al. (1997) Posttraumatic stress disorder, tenderness and fibromyalgia. *J Psychosom Res* 42, 607–613.

Anda RF, Felitti VJ, Walker J et al. (2006) The enduring effects of childhood abuse and related experiences in childhood: A convergence of evidence from neurobiology and epidemiology. *Eur Arch Psychiatr Clin Neurosci* 256, 174–186.

Anda R, Williamson D, Jones D (1993) Depressed affect, hopelessness, and the risk of ischemic heart disease in a cohort of U.S. adults. *Epidemiology* 4, 285–294.

Anstey KJ, Luszcz MA (2002) Mortality risk varies according to gender and change in depressive status in very old adults. *Psychosom Med* 64, 880–888.

APA. (2014) *Diagnostic and Statistical Manual-5* (DSM-5). American Psychiatric Association Press.

Apkarian AV, Sosa Y, Sonty S et al. (2004) Chronic back pain is associated with decreased prefrontal and thalamic gray matter density. *J Neurosci* 24, 10 410–10 415.

Arrighi JA, Burg M, Cohen IS et al. (2000) Myocardial blood-flow response during mental stress in patients with coronary artery disease. *Lancet* 356, 310–311.

Arrighi JA, Burg M, Cohen IS et al. (2003) Simultaneous assessment of myocardial perfusion and function during mental stress in patients with chronic coronary artery disease. *J Nucl Cardiol* 10, 267–274.

Backe EM, Seidler A, Latza U et al. (2012) The role of psychosocial stress at work for the development of cardiovascular diseases: a systematic review. *Int Arch Occup Environ Health* 85, 67–79.

Baker DG, West SA, Nicholson WE et al. (1999) Serial CSF corticotropin-releasing hormone levels and adrenocortical activity in combat veterans with posttraumatic stress disorder. *Am J Psychiatry* 156, 585–588.

Ballenger JC, Davidson, JRT, Lecrubier Y et al. (2001) Consensus statement on depression, anxiety, and functional gastrointestinal disorders. *J Clin Psychiatry* 62(Suppl 8)

Barefoot JC, Helms MJ, Mark DB (1996) Depression and long-term mortality risk in patients with coronary artery disease. *Am J Cardiol* 78, 613–617.

Barefoot J, Schroll M (1996) Symptoms of depression, acute myocardial infarction, and total mortality in a community sample. *Circulation* 93, 1976–1980.

Barsky AJ, Borus JF (1999) Functional somatic syndromes. *Ann Intern Med* 130, 910–921.

Barth J, Schneider S, von Kanel R (2010) Lack of social support in the etiology and the prognosis of coronary heart disease: a systematic review and meta-analysis. *Psychosom Med* 72, 229–238.

Barth J, Schumacher M, Herrmann-Lingen C (2004) Depression as a risk factor for mortality in patients with coronary heart disease: a meta-analysis. *Psychosom Med* 66, 802–813.

Batten SV, Aslan M, Maciejewski PK et al. (2004) Childhood maltreatment as a risk factor for adult cardiovascular disease and depression. *J Clin Psychiatry* 65, 249–254.

Becker LC, Pepine CJ, Bonsall R et al. (1996) Left ventricular, peripheral vascular, and neurohumoral responses to mental stress in normal middle-aged men and women. Reference Group for the Psychophysiological Investigations of Myocardial Ischemia (PIMI) Study. *Circulation* 94, 2768–2777.

Beckham JC (1999) Smoking and anxiety in combat veterans with chronic posttraumatic stress disorder: a review. *J Psychoact Drugs* 31, 103–110.

Beckham JC, Crawford AL, Feldman ME et al. (1997) Chronic posttraumatic stress disorder and chronic pain in Vietnam combat veterans. *J Psychosom Res* 43, 379–389.

Beckham JC, Moore SD, Feldman ME et al. (1998) Health status, somatization, and severity of posttraumatic stress disorder in Vietnam combat veterans with posttraumatic stress disorder. *Am J Psychiatry* 155, 1565–1569.

Blumenthal JA, Jiang W, Waugh RA et al. (1995) Mental stress-induced ischemia in the laboratory and ambulatory ischemia during daily life. *Circulation* 92, 2102–2108.

Boltwood MD, Taylor CB, Boutte Burke M et al. (1993) Anger report predicts coronary artery vasomotor response to mental stress in atherosclerotic segments. *Am J Cardiol* 72, 1361–1365.

Borowicz L, Royall R, Grega M et al. (2002) Depression and cardiac morbidity 5 years after coronary artery bypass surgery. *Psychosomatics* 43, 464–471.

Boscarino JA (2008) A prospective study of PTSD and early-age heart disease mortality among Vietnam veterans: implications for surveillance and prevention. *Psychosom Med* 70, 668–676.

Boyle SH, Samad Z, Becker RC et al. (2013) Depressive symptoms and mental stress-induced myocardial ischemia in patients with coronary heart disease. *Psychosom Med* 75, 822–831.

Bradford K, Shih W, Videlock EJ et al. (2012) Association between early adverse life events and irritable bowel syndrome. *Clin Gastroenterol Hepatol* 10, 385–390.

Bremner JD (2002) *Does Stress Damage the Brain? Understanding Trauma-related Disorders from a Mind-Body Perspective.* WW Norton, New York, NY.

Bremner JD (2006) Traumatic stress from a multiple-levels-of-analysis perspective. In Cicchetti D, Cohen, DJ (eds) *Developmental Psychopathology*, Vol. 2. John Wiley & Sons, Hoboken, NJ, pp. 656–676

Bremner JD (2009) Combat-related psychiatric syndromes. In: Mayer EA, Bushnell MC (eds) *Functional Pain Syndromes: Presentation and Pathophysiology*. IASP Press, Seattle, WA, pp. 169–183.

Bremner JD (2012) Brain and trauma. In Figley, CR (ed.) *Encyclopedia of Trauma: An Interdisciplinary Guide*. SAGE Publishers, Los Angeles, CA.

Bremner JD, Charney DS (2010) Neural circuits in fear and anxiety. In Stein DJ, Hollander E, Rothbaum BO (eds) *Textbook of Anxiety Disorders*, 2nd edn. American Psychiatric Publishing, Arlington, VA, pp. 55–71.

Bremner JD, Elzinga B, Schmahl C et al. (2008) Structural and functional plasticity of the human brain in posttraumatic stress disorder. *Prog Brain Res* 167, 171–186.

Bremner JD, Krystal JH, Southwick SM et al. (1996a) Noradrenergic mechanisms in stress and anxiety: II. Clinical studies. *Synapse* 23, 39–51.

Bremner JD, Krystal JH, Southwick SM et al. (1996b) Noradrenergic mechanisms in stress and anxiety: I. Preclinical studies. *Synapse* 23, 28–38.

Bremner JD, Licinio J, Darnell A et al. (1997) Elevated CSF corticotropin-releasing factor concentrations in posttraumatic stress disorder. *Am J Psychiatry* 154, 624–629.

Bremner JD, Southwick SM, Darnell A et al. (1996c) Chronic PTSD in Vietnam combat veterans: Course of illness and substance abuse. *Am J Psychiatry* 153, 369–375.

Bremner JD, Vermetten E, Kelley ME (2007) Cortisol, dehydroepiandrosterone, and estradiol measured over 24 hours in women with childhood sexual abuse-related posttraumatic stress disorder. *J Nerv Ment Dis* 195, 919–927.

Bremner JD, Vythilingam M, Vermetten E et al. (2003) Cortisol response to a cognitive stress challenge in posttraumatic stress disorder (PTSD) related to childhood abuse. *Psychoneuroendocrinology* 28, 733–750.

Brown RJ, Schrag A, Trimble MR (2005) Dissociation, childhood interpersonal trauma, and family functioning in patients with somatization disorder. *Am J Psychiatry* 162, 899–905.

Buescher JJ (2007) Temporomandibular joint disorders. *Am Fam Physician* 76, 1477–1482.

Burg MM, Benedetto MC, Rosenberg et al. (2003) Presurgical depression predicts medical morbidity at 6-months after coronary artery bypass grafting. *Psychosom Med* 65, 111–118.

Burg MM, Jain D, Soufer R et al. (1993) Role of behavioral and psychological factors in mental stress-induced silent left ventricular dysfunction in coronary artery disease. *J Am Coll Cardiol* 22, 440–448.

Butterfield MI, Forneris CA, Feldman ME, Beckham JC (2000) Hostility and functional health status in women veterans with and without posttraumatic stress disorder: a preliminary study. *J Trauma Stress* 13, 735–741.

Carney RM, Blumenthal JA, Catellier D et al. (2003) Depression as a risk factor for mortality following acute myocardial infarction. *Am J Cardiol* 62, 212–219.

Carney RM, Freedland KE (2003) Depression, mortality, and medical morbidity in patients with coronary heart disease. *Biol Psychiatry* 54, 241–247.

Carney RM, Freedland KE (2009). Depression and heart rate variability in patients with coronary heart disease. *Cleve Clin J Med* 76(Suppl 2), S13–17.

Carney RM, Rich MW, Freedland KE (1988) Major depressive disorder predicts cardiac events in patients with coronary artery disease. *Psychosom Med* 50, 627–633.

Change L, Berman S, Mayer EA et al. (2003) Brain responses to visceral and somatic stimuli in patients with irritable bowel syndrome with and without fibromyalgia. *Am J Gastroenterol* 98, 1354–1361.

Chi JS, Kloner RA (2003) Stress and myocardial infarction. *Heart* 89, 475–476.

Chida Y, Steptoe A (2010) Greater cardiovascular responses to laboratory mental stress are associated with poor subsequent cardiovascular risk status: a meta-analysis of prospective evidence. *Hypertension* 55, 1026–1032.

Ciccone DS, Elliott DK, Chandler HK et al. (2005) Sexual and physical abuse in women with fibromyalgia syndrome: a test of the trauma hypothesis. *Clin J Pain* 21, 378–386.

Clauw DJ, Chrousos GP (1997) Chronic pain and fatigue syndromes: overlapping clinical and neuroendocrine features and potential pathogenic mechanisms. *Neuroimmunomodulation* 4, 134–153.

Clauw DJ, Schmidt M, Radulovic D et al. (1997) The relationship between fibromyalgia and interstitial cystitis. *J Psychiatr Res* 31, 125–130.

Cohen H, Neumann L, Haiman Y et al. (2002) Prevalence of post-traumatic stress disorder in fibromyalgia patients: overlapping syndromes or post-traumatic fibromyalgia syndrome? *Semin Arthritis Rheum* 32, 38–50.

Cohen H, Jotkowitz A, Buskila D et al. (2006) Post-traumatic stress disorder and other co-morbidities in a sample population of patients with irritable bowel syndrome. *Eur J Intern Med* 17, 567–571.

Connerney I, Shapiro PA, McLaughlin JS et al. (2001) Relation between depression after coronary artery bypass surgery and 12-month outcome: a prospective study. *Lancet* 358, 1766–1771.

Croft P (2000) Testing for tenderness: What's the point? *J Rheumatol* 27, 2531–2533.

Culclasure TF, Enzenauer RJ, West SG (1993) Post-traumatic stress disorder presenting as fibromyalgia. *Am J Med* 94, 548–549.

Dakak N, Quyyumi AA, Eisenhofer G et al. (1995) Sympathetically mediated effects of mental stress on the cardiac microcirculation of patients with coronary artery disease. *Am J Cardiol* 76, 125–130.

Danese A, Pariante CM, Caspi A et al. (2007) Childhood maltreatment predicts adult inflammation in a life-course study. *Proc Natl Acad Sci USA* 104, 1319–1324.

Danese A, McEwen BS (2012) Adverse childhood experiences, allostasis, allostatic load, and age-related disease. *Physiol Behav* 106, 29–39.

de Geus EJ (2006) Genetic pleiotropy in depression and coronary artery disease. *Psychosom Med* 68, 185–186.

de Jonge P, van der Brink RHS et al. (2006) Only incident depressive episodes after myocardial infarction are associated with new cardiovascular events. *J Am Coll Cardiol* 48, 2204–2208.

Deanfield JD, Shea, M, Kensett M et al. (1984) Silent myocardial ischaemia due to mental stress. *Lancet* 2, 1001–1005.

DeCarvalho LT, Whealin JM (2006) What pain specialists need to know about posttraumatic stress disorder in Operation Iraqi Freedom and Operation Enduring Freedom returnees. *J Musculoskel Pain* 14, 37–45.

Derbyshire SWG, Bremner JD (2009) Impact of functional visceral and somatic pain/stress syndromes on cingulate cortex. In: Vogt B (ed.) *Cingulate Neurobiology and Disease*. Oxford University Press, Oxford, UK, pp. 499–518.

Derbyshire SWG, Jones AKP et al. (2002) Cerebral responses to noxious thermal stimulation in chronic low back pain patients and normal controls. *NeuroImage* 16, 158–168.

Derbyshire SWG, Whalley MG, Stenger VA et al. (2004) Cerebral activation during hypnotically induced and imagined pain. *NeuroImage* 23, 392–401.

Dimsdale JE (2008) Psychological stress and cardiovascular disease. *J Am Collof Cardiol* 51, 1237–1246.

Drossman DA, Corazziari E, Talley NJ et al. (2000) *Rome II. The Functional Gastrointestinal Disorders: Diagnosis Pathophysiology and Treatment A Multinational Consensus*, 2nd edn. Degnon and Associates, McLean, VA.

Drossman DA, Camilleri M, Mayer EA et al. (2002) AGA technical review on irritable bowel syndrome. *Gastroenterology* 123, 2108–2131.

Dube SR, Felitti VJ, Dong M et al. (2003) The impact of adverse childhood experiences on health problems: evidence from four birth cohorts dating back to 1900. *Prev Med* 37, 268–277.

Edmondson D, Richardson S, Falzon L et al. (2012) Posttraumatic stress disorder prevalence and risk of recurrence in acute coronary syndrome patients: a meta-analytic review. *PlosS one* 7, e38915.

Ehlert U, Heim C, Hellhammer DH (1999) Chronic pelvic pain as a somatoform disorder. *Psychother Psychosom* 68, 87–94.

Ellingson BM, Mayer E, Harris RJ et al. (2013) Diffusion tensor imaging detects microstructural reorganization in the brain associated with chronic irritable bowel syndrome. *Pain* 154, 1528–1541.

Elzinga BM, Schmahl CS, Vermetten E et al. (2003) Higher cortisol levels following exposure to traumatic reminders in abuse-related PTSD. *Neuropsychopharmacology* 28, 1656–1665.

Evans DL, Charney DS, Lewis L et al. (2005) Mood disorders in the medically ill: Scientific review and recommendations. *Biol Psychiatry* 58, 175–189.

Flaa A, Eide IK, Kjeldsen SE et al. (2008) Sympathoadrenal stress reactivity is a predictor of future blood pressure: an 18-year follow-up study. *Hypertension* 52, 336–341.

Ford DE, Mead LA, Chang PP et al. (1998) Depression is a risk factor for coronary artery disease in men. *Arch Intern Med* 158, 54–59.

Francati V, Vermetten E, Bremner JD (2007) Functional neuroimaging studies in posttraumatic stress disorder: review of current methods and findings. *Depress Anxiety* 24, 202–218.

Frasure-Smith N, Lesperance F, Juneau M et al. (1999) Gender, depression and one-year prognosis after myocardial infarction. *Psychosom Med* 61, 26–37.

Frasure-Smith N, Lesperance F, Talajic M (1993) Depression following myocardial infarction. *JAMA* 270, 1819–1825.

Fredman L, Magaziner J, Hebel JR et al. (1999) Depressive symptoms and 6-year mortality among elderly community-dwelling women. *Epidemiology* 10, 54–59.

Gabbay FH, Krantz DS, Kop WJ et al. (1996) Triggers of myocardial ischemia during daily life in patients with coronary artery disease: Physical and mental activities, anger and smoking. *J Am Coll Cardiol* 27, 585–592.

Geuze E, Vermetten E, Jochims A et al. (2006) Neuroimaging of pain perception in Dutch veterans with and without posttraumatic stress disorder: preliminary results. *Ann NY Acad Sci* 1071, 401–404.

Geuze E, Westenberg HG, Jochims A et al. (2007) Altered pain processing in veterans with posttraumatic stress disorder. *Arch Gen Psychiatry* 64, 76–85.

Goldberg AD, Becker LC, Bonsall R et al. (1996) Ischemic, hemodynamic, and neurohormonal responses to mental and exercise stress: Experience from the Psychophysiological Investigations of Myocardial Ischemia Study (PIMI) *Circulation* 94, 2402–2409.

Goldenberg DL, Sandhu HS (2002) Fibromyalgia and post-traumatic stress disorder: another piece in the biopsychosocial puzzle. *Semin Arthritis Rheum* 32, 1–2.

Gracely RH, Geisser ME, Giesecke T et al. (2004) Pain catastrophizing and neural responses to pain among persons with fibromyalgia. *Brain* 127, 835–843.

Gracely RH, Petzke F, Wolf JM et al. (2002) Functional magnetic resonance imaging evidence of augmented pain processing in fibromyalgia. *Arthritis Rheum* 46, 1333–1343.

Griep EN, Boersma JW, Lentjes et al. (1998) Function of the hypothalamic-pituitary-adrenal axis in patients with fibromyalgia and low back pain. *J Rheumatol* 25, 1374–1382.

Gullette ECD, Blumenthal JA, Babyak M (1997). Effect of mental stress on myocardial ischemia during daily life. *JAMA* 277, 1521–1526.

Hadler NM (1994) The injured worker and the internist. *Ann Intern Med* 120, 163–164.

Haley WE, Roth DL, Howard G et al. (2010) Caregiving strain and estimated risk for stroke and coronary heart disease among spouse caregivers: differential effects by race and sex. *Stroke* 41, 331–336.

Hamer M, Endrighi R, Venuraju SM et al. (2012) Cortisol responses to mental stress and the progression of coronary artery calcification in healthy men and women. *Plos One* 7, e31356.

Hamer M, Steptoe A (2012) Cortisol responses to mental stress and incident hypertension in healthy men and women. *J Clin Endocrinol Metab* 97, E29–34.

Heim C, Ehlert U, Hanker JP, Hellhammer DH (1998) Abuse-related posttraumatic stress disorder and alterations of the hypothalamic-pituitary-adrenal axis in women with chronic pelvic pain. *Psychosom Med* 60, 309–318.

Heim C, Ehlert U, Rexhausen J et al. (1997) Psychoendocrinological observations in women with chronic pelvic pain. *Ann NY Acad Sci* 821, 456–458.

Hippisley-Cox J, Fielding K, Pringle M (1998) Depression as a risk factor for ischemic heart disease in men: population based case-control study. *Brit Med J* 316, 1714–1719.

Holmes SD, Krantz DS, Rogers H et al. (2006) Mental stress and coronary artery disease: a multidisciplinary guide. *Progr Cardiovasc Dis* 49, 106–122.

Hong JY, Kilpatrick LA, Labus J et al. (2013) Patients with chronic visceral pain show sex-related alterations in intrinsic oscillations of the resting brain. *J Neurosci* 33, 11994–12002.

Hudson JI, Goldenberg DL, Pope et al. (1992) Comorbidity of fibromyalgia with medical and psychiatric disorders. *Am J Med* 92, 363–367.

Hudson JI, Pope HG (1989) Fibromyalgia and psychopathology: is fibromyalgia a form of "affective spectrum disorder"? *J Rheumatol Suppl*, 15–22.

Iowa (1997) Self-reported illness and health status among Gulf War veterans: a population-based study. (Iowa Persian Gulf Study Group). *JAMA* 277, 238–245.

Jain D, Burg M, Soufer R et al. (1995) Prognostic implications of mental stress-induced silent left ventricular dysfunction in patients with stable angina pectoris. *Am J Cardiol* 76, 31–35.

Jain D, Shaker SM, Burg M et al. (1998) Effects of mental stress on left ventricular and peripheral vascular performance in patients with coronary artery disease. *J Am Coll Cardiol* 31, 1314–1322.

Jenkins CD, Stanton, B, Jono RT (1994) Quantifying and predicting recovery after heart surgery. *Psychosom Med* 56, 203–212.

Jensen MC, Brant-Zawadzki MN, Obuchowski N et al. (1994) Magnetic resonance imaging of the lumbar spine in people without back pain. *N Engl J Med* 331, 69–73.

Jiang W, Babyak M, Krantz DS et al. (1996) Mental stress-induced myocardial ischemia and cardiac events. *JAMA* 275, 1651–1656.

Jiang Z, Dinov ID, Labus J et al. (2013) Sex-related differences of cortical thickness in patients with chronic abdominal pain. *PLoS One* 8, e73932.

Kaplan JR, Chen H, Manuck SB (2009) The relationship between social status and atherosclerosis in male and female monkeys as revealed by meta-analysis. *Am J Primatol* 71, 732–741.

Kent LK, PA., Shapiro. (2009) Depression and related psychological factors in heart disease. *Harvard Review of Psychiatry* 17, 377–388.

Kivimäki M, Virtanen M, Elovainio M et al. (2006) Work stress in the etiology of coronary heart disease – a meta-analysis. *Scand J Work Env Health* 32, 431–442.

Kloner RA (2006) Natural and unnatural triggers of myocardial infarction. *Progr Cardiovasc Dis* 48, 285–300.

Kloner RA, McDonald S, Leeka J et al. (2009) Comparison of total and cardiovascular death rates in the same city during a losing versus winning super bowl championship. *Am J Cardiol* 103, 1647–1650.

Kop WJ, Krantz DS, Nearing BD et al. (2004) Effects of acute mental stress and exercise on T-wave alternans in patients with implantable cardioverter defibrillators and controls. *Circulation* 109, 1864–1869.

Kop WJ, Krantz DS, Howell RH et al. (2001) Effects of mental stress on coronary epicardial vasomotion and flow velocity in coronary artery disease: Relationship with hemodynamic stress responses. *J Am Coll Cardiol* 37, 1359–1366.

Krantz DS, Helmers KF, Bairey CN et al. (1991) Cardiovascular reactivity and mental stress-induced myocardial ischemia in patients with coronary artery disease. *Psychosom Med* 53, 1–12.

Krantz DS, Santiago HT, Kop WJ et al. (1999) Prognostic value of mental stress testing in coronary artery disease. *Am J Cardiol* 84, 1292–1297.

Kubzansky LD, Koenen KC, Spiro A 3rd et al. (2007) Prospective study of posttraumatic stress disorder symptoms and coronary heart disease in the Normative Aging Study. *Arch Gen Psychiatry* 64, 109–116.

Kumari M, Badrick E, Chandola T, al., et. (2010) Measures of social position and cortisol secretion in an aging population: findings from the Whitehall II study. *Psychosom Med* 72, 27–34.

Labus JS, Gupta A, Coveleskie K et al. (2013a) Sex differences in emotion-related cognitive processes in irritable bowel syndrome and healthy control subjects. *Pain* 154, 2088–2099.

Labus JS, Dinov ID, Jiang Z et al. (2014) Irritable bowel syndrome in female patients is associated with alterations in structural brain networks. *Pain* 155, 137–149.

Labus JS, Hubbard CS, Bueller J et al. (2013b) Impaired emotional learning and involvement of the corticotropin-releasing factor signaling system in patients with irritable bowel syndrome. *Gastroenterology* 145,e1251–1253.

Lacy CR, Contrada RJ, Robbins ML et al. (1995) Coronary vasoconstriction induced by mental stress (simulated public speaking) *Am J Cardiol* 75, 503–505.

Lampert R, Ickovics J, Viscoli C et al. (1998) Inter-relationship between effect on heart rate variability and effect on outcome by beta-blockers in the Beta Blocker Heart Attack Trial (BHAT) *Circulation* 98, 1–80.

Lampert R, Joska T, Burg MM et al. (2002) Emotional and physical precipitants of ventricular arrhythmia. *Circulation* 106, 1800–1805.

Lane RD, Laukes C, Marcus FI et al. (2005) Psychological stress preceding idiopathic ventricular fibrillation. *Psychosom Med* 67, 359–365.

Lane RD, Waldstein SR, Critchley HD et al. (2009) The rebirth of neuroscience in psychosomatic medicine, part II: Clinical applications and implications for research. *Psychosom Med* 71, 135–151.

LaVeau PJ, Rozanski A, Krantz DS et al. (1989) Transient left ventricular dysfunction during provocative mental stress in patients with coronary artery disease. *Am Heart J* 118, 1–8.

Legault SE, Langer A, Armstong P (1995) Usefulness of ischemic response to mental stress in predicting silent myocardial iscemia during ambulatory monitoring. *Am J Cardiol* 75, 1007–1011.

Lemrow N, Adams D, Coffey R et al. (1990) The 50 Most Frequent Diagnosis-Related Groups (DRGs), Diagnoses, and Procedures: Statistics by Hospital Size and Location (DHHS Publication No. (PHS) 90–3465 - Hospital Studies Program Research Note 13) Agency for Health Care Policy and Research, Rockville, MD.

Libby P, Ridker PM, Hansson GK (2009) Inflammation in atherosclerosis: from pathophysiology to practice. *J Am Coll Cardiol* 54, 2129–2138.

Liebschutz J, Saitz R, Brower V et al. (2007) PTSD in urban primary care: high prevalence and low physician recognition. *J Gen Intern Med* 22, 719–726.

Lipovetzky N, Hod H, Roth A et al. (2007) Emotional events and anger at the workplace as triggers for a first event of the acute coronary syndrome: a case-crossover study. *Israel Med Assoc J* 9, 310–315.

Longstreth GF, Thompson WG, Chey WD et al. (2006) Funtional bowel disorders. *Gastroenterology* 130, 1480–1491.

Mallik S, Krumholz HM, Lin ZQ et al. (2005) Patients with depressive symptoms have lower health status benefits after coronary artery bypass surgery. *Circulation* 111, 271–277.

Mayer EA, Craske M, Naliboff BD (2001a). Depression, anxiety, and the gastrointestinal system. *J Clin Psychiatry* 62 Suppl8, 28–36; discussion 37.

Mallik S, Spertus JA, Reid KJ et al. (2006) Depressive symptoms after acute myocardial infarction: evidence for highest rates in younger women. *Arch Intern Med* 166, 876–883.

Mayer EA, Collins SM (2002) Evolving pathophysiologic models of functional gastrointestinal disorders. *Gastroenterology* 122, 2032–2048.

Mayer EA (2000) The neurobiology of stress and gastrointestinal disease. *Gut* 47, 861–869.

Mayer EA, Bushnell CM (2009a). Functional pain disorders: time for a paradigm shift? In: Mayer EA, Bushnell CM (eds), *Functional Pain Syndromes: Presentation and Pathophysiology.* (pp. 531–566) IASP Press, Seattle, WA.

Mayer EA, Bushnell MC (eds) (2009b) *Functional Pain Syndromes: Presentation and Pathophysiology.* IASP Press, Seattle, WA.

Mayer EA, Gupta A, Kilpatrick LA et al. (2015) Brain mechanisms in chronic visceral pain. *Pain* (in press)

Mayer EA, Naliboff BD, Chang L et al. (2001b). Stress and the gastrointestinal tract V. Stress and irritable bowel syndrome. *Am J Physiol Gastrointest Liver Physiol* 280, G519–G524.

McEwen, B.S (2012) Brain on stress: How the social environment gets under the skin. *Proc Natl Acad Sci USA* 109(Suppl 2), 17180–17185.

McFall ME, Murburg, M.M, Ko GN, Veith RC (1990) Autonomic responses to stress in Vietnam combat veterans with posttraumatic stress disorder. *Biol Psychiatry* 27, 1165–1175.

McLean SA, Clauw DJ, Abelson JL et al. (2005) The development of persistent pain and psychological morbidity after motor vehicle collision: integrating the potential role of stress response systems into a biopsychosocial model. *Psychosom Med* 67, 783–790.

Meijer A, Conradi HJ, Bos EH et al. (2011) Prognostic association of depression following myocardial infarction with mortality and cardiovascular events: a meta-analysis of 25 years of research. *Gen Hosp Psychiatry* 33, 203–216.

Mendes de Leon CF, Krumholz HM, Seeman TS et al. (1998) Depression and risk of coronary heart disease in elderly men and women: prospective evidence from the New Haven E.P.E.S.E. *Arch Intern Med* 158, 2341–2348.

Mittleman MA, Maclure M, Sherwood JB et al. (1995) Triggering of acute myocardial infarction onset by episodes of anger. *Circulation* 92, 1720–1725.

Mostofsky E, Maclure M, Sherwood JB et al. (2012a). Risk of acute myocardial infarction after the death of a significant person in one's life: the Determinants of Myocardial Infarction Onset Study. *Circulation* 125, 491–496.

Mostofsky E, Maclure M, Sherwood JB et al. (2012b). Risk of acute myocardial infarction after the death of a significant person in one's life: the Determinants of Myocardial Infarction Onset Study. *Circulation* 125, 491–496.

Mostofsky E, Maclure M, Tofler GH et al. (2013a). Relation of outbursts of anger and risk of acute myocardial infarction. *Am J Cardiol* 112, 343–348.

Mostofsky E, Maclure M, Tofler GH et al. (2013b). Relation of outbursts of anger and risk of acute myocardial infarction. *Am J Cardiol* 112, 343–348.

Mulle JG, Vaccarino V (2013) Cardiovascular disease, psychosocial factors, and genetics: the case of depression. *Progr Cardiovasc Dis* 55, 557–562.

Naliboff BD, Derbyshire SW, Munakata J et al. (2001) Cerebral activation in patients with irritable bowel syndrome and control subjects during rectosigmoid stimulation. *Psychosom Med* 63, 365–375.

Nice S, Garland CF, Hilton SM et al. (1996) Long-term health outcomes and medical effects of torture among US Navy prisoners of war in Vietnam. *JAMA* 276, 375–381.

Nicholson A, Kuper H, Hemingway H (2006) Depression as an aetiologic and prognostic factor in coronary heart disease: a meta-analysis of 6362 events among 146 538 participants in 54 observational studies. *Eur Heart J* 27, 2763–2774.

Orr SP, Pitman RK, Lasko NB et al. (1993) Psychophysiological assessment of posttraumatic stress disorder imagery in World War II and Korean combat veterans. *J Abnorm Psychology* 102, 152–159.

Orth-Gomér K (2007) Psychosocial and behavioral aspects of cardiovascular disease prevention in men and women. *Curr Opin Psychiatry* 20, 147–151.

Parashar S, Rumsfeld JS, Spertus JA et al. (2006) Time course of depression and outcome of myocardial infarction. *Arch Intern Med* 166, 2035–2043.

Perski A, Feleke E, Anderson G et al. (1998) Emotional distress before coronary bypass grafting limits the benefits of surgery. *Am Heart J* 136, 510–517.

Pitman RK, Orr SP (1990) Twenty-four hour urinary cortisol and catecholamine excretion in combat-related posttraumatic stress disorder. *Biol Psychiatry* 27, 245–247.

Pitman RK, Orr SP, Forgus DF et al. (1987) Psychophysiologic assessment of posttraumatic stress disorder imagery in Vietnam combat veterans. *Arch Gen Psychiatry* 44, 970–975.

Plantinga L, Bremner JD, Miller AH et al. (2013) Association between posttraumatic stress disorder and inflammation: a twin study. *Brain Behav Immun* 30, 125–132.

Pratt LA, Ford DE, Crum RM et al. (1996) Depression, psychotropic medication, and risk of myocardial infarction: prospective data from the Baltimore ECA follow-up. *Circulation* 94, 3123–3129.

Proctor SP, Harley R, Wolfe J et al. (2001) Health-related quality of life in Persian Gulf War veterans. *Mil Med* 166, 510–519.

Proctor SP, Heeren T, White RF et al. (1998) Health status of Persian Gulf War veterans: self-reported symptoms, environmental exposures, and the effect of stress. *Int J Epidemiol* 27, 1000–1010.

Ramachandruni S, Fillingim RB, McGorray SP et al. (2006) Mental stress provokes ischemia in coronary artery disease subjects without exercise- or adenosine-induced ischemia. *J Am Coll Cardiol* 47, 987–991.

Ramadan R, Sheps D, Esteves F et al. (2013) Myocardial ischemia during mental stress: role of coronary artery disease burden and vasomotion. *J Am Heart Assoc* 2, e000321.

Rich-Edwards JW, Mason, S, Rexrode K et al. (2012) Physical and sexual abuse in childhood as predictors of early-onset cardiovascular events in women. *Circulation* 126, 920–927.

Rosengren A, Hawken S, Ounpuu S et al. (2004) Association of psychosocial risk factors with risk of acute myocardial infarction in 11 119 cases and 13 648 controls from 52 countries (the INTERHEART study): case-control study. *Lancet* 364, 953–962.

Rozanski A, Bairey CN, Krantz DS et al. (1988) Mental stress and the induction of silent myocardial ischemia in patients with coronary artery disease. *N Engl J Med* 318, 1005–1012.

Rozanski A, Blumenthal JA, Davidson KW et al. (2005) The epidemiology, pathophysiology, and management of psychosocial risk factors in cardiac practice: the emerging field of behavioral cardiology. *J Am Coll Cardiol* 45, 637–651.

Russ TC, Stamatakis E, Hamer M et al. (2012) Association between psychological distress and mortality: individual participant pooled analysis of 10 prospective cohort studies. *BMJ* 345, e4922.

Rutledge T, Reis SE, Olson MB et al. (2006) Depression symptom severity and reported treatment history in the prediction of cardiac risk in women with suspected myocardial ischemia: The NHLBI-sponsored WISE study. *Arch Gen Psychiatry* 63, 874–880.

Savas LS, White DL, Wieman M et al. (2009) Irritable bowel syndrome and dyspepsia among women veterans: Prevalence and association with psychological distress. *Aliment Pharmacol Ther* 29, 115–125.

Schang SJ, Pepine CJ (1977) Transient asymptomatic S-T segment depression during daily activity. *Am J Cardiol* 39, 396–402.

Schiffer F, Hartley LH, Schulman CL et al. (1980) Evidence for emotionally-induced coronary arterial spasm in patients with angina pectoris. *Br Heart J* 44, 62–66.

Schnurr PP, Spiro A (1999) Combat exposure, posttraumatic stress disorder symptoms, and health behaviors as predictors of self-reported physical health in older veterans. *J Nerv Ment Dis* 187, 353–359.

Schur EA, Afari N, Furberg H et al. (2007) Feeling bad in more ways than one: comorbidity patterns of medically unexplained and psychiatric conditions. *J Gen Intern Med* 22, 818–821.

Shah AJ, Lampert R, Goldberg J et al. (2013) Posttraumatic stress disorder and impaired autonomic modulation in male twins. *Biol Psychiatry* 73, 1103–1110.

Shah AJ, Veledar E, Hong Y et al. (2011) Depression and history of attempted suicide as risk factors for heart disease mortality in young individuals. *Arch Gen Psychiatry* 68, 1135–1142.

Shalev AY, Orr SP, Peri T et al. (1992) Physiologic responses to loud tones in Israeli patients with posttraumatic stress disorder. *Arch Gen Psychiatry* 49, 870–875.

Shalev AY, Orr SP, Pitman RK (1993) Psychophysiologic assessment of traumatic imagery in Israeli civilian patients with posttraumatic stress disorder. *Am J Psychiatry* 150, 620–624.

Sheps DS, McMahon RP, Becker L et al. (2002) Mental stress-induced ischemia and all-cause mortality in patients with coronary artery disease: Results from the Psychophysiological Investigations of Myocardial Ischemia Study. *Circulation* 105, 1780–1784.

Sherman JJ, Carlson CR, Wilson JF et al. (2005) Post-traumatic stress disorder among patients with orofacial pain. *J Orofac Pain* 19, 309–317.

Sherman JJ, Turk DC, Okifuji A (2000) Prevalence and impact of posttraumatic stress disorder-like symptoms on patients with fibromyalgia syndrome. *Clin J Pain* 16, 127–134.

Sherwood A, Hinderliter AL, Watkins LL et al. (2005) Impaired endothelial function in coronary heart disease patients with depressive symptomatology. *J Am Coll Cardiol* 46, 656–659.

Sherwood A, Johnson, K, Blumenthal JA et al. (1999) Endothelial function and hemodynamic responses during mental stress. *Psychosom Med* 61, 365–370.

Shishehbor MH, Litaker D, Pothier CE et al. (2006) Association of socioeconomic status with functional capacity, heart rate recovery, and all-cause mortality. *JAMA* 295, 784–792.

Shively CA, Register TC, Clarkson TB (2009) Shively CA, Register TC, Clarkson TB. Social stress, visceral obesity, and coronary artery atherosclerosis: product of a primate adaptation. *Am J Primatol* 71, 742–751.

Soufer R (2004) Neurocardiac interaction during stress-induced myocardial ischemia: How does the brain cope? *Circulation* 110, 1710–1713.

Soufer R, Bremner JD, Arrighi JA et al. (1998) Cerebral cortical hyperactivation in response to mental stress in patients with coronary artery disease. *Proc Natl Acad Sci USA* 95, 6454–6459.

Soufer R, Jain H, Yoon AJ (2009) Heart-brain interactions in mental stress-induced myocardial ischemia. *Curr Cardiol Reports* 11, 133–140.

Spiller, R, Garsed K (2009) Postinfectious irritable bowel syndrome. *Gastroenterology* 136, 1979–1988.

Spinhoven P, Roelofs K, Moene F et al. (2004) Trauma and dissociation in conversion disorder and chronic pelvic pain. *Int J Psychiatry Med* 34, 305–318.

Spitzer WO, Leblanc FE, Dupuis M (1987) Scientific approach to the assessment and management of activity-related spinal disorders. Report of the Quebec Task Force on Spinal Disorders. *Spine* 12, 7S.

Steptoe A, Brydon L (2009) Emotional triggering of cardiac events. *Neurosci Biobehav Rev* 33, 63–70.

Steptoe A, Hamer M, Chida Y (2007) The effects of acute psychological stress on circulating inflammatory factors in humans: A review and meta-analysis. *Brain Behav Immun* 21, 901–912.

Steptoe A, Kivimaki M (2012) Stress and cardiovascular disease. Nature reviews. *Nat Rev* 9, 360–370.

Steptoe A, Strike PC, Perkins-Porras L et al. (2006) Acute depressed mood as a trigger of acute coronary syndromes. *Biol Psychiatry* 60, 837–842.

Stone PH, Krantz DS, McMahon RP et al. (1999) Relationship among mental stress-induced ischemia and ischemia during daily life and during exercise: The Psychophysiologic Investigations of Myocardial Ischemia (PIMI) study. *J Am Coll Cardiol* 33, 1476–1484.

Strike PC, Perkins-Porras L, Whitehead DL et al. (2006) Triggering of acute coronary syndromes by physical exertion and anger: clinical and sociodemographic characteristics. *Heart* 92, 1035–1040.

Strike PC, Steptoe A (2005) Behavioral and emotional triggers of acute coronary syndromes: a systematic review and critique. *Psychosom Med* 67, 179–186.

Thayer JF, Lane RD (2007) The role of vagal function in the risk for cardiovascular disease and mortality. *Biol Psychiatry* 74, 224–242.

Thieme K, Turk DC, Flor H (2004) Comorbid depression and anxiety in fibromyalgia syndrome: relationship to somatic and psychosocial variables. *Psychosom Med* 66, 837–844.

Turk DC, Rudy TE (1992) Cognitive factors and persistent pain: A glimpse into Pandora's Box. *Cogn Ther Res* 16, 99–122.

Turk DC (2003) Cognitive-behavioral approach to the treatment of chronic pain patients. *Reg Anesth Pain Med* 28, 573–579.

Vaccarino V, Bremner JD (2011) Psychiatric and behavioral aspects of cardiovascular disease. In R.O. Bonow, D.L. Mann, D.P. Zipes & P. Libby (Eds.), *Braunwald's Heart Disease: A Textbook of Cardiovascular Medicine 9th Edition* (9 ed., Vol. 2, pp. 1904–1915) Philadelphia, PA: Saunders.

Vaccarino V, Goldberg J, Rooks C et al. (2013) Post-traumatic stress disorder and incidence of coronary heart disease: a twin study. *J Am Coll Cardiol* 62, 970–978.

Vaccarino V, Johnson BD, Sheps DS et al. (2007) Depression, inflammation and incident cardiovascular disease in women with suspected coronary ischemia: The NHLBI-Sponsored WISE Study. *J Am Coll* Cardiol, in press.

Vaccarino V, Kasl SV, Abramson J et al. (2001) Depressive symptoms and risk of functional decline and death in patients with heart failure. *J Am Coll Cardiol* 38, 199–205.

Vaccarino V, Votaw J, Faber T et al. (2009) Major depression and coronary flow reserve detected by positron emission tomography. *Arch Intern Med* 169, 1668–1676.

van Melle JP, de Jonge P, Spijkerman TA et al. (2004) Prognostic association of depression following myocardial infarction with mortality and cardiovascular events: a meta-analysis. *Psychosom Med* 66, 814–822.

Vermetten E, Bremner JD (2002a). Circuits and systems in stress. I. Preclinical studies. *Depress Anxiety* 15, 126–147.

Vermetten E, Bremner JD (2002b). Circuits and systems in stress. II. Applications to neurobiology and treatment of PTSD. *Depress Anxiety* 16, 14–38.

Virtanen M, Nyberg ST, Batty. G.D. et al. (2013) Perceived job insecurity as a risk factor for incident coronary heart disease: systematic review and meta-analysis. *BMJ* 8, 347.

Wagner AW, Wolfe J, Rotnitsky A et al. (2000) An investigation of the impact of posttraumatic stress disorder on physical health. *J Trauma Stress* 13, 41–55.

Walker EA, Keegan D, Gardner G et al. (1997) Psychosocial factors in fibromyalgia compared with rheumatoid arthritis: II. Sexual, physical, and emotional abuse and neglect. *Psychosom Med* 59, 572–577.

Wang HX, Leineweber C, Kirkeeide R et al. (2007) Psychosocial stress and atherosclerosis: family and work stress accelerate progression of coronary disease in women. The Stockholm Female Coronary Angiograpy Study. *J Int Med* 261, 245–254.

Wegman HL, Stetler C (2009) A meta-analytic review of the effects of childhood abuse on medical outcomes in adulthood. Psychosom. Med. *Psychosom Med* 71, 805–812.

Weissbecker I, Floyd A, Dedert E et al. (2006) Childhood trauma and diurnal cortisol disruption in fibromyalgia syndrome. *Psychoneuroendocrinology* 31, 312–324.

Wessely S, Nimnuan C, Sharpe M (1999) Functional somatic syndromes: one or many? *Lancet* 354, 936–939.

White DL, Savas LS, Daci K et al. (2010) Trauma history and risk of irritable bowel syndrome in women veterans. *Aliment Pharmacol Ther* 32, 551–561.

White KP, Speechley M, Harth M et al. (1999) The London Fibromyalgia Epidemiology Study: the prevalence of fibromyalgia syndrome in London, Ontario. *J Rheumatol* 26, 1570–1576.

Whooley MA, de Jonge, P et al. (2008) Depressive symptoms, health behaviors, and risk of cardiovascular events in patients with coronary heart disease. *JAMA* 300, 2379–2388.

Wilbert-Lampen U, Leistner D, Greven S et al. (2008) Cardiovascular events during World Cup soccer. *N Engl J Med* 358, 475–483.

Williamson DF, Thompson TJ, Anda RF et al. (2002) Body weight and obesity in adulthood and self-reported abuse in childhood. *Int J Obesity Related Metab Disord* 26, 1075–1082.

Wittstein IS, Thiemann DR, Lima et al. (2005) Neurohormonal features of myocardial stunning due to sudden emotional stress. *N Engl J Med* 352, 539–548.

Wolfe F, Smythe HA, Yunus MB et al. (1990) The American College of Rheumatology 1990 criteria for the classification of fibromyalgia. Report of the multicenter criteria committee. *Arthritis Rheum* 33, 160–172.

Wulsin LR, Vaillant GE, Wells VE (1999) A systematic review of the mortality of depression. *Psychosom Med* 61, 6–17.

Wyman L, Crum RM, Celentano D (2012) Depressed mood and cause-specific mortality: a 40-year general community assessment. *Ann Epidemiol* 22, 638–643.

Yehuda R, Southwick SM, Nussbaum EL et al. (1991) Low urinary cortisol in PTSD. *J Nerv Ment Dis* 178, 366–369.

Yehuda R, Teicher MH, Levengood RA et al. (1994) Circadian regulation of basal cortisol levels in posttraumatic stress disorder. *Ann NY Acad Sci*, 378–380.

Yeung AC, Vekshtein VI, Krantz DS et al. (1991) The effect of atherosclerosis on the vasomotor response of coronary arteries to mental stress. *N Engl J Med* 325, 1551–1556.

Zatzick DF, Marmar CR, Weiss DS et al. (1997) Posttraumatic stress disorder and functioning and quality of life outcomes in a nationally representative sample of male Vietnam veterans. *Am J Psychiatry* 154, 1690–1695.

SECTION IV

PTSD: from neurobiology to treatment

CHAPTER 16

Pharmacotherapy for PTSD: effects on PTSD symptoms and the brain

Lori Davis[1], Mark Hamner[2] & J. Douglas Bremner[3]

[1] *Department of Psychiatry, University of Alabama-Birmingham and the Tuscaloosa VA Medical Center, Tuscaloosa, AL, USA*
[2] *Department of Psychiatry, Medical University of South Carolina, and The Charleston VA Medical Center, Charleston, SC, USA*
[3] *Departments of Psychiatry & Behavioral Sciences and Radiology, Emory University School of Medicine, and the Atlanta VA Medical Center, Atlanta, GA, USA*

16.1 Introduction

As outlined in previous chapters of this book, posttraumatic stress disorder (PTSD) is associated with changes in brain and neurobiology that can potentially be the target of treatment. In an ideal world, alterations in a particular neurochemical or brain circuit would be targeted by a medication that specifically "fixed" the deficit. In reality, the brain is a much more complex organ for that, and it isn't always possible to create such compounds. In fact, the story of the development of medications for the treatment of psychiatric disorders such as PTSD has often been one of serendipity. This in turn leads to the opportunity to work backwards from the known action of effective medications to a greater understanding of the neurobiology of the disease. Some medications, however, such as the corticotropin-releasing factor antagonists, were developed in order to target a specific neurohormonal system based on knowledge of neurobiology. This chapter reviews pharmacotherapy for PTSD (Cooper et al., 2005; Davis et al., 2006a; Fani et al., 2006; Leon & Davis, 2010; Schoenfeld et al., 2004; Seedat et al., 2002; Spaulding, 2012) and touches on the effects of medication on the brain.

Antidepressants were originally discovered by accident, when someone noticed that patients treated with these medications for tuberculosis also became less depressed (Healy, 1999). The first generation of antidepressants, the tricyclics, which include imipramine and amitriptyline, were assessed originally for their efficacy in the treatment of depression. Later, medications used in the treatment of epilepsy were found to have mood-stabilizing effects, and so

Posttraumatic Stress Disorder: From Neurobiology to Treatment, First Edition.
Edited by J. Douglas Bremner.
© 2016 John Wiley & Sons, Inc. Published 2016 by John Wiley & Sons, Inc.

they were also used in the treatment of bipolar disorder, and eventually PTSD. Antipsychotic medications originally used for the treatment of schizophrenia were later applied to PTSD as well. We review these medications classes in more detail in this chapter.

Much of the history of the development of pharmacotherapy for PTSD and the other anxiety disorders involved testing to see if antidepressant medications found efficacious for the treatment of depression were also effective for anxiety disorders. The fact that antidepressants were found to effectively treat PTSD is at least partly a reflection of the fact that there is overlapping symptomatology between depression and PTSD. In addition, stress exposure is an important factor in the etiology of both disorders. The mood lability seen in many patients with PTSD led to an extension of mood-stabilizing agents developed for the treatment of epilepsy and later applied to bipolar disorder and then tested in PTSD. In a similar way, the atypical "psychotic" symptoms, which typically involve things like visions of dead comrades from war, in contradistinction to the psychotic symptoms seen in schizophrenia, such as auditory hallucinations involving a foreign other making derogatory comments about the individual, led to the application of neuroleptic medication in the treatment of PTSD, often as an adjunct. Neuroleptics have also been shown to have efficacy in the treatment of depression when used as an adjunct to antidepressants, which also supports the idea of testing these medications in the treatment of PTSD.

Specific symptom areas in PTSD also suggest specific targets of treatment. PTSD has been conceptualized as a disorder of memory, which can include both an inability to learn and retain information, and disordered fear learning (Bryant et al., 2005; Elzinga & Bremner, 2002; van Praag, 2004; Williams et al., 2006). Fear learning that was appropriate to the original condition may be resistant to extinction and persist for many years after the trauma. The original context of the fear learning may also be lost or over-generalized. Emotional memories are subject to a consolidation/reconsolidation process (McGaugh, 2004); during reconsolidation phases, memories are labile and subject to alteration, including either strengthening or extinction. Interventions designed to facilitate extinction during this reconsolidation phase could potentially prevent the development of chronic symptoms of PTSD (Davis et al., 2006b).

Early intervention for PTSD, whether psychopharmacological or otherwise, may be helpful in the prevention of chronic PTSD (Davidson, 2006 ; Elsesser et al., 2005; Morgan et al., 2003; Shalev, 2002). With time, traumatic memories become indelible as they move from short-term storage in the hippocampus and associated regions to long-term storage in the cerebral cortex (Bremner & Charney, 2010). When this happens, clinical and neurobiological evidence suggests that PTSD symptoms are more resistant to intervention.

What follows is a review of the literature on the pharmacotherapy of PTSD with an eye toward the implications for the neurobiology of trauma and stress, followed by a review of findings related to the effects of treatment on the brain.

16.2 Agents acting on the GABA–benzodiazepine receptor complex

Benzodiazepines act on the gamma-aminobutyric acid (GABA)–benzodiazepine receptor complex and are associated with a reduction in anxiety (see Chapter 5). The different benzodiazepines all have a similar mechanism of action and differ only in the time course of action. As symptoms of anxiety are prominently seen in PTSD, it was assumed that they would be beneficial in their treatment. However, clinical trials had mixed results.

Five nights of open-label treatment with the benzodiazepine, temazepam (Restoril), followed by a taper and discontinuation in four patients with PTSD related to a recent traumatic event resulted in improvements in sleep and PTSD symptoms (Mellman et al., 1998). Five weeks of alprazolam (Xanax) compared with placebo resulted in an improvement in anxiety but not PTSD symptoms in 10 patients with PTSD (Braun et al., 1990; Shalev et al., 1998). One study suggested that early treatment with alprazolam in the setting of the emergency room actually led to a worsening in the long-term course of PTSD symptoms (Gelpin et al., 1996). The authors interpreted these results as being related to the fact that benzodiazepines interfere with memory consolidation, and might be interrupting the natural process of processing of traumatic memories that can lead to spontaneous recovery.

Gabapentin (Neurontin) is an analog of GABA. Several case report and chart review studies found that gabapentin is beneficial for the treatment of PTSD symptoms (Brannon et al., 2000; Hamner et al., 2001). The GABA agonist, baclofen, given to 14 PTSD patients on an open-label basis, resulted in a significant improvement in PTSD symptoms (Drake et al., 2003). No placebo-controlled studies have evaluated the efficacy of gabapentin in the treatment of PTSD.

16.3 Agents acting on norepinephrine and serotonin receptors

Because of the role of norepinephrine in the stress response and evidence from both pre-clinical and clinical studies that alterations in noradrenergic function are associated with chronic stress and PTSD, and because of the role of serotonin in anxiety demonstrated in animal studies, there has long been an interest in the development of pharmacological approaches that target these systems (Vermetten & Bremner, 2002a,b). Norepinephrine release during stress results in increased arousal as well as modulation of the encoding of memory. This has led to an interest in modifying the encoding of traumatic memory through agents that target this neurochemical system. Along this vein, the noradrenergic β_2-receptor blocker, propranolol, was shown to result in a significant reduction in PTSD symptoms when administered to 11 children with abuse-related PTSD in an on–off–on design (Famularo et al., 1988). When given in the acute aftermath of a trauma, propanolol ($N = 18$) compared with placebo ($N = 23$) resulted in a decrease in physiological responding to trauma scripts, but not a significant reduction in PTSD symptoms, although there was a trend towards greater reduction in the PTSD group after 1 month of treatment (Pitman et al., 2002). Eleven patients were treated for PTSD symptoms in the immediate aftermath of trauma with a week of propanolol followed by a 1-week taper. Propanolol-treated patients had a significant reduction in PTSD symptoms following treatment when compared with eight patients who refused treatment and were followed longitudinally (Vaiva et al., 2003). These studies suggest that propanolol might be promising in the treatment of acute trauma victims, although more controlled trials are needed.

Agents acting on the α_2-noradrenergic receptor have also been assessed for their efficacy in treating PTSD. The α_2-receptor agonist, clonidine, which decreases firing of norepinephrine cell bodies in the locus coeruleus by acting on the α_2 autoreceptor, decreases norepinephrine release centrally in the brain (Siever et al., 1982). A case study in a child with PTSD showed improvement in PTSD symptoms with clonidine (Horrigan & Barnhill, 1996). PTSD symptoms improved in six out of nine PTSD patients treated with a combination of the antidepressant imipramine and clonidine as measured with a PTSD checklist, a result that was better than imipramine alone (Kinzie & Leung, 1989). Treatment with the α_2-receptor agonist, guanfacine, resulted in no change in combat veterans with PTSD ($N = 29$) compared with subjects treated with placebo ($N = 34$) in a double-blind, randomized trial (Neylan et al., 2006).

The α_1-noradrenergic system has also been the target of pharmacotherapy for PTSD. The α_1 noradrenergic antagonist, prazosin, was originally developed as a treatment for hypertension. Stimulation of the norepinephrine system induces a decrease in frontal lobe metabolism in PTSD (Bremner et al., 1997), so it is reasonable to hypothesize that medications acting at this receptor could be efficacious in the treatment of PTSD (Raskind et al., 2000). Several double blind, placebo-controlled trials have indeed shown that prazosin reduces PTSD symptoms and nightmares in both combat-related (Germain et al., 2012; Raskind et al., 2000, 2003, 2013) and civilian PTSD (Taylor et al., 2008). Based on this, prazosin should be included in the psychopharmacological approach to the treatment of

PTSD when indicated for specific patients, especially for those with nightmares and sleep disturbance.

The anti-anxiety drug, buspirone (Buspar), is an agonist of the serotonin 5-hydroxytryptamine 1 (5-HT$_1$) receptor. Case reports have reported improvement in PTSD symptoms and anxiety after treatment with buspirone (Wells et al., 1991).

Cyproheptadine is an antihistamine used in the treatment of allergies that also has antagonist effects on the serotonin 5-HT$_{2A}$, 5-HT$_{2B}$, and 5-HT$_{2C}$ receptors. Open-label studies have shown that cyproheptidine is useful for nightmares (Clark et al., 1999; Gupta et al., 1998; Rijnders et al., 2000).

16.4 Tricyclic and monoamine oxidase inhibitor antidepressants

The first studies of pharmacotherapy in PTSD involved the medications available at the time, the tricyclic antidepressants and the monoamine oxidase inhibitors (MAOIs). Tricyclics work primarily on the norepinephrine system, and also can have anticholinergic effects that cause the side-effects of dry mouth and blurred vision. MAOIs inhibit the enzyme that breaks down monoamines, resulting in higher concentrations of serotonin, norepinephrine, and other monoamines. Several open-label studies in PTSD patients showed positive responses to the MAOI, phenelzine, for treatment of PTSD symptoms (Davidson et al., 1987; Hogben & Cornfield, 1981; Milanes & Mack, 1984). In a controlled study, 13 patients with PTSD were started on phenelzine or placebo, and then crossed over after 4 weeks of treatment. There was no difference between phenelzine or placebo in PTSD symptom response, although this could be related to short treatment duration and small sample size (Shestatzky et al., 1988). Another double-blind study comparing phenelzine and imipramine with placebo in PTSD did show symptom improvement for phenelzine as well as imipramine (Frank et al., 1988; Kosten et al., 1991). An open trial in PTSD of moclobemide, a reversible MAOI that is not available in the US, showed a significant reduction in PTSD symptom severity after 12 weeks of treatment (Neal et al., 1997).

The tricyclic, imipramine, had also been found to be useful in the treatment of PTSD. Open-label studies in PTSD showed efficacy for the treatment of PTSD symptoms with imipramine (Blake, 1986; Bleich et al., 1986; Burnstein, 1984). In a study of 38 patients with combat-related PTSD randomized to the tricyclic imipramine, the MAOI phenelzine, or placebo, and treated in a double-blind fashion, both imipramine and phenelzine treatment resulted in a decrease in PTSD symptoms compared with placebo (Frank et al., 1988; Kosten et al., 1991). A randomized, double-blind trial failed to show a difference in PTSD symptoms in PTSD patients treated with the MAOI, brofaromine, and placebo (Baker et al., 1995). This medication is not commercially available.

A randomized, placebo-controlled double-blind study of the tricyclic, amitriptyline, in 46 patients with combat-related PTSD showed improvements in symptoms of anxiety and depression, but not PTSD, in comparison to placebo (Davidson et al., 1990).

In summary, imipramine and the MAOIs, may be useful in the treatment of PTSD.

16.5 Medications with other mechanisms of action

A range of antidepressant medications have been developed with alternative mechanisms of action from the tricyclics and MAOIs. They work on other brain chemical systems, such as dopamine, in addition to acting on norepinephrine and serotonin to varying degrees. Bupropion (Wellbutrin) primarily acts on dopamine, and lacks the sexual side effects that can be associated with treatment with serotonin reuptake inhibitors (SSRIs) (reviewed later). An open-label study of 17 PTSD patients treated with bupropion showed improvement in global severity, hyperarousal PTSD symptoms, and depressive symptoms, but not in avoidance or intrusion symptoms (Canive et al., 1998). Trazodone (Desyrel) is often used for PTSD symptoms and/or to help with sleep. An open-label study of six patients treated with trazodone showed improvement in PTSD symptoms measured with objective rating scales (Hertzberg et al., 1996). Mirtazapine (Remeron) is another antidepressant that, like bupriopion, doesn't have as many anticholinergic side-effects and effects on the heart and blood pressure as tricyclics, and doesn't have as many sexual side-effects. An open-label comparison of mirtazapine and sertraline showed a reduction in PTSD symptoms after 6 weeks of treatment that was greater in the mirtazapine group than in the sertraline group (Chung et al., 2004). Two other open-label study showed improvements in PTSD symptoms in PTSD patients treated with mirtazapine (Bakh et al., 2002; Connor et al., 1999a). A double-blind, placebo-controlled study of 29 patients with PTSD showed significant improvement in PTSD symptoms with mirtazapine vs. placebo (Davidson et al., 2003).

Mirtazapine, an antidepressant, is efficacious in the treatment of PTSD. Trazodone and bupropion may also represent useful treatment alternatives in select patients. Trazodone is often used by clinicians as a fairly safe alternative for the treatment of insomnia in PTSD patients.

16.6 Selective norepinephrine reuptake inhibitors

The selective norepinephrine reuptake inhibitors (SNRIs) are antidepressants that work by blocking reuptake of norepinephrine into the neuron. An open-label trial of the SNRI, desipramine (Norpramin), in a small group of PTSD patients showed no difference between desipramine and placebo (Kauffmann et al., 1987). Another study involved treatment of 18 patients with PTSD with desipramine or placebo for 4 weeks in a randomized, double-blind fashion, followed by a crossover of treatment and another 4 weeks of treatment. There was no difference between desipramine or placebo in the effect on PTSD symptoms (Reist et al., 1989). This could be due to small sample size and short duration of treatment. Nevertheless, desipramine is not commonly used for the treatment of PTSD, probably based in part on these results.

16.7 Selective serotonin reuptake inhibitors

The SSRIs increase serotonin levels in the brain by blocking reuptake from the synapse (Mandrioli et al., 2012). SSRIs include paroxetine (Paxil), fluoxetine (Prozac, Sarafem), sertraline (Zoloft), fluvoxamine (Luvox), citalopram (Celexa), and escitalopram (Lexapro) (Mandrioli et al., 2012). Paroxetine and sertraline are approved for the treatment of PTSD by the Food and Drug Administration (FDA). All of them are approved for the treatment of depression. The SSRIs have fewer anticholinergic side-effects than the tricyclics, but a higher prevalence of sexual side-effects. Consensus guidelines and meta-analyses support SSRIs as first-line treatment for PTSD (Ballenger et al., 2000; Foa et al., 1999; Stein et al., 2000a,b).

Early open-label studies of fluoxetine for the treatment of PTSD showed promising results, with an observation of reductions in PTSD symptoms (Davidson et al., 1991; McDougle et al., 1991; Nagy et al., 1993). An initial placebo-controlled, double-blind study of 64 PTSD patients showed a significant reduction in PTSD symptoms at 6 weeks in comparison to placebo (Van der Kolk et al., 1994). Another placebo-controlled, double-blind study of 53 patients with PTSD showed significant reductions in PTSD symptoms at 12 weeks (Connor et al., 1999b; Meltzer-Brody et al., 2000). Another study of 12 patients with combat-related PTSD showed no difference between fluoxetine and placebo at 12 weeks (Hertzberg et al., 2000). Fluoxetine was well tolerated, however, with few side-effects in these last two studies (Barnett et al., 2002). A multinational study randomized 226 patients to fluoxetine and 75 to placebo. There was a significant reduction in PTSD symptoms with fluoxetine vs. placebo after 12 weeks of treatment (Martenyi et al., 2002b). Patients continued on fluoxetine for an additional 24 weeks had significantly lower rates of relapse than those switched to placebo (Martenyi et al., 2002a). A larger randomized, placebo-controlled trial of mostly women with PTSD failed to show a difference between fluoxetine and placebo after 12 weeks of treatment (Martenyi et al., 2007). Review of all of the studies shows a pattern of better response in patients closer to the onset of the trauma, and in civilian vs. combat-related PTSD. It is possible that the later studies were negative because they occurred at a time when combat veterans were farther out from the trauma of the Vietnam War. Based on these studies FDA approval was never obtained for the use of fluoxetine in PTSD.

Paroxetine (Paxil, Seroxat) has also been extensively studied in PTSD. Initial open-label studied showed improvement in PTSD symptoms after treatment with paroxetine (Marshall et al., 1998). It was proposed that, as paroxetine had some actions at the norepinephrine receptor in addition to the serotonin reuptake site, it might be better for symptoms of anxiety than other SSRIs. In a double-blind trial, PTSD patients were randomized to placebo ($N = 186$), 20 mg/day of paroxetine ($N = 183$) or 40 mg/day of paroxetine ($N = 182$). There was a significant improvement in PTSD symptoms at 12 weeks for both doses of paroxetine vs. placebo, but no extra efficacy at the higher dose (Marshall et al., 2001). A second study of variable dosing of paroxetine 20–50 mg/day or placebo in 306 PTSD patients also showed a reduction in PTSD with paroxetine vs. placebo. Treatment response began as early as 4 weeks (Tucker et al., 2001). Long-term treatment led to an increase in PTSD patients with long-term remission (Ballenger, 2004). These results led to approval of paroxetine for the treatment of PTSD by the FDA.

Two randomized double-blind trials in civilian PTSD patients showed that 12 weeks of sertraline (Zoloft) treatment were superior to placebo in the treatment of PTSD symptoms (Brady et al., 2000; Davidson et al., 2001a). PTSD symptoms continued to remain in remission with an additional 24 weeks of treatment, and some initial non-responders converted to responders (Davidson et al., 2001b; Londborg et al., 2001; Rapaport et al., 2002). Sertraline was also associated with a decrease in alcohol intake in patients with PTSD and co-occurring alcohol dependence (Brady et al., 2005b). A study of 42 patients with combat-related PTSD showed improvements in the Clinical Global Impressino (CGI) scale but not a statististically significant improvement in PTSD symptoms (Zohar et al., 2002). Additional studies have demonstrated a particular reduction in anger soon after sertraline doses are initiated (Davidson et al., 2002) and an improvement in the comorbid conditions of depression and anxiety (Brady & Clary, 2003) and excess alcohol consumption (Brady et al., 2005a). Positive early response for anger symptoms predicted eventual reduction in PTSD symptoms (Davidson et al., 2004). Based on these studies, sertraline was approved by the FDA for the treatment of PTSD.

Open-label studies of fluvoxamine (Luvox) showed significant improvements in PTSD symptoms (De Boer et al., 1988; Escalona et al., 2002; Marmar et al., 1996; Neylan et al., 2001; Tucker et al., 2000). Open-label studies of escitalopram

(Celexa) were also efficacious in reducing PTSD symptoms (Hamner et al., 2006; Robert et al., 2006).

These studies show that sertraline and paroxetine are effective treatments for PTSD. Some patients may also benefit from fluvoxamine or escitalopram.

16.8 Antidepressants with actions on norepinephrine and epinephrine reuptake

Nefazodone is a reuptake inhibitor for both serotonin and norepinephrine as well as having some serotonin 5-HT_2 antagonist properties. Several open-label studies in both civilian and veteran PTSD patients showed that nefazodone was efficacious in the treatment of PTSD symptoms (Garfield et al., 2001), depressive symptoms, nightmares, and sleep after 6–12 weeks (Davidson et al., 1998; Davis et al., 2000; Gillin et al., 2001; Hertzberg et al., 1998; Hidalgo et al., 1999; Mellman et al., 1999; Neylan et al., 2003; Zisook et al., 2000) with sustained improvement at up to 3–4 years (Hertzberg et al., 2002). A randomized, double-blind, placebo-controlled trial of nefazodone in 41 patients with mostly combat-related PTSD showed significant improvements in PTSD and depressive symptoms in the nefazodone group vs. placebo at 12 weeks (Davis et al., 2004). Bristol-Myers Squibb removed nefazodone from the US market in 2004 after reports of liver failure associated with treatment.

Venlafaxine (Effexor) and duloxetine (Cymbalta) are part of a new class of antidepressants known as dual-uptake inhibitors that block reuptake of both serotonin and norepinephrine (Silverstone, 2004). Studies in depressed patients suggest great efficacy for venlafaxine than earlier antidepressants but also a possible increase in risk of suicidality (Einarson et al., 1999; Thase et al., 2001; Rubino et al., 2006). Duloxetine is also efficacious for the treatment of PTSD (Lieberman et al., 2005). A 6-month double-blind, placebo-controlled multisite study of 329 PTSD patients showed significant improvement in PTSD and depressive symptoms with venlafaxine in comparison to placebo (Davidson et al., 2006). No studies to date have looked at the effect of duloxetine on PTSD symptoms. An open-label trial of the weight loss drug sibutramine (Meridia) showed improvement within 1 day in 13 PTSD patients, with further improvement at 1 week (Annitto & Mueller, 2005).

16.9 Mood stabilizers

Anticonvulsant medications have also been evaluated for the treatment of PTSD (Keck et al., 1992). These medications were initially developed for the treatment of epilepsy and have imperfectly understood mechanisms of action. They were later used to target mood instability in bipolar disorder. For PTSD, they have been used to target symptoms of irritability, intrusive thoughts, sleep disturbance, and mood lability. Open-label and chart review studies of valproic acid (divalproate) in combat veterans with PTSD showed improvements in symptoms of hyper-arousal and avoidance and global function (Davis et al., 2005; Fesler, 1991). Randomized controlled trials of combat-related PTSD with 29 patients treated for 10 weeks with divalproate (Hamner et al., 2009) and 85 patients treated for 8 weeks with divalproex (Davis et al., 2008) showed no difference in PTSD symptoms in comparison to placebo. Based on these studies, there is no good evidence to support the use of valproic acid in the treatment of PTSD.

Other studies have examined the mood-stabilizing agents carbamazepine, topiramate, and tiagabine. Open-label carbamazepine resulted in improvement in global function and intrusive symptoms (Lipper et al., 1986). Treatment of PTSD with open-label tiagabine resulted in significant improvements in PTSD and/or depressive symptoms in several studies (Berigan, 2002; Connor et al., 2006; Taylor, 2003). Open-label topiramate treatment of PTSD patients resulted in improvements in all three symptom clusters of PTSD (Berlant & van Kammen, 2002). A study of 14 PTSD patients randomized to lamotrigine or placebo showed a pattern of improvement with lamotrigine, although the sample size was too small for statistical comparison (Hertzberg et al., 1999). Open-label treatment with levetiracetam resulted in improvements in PTSD symptoms in a group of treatment-refractory PTSD patients (Kinrys et al., 2006).

Phenytoin (Dilantin) is another anticonvulsant that acts on the glutamate system and has been shown to block the effects of stress on the hippocampus in animal studies (Watanabe et al., 1992a). Open-label phenytoin treatment in civilian PTSD resulted in significant improvement in all three PTSD clusters following 3 months of treatment (Bremner et al., 2004).

16.10 Antipsychotic medications

Atypical antipsychotics may be considered in treatment-refractory patients or in those with comorbid psychotic symptoms. Atypical antipsychotic medications bind to both dopamine and serotonin receptors. They are not considered first-line agents due to concerns about metabolic effects and other potential side-effects. Positive symptoms of psychosis have been described in PTSD and may include hallucinations or delusions that are often referable to the traumatic experience (Hamner, 2011). Psychotic symptoms can be the target of treatment with these agents, as well as symptoms of depression, irritability, anger and aggression. The psychotic symptoms in PTSD patients tend to be less complex or severe than those of other psychoses, e.g., schizophrenia (Hamner et al., 2000; Stefanovics et al., 2014).

A number of studies have assessed the ability of the atypical neuroleptic, risperidone, to treat PTSD symptoms and associated psychotic symptoms. Initial open-label studies showed that risperidone was efficacious for the treatment of both PTSD and associated psychotic symptoms, with particular efficacy for intrusive symptoms (Eidelman et al., 2000; Kozaric-Kovacic et al., 2005; Krashin & Oates, 1999; Leyba & Wampler, 1998). In a controlled study, 15 patients with combat-related PTSD were assigned to 6 weeks of adjunctive risperidone or placebo given in a double-blind fashion. There were significant improvements with risperidone compared with placebo in total PTSD symptoms as well as intrusions and irritability (Monnelly, 2003). Twenty-one women with childhood abuse-related PTSD treated in a blinded fashion for 8 weeks showed a greater improvement in global PTSD symptoms, as well as symptoms in the intrusion and arousal clusters, with risperidone treatment vs. placebo (Reich et al., 2004). A study of 65 veteran PTSD patients on stable psychotropic therapy randomized to receive adjunctive risperidone or placebo showed greater improvements in PTSD symptoms at 4 months in the risperidone group (Bartzokis et al., 2004). A study of 40 PTSD patients with comorbid psychotic symptoms assigned to double-blind risperidone or placebo for 5 weeks showed significant reductions in psychotic symptoms, but not PTSD symptoms, in risperidone compared with placebo (Hamner et al., 2003). A multi-site study of 247 veterans with combat-related PTSD in the Veterans Administration (VA) healthcare system who had failed two SSRI trials compared 6 months of treatment with risperidone or placebo. Risperidone was not associated with a statistically significant reduction in PTSD or depressive symptoms (Krystal et al., 2011). Based on these studies, risperidone may be useful in some patients, although there is not good evidence for efficacy in VA populations with chronic combat-related PTSD.

Clozapine, olanzapine, and quetiapine are three other atypical neuroleptics that have been evaluated for the treatment of PTSD. An open-label study of adolescents with PTSD and associated psychotic symptoms suggested that clozapine was helpful for the treatment of PTSD symptoms (Wheatley et al., 2004). Initial case reports also showed promising results for the treatment of PTSD with olanzapine (Labbate & Douglas, 2000). An open-label study of 20 patients with combat-related PTSD showed significant improvements in PTSD, depressive, and psychotic symptoms after 6 weeks of treatment of quetiapine (Hamner et al., 2003; Robert et al., 2005). An open-label study of 55 veterans with combat-related PTSD treated with olanzapine or fluphenazine for 6 weeks showed that olanzapine was superior for the treatment of psychotic symptoms, and also for the treatment of PTSD symptoms in the intrusion and arousal symptom clusters (Pivac et al., 2004). A placebo-controlled, double-blind randomized trial in 15 patients with PTSD treated for 10 weeks showed no difference between olanzapine and placebo in the effect on PTSD symptoms (Butterfield et al., 2001). A chart review study showed improvement in PTSD symptoms following treatment with quetiapine in treatment-refractory PTSD patients (Sokolski, 2003). The potential treatment response of these symptoms in the context of PTSD needs further study in prospective, randomized controlled trials.

16.11 Glutamatergic agents

D-cycloserine, a partial agonist of the glycine site of the N-methyl-D-aspartate (NMDA) glutamatergic receptor, has been shown in animal studies to facilitate extinction to fear (Rothbaum & Davis, 2003). Based on this, it has been a compound of interest for the treatment of PTSD. A study of 11 PTSD patients treated with D-cycloserine or placebo for 4 weeks, followed by crossover treatment, showed no difference in effects on PTSD symptoms between D-cycloserine or placebo (Heresco-Levy et al., 2002).

16.12 MDMA

±3,4-Methylenedioxymethamphetamine (MDMA), known by the name "ecstasy" when used as a street drug, inhibits the monoamine transporter, leading to increased release of monoamines serotonin, norepinephrine, and dopamine. MDMA has psychotomimetic properties and has been suggested for use in PTSD patients as an adjunct to psychotherapy. A study of 11 patients with PTSD randomized to low-dose or high-dose MDMA in a double-blind fashion, administered in conjunction with three psychotherapy sessions, showed no statistically significant decrease in PTSD symptoms or differences between doses (Oehen et al., 2012). A placebo-controlled, double-blind randomized trial of MDMA given in conjunction with two 8-hour psychotherapy sessions showed significant reductions in PTSD symptoms in the MDMA group compared with the placebo group (Mithoefer et al., 2011). The effects persisted at the 3-year follow-up with no adverse effects on memory or subsequent substance abuse (Mithoefer et al., 2013). Further studies are needed to evaluate the efficacy and safety of MDMA in the treatment of PTSD.

16.13 Effect of pharmacotherapy on the brain and neurobiology in PTSD

Research in animals outlined in other chapters of this book on the neurobiology of stress and the effects of pharmacotherapy on brain areas affected by stress has led to an effort to understand changes in the brain following pharmacotherapy of PTSD patients. This research is also motivated by a desire to document objective changes in the brain with treatment to augment data on the effect on symptoms, and to understand the neuroscience of treatment response in order to develop new treatments in the future that may be superior to currently available treatments.

As reviewed elsewhere in this book, studies in animals have shown that treatment with antidepressants is associated with changes in brain structure and function (see Chapter 6). Antidepressants promote growth of neurons (neurogenesis) and block or reverse the negative effects of stress on hippocampal neurons and hippocampal function, including molecular processes of memory (Czeh et al., 2001; Diamond et al., 1996; Duman et al., 2001; Huang & Herbert, 2006; Lucassen et al., 2004; Manji et al., 2003; Namestkova et al., 2005; Santarelli et al., 2003; Warner-Schmidt & Duman, 2006; Watanabe et al., 1992a,b). Antidepressant-induced neurogenesis may be responsible for the behavioral effects of antidepressants in reducing mental symptoms (Santarelli et al., 2003). Evidence indicates that the new cells become integrated and functional in memory processes. These findings indicate that pharmacotherapy not only reduces symptoms of PTSD, but also helps in the structural recovery of the hippocampus, frontal cortex and possibly other structures following exposure to traumatic stress (Bremner, 2010).

A number of studies in PTSD patients have found cognitive deficits measured with neuropsychological testing, smaller hippocampal volume as measured with magnetic resonance imaging (MRI), and alterations in a circuit of brain areas, including hippocampus, frontal cortex and amygdala, in PTSD measured with positron emission tomography (PET) and functional MRI (fMRI) (Bremner, 2011). In addition, research in animals regarding the effects of pharmacotherapy on the brain have also been extended to clinical neuroscience studies that have looked at the effects of pharmacological treatment on brain, cognition, neurobiology and neurophysiology in PTSD (Bremner, 2011).

Pharmacotherapy in PTSD patients leads to improvements in cognitive function that are probably mediated by the hippocampus and frontal cortex as well as other brain structures. Treatment of PTSD patients with D-cycloserine resulted in a reduction of perseverative errors on the Wisconsin Card Sort Test (WCST), an effect not seen with placebo (Heresco-Levy et al., 2002). Patients treated with prazosin in comparison to placebo had a decrease in measures of affective disturbance and emotional distress in response to trauma-related words used in the emotional Stroop task (naming the color of trauma-related words under time pressure), but no change in completion time of the task (Taylor et al., 2006). Treatment with paroxetine on an open-label basis for up to a year in PTSD patients resulted in a significant 35% improvement in verbal declarative memory (Vermetten et al., 2003). A placebo-controlled, double-blind study found improvements in verbal declarative memory with paroxetine, but not placebo, in patients with primarily civilian PTSD (Fani et al., 2009).

Pharmacotherapy of PTSD patients with antidepressants results in decreased neurohormonal responsiveness, at least for antidepressants. Treatment of PTSD patients with alprazolam did not result in a reduction in physiological reactivity to loud tones as measured by eye-blink response, heart rate, or galvanic skin conductance (Shalev et al., 1998). Ten weeks of treatment of PTSD patients with open-label fluvoxamine resulted in decreased physiological responsivity (heart rate and blood pressure) to individualized traumatic scripts. Elevated at baseline, reactivity fell to levels equivalent to traumatized individuals without PTSD following treatment (Tucker et al., 2000). Open-label paroxetine given to patients with comorbid PTSD and depression resulted in a decrease in physiological reactivity (heart rate and blood pressure) to individualized traumatic script, but no change in diurnal salivary cortisol measured over multiple time points (Tucker et al., 2004). Treatment of PTSD patients for up to 1 year with open-label paroxetine resulted in a decrease in heart rate and cortisol response to a mental stress challenge (mental arithmetic and problem-solving under time pressure with negative feedback) (Vermetten et al., 2006). One month with propanolol in the acute aftermath of trauma led to a reduction in the number of patients with increased physiological reactivity as measured with galvanic skin response in comparison to those treated with placebo (Pitman et al., 2002). These studies consistently show that antidepressants result in a decrease in physiological reactivity in PTSD assessed with objective measures.

In addition to improvements of subjective assessments of sleep and reductions in nightmares, objective assessments of sleep using polysomnography have shown improvements in parameters of sleep with pharmacotherapy in PTSD. Nefazodone was associated with a total increase in sleep time based on objective measures, as well as sleep maintenance, stage 2 sleep time, and delta sleep time (Neylan et al., 2003). Prazosin when compared with placebo in civilian PTSD resulted in an increase in total sleep time by 94 minutes, increased rapid eye movement (REM) sleep time and REM period duration, and reduced distressed awakenings (Taylor et al., 2008). A study in veterans with PTSD showed increases in objectively measured sleep time for both prazosin and cognitive behavioral therapy, but not placebo (Germain et al., 2012). These studies show that pharmacotherapy has effects on the physiology of sleep.

Studies have also shown that pharmacotherapy has effects on the brain in patients with PTSD. Treatment with paroxetine on an open-label basis for up to a year in PTSD patients resulted in significant improvements in verbal declarative memory and a 4.6% increase in mean hippocampal volume (Vermetten et al., 2003). A placebo-controlled, double-blind study found improvements in verbal declarative memory with paroxetine, but not placebo, in patients with primarily civilian PTSD (Fani et al., 2009). Another study showed an increase in hippocampal volume with sertraline treatment in PTSD patients (Bossini et al., 2007). Studies have also shown an increase in right hippocampal and cerebral cortical brain volume, but no effect on cognitive function, following treatment with open-label phenytoin in PTSD (Bremner et al., 2005).

Pharmacological treatment has also been associated with changes in brain function. One case report showed decreased inferior frontal, prefrontal, and insula blood flow measured with PET in response to war-related sounds. These changes normalized with successful treatment with the SSRI fluoxetine (Fernandez et al., 2001). Another study assessed resting brain blood flow with single-photon emission computed tomography with technetium-99m hexamethylpropyleneamine oxime before and after 8 weeks of open-label treatment with the SSRI citalopram in 11 adult patients with PTSD. Treatment resulted in a decrease in left medial temporal cortex blood flow; decreased PTSD symptoms as measured with the Clinician-Administered PTSD Scale were correlated with increased function in the medial prefrontal cortex (Seedat et al., 2003). In patients with PTSD randomized in a double-blind fashion to paroxetine or placebo, treatment with paroxetine, but not placebo, resulted in an increase in frontal cortical function in response to exposure to traumatic scripts of the individual's traumatic experience (Fani et al., 2011). In summary, successful treatment of PTSD is associated with changes in brain areas that have been implicated in PTSD, including the hippocampus and prefrontal cortex.

16.14 Conclusions

Advances in preclinical and clinical studies have informed the development of pharmacotherapy for PTSD. In addition, clinical trials have delineated treatments that are effective from those that are not, and have added to the knowledge base about the effects of these treatments on cognition, physioclogy, brain, and neurobiology, in addition to the primary measures of PTSD symptom response.

Future studies will need to continue to combine information learned from clinical trials with that derived from basic science research on the neurobiology of the stress response as well as clinical neuroscience studies of physiological and neural correlates of response to pharmacotherapeutic treatment in PTSD. Combining these approaches, as described in the other chapters in this book, will show great promise in advancing treatment options for those suffering from PTSD and other stress-related mental disorders.

References

Annitto W, Mueller PS (2005) Rapid treatment of posttraumatic stress disorder with sibutramine. *Epilepsy Behav* 7, 565–566.

Baker DG, Diamond BI, Gillette G et al. (1995) A double-blind, randomized, placebo-controlled, multi-center study of brofaromine in the treatment of post-traumatic stress disorder. *Psychopharmacology* 122, 386–389.

Bakh W-M, Pae C-U, Tsoh J et al. (2002) Effects of mirtazapine in patients with post-traumatic stress disorder in Korea: A pilot study. *Hum Psychopharmacol* 17, 341–344.

Ballenger JC (2004) Remission rates in patients with anxiety disorders treated with paroxetine. *J Clin Psychiatry* 65, 1696–1707.

Ballenger JC, Davidson JR, Lecrubier Y et al. (2000) Consensus statement on posttraumatic stress disorder from the International Consensus Group on Depression and Anxiety. *J Clin Psychiatry* 61, 60–66.

Barnett SD, Tharwani HM, Hertzberg MA et al. (2002) Tolerability of fluoxetine in posttraumatic stress disorder. *Prog Neuropsychopharmacol Biol Psychiatry* 26, 363–367.

Bartzokis G, Lu PH, Turner J (2004) Adjunctive risperidone in the treatment of chronic post-traumatic stress disorder. *Biol Psychiatry* 57, 474–479.

Berigan T (2002) Treatment of posttraumatic stress disorder with tiagabine [letter]. *Can J Psychiat* 47, 788.

Berlant J, van Kammen DP (2002) Open-label topiramate as primary or adjunctive therapy in chronic civilian posttraumatic stress disorder. *J Clin Psychiatry* 63, 15–20.

Blake DJ (1986) Treatment of acute post-traumatic stress disorder. *South Med J* 79.

Bleich A, Siegal B, Garb R et al. (1986) PTSD following combat exposure: Clinical features and psychopharmacological treatment. *Br J Psychiatry* 149, 365–369.

Bossini L, Tavanti M, Lombardelli A et al. (2007) Changes in hippocampal volume in patients with post-traumatic stress disorder after sertraline treatment. *J Clin Psychopharmacol* 27, 233–235.

Brady KT, Clary CM (2003) Affective and anxiety comorbidity in post-traumatic stress disorder treatment trials of sertraline. *Comp Psychiatry* 44, 360–369.

Brady KT, Pearlstein T, Asnis GM et al. (2000) Efficacy and safety of sertraline treatment of posttraumatic stress disorder: a randomized controlled trial. *JAMA* 283, 1837–1844.

Brady KT, Sonne S, Anton RF et al. (2005a) Sertraline in the treatment of co-occurring alcohol dependence and posttraumatic stress disorder. *Alcohol Clin Exp Res* 29, 395–401.

Brady KT, Sonne S, Anton RF et al. (2005b) Sertraline in the treatment of co-occurring alcohol dependence and posttraumatic stress disorder. *Alcohol Clin Exp Res* 29, 395–401.

Brannon N, Labbate L, Huber M (2000) Gabapentin treatment for posttraumatic stress disorder. *Can J Psychiat* 45, 84.

Braun P, Greenberg D, Dasberg H et al. (1990) Core symptoms of posttraumatic stress disorder unimproved by alprazolam treatment. *J Clin Psychiatry* 51, 236–238.

Bremner JD (2010) Imaging in CNS Disease States: PTSD. In: Borsook D, Beccera L, Bullmore E et al. (eds) *Imaging in CNS Drug Discovery and Development: Implications for Disease and Therapy.* Springer, Basel, Switzerland, pp. 339–360.

Bremner JD (2011) Stress and human neuroimaging studies. In: Conrad CD (ed.) *The Handbook of Stress: Neuropsychological Effects on the Brain.* Wiley-Blackwell.

Bremner JD, Charney DS (2010) Neural circuits in fear and anxiety. In: Stein DJ, Hollander E, Rothbaum BO (eds) *Textbook of Anxiety Disorders*, 2 edn. American Psychiatric Publishing, Arlington, VA, pp. 55–71.

Bremner JD, Innis RB, Ng CK et al. (1997) PET measurement of cerebral metabolic correlates of yohimbine administration in posttraumatic stress disorder. *Arch Gen Psychiatry* 54, 246–256.

Bremner JD, Mletzko T, Welter S et al. (2005) Effects of phenytoin on memory, cognition and brain structure in posttraumatic stress disorder: A pilot study. *J Psychopharmacol* 19, 159–165.

Bremner JD, Mletzko T, Welter S et al. (2004) Treatment of posttraumatic stress disorder with phenytoin: An open label pilot study. *J Clin Psychiatry* 65, 1559–1564.

Bryant RA, Felmingham KL, Kemp AH et al. (2005) Neural networks of information processing in posttraumatic stress disorder: a functional magnetic resonance imaging study. *Biol Psychiatry* 58, 111–118.

Burnstein A (1984) Treatment of post-traumatic stress disorder with imipramine. *Psychosomatics* 25, 3681–3687.

Butterfield MI, Becker ME, Connor KM et al. (2001) Olanzapine in the treatment of post-traumatic stress disorder: a pilot study. *Int Clin Psychopharmacol* 16, 197–203.

Canive JM, Clark RD, Calais LA et al. (1998) Bupropion treatment in veterans with posttraumatic stress disorder: an open study. *J Clin Psychopharmacol* 18, 379–383.

Chung MY, Min KH, Jun YJ et al. (2004) Efficacy and tolerability of mirtazapine and sertraline in Korean veterans with posttraumatic stress disorder: a randomized open label trial. *Human Psychopharmacology* 19, 489–494.

Clark RD, Canive JM, Calais LA et al. (1999) Cyproheptadine treatment of nightmares associated with posttraumatic stress disorder. *J Clin Psychopharmacol* 19, 486–487.

Connor KM, Davidson JR, Weisler RH et al. (1999a) A pilot study of mirtazapine in post-traumatic stress disorder. *Int Clin Psychopharmacol* 14, 29–31.

Connor KM, Davidson JRT, Weisler RH et al. (2006) Tiagabine for posttraumatic stress disorder: Effects of open-label and double-blind discontinuation treatment. *Psychopharmacologia* 184, 21–25.

Connor KM, Sutherland SM, Tupler LA et al. (1999b) Fluoxetine in post-traumatic stress disorder. Randomised, double-blind study. *Br J Psychiatry* 175, 17–22.

Cooper J, Carty J, Creamer M (2005) Pharmacotherapy for posttraumatic stress disorder: Empirical review and clinical recommendations. *Aus NZ J Psychiatry* 39, 674–682.

Czeh B, Michaelis T, Watanabe T et al. (2001) Stress-induced changes in cerebral metabolites, hippocampal volume, and cell proliferation are prevented by antidepressant treatment with tianeptine. *Proc Natl Acad Sci USA* 98, 12796–12801.

Davidson J, Baldwin D, Stein DJ et al. (2006) Treatment of posttraumatic stress disorder with venlafaxine extended release: a 6-month randomized controlled trial. *Arch Gen Psychiatry* 63, 1158–1165.

Davidson J, Kudler H, Smith R et al. (1990) Treatment of posttraumatic stress disorder with amitriptyline and placebo. *Arch Gen Psychiatry* 47, 259–266.

Davidson J, Landerman LR, Clary CM (2004) Improvement of anger at one week predicts the effects of sertraline and placebo in PTSD. *J Psychiatr Res* 38, 497–502.

Davidson J, Roth S, Newman E (1991) Fluoxetine in post-traumatic stress disorder. *J Trauma Stress* 4, 419–423.

Davidson J, Walker I, Kilts C (1987) A pilot study of phenelzine in the treatment of post-traumatic stress disorder. *Br J Psychiatry* 150, 252–255.

Davidson JR (2006) Pharmacologic treatment of acute and chronic stress following trauma: 2006. *J Clin Psychiatry* 67 Suppl 2, 34–39.

Davidson JR, Rothbaum BO, van der Kolk BA (2001a) Multicenter, double-blind comparison of sertraline treatment of posttraumatic stress disorder. *Arch Gen Psychiatry* 58, 485–492.

Davidson JR, Weisler RH, Malik ML et al. (1998) Treatment of posttraumatic stress disorder with nefazodone. *Int Clin Psychopharmacol* 13, 111–113.

Davidson JRT, Landerman LR, Farfel GM et al. (2002) Characterizing the effects of sertraline in posttraumatic stress disorder. *Psychol Med* 32, 661–670.

Davidson JRT, Pearlstein T, Londborg P et al. (2001b) Efficacy of sertraline in preventing relapse of posttraumatic stress disorder: results of a 28-week double-blind, placebo-controlled study. *Am J Psychiatry* 158, 1974–1981.

Davidson JRT, Weisler RH, Butterfield MI et al. (2003) Mirtazapine vs. placebo in posttraumatic stress disorder: a pilot trial. *Biol Psychiatry* 53, 188–191.

Davis LL, Ambrose S, Newell J et al. (2005) Divalproex for the treatment of PTSD: a retrospective chart review. *Int J Psychiatry Clini Pract* 9, 278–283.

Davis LL, Davidson JRT, Ward LC et al. (2008) Divalproex in the treatment of posttraumatic stress disorder: A randomized, double-blind, placebo-controlled trial in a veteran population. *J Clin Psychopharmacol* 21, 84–88.

Davis LL, Frazier EC, Williford RB et al. (2006a) Long-term pharmacotherapy for posttraumatic stress disorder. *CNS Drugs* 20, 465–476.

Davis LL, Jewell M, Ambrose S et al. (2004) A placebo-controlled study of nefazodone for the treatment of posttraumatic stress disorder: A preliminary study. *J Clin Psychopharmacol* 24, 291–297.

Davis LL, Nugent A, Murray J et al. (2000) Nefazodone treatment for chronic posttraumatic stress disorder: an open trial. *J Clin Psychopharmacol* 20, 159–164.

Davis M, Myers KM, Chhatwal JP et al. (2006b) Pharmacological treatments that facilitate extinction of fear: relevance to psychotherapy. *NeuroRx: J Am Soc Exp NeuroTherapeutics* 3, 82–96.

De Boer M, Op den Velde W, Falger PJ et al. (1988) Fluvoxamine treatment for chronic PTSD: a pilot study. *Psychother Psychosom* 57, 158–163.

Diamond DM, Fleshner M, Ingersoll N et al. (1996) Psychological stress impairs spatial working memory: Relevance to electrophysiological studies of hippocampal function. *Behav Neurosci* 110, 661–672.

Drake RG, Davis LL, Cates ME et al. (2003) Baclofen treatment for chronic posttraumatic stress disorder. *Ann Pharmacother* 37, 1177–1181.

Duman RS, Malberg JE, Nakagawa S (2001) Regulation of adult neurogenesis by psychotropic drugs and stress. *J Pharmacol Exp Ther* 299, 401–407.

Eidelman I, Seedat S, Stein DJ (2000) Risperidone in the treatment of acute stress disorder in physically traumatized in-patients. *Depress Anxiety* 11, 187–188.

Einarson TR, Arikian SR, Casciano J et al. (1999) Comparison of extended-release venlafaxine, selective serotonin reuptake inhibitors, and tricycli antidepressants in the treatment of depression: A meta-analysis of randomized controlled trials. *Clin Therap* 21, 296–308.

Elsesser K, Sartory G, Tackenberg A (2005) Initial symptoms and reactions to trauma-related stimuli and the development of posttraumatic stress disorder. *Depression Anxiety* 21, 61–70.

Elzinga BM, Bremner JD (2002) Are the neural substrates of memory the final common pathway in posttraumatic stress disorder (PTSD)? *J Affect Disord* 70, 1–17.

Escalona R, Canive JM, Calais LA et al. (2002) Fluvoxamine treatment in veterans with combat-related post-traumatic stress disorder. *Depress Anxiety* 15, 29–33.

Famularo R, Kinscherff R, Fenton T (1988) Propranolol treatment for childhood posttraumatic stress disorder, acute type: A pilot study. *Am J Dis Child* 142, 1244–1247.

Fani N, Ashraf A, Afzal N et al. (2011) Increased neural response to trauma scripts in post-traumatic stress disorder following paroxetine treatment: A pilot study. *Neurosci Lett* 491, 196–201.

Fani N, Hampstead BM, Bremner JD (2006) Pharmacotherapies for acute and chronic responses to trauma. *Psychiatr Issues Emerg Care Sett* 5, 10–16.

Fani N, Kitayama N, Ashraf A et al. (2009) Neuropsychological functioning in patients with posttraumatic stress disorder following short-term paroxetine treatment. *Psychopharmacol Bull* 42, 53–68.

Fernandez M, Pissiota A, Frans O et al. (2001) Brain function in a patient with torture related post-traumatic stress disorder before and after fluoxetine treatment: a positron emission tomography provocation study. *Neurosci Lett* 297, 101–104.

Fesler FA (1991) Valproate in combat-related posttraumatic stress disorder. *J Clin Psychiatry* 52, 361–364.

Foa EB, Davidson JRT, Frances A et al. (1999) The expert consensus guideline series: treatment of posttraumatic stress disorder. *J Clin Psychiatry* 60, 4–76.

Frank JB, Kosten TR, Giller EL et al. (1988) A randomized clinical trial of phenelzine and imipramine for posttraumatic stress disorder. *Am J Psychiatry* 145, 1289–1291.

Garfield DAS, Fichtner CG, Leveroni C et al. (2001) Open trial of nefazodone for combat veterans with posttraumatic stress disorder. *J Trauma Stress* 14, 453–460.

Gelpin E, Bonne O, Peri T et al. (1996) Treatment of recent trauma survivors with benzodiazepines: A prospective study. *J Clin Psychiatry* 57, 390–394.

Germain A, Richardson R, Moul DE et al. (2012) Placebo-controlled comparison of prazosin and cognitive-behavioral treatments for sleep disturbances in US Military Veterans. *J Psychosom Res* 72, 89–96.

Gillin JC, Smith-Vaniz A, Schnierow B et al. (2001) An open-label, 12-week clinical and sleep EEG study of nefazodone in chronic combat-related posttraumatic stress disorder. *J Clin Psychiatry* 62, 789–796.

Gupta S, Austin R, Cali LA et al. (1998) Nightmares treated with cyproheptadine. *J Am Acad Child Adolesc Psychiatry* 37, 570–572.

Hamner MB (2011) Psychotic symptoms in PTSD. *Focus* 9, 278–285.

Hamner MB, Brodrick PS, Labbate LA (2001) Gabapentin in PTSD: A retrospective, clinical series of adjunctive therapy. *Ann Clin Psychiatry* 13, 141–147.

Hamner MB, Deitsch SE, Brodrick PS et al. (2003a) Quetiapine treatment in patients with posttraumatic stress disorder: an open trial of adjunctive therapy. *J Clin Psychopharmacol* 23, 15–20.

Hamner MB, Faldowski RA, Robert S et al. (2009) A preliminary controlled trial of divalproex in posttraumatic stress disorder. *Ann Clin Psychiatry* 21, 89–94.

Hamner MB, Faldowski RA, Ulmer HG et al. (2003b) Adjunctive risperidone treatment in post-traumatic stress disorder: a preliminary controlled trial of effects on comorbid psychotic symptoms. *Int Clin Psychopharmacol* 18, 1–8.

Hamner MB, Frueh BC, Ulmer HG et al. (2000) Psychotic features in chronic PTSD and schizophrenia: comparative severity. *J Nerv Ment Dis* 188, 217–221.

Hamner MB, Ulmer HG, Lorberbaum JP et al. (2006) Open-label trial of escitalopram in the treatment of posttraumatic stress disorder. *J Clin Psychiatry* 67, 1522–1526.

Healy D (1999) *The Antidepressant Era.* Harvard University Press, Cambridge, MA.

Heresco-Levy U, Kremer I, Javitt DC et al. (2002) Pilot-controlled trial of D-cycloserine for the treatment of post-traumatic stress disorder. *Int J Neuropsychopharmacol* 5, 301–307.

Hertzberg MA, Butterfield MI, Feldman ME et al. (1999) A preliminary study of lamotrigine for the treatment of posttraumatic stress disorder. *Biol Psychiatry* 45, 1226–1229.

Hertzberg MA, Feldman ME, Beckham JC et al. (1996) Trial of trazodone for posttraumatic stress disorder using a multiple baseline group design. *J Clin Psychopharmacol* 16, 294–298.

Hertzberg MA, Feldman ME, Beckham JC et al. (2000) Lack of efficacy for fluoxetine in PTSD: a placebo controlled trial in combat veterans. *Ann Clin Psychiatry* 12, 101–105.

Hertzberg MA, Feldman ME, Beckham JC et al. (1998) Open trial of nefazodone for combat-related posttraumatic stress disorder. *J Clin Psychiatry* 59, 460–464.

Hertzberg MA, Feldman ME, Beckham JC et al. (2002) Three- to four-year follow-up to an open trial of nefazodone for combat-related posttraumatic stress disorder. *Ann Clin Psychiatry* 14, 215–221.

Hidalgo R, Hertzberg MA, Mellman T et al. (1999) Nefazodone in post-traumatic stress disorder: results from six open-label trials. *Int Clin Psychopharmacol* 14, 61–68.

Hogben G, Cornfield R (1981) Treatment of traumatic war neurosis with phenelzine. *Arch Gen Psychiatry* 38, 440–445.

Horrigan JP, Barnhill LJ (1996) The suppression of nightmares with guanfacine. *J Clin Psychiatry* 57, 371.

Huang G-J, Herbert J (2006) Stimulation of neurogenesis in the hippocampus of the adult rat by fluoxetine requires rhythmic change in corticosterone. *Biological Psychiatry* 59, 619–624.

Kauffmann CD, Reist C, Djenderedjian A (1987) Biological markers of affective disorders and PTSD: A pilot study with desipramine. *J Clin Psychiatry* 48, 366–367.

Keck PE, McElroy SL, Friedman LM (1992) Valproate and carbamazepine in the treatment of panic and posttraumatic stress disorders, withdrawal states, and behavioral dyscontrol syndromes. *J Clin Psychopharmacol* 12, 36–41.

Kinrys G, Wygant LE, Pardo TB et al. (2006) Levitiracetam for treatment-refractory posttraumatic stress disorder. *J Clin Psychiatry* 67, 211–214.

Kinzie JD, Leung P (1989) Clonidine in Cambodian patients with posttraumatic stress disorder. *J Nerv Ment Dis* 177, 546–550.

Kosten TR, Frank JB, Dan E et al. (1991) Pharmacotherapy for posttraumatic stress disorder using phenelzine or imipramine. *J Nerv Ment Dis* 179, 366–370.

Kozaric-Kovacic D, Pivac N, Muck-Seler D et al. (2005) Risperidone in psychotic combat-related posttraumatic stress disorder: An open trial. *J Clin Psychiatry* 66, 922–927.

Krashin D, Oates EW (1999) Risperidone as an adjunct therapy for post-traumatic stress disorder. *Mil Med* 164, 605–606.

Krystal JH, Rosenheck RA, Cramer JA et al. (2011) Adjunctive risperidone treatment for antidepressant-resistant symptoms of chronic military service-related PTSD: A randomized trial. *JAMA* 306, 493–502.

Labbate LA, Douglas S (2000) Olanzapine for nightmares and sleep disturbance in posttraumatic stress disorder (PTSD). *Can J Psychiat* 45, 667–668.

Leon AC, Davis LL (2010) Enhancing clinical trial design of interventions for posttraumatic stress disorder. *J Trauma Stress* 22, 603–611.

Leyba CM, Wampler TP (1998) Risperidone in PTSD. *Psychiatr Serv* 49, 245–246.

Lieberman JA, Greenhouse J, Hamer RM et al. (2005) Comparing the effects of antidepressants: Consensus guidelines for evaluating quantitative reviews of antidepressant efficacy. *Neuropsychopharmacology* 30, 445–460.

Lipper S, Davidson JR, Grady TA et al. (1986) Preliminary study of carbamazepine in the treatment of posttraumatic stress disorder. *Psychosomatics* 27, 849–854.

Londborg PD, Hegel MT, Goldstein S et al. (2001) Sertraline treatment of posttraumatic stress disorder: results of 24 weeks of open-label continuation treatment. *J Clin Psychiatry* 62, 325–331.

Lucassen PJ, Fuchs E, Czeh B (2004) Antidepressant treatment with tianeptine reduces apoptosis in the hippocampal dentate gyrus and temporal cortex. *Eur J Neurosci* 14, 161–166.

Mandrioli R, Mercolini L, Saracino MA et al. (2012) Selective serotonin reuptake inhibitors (SSRIs): therapeutic drug monitoring and pharmacological interactions. *Curr Med Chem* 19, 1846–1863.

Manji HK, Quiroz JA, Sporn J et al. (2003) Enhancing neuronal plasticity and cellular resilience to develop novel, improved therapeutics for difficult-to-treat depression. *Biol Psychiatry* 53, 707–742.

Marmar CR, Schoenfeld FB, Weiss DS (1996) Open trial of fluvoxamine treatment for combat-related posttraumatic stress disorder. *J Clin Psychiatry* 57, 66–72.

Marshall RD, Beebe KL, Oldham M et al. (2001) Efficacy and safety of paroxetine treatment for chronic PTSD: A fixed-dose, placebo-controlled study. *Am J Psychiatry* 158, 1982–1988.

Marshall RD, Schneier FR, Fallon BA et al. (1998) An open trial of paroxetine in patients with noncombat-related, chronic posttraumatic stress disorder. *J Clin Psychopharmacol* 18, 10–18.

Martenyi F, Brown EB, Caldwell CD (2007) Failed efficacy of fluoxetine in the treatment of posttraumatic stress disorder: results of a fixed-dose, placebo-controlled study. *J Clin Psychopharmacol* 27, 166–170.

Martenyi F, Brown EB, Zhang H (2002a) Fluoxetine versus placebo in prevention of relapse in post-traumatic stress disorder. *Br J Psychiatry* 181, 315–320.

Martenyi F, Brown EB, Zhang H et al. (2002b) Fluoxetine versus placebo in posttraumatic stress disorder. *J Clin Psychiatry* 63, 199–206.

McDougle CJ, Southwick SM, Charney DS et al. (1991) An open trial of fluoxetine in the treatment of posttraumatic stress disorder (letter). *J Clin Psychiatry* 11, 325–327.

McGaugh JL (2004) The amygdala modulates the consolidation of memories of emotionally arousing experiences. *Ann Rev Neurosci* 27, 1–28.

Mellman TA, Byers PM, Augenstein JS (1998) Pilot evaluation of hypnotic medication during acute traumatic stress response. *J Trauma Stress* 11, 563–569.

Mellman TA, David D, Barza L (1999) Nefazodone treatment and dream reports in chronic PTSD. *Depress Anxiety* 9, 146–148.

Meltzer-Brody S, Connor KM, Churchill E et al. (2000) Symptom-specific effects of fluoxetine in post-traumatic stress disorder. *Int Clin Psychopharmacol* 15, 227–231.

Milanes F, Mack C (1984) Phenelzine treatment of post-Vietnam stress syndrome. *VA Practitioner* 1, 40–49.

Mithoefer MC, M.T. W, Mithoefer AT et al. (2013) Durability of improvement in post traumatic stress disorder symptoms and absence of harmful effects or drug dependency after 3,4-methylenedioxymethamphetamineassisted psychotherapy: a prospective longterm follow-up study. *J Psychopharmacol* 27, 28–39.

Mithoefer MC, Wagner MT, Mithoefer AT et al. (2011) The safety and efficacy of {+/-}3,4-methylenedioxymethamphetamine-assisted psychotherapy in subjects with chronic, treatment-resistant posttraumatic stress disorder: the first randomized controlled pilot study. *J Psychopharmacol* 25, 439–452.

Monnelly EP, Ciraulo DA, Knapp C et al. (2003). Low-dose risperidone as adjunctive therapy for irritable aggression in posttraumatic stress disorder. *J Clin Psychopharmacol* 23, 193–196.

Morgan CA, Krystal JH, Southwick SM (2003) Toward early pharmacological posttraumatic stress intervention. *Biol Psychiatry* 53, 834–843.

Nagy LM, Morgan CA, Southwick SM et al. (1993) Open prospective trial of fluoxetine for posttraumatic stress disorder. *J Clin Psychopharmacol* 13, 107–113.

Namestkova K, Simonova Z, Sykova E (2005) Decreased proliferation in the adult rat hippocampus after exposure to the Morris water maze and its reversal by fluoxetine. *Behav Brain Res* 163, 26–32.

Neal LA, Shapland W, Fox C (1997) An open trial of moclobemide in the treatment of posttraumatic stress disorder. *Int Clin Psychopharmacol* 12, 231–237.

Neylan TC, Lenoci M, Maglione ML et al. (2003) The effect of nefazodone on subjective and objective sleep quality in posttraumatic stress disorder. *J Clin Psychiatry* 61, 40–43.

Neylan TC, Lenoci M, Samuelson KW et al. (2006) No improvement of posttraumatic stress disorder symptoms with guanfacine treatment. *Am J Psychiatry* 163, 2186–2188.

Neylan TC, Metzler TJ, Schoenfeld FB et al. (2001) Fluvoxamine and sleep disturbances in posttraumatic stress disorder. *J Trauma Stress* 14, 461–467.

Oehen P, Traber R, Widmer V et al. (2012) A randomized, controlled pilot study of MDMA (±3,4-Methylenedioxymethamphetamine)-assisted psychotherapy for treatment of resistant, chronic Post-Traumatic Stress Disorder (PTSD). *J Psychopharmacol* 27, 40–52.

Pitman RK, Sanders KM, Zusman RM et al. (2002) Pilot study of secondary prevention of posttraumatic stress sisorder with propranolol. *Biol Psychiatry* 51, 189–192.

Pivac N, Kozaric-Kovacic D, Muck-Seler D (2004) Olanzapine versus fluphenazine in an open trial in patients psychotic combat-related post-traumatic stress disorder. *Psychopharmacology* 175, 451–456.

Rapaport MH, Endicott J, Clary CM (2002) Posttraumatic stress disorder and quality of life: results across 64 weeks of sertraline treatment. *J Clin Psychiatry* 63, 59–65.

Raskind MA, Dobie DJ, Kanter ED et al. (2000) The a1-adrenergic antagonist prazosin ameliorates combat trauma nightmares in veterans with posttraumatic stress disorder: a report of 4 cases. *J Clin Psychiatry* 61, 129–133.

Raskind MA, Peskind ER, Kanter ED et al. (2003) Reduction of nightmares and other PTSD symptoms in combat veterans by prazosin: a placebo-controlled study. *Am J Psychiatry* 160, 371–373.

Raskind MA, Peterson K, Williams T et al. (2013) A Trial of Prazosin for Combat Trauma PTSD With Nightmares in Active-Duty Soldiers Returned From Iraq and Afghanistan. *Am J Psychiatry* 170, 1003–1010.

Reich DB, Winternitz S, Hennen J et al. (2004) A preliminary study of risperidone in the the treatment of posttraumatic stress disorder related to childhood abuse in women. *J Clin Psychiatry* 65, 1601–1606.

Reist C, Kauffmann CD, Haier RJ et al. (1989) A controlled trial of desipramine in 18 men with posttraumatic stress disorder. *Am J Psychiatry* 146, 513–516.

Rijnders RJ, Laman DM, Van Duijn H (2000) Cyproheptadine for posttraumatic nightmares. *Am J Psychiatry* 157, 1524–1525.

Robert R, Hamner MB, Kose S et al. (2005) Quetiapine improves sleep disturbances in combat veterans with PTSD: Sleep data from a prospective, open-label study. *J Clin Psychopharmacol* 25, 387–388.

Robert S, Hamner MB, Ulmer HG et al. (2006) Open-label trial of escitalopram in the treatment of posttraumatic stress disorder. *J Clin Psychiatry* 67, 1522–1526.

Rothbaum BO, Davis M (2003) Applying learning principles to the treatment of post-trauma reactions. *Ann NY Acad Sci* 1008, 112–121.

Rubino A, Roskell N, Tennis P et al. (2006) Risk of suicide during treatment with venlafaxine, citalopram, fluoxetine, and dothiepin: retrospective cohort study. *Br Med J* 334, 242.

Santarelli L, Saxe M, Gross C et al. (2003) Requirement of hippocampal neurogenesis for the behavioral effects of antidepressants. *Science* 301, 805–809.

Schoenfeld FB, Marmar CR, Neylan TC (2004) Current concepts in pharmacotherapy for post-traumatic stress disorder. *Psychiatr Serv* 55, 519–529.

Seedat S, Stein DJ, Ziervogel G (2002) Comparison of response to a selective serotonin reuptake inhibitor in children, adolescents, and adults with posttraumatic stress disorder. *J Child Adolescent Psychopharmacol* 12, 37–46.

Seedat S, Warwick J, van Heerden B et al. (2003) Single photon emission computed tomography in posttraumatic stress disorder before and after treatment with a selective serotonin reuptake inhibitor. *J Affect Disord* 80, 45–53.

Shalev AY (2002) Acute stress reactions in adults. *Biol Psychiatry* 51, 532–543.

Shalev AY, Bloch M, Peri T et al. (1998) Alprazolam reduces response to loud tones in panic disorder but not in posttraumatic stress disorder. *Biol Psychiatry* 44, 64–68.

Shestatzky M, Greenberg D, Lerer B (1988) A controlled trial of phenelzine in posttraumatic stress disorder. *Psychiatry Res* 24, 149–155.

Siever LJ, Uhde TW, Silberman EK et al. (1982) Evaluation of alpha-adrenergic responsiveness to clonidine challenge and noradrenergic metabolism in the affective disorders and their treatment. *Psychopharmacol Bull* 18, 118–119.

Silverstone PH (2004) Qualitative review of SNRIs in anxiety. *J Clin Psychiatry* 65, 19–28.

Sokolski KN, Denson TF, Lee RT et al. (2003) Quetiapine for treatment of refractory symptoms of combat-related post-traumatic stress disorder. *Military Med* 168, 486–489.

Spaulding AM (2012) A pharmacotherapeutic approach to the management of chronic post-traumatic stress disorder. *J Pharm Practice* 25, 541–551.

Stefanovics EA, Krystal JH, Rosenheck RA (2014) Symptom structure and severity: a comparison of responses to the positive and negative syndrome scale (PANSS) between patients with PTSD or schizophrenia. *Compr Psychiat* 55, 887–895.

Stein DJ, Seedat S, van der Linden GJ et al. (2000a) Selective serotonin reuptake inhibitors in the treatment of posttraumatic stress disorder: a meta-analysis of randomized controlled trials. *Int Clin Psychopharmacol* 15, S31–S39.

Stein DJ, Zungu-Dirwayi N, van der Linden GJ et al. (2000b) Pharmacotherapy for posttraumatic stress disorder. *Cochrane Database Systematic Review* 4, CD002795.

Taylor FB (2003) Tiagabine for posttraumatic stress disorder: a case series of 7 women. *J Clin Psychiatry* 64, 1421–1425.

Taylor FB, Lowe K, Thompson C et al. (2006) Daytime prazosin reduces psychological distress to trauma specific cues in civilian trauma posttraumatic stress disorder. *Biol Psychiatry* 59, 577–581.

Taylor FB, Martin P, Thompson C et al. (2008) Prazosin effects on objective sleep measures and clinical symptoms in civilian trauma posttraumatic stress disorder: A placebo-controlled study. *Biol Psychiatry* 63, 629–632.

Thase ME, Entsuah AR, Rudolph RL (2001) Remission rates during treatment with venlafaxine or selective serotonin reuptake inhibitors. *Br J Psychiatry* 178, 234–241.

Tucker P, Beebe KL, Burgin C et al. (2004) Paroxetine treatment of depression with posttraumatic stress disorder: effects on autonomic reactivity and cortisol secretion. *J Clin Psychopharmacol* 24, 131–140.

Tucker P, Smith KL, Marx B et al. (2000) Fluvoxamine reduces physiologic reactivity to trauma scripts in posttraumatic stress disorder. *J Clin Psychopharmacol* 20, 367–372.

Tucker P, Zaninelli R, Yehuda R et al. (2001) Paroxetine in the treatment of chronic posttraumatic stress disorder: results of a placebo-controlled flexible-dosage trial. *J Clin Psychiatry* 62, 860–868.

Vaiva G, Ducrocq F, Jezequel K et al. (2003) Immediate treatment with propranolol decreases posttraumatic stress disorder two months after trauma. *Biol Psychiatry* 54, 947–949.

Van der Kolk BA, Dreyfuss D, Michaels M et al. (1994) Fluoxetine in posttraumatic stress disorder. *J Clin Psychiatry* 55, 517–522.

van Praag HM (2004) The cognitive paradox in posttraumatic stress disorder: a hypothesis. *Progr Neuro-Psychopharmacol Biol Psychiatry* 28, 923–935.

Vermetten E, Bremner JD (2002a) Circuits and systems in stress. I. Preclinical studies. *Depress Anxiety* 15, 126–147.

Vermetten E, Bremner JD (2002b) Circuits and systems in stress. II. Applications to neurobiology and treatment of PTSD. *Depress Anxiety* 16, 14–38.

Vermetten E, Vythilingam M, Schmahl C et al. (2006) Alterations in stress reactivity after long-term treatment with paroxetine in women with posttraumatic stress disorder. *Ann NY Acad Sci* 1071, 80–86.

Vermetten E, Vythilingam M, Southwick SM et al. (2003) Long-term treatment with paroxetine increases verbal declarative memory and hippocampal volume in posttraumatic stress disorder. *Biol Psychiatry* 54, 693–702.

Warner-Schmidt JL, Duman RS (2006) Hippocampal neurogenesis: Opposing effects of stress and antidepressant treatment. *Hippocampus* 16, 239–249.

Watanabe Y, Gould E, Daniels DC et al. (1992a) Tianeptine attenuates stress-induced morphological changes in the hippocampus. *Eur J Pharmacol* 222, 157–162.

Watanabe YE, Gould H, Cameron D et al. (1992b) Phenytoin prevents stress and corticosterone induced atrophy of CA3 pyramidal neurons. *Hippocampus* 2, 431–436.

Wells BG, Chu CC, Johnson R et al. (1991) Buspirone in the treatment of posttraumatic stress disorder. *Pharmacotherapy* 152, 137–139.

Wheatley M, Reader H, Brown G et al. (2004) Clozapine treatment of adolescents with post-traumatic stress disorder and psychotic symptoms. *J Clin Psychopharmacol* 24, 167–173.

Williams LM, Kemp AH, Felmingham K et al. (2006) Trauma modulates amygdala and medial prefrontal responses to consciously attended fear. *Neuroimage* 29, 347–357.

Zisook S, Chentsova-Dutton YE, Smith-Vaniz A et al. (2000) Nefazodone in patients with treatment-refractory posttraumatic stress disorder. *J Clin Psychiatry* 61, 203–208.

Zohar J, Amital D, Miodownik C (2002) Double-blind placebo-controlled pilot study of sertraline in military veterans with posttraumatic stress disorder. *J Clin Psychopharmacol* 22, 190–195.

CHAPTER 17

Effects of psychotherapy for psychological trauma on PTSD symptoms and the brain

J. Douglas Bremner[1] & Carolina Campanella[2]

[1] *Departments of Psychiatry & Behavioral Sciences and Radiology, Emory University School of Medicine, and the Atlanta VA Medical Center, Atlanta, GA, USA*

[2] *Department of Psychiatry & Behavioral Sciences, Emory University, Atlanta, GA, USA*

17.1 Psychotherapy for psychological trauma

Evidence supports the idea that psychotherapy for psychological trauma can affect the brain as well as alleviate symptoms of PTSD. The same brain regions and neurochemical systems that underlie the symptoms of PTSD also play a role in recovery (see Chapters 9 and 12). These brain areas include the amygdala, hippocampus and medial prefrontal cortex, and neurochemical systems including norepinephrine, serotonin, and the hypothalamic–pituitary–adrenal (HPA) axis. There are a number of models of psychotherapy that are utilized in the treatment of PTSD, including cognitive behavioral therapy (CBT), supportive therapy, systematic desensitization and imaginal exposure, or psychologically focused psychotherapy. These different treatments, however, are all felt to work on the same brain regions and systems in the course of a successful treatment.

Most psychological treatments for PTSD involve talking about traumatic events and changing negative cognitions, as well as decreasing levels of arousal and anxiety associated with thinking about the traumatic event.

17.2 The neuroscience of early interventions for trauma

Appropriate treatment of trauma victims may require rapid interventions soon after the trauma. Animal studies show that memories are not immediately engraved in the mind – it can take a month or more before they become

Posttraumatic Stress Disorder: From Neurobiology to Treatment, First Edition.
Edited by J. Douglas Bremner.
© 2016 John Wiley & Sons, Inc. Published 2016 by John Wiley & Sons, Inc.

indelible. For instance, animals that undergo lesions of the hippocampus within the first month after an aversive memory lose memory for the event (Kim & Fanselow, 1992; Phillips & LeDoux, 1992). During this period of memory consolidation, memories continue to be susceptible to modification. After a month or more, lesions of the hippocampus no longer erase the negative memory. Memory becomes engraved in the long-term memory storage areas in the cerebral cortex.

Animal studies show that early interventions before memories become firmly engraved in the mind can be beneficial. Medications given before exposure to trauma – including benzodiazepines, antidepressants, opiates, and alcohol – can diminish or prevent the long-term behavioral effects of stressors.

17.3 Psychological therapy for psychological trauma

Most psychological therapies for PTSD involve some degree of mental exposure to the traumatic event in a safe, controlled environment, with an evaluation of personal response to the exposure. Patients are asked to recount their traumatic event, and talk about their thoughts, feelings, and understandings (or misunderstandings) about the event.

Cognitive behavioral therapy involves a focus on the thoughts, feelings, and cognitions related to the traumatic event. CBT focuses on correcting negative or distorted thoughts or cognitions about the trauma. In CBT the therapist will take one element of the trauma at a time (known as "desensitization") so that the traumatic event is not too overwhelming. Other relaxation techniques (deep breathing, muscle stretching, and relaxation) are used in conjunction with CBT, and can be used to help a client get through the imagery of a traumatic memory. Guided imagery involves developing a mental image of a safe and happy place, perhaps at the beach, or up a mountain. These images are used if the client becomes too overwhelmed with traumatic images. In CBT, exposure to the imagery of the traumatic event occurs repeatedly over the course of the sessions, with gradual desensitization to the traumatic memory. Multiple studies have shown CBT to be effective for treatment of PTSD (Foa & Kozak, 1986; Foa & Rothbaum, 1998; Foa et al., 1991; Marks et al., 1998; Resick et al., 2002; Tarrier et al., 1999).

Two techniques closely related to CBT and often used together include systematic desensitization and imaginal exposure therapies (Keane & Kaloupek, 1982). In systematic desensitization, there is pairing of a reminder of the trauma with relaxation. In imaginal exposure therapy, clients are asked to imagine the event in their mind and focus on thoughts and emotions as if the event were happening in the present (Fairbank et al., 1982). These techniques are also useful in the treatment of PTSD (Boudewyns et al., 1990; Bryant et al., 2003; Cooper & Clum, 1989; Foa et al., 2005; Keane et al., 1989; Saigh, 1987a,b).

Stress inoculation training involves several anxiety management techniques, including psychoeducation, muscle relaxation training, breathing retraining, role playing, covert modeling, guided self-dialogue, and thought stopping. This treatment program has been shown to be effective in the treatment of PTSD (Foa et al., 1999).

Eye movement desensitization and reprocessing (EMDR) therapy involves having patients follow a moving finger while visualizing their trauma (Grant, 2000). Newer versions of EMDR involve other methods such as tapping on alternative shoulders during re-exposure to the trauma. Controlled studies have shown the usefulness of this technique for treating trauma (Taylor et al., 2003).

Although hypnosis has had a controversial place in the treatment of stress-related psychiatric disorders, in the hands of competent and trained professionals, it does serve a potentially useful role. Memories not available to consciousness due to processes such as dissociative amnesia may be accessed through hypnosis. Studies have shown that hypnosis may lead to an improvement in PTSD.

Psychodynamic therapy typically involves meeting one-on-one with a therapist for once a week and talking about things related to the trauma, as well as things in the here and now and how they are connected to the original trauma. It also involves evaluating the thoughts and feelings the client develops about the therapist and the therapy itself.

17.4 Effects of psychotherapy on the brain

Psychological therapies are felt to be effective by acting on brain areas affected by trauma. As discussed in Chapter 4, psychological trauma involves an inability to extinguish fear responses with reminders of the trauma. This can become very disabling, to the point where it interferes with daily activities. Dysfunction in the prefrontal cortex leads to an inability to extinguish traumatic memories through inhibition of activity in the amygdala. The model states that one of the roles of psychotherapy is to help the brain to inhibit or extinguish traumatic memories through techniques such as gradual exposure to traumatic reminders in the supportive context of therapy, with a parallel increase in prefrontal function and reduced responsiveness of the amygdala.

The animal model of conditioned fear is used to understand neuroanatomical correlates of fear learning. In conditioned fear, pairing an unconditioned stimulus (e.g., an electric shock) with a conditioned stimulus (e.g., a bright light) leads to a fear reaction to the conditioned stimulus (bright light) alone. With repeated exposure to the conditioned stimulus, there is a decrease in fear responding, related to an inhibition of the amygdala (which plays a critical role in learning fear) by the prefrontal cortex (Quirk et al., 2003, 2006). In PTSD patients, dysfunction in the prefrontal cortex leads to an inability to extinguish traumatic memories through inhibition of activity in the amygdala.

Behavioral therapies facilitate the ability of the brain to inhibit or extinguish traumatic memories by taking advantage of techniques such as gradual exposure to traumatic reminders, in the supportive context of a therapeutic environment.

17.5 Brain imaging of psychotherapy in PTSD

Brain imaging studies have shown that psychotherapy affects brain areas involved in PTSD that are also affected by pharmacotherapy, including the hippocampus, amygdala, and prefrontal cortex. One study of eclectic psychotherapy showed smaller hippocampal volume measured with magnetic resonance imaging in PTSD, but no effects of treatment on hippocampal volume (Lindauer et al., 2005).

These brain areas can also be used to predict who will and will not respond to therapy. For instance, patients who did not respond to EMDR therapy showed lower gray matter density compared with patients who responded to EMDR in the bilateral posterior cingulate, anterior insula, anterior parahippocampal gyrus, and amygdala in the right hemisphere (Nardo et al., 2009).

Functional imaging studies have looked at neural correlates of successful treatment response. PTSD patients treated with brief eclectic psychotherapy showed an increase in left superior temporal and superior/middle frontal gyrus during exposure to traumatic scripts that was correlated with response to treatment (Lindauer et al., 2008). Successful CBT treatment resulted in decreased amygdala response and increased anterior cingulate response to fearful faces in PTSD patients (Felmingham et al., 2007), demonstrating that successful CBT is important for reducing fear responses. Patients with PTSD who responded to CBT had larger rostral anterior cingulate volumes than did non-responders (Bryant et al., 2008b), whereas those who did not respond well to CBT showed increased amygdala and ventral anterior cingulate cortex activation to masked fearful faces relative to patients who did respond well (Bryant et al., 2008a). More recently, it has been shown that greater activity in left dorsal striatal and frontal networks during an inhibitory task was associated with lower PTSD symptom severity after treatment, suggesting that circuits involved in inhibitory control may play a role in the outcome of CBT in PTSD patients (Falconer et al., 2013). Single-photon emission computed tomography (SPECT) studies also showed that patients with sub-threshold PTSD had significant increases in perfusion following psychotherapy as measured with SPECT hexamethylpropyleneamine oxime

(HMPAO) in parietal lobes, left hippocampus, thalamus, and left prefrontal cortex during memory retrieval (Peres et al., 2007).

Studies have also measured neural correlates of response to EMDR. PTSD patients who responded to EMDR treatment showed decreased frontal and hippocampal perfusion with SPECT HMPAO, compared with controls (Pagani et al., 2007). Treatment of PTSD with EMDR also resulted in decreases in perfusion in the left and right occipital lobes, left parietal lobe, and right precentral frontal lobe, and increased perfusion in the left inferior frontal gyrus as measured with SPECT HMPAO (Felmingham et al., 2007). These studies show that successful treatment of PTSD is associated with changes in brain areas, including the hippocampus, amygdala and prefrontal cortex, that have been implicated in the pathophysiology of PTSD.

17.6 Conclusions

This chapter reviewed the evidence for changes in the brain with successful psychotherapy in PTSD. Studies showing brain correlates that predict response to treatment were also reviewed. Both studies from preclinical science and neuroimaging studies in PTSD support the idea that interventions and treatments can affect brain function. Studies have implicated the hippocampus, amygdala and prefrontal cortex both in the pathophysiology of PTSD and in the successful response to psychotherapy treatment. These results parallel findings of the effects of pharmacotherapy on the brain in PTSD. Our model states that changes in these brain areas underlie the relief of symptoms in PTSD patients. Changes in brain areas that inhibit the fear response, such as the prefrontal cortex and hippocampus, seem to be an important factor in determining treatment outcome. Increased reactivity in the amygdala, on the other hand, may be a predictor of poor responsivity to CBT.

References

Boudewyns PA, Hyer LA, Woods MG et al. (1990) PTSD among Vietnam veterans: An early look at treatment outcome using direct therapeutic exposure. *J Trauma Stress* 3, 359–368.

Bryant RA, Felmingham K, Kemp A et al. (2008a) Amygdala and ventral anterior cingulate activation predicts treatment response to cognitive behaviour therapy for post-traumatic stress disorder. *Psychol Med* 38, 555–561.

Bryant RA, Felmingham K, Whitford TJ et al. (2008b) Rostral anterior cingulate volume predicts treatment response to cognitive-behavioural therapy for posttraumatic stress disorder. *J Psychiatry Neurosci* 33, 142–146.

Bryant RA, Moulds ML, Guthrie RM et al. (2003) Imaginal exposure alone and imaginal exposure with cognitive restructuring in treatment of posttraumatic stress disorder. *J Consult Clin Psychol* 71, 706–712.

Cooper NA, Clum GA (1989) Imaginal flooding as a supplementary treatment for PTSD in combat veterans: A controlled study. *Behav Therap* 3, 381–391.

Fairbank JA, DeGood DD, Jenkins CW (1982) Behavioral treatment of a persistent post-traumatic startle response. *J Behav Therap Exp Psychiatry* 12, 321–324.

Falconer E, Allen A, Felmingham KL et al. (2013) Inhibitory neural activity predicts response to Cognitive-Behavioral Therapy for posttraumatic stress disorder. *J Clin Psychiatry* 74, 895–901.

Felmingham K, Kemp A, Williams L et al. (2007) Changes in anterior cingulate and amygdala after cognitive behavior therapy of posttraumatic stress disorder. *Psychol Sci* 18, 127–129.

Foa EB, Dancu CV, Hembree EA et al. (1999) A comparison of exposure therapy, stress inoculation training, and their combination for reducing posttraumatic stress disorder in female assault victims. *J Consult Clin Psychol* 67, 194–200.

Foa EB, Hembree EA, Cahill SP (2005) Randomized trial of prolonged exposure for posttraumatic stress disorder with and without cognitive restructuring: outcome at academic and community clinics. *J Consult Clin Psychol* 73, 953–964.

Foa EB, Kozak MJ (1986) Emotional processing of fear: Exposure to corrective information. *Psychol Bull* 99, 20–35.

Foa EB, Rothbaum BO (1998) *Treating the Trauma of Rape: Cognitive-behavioral Therapy for PTSD.* The Guilford Press, New York

Foa EB, Rothbaum BO, Riggs D et al. (1991) Treatment of posttraumatic stress disorder in rape victims: A comparison between cognitive behavioral procedures and counseling. *J Consult Clin Psychol* 59, 715–723.

Grant M (2000) EMDR: a new treatment for trauma and chronic pain. *Complement Ther Nurs Midwifery* 6, 91–94.

Keane TM, Fairbank JA, Caddell JM et al. (1989) Implosive (flooding) therapy reduces symptoms of PTSD in Vietnam combat veterans. *Behav Therap* 20, 245–260.

Keane TM, Kaloupek DG (1982) Imaginal flooding in the treatment of post-traumatic stress disorder. *J Consult Clin Psychol* 50, 138–140.

Kim JJ, Fanselow MS (1992) Modality-specific retrograde amnesia of fear. *Science* 256, 675–677.

Lindauer RJ, Booij J, Habraken JB et al. (2008) Effects of psychotherapy on regional cerebral blood flow during trauma imagery in patients with post-traumatic stress disorder: a randomized clinical trial. *Psychol Med* 38, 543–554.

Lindauer RJ, Vlieger EJ, Jalink M et al. (2005) Effects of psychotherapy on hippocampal volume in out-patients with post-traumatic stress disorder: an MRI investigation. *Psychol Med* 35, 1421–1431.

Marks I, Lovell K, Noshirvani H et al. (1998) Treatment of post-traumatic stress disorder by exposure and/or cognitive restructuring: a controlled study. *Arch Gen Psychiatry* 55, 317–325.

Pagani M, Hogberg G, Salmaso D et al. (2007) Effects of EMDR psychotherapy on 99mTc-HMPAO distribution in occupation-related post-traumatic stress disorder. *Nucl Med Commun* 28, 757–765.

Peres JFP, Newberg AB, Mercante JP et al. (2007) Cerebral blood flow changes during retrieval of traumatic memories before and after psychotherapy: a SPECT study. *Psychol Med* 37, 1481–1491.

Phillips RG, LeDoux JE (1992) Differential contribution of amygdala and hippocampus to cued and contextual fear conditioning. *Behav Neurosci* 106, 274–285.

Quirk GJ, Garcia R, Gonzalez-Lima F (2006) Prefrontal mechanisms in extinction of conditioned fear. *Biol Psychiatry* 60, 337–343.

Quirk GJ, Likhtik E, Pelletier JG et al. (2003) Stimulation of medial prefrontal cortex decreases the responsiveness of central amygdala output neurons. *J Neurosci* 23, 8800–8807.

Resick PA, Nishith P, Weaver TL et al. (2002) A comparison of cognitive-processing therapy with prolonged exposure and a waiting condition for the treatment of chronic posttraumatic stress disorder in female rape victims. *J Consult Clin Psychol* 70, 867–879.

Saigh PA (1987a) In vitro flooding of a childhood posttraumatic stress disorder. *J Clin Child Psychol* 16, 147–150.

Saigh PA (1987b) In vitro flooding of childhood posttraumatic stress disorders: A systematic replication. *Prof School Psychol* 2, 133–145.

Tarrier N, Pilgrim H, Somerfield C et al. (1999) A randomized trial of cognitive therapy and imaginal exposure in the treatment of chronic posttraumatic stress disorder. *J Consult Clin Psychol* 67, 13–18.

Taylor S, Thordarson DS, Maxfield L et al. (2003) Comparative efficacy, speed, and adverse effects of three PTSD treatments: Exposure therapy, EMDR, and relaxation training. *J Consult Clin Psychol* 71, 330–338.

Index

A

acetylcholine, 189, 305, 329, 367
acute coronary syndrome, *see* cardiovascular disease (CVD)
acute stress disorder, 347
addiction, 113, 114, 200, 201
addicts, *see* addiction
adrenal glands
  adrenal cortex, 12, 62, 127, 161, 181, 182, 185, 193, 207, 266, 267, 270
  adrenal gland weight, 132, 136
  adrenal medulla, 160
adrenaline, *see* epinephrine
adrenal steroids, 181, 206
adrenocorticotropic hormone (ACTH), *see* hypothalamic-pituitary-adrenal (HPA) axis
Afghanistan combat, 253, 321–323, 330, 331, 333
aggression, 63–65, 193, 196, 398
agoraphobia, 44
akathisia, *see* side effects
alcohol, 65, 108, 112, 114, 115, 183, 198, 414
alcohol dependence, 9, 10, 18, 113, 116, 117, 125, 242, 243, 396
alcoholic, *see* alcohol dependence
alcoholism, *see* alcohol dependence
alpha-2 adrenergic receptor agonists, clonidine, 135, 183, 392
alpha-2 adrenergic receptor antagonists, yohimbine, 127, 128, 132, 166, 168, 184, 185, 195, 203, 204
alpha-1 adrenergic receptors, 392
alpha-2 adrenergic receptors, 183–185, 268
alpha-amino-3-hydroxy-5-methyl-4-isoxazole-propionic acid (AMPA) receptor, 90, 91
alprazolam, 391, 402, *see also* benzodiazepines
amitriptyline, 18, 135, 281, *see also* antidepressants
amnesia, 95, 322, 331, *see also* dissociative amnesia
AMPA receptor, alpha–amino–3–hydroxy–5–methyl–4–isoxazolepropionic acid (AMPA) receptor
amphetamines, 113, 183
amygdala, 12–17, 62–64, 67, 68, 70–72, 81–100, 115, 128, 130, 131, 136, 146, 159–172, 182, 183, 185, 186, 189, 190, 192–194, 199, 201–205, 207, 209, 210, 239, 246, 251, 271, 293–297, 299, 301–305, 322, 326–328, 332, 333, 347, 352, 353, 370, 401, 413–417
analgesia, 106, 113, 193, 195, 200, 201

B

androgen, 206, 207, 263
anhedonia, 63, 191
anorexia nervosa, 345, 349–351
anterior cingulate, *see* cingulate, anterior
anticholinergic side effects, 393–395, *see also* side effects, anticholinergic
antidepressants
  bupropion (Wellbutrin), 394
  monoamine oxidase inhibitors (MAOI), 393, 394
  serotonin and norepinephrine reuptake inhibitors (SNRIs), 395
  tricyclics, 393, 394
antipsychotics, 349, 364, 390, 398
  fluphenazine, 399
  olanzapine, 399
  risperidone, 399
anxiety, 3, 5, 9–11, 30, 42–44, 48, 63, 65, 66, 68, 81, 82, 92–94, 98, 115–117, 125–128, 130, 132, 136, 137, 165–167, 183, 185, 186, 193, 194, 196–199, 202–207, 210, 234, 235, 242, 270, 278, 300, 305, 363, 371–373, 390–394, 396, 413, 415
anxiolytics, buspirone, 194, 197, 393
appetite, 197, 204
arrhythmia, 366, 367
atherosclerosis, 364, 368
attachment theory, 65
atypical antipsychotics, 399
autonomic function, 367
avoidance, 4–6, 10, 72, 81, 82, 94, 95, 99, 105, 201, 206, 266, 269, 280, 292, 328, 329, 373, 394, 398

barbiturates, 198
basal ganglia, 203, 226, 297
BDNF, *see* brain-derived neurotrophic factor (BDNF)
benzodiazepines, 106–117
  alprazolam, 391, 402
  chlordiazepoxide, 106
beta adrenergic receptors, 91
bicuculline, 107, 108
bipolar disorder, 243, 390, 398
birds, stress response of, 145–156
blood pressure, 127, 181, 183, 184, 197, 298, 345, 347, 350, 362, 363, 366, 367, 369, 402

Posttraumatic Stress Disorder: From Neurobiology to Treatment, First Edition.
Edited by J. Douglas Bremner.
© 2016 John Wiley & Sons, Inc. Published 2016 by John Wiley & Sons, Inc.